Trauma Care:
A Team Approach

Edited by

Deborah Langstaff
MBA RN FETC ONC

Service Delivery Unit Manager – Trauma Service, Oxford Radcliffe Hospitals Trust, Oxford, UK

and

Jane Christie
MSc PGDE RN

Lecturer Practitioner, Oxford Radcliffe Hospitals Trust, Oxford, UK

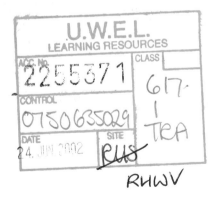

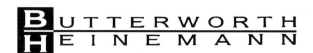

BUTTERWORTH
HEINEMANN

OXFORD AUCKLAND BOSTON JOHANNESBURG MELBOURNE NEW DELHI

Butterworth-Heinemann
Linacre House, Jordan Hill, Oxford OX2 8DP
225 Wildwood Avenue, Woburn, MA 01801-2041
A division of Reed Educational and Professional Publishing Ltd

ℜ A member of the Reed Elsevier plc group

First published 2000

Reed Educational and Professional Publishing Ltd 2000

Every effort has been made to obtain permission for reproduction of the cover design
(reproduced design based upon detail from Classical Greek bowl, Arboreo Mella, Milan.)

British Library Cataloguing in Publication Data
Trauma care: a team approach
  1   Wounds and injuries – Nursing 2. Traumatology
  I   Langstaff, Deborah   II   Christie, Jane
  617.1

ISBN 0 7506 3502 9

Library of Congress Cataloguing in Publication Data
A catalogue record for this book is available from the Library of Congress

Typeset by Bath Typesetting
Printed and bound by MPG Books Ltd, Bodmin, Cornwall

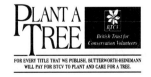

Trauma Care

In memory of Tess Evans, a nurse dedicated to trauma care, who died tragically in a road traffic accident in September 1998. May she be remembered for her supportive, fun-loving nature and her commitment to the speciality.

Senior commissioning editor: Mary Seager
Editorial assistant: Caroline Savage
Production controller: Anthony Read
Desk editor: Angela Davies
Cover designer: Alan Studholme

Contents

Acknowledgements

Although this book has been written by 'the few', it is representative of the efforts of 'the many' who over the years have worked to promote trauma as a unique speciality. We acknowledge and are grateful to all those staff who have worked in the Oxford Trauma Service. It is the distillation of their knowledge, skills and effort that has culminated in the publication of this book, and it is their endeavours we applaud.

We must also thank the following:
Lisa Johnson for her meticulous preparation of the manuscript and advice on layout, together with Sally Carr and Kerry Lavelle for their administrative and secretarial support. Also, thanks must go to Bryon Davidson for his photographic contribution. Finally, we extend our gratitude to family and friends for their patience, support and advice, without which our labours may well not have reached fruition.

Contributors

Peter Austin Former patient of the Oxford Radcliffe Trauma Service.

Sarah Banner BA(Hons) Formerly Staff Nurse, The Radcliffe Infirmary, Oxford.

Helen Barnett BA(Hons) Formerly Associate Nurse, Trauma Service, Oxford Radcliffe Hospitals Trust, Oxford.

Mary Burrows MBE(Hon) BSc MBA Assistant Director, Risk Management, Oxford Radcliffe Hospitals Trust, Oxford.

Philip Chapman-Sheath BSc MBBS FRCS Specialist Registrar in Trauma and Orthopaedic Surgery, Oxford Regional Training Programme, Oxford.

Jane Christie MSc PGDE RN Lecturer Practitioner, Oxford Radcliffe Hospitals Trust, Oxford.

Sharon Christie RGN ENB219 ENB998 DipHE (Geratology) Oxford Radcliffe Hospitals Trust, Oxford.

Maureen Coombs RGN DN(Lond) BSc (Hons) PGDipEd MSC SDU Manager, ITU, Oxford Radcliffe Hospitals Trust, Oxford.

Kerry Davidson RGN ENB219 ENB998 DipHE (Orth & Trauma Care) Team Leader, Trauma Service, Oxford Radcliffe Hospitals Trust, Oxford.

Sally Davis RGN MSc PGCEA DipMan, Senior Lecturer, Rehabilitation SHC, Oxford Brookes University, Oxford.

Ann Dillon RGN ENB100 BSc(Hons) Senior Nurse, Intensive Care Unit, Queen Alexandra Hospital, Portsmouth.

Helen Disley (née Sampson) BA(Hons) DipHE RGN ENB199 ENB998 Team Leader, Trauma Service, Oxford Radcliffe Hospitals Trust, Oxford.

Stephen Double Huntingdon Ambulance Service, Huntingdon, Cambs.

Mary Duncan Llb(Exon) Member of the Law Society Personal Injury Panel and AVMA Panel, Henmans (Solcrs), St Aldates, Oxford.

Liz Ellis MCSP SRP Formerly Senior Physiotherapist, Trauma Service, Oxford Radcliffe Hospitals Trust, Oxford

Tracy-Anne Enoch BA(Hons) RGN ONC DipN(Lon) FEATC Team Leader, Trauma Service, Oxford Radcliffe Hospitals Trust, Oxford.

Catherine Evans BSc MSc DipHE RN Primary Nurse, Trauma Service, Oxford Radcliffe Hospitals Trust, Oxford.

Claire Granville (née Scholes) BSc(Hons) RGN Associate Nurse, Trauma Service, Oxford Radcliffe Hospitals Trust, Oxford.

Bridget Gray BA (Pall-Care) RGN   Primary Nurse, Trauma Service, Oxford Radcliffe Hospitals Trust, Oxford.

Lisa Hadfield-Law RGN A&E Cert   Chair, Advanced Trauma Nursing Course Committee, Baileys Consulting, Charlbury, Oxon.

Judith Harris RGN ENB219 ENB998   Primary Nurse, Trauma Service, Oxford Radcliffe Hospitals Trust, Oxford

Julian Heath RGN   Primary Nurse, Trauma Service, Oxford Radcliffe Hospitals Trust, Oxford.

Mike Hobbs MA MB BChir MSc FRCPsych Consultant Psychotherapist, Oxfordshire Mental Healthcare NHS Trust, Psychotherapy Department, Warneford Hospital, Oxford.

Sally Lamb DPhil MSC(Rehab) MCSP SRP Research Professor in Physiotherapy, Coventry University, Coventry.

Deborah Langstaff MBA FRN FETC ONC - Service Delivery Unit Manager, Trauma Service, Oxford Radcliffe Hospitals Trust, Oxford.

Ronald Langstaff MA FRCSEd   Consultant Orthopaedic Surgeon, Hillingdon Hospital, Uxbridge, Middlesex

Anna Leeman RN BA(Hons) ENB219   Team Leader, Trauma Service, Oxford Radcliffe Hospitals Trust, Oxford.

Kathryn Lewis BA(Hons) RN(Adult) ENB998   Team Leader, Trauma Service, Oxford Radcliffe Hospitals Trust, Oxford

Helen McDermott RN DipHE(Trauma Practice) ENB998   Primary Nurse, Trauma Service, Oxford Radcliffe Hospitals Trust, Oxford.

Heather McDowell BSc(Hons) SROT   Senior Occupational Therapist in Trauma and Orthopaedics

David McMillan   226 The Strand, London WC2 1BA.

Martin McNally MD FRCSEd FRCS(Orth) Consultant in Trauma Surgery, Oxford Radcliffe Hospitals Trust, Oxford.

Duncan Moore   Cambridge Ambulance Station, Addenbrookes Hospital, Cambridge

Marie-Noelle Orzel MSc PGDE RGN RSCN Assistant Director of Nursing, Oxford Radcliffe Hospitals Trust, Oxford.

Lynn Pilgrim RGN ONC IMPS Development Co-ordinator, John Radcliffe Hospital, Oxford.

Liz Purcell BSc(Hons) Dietetics, Accredited Sports Dietician, Oxford Radcliffe Hospitals Trust, Oxford.

Kerri Rance BA(Hons)   Primary Nurse, Trauma Service, Oxford Radcliffe Hospitals Trust, Oxford.

Mike Redrup DipHE (Nursing Studies) Primary Nurse, Trauma Service, Oxford Radcliffe Hospitals Trust, Oxford.

Sarah Richards Dip(Adv Nursing) RGN   Clinical Nurse Specialist in Acute Pain, Nuffield Orthopaedic Centre, Oxford.

Jacqueline Scott BEd(Hons) RGN DipN (Lon) RNT RCNT ONC MIHSM   Formerly Chief Executive and Director of Nursing, St Vincent's Hospital, Middlesex; Co-director, Harrow & Hillingdon Community Trust.

Rachel Steel BN(Hons) RN Dip(Palliative Care) Formerly Staff Nurse, Oncology, Royal Marsden Hospital, London.

Julie Stewart-Smith RN DPSN(Tissue Viability) EN8264 ENB998   Primary Nurse, Trauma Service Oxford Radcliffe Hospitals Trust, Oxford.

Keith Willett FRCS   Consultant Trauma Surgeon, Oxford Radcliffe Hospitals Trust, Oxford.

Julie Wright BN FETC EN988   Team Leader, Trauma Service, Oxford Radcliffe Hospitals Trust, Oxford.

Tracy Wright RGN   Associate Nurse, Trauma Service, Oxford Radcliffe Hospitals trust, Oxford.

Preface

Trauma is in essence a composite speciality. Its sphere encompasses not only the immediate manifestations of injury – musculoskeletal, neurovascular and head injury – but also the associated psychological sequelae which affect both patient and family. The clinical skills most commonly associated with this speciality are usually cited as those to be found within orthopaedic trauma, plastic surgery and intensive care. Perhaps less readily associated, but equally relevant, are the skills accessed from specialities such as gerontology, palliative care and mental health. Those who practice within the speciality must therefore be aware of and ready to accommodate the diversity of professional's expertise required to meet the needs of such a unique patient population.

Trauma can intrude into all our lives, its advent unexpected, and our ability to cope often untested. Pre-admission preparation which has become such a valuable part of the 'hospital experience' for many individuals, particularly those undergoing elective procedures, can never become part of the care process in trauma – although a previous injury might afford some insight.

It is not only important to recognize and understand the effect of trauma on patients and families, but also that it can take its toll on those who provide care. It has been recognized for some time that exposure to 'traumatic events' in both accident and emergency departments and intensive care units can affect the mental health of staff. Less well recognized is the cumulative effect experienced by ward staff who provide care for traumatized patients and families over periods of many weeks. Some pay a high price for their contribution to the healing of others.

Much has been written in relation to the needs of trauma patients in specialities such as accident and emergency and critical care. This book is different. In it we aim to explore the breadth of trauma, describing the demands and challenges of the speciality, but including the patient's perspective wherever possible. The detailed management of paediatric trauma and the special needs of children are beyond the scope of this book, and therefore we have chosen to focus on the needs of the adult.

The approach we have taken is to divide the text into five parts. In Part I the patient's experience of trauma is detailed, highlighting the fact that the causes and effects of trauma vary with age. The continuum of trauma care Part II covers the patient's journey from the pre-hospital phase, through the critical period, to stabilization and rehabilitation. In this section also we have chosen to focus on one unique programme, the 'Injury Minimization Programme for Schools', an accident prevention initiative which specifically targets 10- and 11-year-old children. 'Trauma and Mental Health' provides the concluding chapter, summarizing key issues for both patients and professionals. In Part III, meeting the needs of the injured person focuses on care needs, addressing both principles and specifics. Role clarification and teamwork are covered in Part IV; individual chapters explore both the roles of different disciplines and issues arising from collaborative practice. Finally, Part V attempts to give the reader insight into some of the current political, environmental and organizational issues which impact on the provision of trauma care. It is by no means exhaustive, seeking only to identify certain constraints, legislation and resource issues, all of which influence not only treatment options but also the quality of care that healthcare professionals can provide. The chapter on legal issues high-lights the patient's experience when seeking compensation following injury, a journey which for many must also be seen as part of the healing process.

The conclusion has been written by a patient. It is a series of poems penned during the two months he spent in hospital following a road traffic accident. The subject matter he has chosen may seem surprising to some, yet it affords us all food for thought.

Part I

The patient's experience of trauma

1

What is trauma?

Jane Christie (with a contribution by David McMillan)

Introduction

Trauma has been defined as 'the condition caused by wound or injury which can lead to shock' (Swannell, 1992). While this provides a somewhat superficial description of the physical response to injury, trauma has psychological and social implications as well – it is holistic in nature (Beachley, 1988). Trauma results in severe psychological as well as physical disruption, and a loss of lifelong productivity for many (Howell *et al.*, 1988). It is the main cause of death in young people (Department of Health, 1998).

Examples

> A business man driving home in his car and has an accident – in a matter of seconds he is transformed from being fit and healthy to having life-threatening injuries.
>
> An older person who enjoys independence and cycles daily to his pensioners' club is knocked from his bicycle, breaks his hip and has to adapt to a new life with help from carers.
>
> A young girl survives extensive self-inflicted injury and has to cope with a resultant lifelong disability.

Trauma is far more complex than descriptors of fracture, soft tissue and organ damage would suggest. The psychological sequelae emanate from the affected individual like ripples on a pond, spreading out to incorporate loved ones, friends and colleagues. The significance of any injury, however minor, can only be viewed in the context in which the injured person functions. Consider the consequences of a broken finger to a concert pianist – such an injury would be devastating and might herald the end of a career. The same injury may merely be viewed as a temporary inconvenience to someone of another profession.

The aim of this chapter is to give an overview of the meaning of trauma considering the causes, the incidence, the development of the speciality, the nature, the effects and the different phases of recovery.

Table 1.1 Circumstances that contribute to accidents (Adapted from Smeltzer, 1988).

Increased stress levels or emotional problems	
Effective coping mechanisms	• Anger • Blame • Drugs and alcohol
High risk-taking behaviours	• Excess drinking • Speeding • Careless driving • Not wearing a seat belt or crash helmet

The causes of injury

Injury happens suddenly and for many reasons (Table 1.1). Accidents tend to happen to those who are under emotional pressure, those who drink or take drugs, or those who seek pleasure in high-risk behaviours. Some accidents are caused by those who are ignorant of safe practice or simply make an error of judgement. Sadly, there are many who suffer injury as the result of the mistakes or reckless behaviour of others. Trauma may also result from a medical condition such as a transient ischaemic attack or cancer. Older people are susceptible to falls due to visual defects, health problems and some degree of isolation in their living conditions (Table 1.2).

Table 1.2 Health problems experienced by the elderly which may increase the risk of trauma (Adapted from Craven and Bruno, 1986)

Dizziness
Hypertension
Infection
Cognitive impairment
Impaired mobility

The incidence of trauma

Trauma is the most common cause of death in those under 35 years old, and accounts for 14 500 deaths per year, with road accidents responsible for one-third of this number (Paynter, 1990; Driscoll, 1992). In England alone, 630 000 people are admitted to hospital each year following injury or poisoning. The mean duration of each hospital stay is calculated as 8.5 days (Department of Health, 1994). This means that the injured are incapacitated for a total of 25 million potential working days (Department of Trade and Industry, 1987). Although statistically there has been a decrease in the incidence of trauma, caring for injured people still costs the healthcare services at least £300 million per year (Central Statistics Office, 1994). Most people believe they are immune to injury; they are careful and practised in what they do (Beachley, 1989). Others feel helpless to prevent its intrusion, which is unexpected, unplanned, unwanted and life-threatening (Frese, 1985). In order to reduce the number of injuries, society has created legislation that provides clear safety measures, for example the compulsory wearing of seat belts, helmets and protective eye gear, and the drink-driving laws (Hill, 1990). There is no lack of information for the consumer who chooses a safer lifestyle, but in a democracy where risk-taking behaviour is viewed as a positive characteristic, these laws are not always adhered to (Feist and Brannon,

1988). Consequently accidents happen and the resulting injuries lead to a loss of working days, loss of national talent and loss of tax revenue, not to mention the extensive emotional and material consequences for the victim and their family (Driscoll, 1992).

It has been suggested that traumatic injury is the neglected surgical disease of the twentieth century (London, 1987). In 1988 Anderson and colleagues looked at 1000 deaths from trauma in England and Wales and found that 33% of the deaths were judged preventable. These statistics illustrate the tremendous health problem facing the healthcare system both in financial terms and in terms of human suffering, pain, loss and disability (Hadfield, 1993). Ignorance of the size of the problem has led to poor financial support for research and development in trauma care (Driscoll, 1992). More recently the government has published national targets in an effort to create a 20% reduction in the number of accidents by the year 2010 (Department of Health, 1998). This is a small step towards addressing the problem. However, more needs to be done to manage the care of the injured, helping them back to a lifestyle in which they can meet both their personal and social needs.

The development of trauma care as a speciality

Until recently, specialist trauma care has not been available in the UK. The nation has shown little interest in the statistics relating to trauma and, unfortunately, to many healthcare professionals traumatic injury is still considered to be synonymous with orthopaedics (Driscoll, 1992). Traditionally, caring for the injured person has been task orientated and influenced by the medical model (Miller and Miller, 1985; Smith, 1989). Consequently, the injured were cared for in the area where their medical condition dictated, e.g. general surgery, neurosurgery, orthopaedics, maxillofacial surgery. Little provision had been made for rehabilitation following injury, as the need was not recognized and, sadly, people rarely survived major injuries.

It has been shown that the concentration of trauma patients at specialist hospitals helps to improve the outcome for the seriously injured (Lowe *et al.*, 1983; Cales, 1984; Baker *et al.*, 1985; Cales and Trunkey, 1985; Clemmer *et al.*,

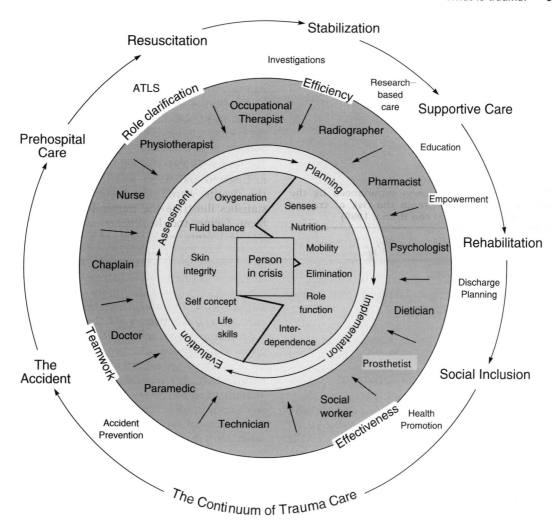

Figure 1.1 The continuum of trauma care

1985; Roy, 1987; Rhodes *et al.*, 1988). The response to this has been the development of trauma systems that can provide a fully educated and integrated team of healthcare professionals to care for the injured person and those close to them (Driscoll *et al.*, 2000). The team members come from many different areas of practice and are encouraged to participate in a holistic approach to care leading to successful outcomes (Dunnum and Bailey, 1991). This holistic approach aims to provide continuous care (Figure 1.1), beginning with prevention and encompassing pre-hospital care, resuscitation, stabilization, supportive care, rehabilitation and reintegration into society (Beachley, 1988). This model depicts a seamless approach

to trauma care, central to which is the injured person and those close to them.

The nature of trauma care

One of the reasons that trauma care is different from other specialities is the sudden, unpredictable nature of injury (Lenehan, 1986). It is unpredictable from the point of view of both patients and staff, and involves caring for someone who one minute has been happily leading a normal life, and the next minute suffers an accident, fall or assault, necessitating admission to hospital, observation, treatment or surgery.

Nursing in the acute hospital setting – the view of a healthcare professional

It's a very changeable environment, so rapidly moving and demanding that you get variety. I think you have to be adaptable and able to respond very quickly. One minute it can be quiet and the next minute you have four admissions coming through the door. It is organized, controlled chaos. You could be looking after six patients: two for rehabilitation; two off to theatre; two just coming through the door. It is quite a unique experience to take someone from a very critical situation right up to discharge and back into normal life.

Trauma involves caring for people who are not expecting to come into hospital and who have injuries that have happened unexpectedly. The more severe the injury is perceived, the more worried an individual will be about the consequences of that injury and how it is going to affect their future (Braulin *et al.*, 1982) (Table 1.3).

Table 1.3 Factors that influence an individual's ability to cope following injury

Perception of the event
Coping mechanisms
Physical health
Situational support

The effects of injury on the individual

The impact of an injury on someone's life is influenced by that individual's response to the accident (Braulin *et al.*, 1982). Every person is different; their injury, the way they cope with the injury, the way the relatives cope, how different age or ethnic groups react to trauma and to death all differ. An injury may be deemed minor by those who encounter trauma as a routine part of their working day, but to the injured person it could signify a major lifestyle change. As injury is always unexpected, its consequences frequently interfere with people's life plans (Craig *et al.*, 1988).

The devastating impact of an injury – a nurse's experience of a patient

A 21-year-old smashed his wrists skiing. Minor injuries he thought – two smashed wrists – but they had to be fused and his dream of becoming a fighter pilot was taken away. He was utterly destroyed and just wanted to die. His family were also destroyed as they had shared in his dream. He had to come to terms with the loss of body image, a change in role and the potential loss of income. He became temporarily dependent where he had been independent. Basically, his whole life had been turned upside down – total devastation.

The need for a body of knowledge for trauma care was first recognized and documented in the 1960s (Committee on Trauma Research, 1985). Since then, much has been written about the care of the trauma victim in the first hour (Buschiazzo *et al.*, 1986; American College of Surgeons, 1990; Beaver, 1990; Gauthier, 1990; Paynter, 1990; Skinner, 1992). However, less has been written about the knowledge required to care for the injured person throughout the continuum of trauma care. During their recovery each injured person goes through the different stages of the continuum at varying time spans, from minutes to months. With this in mind, the healthcare team need to understand the priorities of care at each stage and the effects they have on the injured person and those close to them. These stages provide the framework for this chapter:

Resuscitation

The initial phase is described in the literature as the 'golden hour' (American College of Surgeons, 1990). It is during this phase that emergency treatment is required to save life or limb and stabilize the condition of the injured person. For some the treatment required may be simple, such as elevation and the application of ice packs. For others, such as the multiply-injured, extensive fluid replacement and emergency surgery may be required.

If conscious, the injured person will often be concerned about their plans for that day – the child that needs to be collected from school, the presentation that has to be given or the dog that needs to be fed. They may worry that their family does not know where they are.

The more seriously injured are either unconscious or so shocked that they lie passively as they are being attended to; out of necessity the injury becomes the focus of care. Once their condition has been stabilized care can focus on other needs. At this stage it is the family or close friends who require individual support, information and assurance (Braulin *et al.*, 1982).

As accidents often happen away from home the family may arrive having trekked from the other side of the country, distressed and disorganized by the unexpected emotional impact of the accident. Anger provides temporary reprieve from the helplessness and fear and must not be disregarded (Howell *et al.*, 1988). It is often more safely directed at care-givers and the treatment programme than at those close to them.

Stabilization

As the patient's condition stabilizes, the approach of the team changes. They further assess the injury with its associated problems and help the patient to identify the implications for their own personal lifestyle (Howell *et al.*, 1988).

At this stage the injured person may exhibit a hypervigilant response and will have difficulty in problem-solving and decision-making (Table 1.4). They need information about their situation, as much mobility as possible, information in manageable doses and contact with significant others (Janis and Mann, 1977).

Table 1.4 Signs of a hypervigilant response (Adapted from Janis and Mann, 1977)

Jittery behaviour
Nervousness
Agitation
Preoccupation with frightening images

The injured person is frightened and needs help to overcome this fear. Gently increasing their perception of control over stressful events (Table 1.5), reducing time pressures and getting them to talk about the events as they indicate

their readiness will be of help (McGubbin and Figley, 1983).

Table 1.5 Stressful elements present following traumatic injury (Adapted from McGubbin and Figley, 1983)

Minimal time for preparation
Absence of guidance or previous experience
Few accessible resources for guidance
Limited sense of control
Extreme or overwhelming sense of loss and feelings of anger

The injured person and their family experience a grief reaction that can be severe and prolonged (Parkes and Weiss, 1983). This can be in response to the loss of life of those close to them, loss of a body part or loss of function. This reaction is often accompanied by strong denial which interferes with their ability to understand and make decisions. There is evidence that those who deliberately put the thoughts of loss out of their mind so as to avoid painful feelings have poorer patterns of adjustment than those who confront the loss (Archer, 1991). Relationships with others become unbalanced and significant others cannot always offer the support that is needed, as they need extra support themselves (Howell *et al.*, 1988). Sleep deprivation caused by traumatic injury, pain, nightmares, altered routine and a strange environment all add to the patient's difficulties in coping and adjusting to their changed circumstances (Brewer, 1985).

Support

The injured and those close to them are faced with the unanticipated emotional impact, not only of what has already happened to them, but also the impending treatment. They experience emotional instability related to feelings of being overwhelmed and helpless (Howell *et al.*, 1988). Contact with the family can facilitate acceptance and help an individual move out of the shock stage. It can also reverse their feelings of helplessness to those of being helpful and making a meaningful contribution (Ragiel, 1984).

Immobility, fatigue or pain can compromise an individual's ability to carry out activities of daily living (Howell *et al.*, 1988) and managing all the things we take for granted. Loss is experienced, and expressions of grief such as anger and depression are to be expected; maintaining a balance between privacy and autonomy is essential (Winship, 1995).

Example: Facilitative care

You start with someone who is just lying there post-injury and you gently encourage them to brush their hair, clean their teeth and help them do things for themselves again.

Trauma care involves informal helping behaviours that Gottlieb (1983) suggests arise from the social surroundings. These can be problem-solving or emotion-focused behaviours (Table 1.6).

Table 1.6   Emotion-focused behaviours (Adapted from Gottlieb, 1983)

These involve:

Giving people time to talk about how they feel and to express their fears and anxieties
Providing reassurance and encouragement
Listening
Reflecting respect and concern
Developing a relationship of trust and intimacy
Providing companionship and support

Example: Discussing a problem, offering suggestions, giving information and following through a directive aimed towards a positive outcome

I encouraged her to talk about her experiences, her feelings about the injury, her fears and her worries about the future. I prompted her and encouraged her to seek solutions and set short- or long-term goals for herself. She was frightened of getting up and walking because she was worried that she would get chest pain, so we started her off on a gradual mobilization programme that we worked out together – sitting out in a chair when she was all right, leading to the next one and the next one. Helping her to come to terms with what had happened to her and helping her to lead a positive life again.

Example: Emotion-focused care

The person with multiple injuries needs to build a strong relationship with the nurse as they are going to be in hospital for a long time. You need to build a therapeutic relationship with patients to find out how they feel about their injuries; we need to hold their hands and let them have a good cry; to be aware there are no right or wrong answers. You need to be able to talk to anybody in any situation, to have a rapport and show you are interested in them and that you do understand what they are going through. To allow a patient to achieve his potential you have to give something of yourself. It is important to enable the patient to trust you, so that you can get the best for their recovery.

Rehabilitation

With the increasingly advanced surgical techniques now available the injured person may not be in the acute hospital setting for very long. The hospital trauma team may only continue to see the patient on an outpatient basis. Complaints of problems at this stage should alert members of the healthcare team to explore further such areas as coping mechanisms, family dynamics, role performance and social support. Sometimes those close to the injured person experience a conflict in the change of role. Initially, the distress that a family may experience is due to the physical deficits, but in time it is the rigidity by which the family cling to traditional roles and associated expectations which causes the problems (Howell *et al.*, 1988).

Trauma often causes financial problems for the victim and those close to them. Without social support it is very difficult for the injured person to come to terms with their situation and try to rebuild their life. Until the family can move forward, finding a social network of supportive people with whom they can identify, their social isolation will persist (Koch, 1985).

Example: The experience of a family

The parents refused to accept these injuries had happened to their son; they wouldn't talk about the fact that their house would have to be adapted for him. They were frightened and had lost their identity; they wanted to get back to where they were.

The aim of rehabilitation is to secure social wellbeing or life satisfaction for the injured person and those close to them (Fugi-Meyer *et al.*, 1991). The achievement of this aim requires consideration at all levels of the disease process from pathology to handicap (McGrath and Davies, 1992).

Rehabilitation in a general ward is unsatisfactory for the prolonged care of a patient with a recently acquired disability, because of the conflicting demands of the staff and the inappropriate resources and environment. Ideally, a team of experts in the process of rehabilitation should manage the injured person's care at an agreed stage following acute care. This team of healthcare professionals work together offering tasks and skills of different levels (Evers, 1981), encouraging good communication, mutual trust and respect in order for successful outcomes to be achieved (Harvey *et al.*, 1997).

Reintegration

The aim of trauma care is to help the injured person back to a satisfactory lifestyle, able to integrate with others and contribute to life in a way that is meaningful to them. Trauma care involves more than just the treatment of injuries, it also encompasses a sense of wellbeing and achievement shared by the patient, their family and the healthcare team. The following passage is an example of a patient's experience of trauma from injury through to reintegration.

A patient's eye view of trauma – by David McMillan

Nobody can ever prepare you for coping with trauma because you never plan to be injured in the first place.

I left work on a Friday night in February 1996 expecting to be back at work on the Monday morning. But it was eighteen months before I walked back into my office.

A Sunday morning run preparing for the London Marathon and as I crossed a mist-shrouded country lane I was hit by a car. My lower right leg broken in several places, my right arm broken and nerve almost severed, shoulder blade broken in two places, five fractured ribs

---

and a punctured lung.

But alive. Only just - thanks to some quick thinking from the Oxfordshire paramedic, Graham White, who successfully carried out a thoracotomy in a lay-by in the ambulance on the way to hospital. Without his intervention I would have died and he deservedly won Paramedic of the Year for being the first paramedic in the country to carry out such an operation successfully.

Coming to intensive care, not being able to speak because of tubes down my throat, staring at the ceiling and hallucinating because of the drugs I had been given. I was scared and had a thousand questions to ask. Eventually given a letterboard to try to ask the questions to find out what happened. I still cannot remember everything to this day.

Then I was transferred to the trauma ward and I had to come to terms with my life being turned upside down.

For a start, to a layman, what was trauma? 'Emotional shock' says the dictionary, 'A condition brought on by external wound.'

The answer to coping is that there is no easy solution. You do your best to accept your life may never be the same again.

You are confused, full of mixed emotions. Personally I have cried alone for many hours asking 'Why me?'

I have endured hours of endless pain when nothing seems to stop the agony. There are danger signals here which people should be aware of. You are sent home with countless drugs and at times when you hit rock bottom the temptation to end it all becomes very strong. You become so scared, it seems the only way out. I was lucky to be able to talk to someone on the telephone to reassure me it would get better. But at times I still doubled my intake of pills. Others may not be so lucky. But everyone who fights so hard to put your body back together should remember that your mind also needs a lot of help.

Before you can cope with trauma you have to come to terms with what has happened and accept there is absolutely nothing you can do to change the past. What happened, happened – it's as simple as that.

The important thing is the future. That is all you can hope to change. The past is a *fait accompli*. You need the will and determination to overcome any problems that arise and to fight disappointments if things do not go according to plan.

The easy solution is to give up and blame everyone and everything for what has happened.

But facing up to trauma and beating the odds to resume a normal life is a bit like a top athlete becoming injured and having to fight his way back to fitness. If you want to enough, you can succeed.

You have to accept your limitations at first and then take one step at a time.

Never a truer word was spoken than the old saying 'Don't try to run before you can walk'.

It is frustrating and you can face countless setbacks as I have. There are times when I thought my body had healed only to get first a refracture of the leg which couldn't stand the strain, then, as that was healing, the arm gave way again. I thought I had a season ticket for the operating theatre.

The tears of emotion flowed endlessly. You feel that you will never ever get better. But do not think of it as a weakness. It is a release of pent-up emotion and frustration. But even when you are healed, the fear of breaking down is always with you.

It is important from a patient's point of view to understand what is going on with your body. How the changes might affect you. Whether you will ever walk again or have full use of your limbs.

I was lucky, because the consultants who operated on me took time to explain what was going on. I needed to know and they took time out of their busy schedules to explain what was being done, how it might affect me and whether I might walk, or in my case, run again.

Once I reached the walking stage, every visit to clinic was accompanied by the question 'When can I run?' Only to be answered by 'Not yet'. It was twenty months after the accident that I finally started running again.

The care from the nurses is also vital. When I was confined to bed with tubes all over the place and unable to use my right arm I felt I was totally helpless and reliant on others.

A simple task like buttering a piece of toast becomes a nightmare when you only have one good arm and it is not the one you usually use. You feel stupid asking someone to do it for you. To try and shave left-handed or even write were all gigantic tasks. I needed help and the poor hard-worked nurses were always there to lend a helping hand. That is vital.

Then, when it comes to recuperation, trying to regenerate wasted muscles, you need to rely on the help and understanding of the physios. Of course you have to help yourself, and if you are set tasks to do on your own then you must do them. Many people I saw in hospital couldn't be bothered. The physios did not give up. But they

can only do so much. To conquer the traumatic event that has changed your life forever you have to have the will to want to get better.

One elderly man in the bed beside me who was told after a fall and broken hip that he would not be able to be as active as he was before the fall, simply gave up the will to live. It was sad and he died. I spoke to his wife who said he simply could not face a future unable to do the things he used to be able to. That is a very sad example of what I mean when I say you have to want to get better.

Trauma can affect you deeply and change your attitude to life. I know that when I was unable to get around and spent hours of each and every day thinking how close I came to death, it actually felt wonderful to be alive.

You begin to appreciate little things that you always took for granted. The sun rising in the sky at daybreak, flowers coming into bud, and the birds in song.

And the first time I walked unaided across a room almost eleven months after the accident – the pleasure was unbelievable.

You still need help though, as there is a vast difference between being in a protected hospital environment and going back out into the world at large.

When I first went back to work it was a shock to the system. The pace of life was so much quicker than I had become accustomed to in hospital. I became tired very quickly. I could not work at the speed I had before the accident. I could not do some of the things I had taken for granted.

As a court reporting journalist, shorthand is essential. But I had slowed down and my rebuilt right arm became tired a lot quicker than it used to. The build-up of anger and frustration is enormous. Not anger at anyone else, but anger at yourself for being so incompetent and not being able to do anything about it.

Unfortunately, within a couple of months I was back in hospital with a badly infected leg and the metal plate had to be removed. I spent some eight weeks on antibiotics and some three weeks back in a hospital bed.

One thing that would be useful for patients, is for someone to talk to them to give them some hint as to what they might expect when they are away from the protected environment of the hospital and back out in the real world. The longer you are away the harder it is to re-adapt. Even now, some six months later, there are still problems. You have to accept that life will never be the same again.

Trauma can also have an effect on relationships.

It can be as difficult for your partner to come to terms with as you yourself. It may bring you closer or it may push you further apart.

People ask if I am a different person as a result of what I have been through. I like to think nothing has changed and I am still the same. But in reality I know that isn't true.

When I think how close I came to death it is, in a way, frightening. I try to carry on a normal life. But I still suffer pain as a result of my injuries and I have to accept that my life will never be the same again. I think how lucky I am to be alive. I can walk.

A few months in a wheelchair made me appreciate what those confined permanently to a wheelchair have to go through each day. Unless you are in the position to experience it for yourself, you can never be fully aware of how difficult it is.

I am now running again. The joy of putting on my trainers and going out for that first run in twenty months was bliss. I have even completed my first marathon since the accident.

But I still find it hard to accept my limitations. A game of football with my nephews and I have to be on guard against a flying boot on my shin, which could so easily shatter my leg again.

You become so protective of your own body and there is a built-in mechanism – it's called survival – that comes into play. How, I just don't know. But a good example is when I was out on a run the other day. Running down a lane, across country, some stinging nettles blocked my way. I jumped over them and as I landed my toe caught a tree root and I was sent flying. Normally you would put your arm out to save yourself. But if my right arm had hit the ground first it could have snapped. So I turned in mid-air and landed on my shoulder and then split my lip as my face hit the ground. But my arm was safe. In the split second it happened, how did my brain know to send out all these instructions? By the way – I still finished up stung by the nettles I had tried to avoid in the first place!

So I ask the question again. How do we cope with trauma? Everybody is different. Some people never do cope. Some people never come to terms with what they have been through.

That is why I think it would be good if there was some support available where somebody needing help could talk to another person who has experienced trauma and re-adapted themselves back into society. It isn't easy and it is only by experiencing it yourself that you may be able to help others cope with an emotional shock to the system that none of us is ever prepared for.

Having considered the stages of the continuum of trauma care in relation to the needs of the individual, it is also important to note that the smooth journey to recovery requires skilled teamwork, professional judgement and organizational support for the team members. The value base of the healthcare team must come from an open discussion of ethical principles and professional standards. There must be evidence of commitment towards continually improving professional practice by evaluating the outcome of care from the injured person's perspective and that of the staff and organization. Shared goals, mutual respect, trust, openness and cooperation between disciplines, and an empowering leadership style, all contribute to an effective team (Barr, 1993).

Given the magnitude of the problem of traumatic injury, holistic care of the injured person has developed as one of the greatest clinical challenges in healthcare. The healthcare team must be able to respond quickly and analytically to assist in the restoration of physiological stability. Their aims must go further to focus on psychological development and sociocultural factors important for the wellbeing of the injured person and those close to them (Howell *et al.*, 1988).

References

American College of Surgeons (1990) *Advanced Trauma Life Support Course*. American College of Surgeons.

Anderson, I. D., Woodford, M., Dombal, F. T. and Irving, M. (1988) Retrospective study of 1000 deaths from injury in England and Wales. *British Medical Journal*, **296,** 1305–1308.

Archer, J. (1991) The process of grief: a selective review. *Journal of Advances in Health and Nursing Care*, **1**(2), 9–37.

Baker, C., Degutis, L. and Desantis, J. (1985) Impact of trauma service on trauma care in a university hospital. *American Journal of Surgery*, **149,** 453.

Barr, O. (1993) Reap the benefits of a co-operative approach. Understanding interdisciplinary team work. *Professional Nurse*, April, 473–477.

Beachley, M. L. (1988) Trauma nurse network standards. *Trauma Nurse Newsletter*, **2**(2), 2.

Beachley, M. L. (1989) Trauma nursing is a developing speciality. *Journal of Emergency Nursing*, **15**(5), 372–373.

Beaver, B. M. (1990) Care of the multiple trauma victim: the first hour. *Nursing Clinics of North America*, **25**(1), 11–21.

Braulin, J. L. D., Rook, J. and Sills, G. M. (1982) Families in crisis: the impact of trauma. *Critical Care Nursing*

Quarterly, **5**(3), 38–46.

Brewer, M. J. (1985) To sleep or not to sleep: the consequences of sleep deprivation. *Critical Care Nurse*, **5**(6), 35–41.

Buschiazzo, L., Possanza, C. and LeDent, M. (1986) Co-ordinating your efforts to manage multiple trauma. *Nursing Life*, Sept./Oct., 33–40.

Cales, R. (1984) Regional mortality in orange country: the effect of implementation of a regional trauma system. *Annals of Emergency Medicine*, **13**, 1.

Cales, R. and Trunkey, D. (1985) Preventable trauma deaths. *Journal of the American Medical Association*, **254**, 1059.

Central Statistics Office (1994) *Social Trends 24*. HMSO.

Clemmer, T., Orme, J. and Thomas, F. (1985) Outcome of the critically injured patients treated at Level 1 trauma centres versus full-service community hospitals. *Critical Care Medicine*, **13**, 861.

Committee on Trauma Research (1985) *Injury in America*. National Academy Press.

Craig, M., Copes, W. and Champion, H. (1988) Psychosocial considerations in trauma care. *Critical Care Nursing Quarterly*, **11**(2), 51–58.

Craven, R. and Bruno, P. (1986) Teach the elderly to prevent falls. *Journal of Gerontological Nursing*, **12**(8), 27–33.

Department of Health (1994) *Hospital Episode Statistics*, Vol. 2, *Financial Year 1990–1991*. London: HMSO.

Department of Health (1998) *Our Healthier Nation* (cmd 3852). London: HMSO.

Department of Trade and Industry (1987) Home accident surveillance system. *11th Annual Report, Home and Leisure Accident Research*. Newgate Press.

Driscoll, P. A. (1992) Trauma: today's problems, tomorrow's answers. *Injury*, **23**(3), 151–158.

Driscoll, P. A., Skinner, D. and Earlham, R. (2000) *ABC of Major Trauma*. 3rd edn, BMJ Publishing.

Dunnum, L. and Bailey, K. (1991) Trauma internship: a success story. *Journal of Neuroscience Nursing*, **23**(4), 253–255.

Evers, H. (1981) Multidisciplinary teams in geriatric wards: myth or reality. *Journal of Advanced Nursing*, **6**, 205–214.

Feist, J. and Brannon, L. (1988) *Health Psychology: An Introduction to Behaviour and Health*. Waddesworth.

Frese, S. (1985) Coping with trauma. *Orthopaedic Nursing*, **4**(2), 58–60.

Fugi-Meyer, A., Brannoim, J. and Fugi-Meyer, K. (1991) Happiness and domain-specific life satisfaction in adult northern Swedes. *Clinical Rehabilitation*, **5**, 23–25.

Gauthier, D. K. (1990) The acute response. *AAOHN Journal*, **38**(10), 475–482.

Gottlieb, B. H. (1983) *Social Support Strategies: Guidelines for Mental Health Practices*. Sage Publications.

Hadfield, L. (1993) Preparation for the nurse as part of the trauma team. *Accident and Emergency Nursing*, **1**, 154–160.

Harvey, A., Goodwill, C., Chamberlain, M. and Evans, C. (1997) *Rehabilitation of the Physically Disabled Adult*. Stanley Thomas.

Hill, M. G. (1990) Trauma prevention: puzzlement or possibility? *AAOHN Journal*, **38**(10), 465.

Howell, E., Widra, L. and Hill, M. G. (1988) *Comprehensive Trauma Nursing: Theory and Practice*. Scott Foresman.

Janis, I. L. and Mann, L. (1977) *Decision Making: a Psychological Analysis of Conflict, Choice and Commitment*. Free Press.

Koch, A. (1985) A strategy for prevention: role, flexibility and affective reactivity as factors in family coping. *Family Systems Medical Journal*, **3**, 70–81.

Lenehan, G. P. (1986) Emotional impact of trauma. *Nursing Clinics of North America*, **21**(4), 729–740.

London, P. (1987) A raw deal for the injured person. *Care of the Critically Ill*, **3**, 171.

Lowe, D., Gately, H. and Goss, J. (1983) Patterns of death, complications and error in the management of motor vehicle accident victims: implications for a regional system of trauma care. *Journal of Trauma*, **23**, 503.

McGrath, J. and Davies, A. (1992) Rehabilitation: where are we going and how do we get there? *Clinical Rehabilitation*, **6**, 225–235.

McGubbin, H. I. and Figley, C. R. (1983) *Stress and the Family: Coping with Normative Transition*, Vol 1. Brunner/Mazel.

Miller, M. and Miller, J. (1985) *Orthopaedics and Accidents*. Hodder and Stoughton.

Parkes, C. M. and Weiss, R. S. (1983) *Recovery from Bereavement*. Basic Books.

Paynter, M. (1990) The nurse in trauma care. *Nursing Standard*, **4**(41), 49.

Ragiel, C. A. (1984) The impact of critical injury on patient, family and clinical systems. *Critical Care Quarterly*, **7**, 73–78.

Rhodes, M., Aronson, J. and Moerkirk, G. (1988) Quality of life after the trauma centre. *Journal of Trauma*, **28**, 931.

Roy, P. (1987) The value of trauma centres: a methodological review. *Canadian Journal of Surgery*, **30**, 17.

Skinner, D. V. (1992) Advanced trauma life support. *Care of the Critically Ill*, **8**(3), 98–99.

Smeltzer, S. C. O. (1988) Research in trauma nursing: state of the art and future directions. *Journal of Emergency Nursing*, **14**(3), 145–153.

Smith, C. (1989) *Orthopaedic Nursing*. Heinemann.

Swannell, J. (1992) *The Oxford Modern English Dictionary*. Clarendon Press.

Winship, G. (1995) Patient empowerment – individualism v collectivism. *Therapeutic Communities*, **16**(2), 113–116.

2

Fracture healing and principles of fracture management

Ronald Langstaff

FRACTURE HEALING

Bone healing occurs in nature by the formation of callus. When a bone is fractured the consequence is haemorrhage into surrounding tissues and under the periosteum. Fracture healing may then be divided into the initial inflammatory response and the proliferative phase in which bone is formed.

Initial bridging of the fracture gap is by granulation tissue and then provisional callus, which is a mixture of new bone and cartilage. This provisional callus then undergoes remodelling.

Formation of bone callus depends on the activities of mesenchymal cells controlled by a mixture of physical stimuli, biochemical stimuli and electrical stimuli, together with remodelling of the fracture which depends on local osteoblastic and osteoplastic activity. It was thought that osteoblasts produced the bony healing callus, but this has subsequently been disproved (Frost, 1989). It has become obvious in more recent years that callus formation depends on the recruitment of undifferentiated mesenchymal or stem cells, together with a large number of local factors such as platelet derived growth factor, PPE 1 and 2 and bone morphogenetic protein.

Inflammatory phase

Following a fracture, the normal response is the formation of a haematoma or a blood clot; within this blood clot, and surrounding the fracture site, is an area of necrosis. This necrosis involves soft tissue and the bone itself, and may extend for up to 1 cm on either side of the fracture. This dying back of the ends of a fractured bone is mediated by osteoplastic cells.

As a consequence of haemorrhage and necrosis there is the traditional acute inflammatory response with macrophage migration into the blood clot, together with phagocytosis of the clot and tissue debris. Following this there is an ingrowth of new blood vessels and fibroblasts. This whole process takes any time up to 5 days.

Reparative phase

The reparative phase in fracture healing is marked by organization of the haematoma and ingrowth of granulation tissue. There is a degree of periosteal proliferation, with cells on the inner layer of the periosteum proliferating in the zone overlying the cortex of each fractured bone end. It would seem that it is this periosteal layer which is responsible for the origin of much of the granulation tissue seen in the reparative phase of fracture healing. The early provisional callus previously referred to is formed by proliferation of mesenchymal cells derived from the periosteum. Initially, a surrounding mass of non-calcified fibrous tissue is formed around the ends of the fracture with woven bone spicules anchored to the cortex at right angles to its surface. This irregular meshwork, within which is mixed a variable amount of cartilage, eventually forms a bridge across the fracture helping to immobilize the bone fragments.

Cortical reaction

Simultaneous to the periosteal response to the fracture, there is also osteoplastic resorption of cortical bone at the fracture site. This may be noted on X-rays initially as a widening of the fracture gap.

Medullary reaction

The response to the process of fracture healing within the medullary canal also involves granulation tissue and phagocytosis of necrotic tissue with resorption of dead bone by osteoplastic activity. This produces so-called internal callus with woven bone formation.

Fracture gap

Two bone fragments are united externally by periosteal callus, but this does not directly unite the two ends of the bone. The bone ends are separated by a clot which is eventually replaced by granulation tissue. This granulation tissue may then be replaced by either ossification or fibrous tissue, the fibrous tissue being formed if there is major instability or a poor blood supply. Initial fracture healing takes place due to the presence of calcified external and internal callus within the medullary canal, together with bridging of the fracture gap by calcified bone. Following this restoration of anatomical integrity remodelling occurs, where woven bone is replaced by new bone, i.e. normal bone. This new bone is distributed according to Wolf's law (1892) which states that bone develops a structure most suited to the forces acting upon it. The process of remodelling also removes any callus formed within the medullary canal, thereby allowing reformation of normal bone marrow constituents.

PRINCIPLES OF FRACTURE MANAGEMENT

The management of a fracture is no different from the management of any medical condition. It consists of:

- a clinical history of the injury
- an examination of the patient
- investigation
- diagnosis and classification of the fracture
- treatment of the patient.

Each one of these stages of fracture management would necessitate a textbook in itself, and to cover them comprehensively in a short single chapter is impossible. This chapter will therefore concentrate on the very broad principles of fracture management in adults; no attempt is made to consider fractures in children.

It is sometimes forgotten that trauma surgeons treat people, not X-rays or isolated limbs, and while X-rays of two fractures may have the same appearance, the circumstances surrounding the production of those fractures may be very different. Individuals are unique, and therefore the consequences of injury to those individuals will vary. The corollary of this is that the treatment required by individuals may be very different. This is the art, as opposed to the science, of medical practice; the tailoring of treatment to the needs of the individual.

The objectives in fracture management are to promote bony union and soft tissue healing, together with the restoration of function not only of the injured limb, but also of the individual into society. To do this it is necessary to restore anatomy to as near normal as possible, avoiding both natural and iatrogenic complications. The surgeon must therefore understand the natural history of various fracture patterns and be able to deploy the full range of modern fracture management techniques using a sound understanding of the indications for their application. An inability to do this often results in mismanagement.

It is becoming increasingly clear that some fractures should be managed in specialist centres to allow concentration of expertise. There is no room for the occasional operator in complex fracture management. The consequences of mismanagement are often a lifetime of disability for the patient and, increasingly for the surgeon, an encounter with the legal profession! That is not to say that normality can always be restored following fractures – some cannot be reconstructed and inevitably there will be some functional disability – but the prognosis and treatment options must always be made clear to the patient from the outset. The dictum of informed consent demands no less.

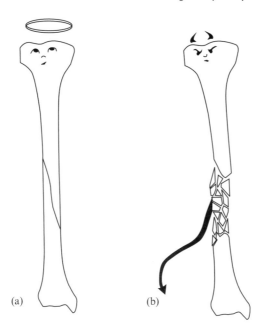

Figure 2.1 a & b The personality of a tibial fracture

History

The taking of a clinical history in fracture management concentrates first on the mechanism of injury. It is important to ascertain the energy involved in the production of the fracture.

The natural history of a high-energy tibial fracture sustained as a consequence of a high-speed road traffic accident is very different from that of a low-energy fracture sustained in a fall. The damage to the soft tissue envelope surrounding the broken bone varies and critically influences the behaviour of the fracture and the likelihood of complications developing. It is often suggested that if fractures were to be considered as soft tissue injuries complicated by a broken bone, a more satisfactory approach to fracture management might ensue. Nicholl (1964) coined the term 'the personality' of the fracture and, like people, some fractures have good personalities – low-energy, closed, simple (Figure 2.1a); and others bad – high-energy, displaced, open, complex or multifragmentary. A fracture with bad personality is less likely to be successfully managed using non-operative techniques and is more likely to require aggressive intervention (Figure 2.1b).

A comprehensive history should also include those aspects of the individual's life which may have a bearing on fracture management. Age, occupation and expectations must be taken into consideration, and treatment must be tailored to individual needs. What is appropriate treatment for a sedentary 70-year-old may not be for a young, manual labourer. It is only by taking a comprehensive clinical history and finding out about the patient as an individual that one can begin to tailor treatment. What must be avoided is the 'cookery book' approach to fracture management, where fractures are all managed in the same fashion depending on the X-ray appearance.

Examination

The examination of an individual with a fracture should always be comprehensive, but the history will dictate the extent of the examination required. There is little point in performing a full neurological examination on a child with a buckle fracture of the distal radius. There is every necessity to perform that examination on a patient with multiple limb fractures following a high-speed road traffic accident and who may have been rendered unconscious at the scene.

Examination of the injured limb involves three stages: (a) look, (b) feel, and (c) move.

Look

Even in closed fractures the diagnosis of a fracture may be straightforward, with obvious swelling and deformity of the limb. In open fractures there may be obvious wounds. However, this may not always be the case, and undisplaced fractures may, in the immediate acute phase, have little in the way of any obvious external physical signs on inspection.

Feel

Palpation of any injured limb with a suspected fracture should be gentle. The patient's face should be watched carefully during any palpation. Crepitus may be felt but should not be sought. If the fracture is in a long bone, assessment of the neurovascular state of the limb distal to the fracture must be assessed, and the presence or absence of pulses and sensation must be recorded in the notes. Paraesthesia or anaesthesia may be a sign of either direct damage to a nerve, the onset of a compartment syndrome, or an early sign of vascular insufficiency secondary to arterial damage.

Move

Movement may be active or passive. The inability of a patient to actively move a limb without pain may be a sign of fracture. Elderly patients who are unable to walk after a fall and complain of pain in the groin on movement of the hip must be considered to have a fracture of the neck of the femur until proved otherwise.

Passive movement in the presence of a suspected fracture should be gentle, but in the case of an obvious fracture dislocation of the ankle where skin viability is threatened, urgent reduction may be necessary.

Investigations

The investigation of patients following injury is covered more comprehensively later in this book, but the whole gamut of modern medical investigative technology is available in the treatment of patients with fractures. This ranges from plain radiography, ultrasound or CT scanning, to MRI scanning and isotope bone scans.

Plain radiography comprises the majority of the routine investigations in fracture management. There are a number of basic rules which should be followed in the use of plain X-rays, and it must be remembered that radiation should be avoided wherever possible as it is potentially hazardous (RCR Working Party, 1993). There are a number of clinical guidelines for the use of X-rays in extremity injuries, and in some circumstances their use is not appropriate (De Lacey and Bradbrooke, 1979).

Classification and fracture patterns

Having investigated the patient and diagnosed the fracture, it is usually possible to describe and classify it. The major descriptive division is into closed or open fractures; the word compound should be avoided – it is meaningless. This simple division is of fundamental importance in management and prognosis; any open fracture has a far worse prognosis than a closed fracture of a similar pattern. It should be remembered that open fractures constitute a surgical emergency and the aim must be to complete the initial surgical debridement and stabilization of the fracture within 6 hours. By this time the majority of open wounds cease to be contaminated only by bacteria, but become frankly infected, and it is infection in the open fracture that is the greatest cause of subsequent morbidity.

In the long bones, fractures (whether open or closed) may be described in terms of their position – intra-articular, metaphyseal, diaphyseal; or by their appearance – transverse, oblique, spiral, butterfly. They can be described as simple with single fracture lines, or complex where there is more than one fragment. Fractures with more than one fragment are called multifragmentary or comminuted. Fractures are described as segmental where there is a double fracture line producing an isolated segment of a long bone.

These various fracture patterns are not solely of academic interest, but give a clue as to the forces producing the injury. For instance, a transverse fracture is produced by a direct blow as seen typically in the isolated, closed, transverse ulnar fracture, the 'night stick' fracture. (A night stick is an American policeman's baton, the ulna being fractured as the arm is raised to ward off a blow.) A spiral fracture is seen following a twisting injury, and multi-fragmentary fractures are associated with high-speed, high-energy injuries. Impacted or crush fractures, in which there is no displacement of the fracture fragments but loss of normal bony contour, may be seen after a high fall, typically in the calcaneum or in a vertebral body.

Pathological fractures occur where an abnormal bone fractures following the application of a physiological load. This fracture type is seen in metastatic disease where normal bone has been replaced by tumour mass. Alternatively, normal bone may fracture following the repeated application of physiological stress. A typical example is the 'march' fracture, so-called because of its prevalence in military recruits, where it is found in the mid-shaft of the second or third metatarsals. These stress fractures may not be immediately apparent on X-ray, but can be seen some weeks later as a periosteal reaction with subperiosteal callus.

More systematic attempts to classify, as opposed to merely describing, fractures exist with almost as many systems as there are fracture types. Some of these are eponymous, such as the Garden classification system of subcapital femoral neck fractures, or Frick's classification of distal radial fractures, and apply to specific sites only. Other fracture classification systems are alpha-numeric, such as the AO Fracture Classification System which makes a claim to be universal.

It should be remembered that fractures are classified for the purpose of producing a guide to treatment. Many fracture classification systems are of academic interest only, and those which are more elaborate inevitably result in a degree of inter- and indeed intra-observer variation, which may render them useless in practical terms as a tool for the working clinician.

Having established a diagnosis and classified a fracture, and confirmed the presence or absence of associated complications, the next stage is choice of definitive treatment.

Treatment

Fracture treatment may be broadly divided into:

- conservative or non-operative management
- operative management.

This is somewhat arbitrary, as the manipulative treatment of a fracture might be considered 'operative'. However, in this discussion 'operative' management will be taken to mean surgical treatment, where the fracture site is opened, or implants are inserted into the limb or around the fracture site.

Within these two broad divisions of treatment the principles are the same:

- reduction of the fracture
- stabilization of the fracture
- mobilization of the limb and the patient.

Conservative or non-operative management

The majority of fractures can, and still should, be treated by non-operative means. When considering non-operative treatment it must be appreciated that there is a likelihood or a possibility of that treatment failing, particularly in the case of the manipulation of forearm fractures in children. It is always wise to obtain consent to allow the operation to proceed from 'non-operative' to 'operative reduction, with internal fixation' if appropriate.

Fracture reduction

A fracture is a break in the continuity of a bone. Displacement of the fragments will result in loss of normal anatomy and subsequently loss of function, either of the limb or of the patient as a whole. Reduction of a fracture may therefore be defined as the restoration of normal anatomy – the length, axial and rotational alignment of the bone.

It is not necessary to reduce anatomically all displaced fractures and the decision as to the necessity, or not, of reduction is one of the skills in fracture management.

The decision as to whether or not to reduce a fracture depends on a number of factors such as the age of the patient and the fracture site.

The age of the patient

Fractures in children show a considerable degree of potential for remodelling after the fracture has united. What may be an unacceptable degree of displacement in an adult would be wholly acceptable in a child, as further growth can result in the gradual loss of the deformity. However, not all fractures remodel in children; there is no potential for remodelling in the rotational plane or in the case of intra-articular fractures. The potential obviously depends on the skeletal maturity of the child, younger children having greater scope for remodelling.

Site of the fracture

As a general rule intra-articular fractures need accurate reduction to avoid joint incongruity after bony union, and to prevent subsequent development of joint stiffness and secondary osteoarthritis. For extra-articular metaphyseal and diaphyseal fractures the requirement varies, depending on which bone is fractured.

In the upper limb, fractures such as those of the humerus or clavicle do not need accurate reduction; a significant amount of residual distortion of normal anatomy can be accepted with surprisingly little functional deficit.

In the forearm accurate reduction is required, as there will be major loss of movement, particularly pronation and supination, should the fracture heal in an abnormal position (mal-union).

In the lower limb, long bone diaphyseal fractures of the femur or tibia need reduction in terms of length, axial and rotational alignment. Failure to achieve this may result in leg length inequality, angulation of the distal joint line at the knee or ankle, or excessive internal or external rotation of the foot.

In other lower limb fractures, such as those of the lateral malleolus of the ankle, there is a requirement for near perfect anatomical reduction. A 1 mm shift of the talus as a consequence of an unreduced, or poorly reduced, fibular fracture increases the talotibial plafond contact pressures by 47%. The consequence may be the onset of early osteoarthritis of the ankle joint, as the articular surface between the talus and the tibia breaks down under the increased load.

Techniques of non-operative fracture reduction

The non-operative reduction of fractures can be achieved in a number of ways by the use of gravity, traction or manipulation. When a fracture is reduced, the aim is to reverse the forces which acted to produce the fracture in the first instance. The choice as to how this is done will involve consideration of the soft tissue attachments to the fracture fragments, the deforming forces they produce, and whether or not the periosteal sleeve surrounding the cortex of the bone is intact or disrupted.

Gravity. With closed fractures it is not always necessary to consider manipulation, and the satisfactory reduction of a fracture may be achieved simply by the use of gravity. The weight of the limb itself is used to overcome muscle forces producing shortening of the fracture. This technique is most commonly used with a collar and cuff sling or hanging cast when treating a humeral shaft or proximal humeral fracture.

Traction. Traction is considered elsewhere in this book and will not be explored further in this chapter. It is listed for completeness as one of the ways to reduce a fracture.

Manipulation. In manipulative treatment an attempt is made to reverse the mechanism of injury which produced the fracture and the consequent malalignment of the fragments.

Manipulation can be performed under local, regional or general anaesthesia. It is usually undertaken as soon as possible after the injury and before any swelling of the limb secondary to haemorrhage or oedema has occurred. It is all too easy to produce secondary injuries to the skin by careless manipulation.

The technique involves, first, the application of gentle traction to the injured limb, with an assistant providing counter-traction. This is done under image intensifier control. The aim is to disimpact the fracture fragments, and overcome any overlap or shortening caused by muscle spasm.

In a fracture where the periosteal hinge is intact, the angulation of the fracture is then increased, allowing relaxation of the soft tissue hinge on the concave side of the deformity, leading to disimpaction of the fracture fragment. Traction and manipulation then align the fragments, tightening up the periosteal hinge and providing a stable fracture configuration, thereby preventing further axial shortening or rotation.

Where the periosteal hinge is not intact there is no need to increase the angulation of the deformity, and simple traction will usually allow restoration of length.

Stabilization

If after reduction it is considered that a fracture is unstable, then some form of stabilization device should be applied. If a fracture has been displaced and subsequently reduced it is usually necessary to consider some form of stabilization because without it, it is likely that the fracture will redisplace. Fractures which have never been displaced, or are only minimally displaced, may not require stabilization. Unstable fractures are typically short oblique, spiral or multifragmentary fractures. In non-operative management, stability may be obtained in a number of ways by the use of gravity, splints or casts.

Gravity. Gravity can be used to stabilize a fracture that was initially undisplaced, or where it is unlikely that a reduced fracture will significantly redisplace. The most common example would be in a transverse humeral fracture. It is often necessary, however, to supplement simple gravity traction by the use of external casts or splints.

Splints. There are a large number of commercially available splints on the market. They may be used acutely, such as in the acute undisplaced humeral fracture, or in the rehabilitation stage of fracture healing when the fracture requires only minimal external support.

Casts. Traditional casting material is plaster of Paris – hydrated calcium sulphate adsorbed onto a bandage. It can be used in slabs or as a complete encircling bandage applied over padding. The padding needs to be thick enough to protect any bony prominence, but not so thick that the cast cannot hold the reduction. There are newer synthetic materials which are lighter in weight and waterproof, but they are harder to mould.

The application of a cast to a freshly reduced fracture requires two people – one to hold the reduction and one to apply the cast. This is then moulded using the principle of three-point fixation described in the classic text *The Closed Treatment of Common Fractures* (Charnley, 1961). A well-applied cast will control angular deformities, but to control any rotatory malalignment it is necessary to include the joints above and below the fracture, such as the wrist and elbow in a forearm fracture.

In some ways it is harder to manage patients conservatively in a cast than it is operatively by internal fixation. It is not enough simply to apply the cast and leave it until, hopefully, the fracture heals. The patient requires careful monitoring with frequent follow-up and X-ray until the fracture has healed. This is to ensure that, with the resolution of any swelling around the fracture following reduction, it does not subsequently slip resulting in mal-union.

The cast should act to control the movement of the fracture, maintaining length, axial and rotational alignment. Stable transverse fractures may be held in a plaster easily. Unstable fractures are much more difficult to control in plaster, and some other method of obtaining stability should be considered. Casts will not control length well in oblique diaphyseal fractures, as the fracture often shortens.

Mobilization

Mobilization of the limb and the patient should begin as soon as possible. One of the most common complications of an otherwise straightforward fracture of the distal radius is shoulder and elbow stiffness resulting from being left in a broad arm sling for 4 weeks. The value of good physiotherapy in the management of patients with fractures cannot be overemphazised.

Operative management of fractures

The decision to operate on a fracture should be considered very carefully. Complications of operative management, if they occur, can be severe.

It was often said by an older generation of surgeons that 'no fracture must be fixed'. That statement is certainly debatable, but operative management should only be used where it is not possible to achieve a satisfactory outcome by the use of conservative management. There are some relative indications for considering operative management, and these are:

- open fractures
- irreducible or unstable fractures
- pathological fractures
- to aid management of soft tissue or neurovascular complications
- multiple fractures
- the presence of a significant head injury.

Having made the decision to manage a fracture operatively, the management follows the same principles as non-operative management, with reduction and stabilization of the fracture followed by mobilization of the limb and the patient.

Operative reduction of fractures

Open reduction should be used only in line with the previously definite indications, or when closed reduction has failed. The operative reduction of fractures may be divided into direct and indirect techniques.

Direct reduction techniques

Direct reduction techniques involve exposure of the fracture site by dissection, and manipulation of the bone ends under direct vision to achieve restoration of the normal anatomy. Such an approach is used in adult forearm fractures, where a failure to restore the normal curvature of the radius and radioulnar relationship results in loss of pronation and supination, or in other situations where normal anatomy is necessary for the restoration of function.

Indirect reduction techniques

Indirect reduction techniques avoid opening of the fracture site and are used when it is not necessary to achieve an exact anatomical reduction, but merely an approximation of the normal anatomy. These techniques rely on the application of forces transmitted to the bony fragments through the soft tissue attachments to give restoration of length and rotation.

Indirect vs. direct reduction techniques

The advantages of indirect, as opposed to direct, reduction techniques relate to the pre-servation of the blood supply to the fracture fragments, something that can be damaged or lost if the fracture site is opened and the fragments dissected to allow their direct manipulation. Loss of blood supply results in death of the bone, delay in healing and, if complicated by infection, disaster.

Direct reduction techniques are important where the restoration of normal anatomy is important for the restoration of function, as already mentioned in the case of forearm fractures or intra-articular fractures. In other sites, where exact reduction of the fracture is not so important and all that is required is restoration of length and alignment, then indirect reduction is to be favoured.

Operative stabilisation of fractures

Techniques of operative stabilization of fractures may be divided into, first, those using internal fixation, secondly those using external fixation, and finally those using a combination of the two. These techniques are described in some detail below.

Internal fixation

Internal fixation in fracture surgery dates back to the nineteenth century, but the devices used were often inadequate, the metallurgy also inadequate and the results of surgery poor. Modern use of plates and screws dates back to the 1960s with the rise of the 'AO' school of fracture surgery in Switzerland.

The AO or Arbeitgemeinschaft für Osteosynthesefragen (Association for the Study of Internal Fixation) were a group of Swiss orthopaedic surgeons who set out to study fracture healing and the response to internal fixation in a scientific manner. Based on the principles first stated by Robert Danis in 1947, they developed a range of surgical implants and laid the foundations of modern fracture surgery. The principles were:

- anatomical reduction of fractures
- rigid internal fixation
- early mobilization
- meticulous care of the soft tissues.

The first two principles are no longer regarded as universally applicable. The concept in fracture surgery is now not of rigidity but of stability. Operative stabilization of fractures can produce a range of stability at the fracture site from absolute to relative. Stability is important because it is this which produces the optimal conditions for the proliferation of callus and fracture healing.

Stability can be absolute, where open reduction and the insertion of plates and screws is the preferred method of treatment (such as in some intra-articular fractures), or relative, with the advent of modern techniques of intramedullary nailing. What is still universally true is that the goal of operative fracture surgery is to create a bone–implant construct that is sufficiently stable to allow early mobilization of the fracture and the patient without the risk of redisplacement of the fracture fragments. The last principle, soft tissue care, remains as vital as always.

Devices for internal fixation of fractures are many and varied. They comprise wire, screws, plates and nails. The majority of implants are manufactured from stainless steel alloy, although titanium is becoming more popular because of its lower modulus of elasticity, which gives less stress shielding of the bone thereby allowing a more physiological response of the bone to load. Recently, interest has revived in absorbable implants manufactured from polylactic or polyglycolic acid.

Wire. Kirshner or 'K' wires have a trocar pointed tip and are used to secure small fragments of metaphyseal bone where compression is not required. They can be used in cortical bone in children, but not in adults.

The other common use of wire fixation is usually to form a figure-of-eight tension band in combination with longitudinal K wires crossing a transverse fracture. This type of fixation is seen most commonly in the fractured olecranon (Figure 2.2) where it is still the most reliable method of fixation, or in a transverse fracture of the patella.

Circlage wiring, where wire is twisted round the shaft of a long bone, can be used to provide temporary intraoperative stability, but it is best avoided as a definitive fracture fixation. It destroys the periosteum and gives insufficient stability for early mobilization.

Screws. Screws come in all shapes and sizes to match the size of bone into which they are to be inserted, but are essentially designed either to

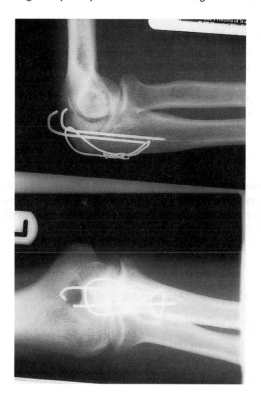

Figure 2.2 Internal fixation of an olecranon fracture

hold a plate against a bone or to apply compression across a fracture site – the so-called 'lag screw effect'. Screws which are used in metaphyseal bone have a different thread characteristic from those used in harder, denser cortical bone. Compression is not an indispensable condition of fracture healing, it simply increases the stability across the fracture site, allowing mobilization.

Plates. Plates have been developed in a variety of sizes and contours to match the differing anatomical sites and fracture configurations for which they are needed, but their usage can be divided into four or possibly five basic mechanical categories. They can be used either as a buttress plate (usually in a metaphyseal fracture), as a compression plate (usually in a diaphyseal fracture), or as a neutralization plate to neutralize torsional forces (such as in the spiral fracture of a long bone fixed with lag screws). They can also be used as a bridging or biological plate across a multifragmentary fracture and, finally, as a reconstruction plate where they are a template to which multiple

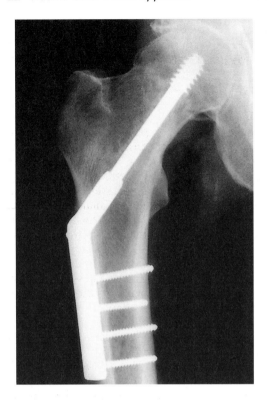

Figure 2.3 Dynamic hip screw

bone fragments are fixed to recreate the anatomical shape of a shattered bone.

The use of screws and plates together can provide extremely stable or 'rigid' fixation. This allows early mobilization of the injured limb or patient. The disadvantage of the use of the plates and screws is, however, the often extensive dissection required in order to position the implant in a mechanically suitable way. The consequence of the dissection is further soft tissue damage and the stripping of the periosteum from the bone resulting in devitalization, compounding the injury already sustained. If infection supervenes the consequences can be disastrous.

In experienced hands, and with very careful attention to detail, plating of fractures produces excellent results (Figure 2.3). However, it demands not only an understanding of the biology of fracture healing, but also the mechanics of stability. Dissatisfaction with the outcome of plating of long-bone fractures, particularly in the femur and in open fractures of the tibia, led in the 1980s to a resurgence of interest in intramedullary nailing.

Intramedullary nailing

Early Aztec writings on the management of fractures describe the use of intramedullary nails fashioned from pine wood. The modern scientific era of intramedullary nailing began with Hay-Groves in 1916, but was extended and popularized by Otto Kuntschner, a German Air Force surgeon, during World War II. A *Lancet* editorial in 1946 suggested that this 'new fangled' method of treatment would 'never catch on'! Fortunately the editorial proved to be wrong, and intramedullary nailing is now the preferred management of both closed, and probably open, long-bone fractures.

Intramedullary nails act as internal splints. When inserted into the medullary canal they give fracture fixation which is relatively, but not absolutely stable, allowing a degree of movement at the fracture site. The fracture heals by the formation of external callus.

An intramedullary nail acts as a load-sharing device, taking up torsional and bending forces normally carried by the bone. These forces are transmitted to the nail until the fracture has healed. The forces transmitted to the nail depend on the grip between the nail and the bone, and the efficiency of rigid nails is dependent on their so-called 'working length', which is the length of the nail not protected by intact bone, i.e. the length between the two points where the nail has no purchase on the bone. This varies, depending on the nature of the fracture. A multifragmentary fracture where the nail grips the bone at the top and bottom of the shaft only will impose a greater working length on the bone than a simple transverse fracture. The greater the forces carried by the nail, the stronger and more rigid it must be. Too much movement as a consequence of a lack of stability at the fracture site will result in a non-union, where fibrous tissue forms instead of callus.

The rigidity and strength of intramedullary nails depend on a number of mechanical factors, the most important being size and cross-sectional characteristics.

Size. The larger the nail, the more rigid and stronger it is. The strength of the nail depends on its diameter, and its bending rigidity is proportional to the fourth power of its radius.

Cross-section. A nail may be solid or hollow.

Solid nails are more rigid than hollow nails of equivalent size. If the nail is hollow, the cross-section can be either closed, or have an incomplete section with a slot, like the traditional Kuntschner nail (K-nail) which is cloverleafed. The effect of this longitudinal slot along the length of the nail gives an open section nail, which is less stiff than a closed section nail. The significant reduction in the stiffness of the nail not only makes it easier to insert, but also allows it to expand in the medullary canal to grip the sides of the bone.

Intramedullary nails are therefore somewhat arbitrarily divided into rigid and flexible nails. Rigid nails may be cannulated or solid, and are inserted into the medullary canal in either a reamed or an unreamed fashion. Flexible nails are small solid nails which are inserted across the fracture site in an unreamed fashion.

Rigid cannulated intramedullary nails

The majority of rigid intramedullary nails are cannulated and designed to be introduced in a reamed fashion over a guidewire. In lower limb fractures, where nails are most commonly used, the guidewire is passed through the greater trochanter of the femur or through the anterior tibial eminence under X-ray. A series of powered reamers is then used to increase the size of the medullary canal allowing the insertion of a larger nail than would otherwise be possible. This is inserted over the same guidewire.

Reamed intramedullary nails control the fracture by achieving an interference fit, and are gripped by the bony medullary canal over an area proximal and distal to the fracture. This area of contact is enhanced by reaming. The tighter the fit between the nail and the medullary canal, the less chance there is of rotational instability.

Rigid solid intramedullary nails

Rigid solid nails have no lumen and are inserted into a fractured long bone usually without reaming, although they can be inserted in a reamed fashion. They have a smaller diameter than the hollow nails and, because they are solid, are more rigid than the cannulated slotted nails.

The development of the unreamed nail evolved from consideration of the biological disadvantages of reaming, which include embolization of medullary contents together with damage to the endosteal blood supply (Haas *et al.*, 1993; Renner *et al.*, 1993).

Experiments have shown that reamed tibial nailing may reduce cortical blood flow by 70%, as compared with 30% in unreamed nailing. Given the importance of the blood supply for fracture healing, it appears from a biological point of view more sensible to consider the use of unreamed nailing in fractures. More recently, however, clinical studies have suggested that reaming of the medullary canal may in fact divert blood supply into the periosteum and, as has already been discussed, it is the periosteal layer which is the most important tissue in fracture healing. There may therefore be a paradoxical beneficial effect of medullary reaming with some advantages in using reamed as opposed to unreamed nailing.

A recent important clinical paper (Court-Brown *et al.*, 1996), comparing reamed or unreamed nailing for closed tibial fractures, appears to bear this out. It was shown that reamed nailing was associated with a significantly lower time to bony union that that in unreamed nailing. It is now suggested that the use of unreamed nails in closed fractures is probably contraindicated.

The situation in the open fracture may however be different, and further studies are needed. The only prospective randomized study comparing reamed and unreamed nailing in the management of open tibial fractures showed no difference between the two methods of treatment.

Interlocking nails

Rigid cannulated and later the rigid solid intramedullary nails developed the capacity to be interlocked. The interlocking nail has holes proximally and distally, allowing the insertion of screws through the bone into the nail. This allows control of rotation and length at the fracture site, and has dramatically extended the indication for their use. Prior to interlocking, the use of intramedullary nails was confined to fractures in the isthmus of the long bones where the nail could get a grip. With the advent of locking, their use has extended to virtually the whole of the length of long bones.

Nails may be interlocked in either a static or dynamic fashion. Where nails are locked statically they are locked rigidly to both fragments; where they are locked dynamically they are either locked rigidly to one fragment only and to the second fragment not at all, or the screw is passed through an oval hole in the nail, allowing a degree of movement. It is this movement which is important in the formation of callus. The decision as to whether to lock a nail statically or dynamically depends on the configuration of the fracture and the degree of contact between the cortical fragments. If the fracture is multifragmentary and likely to shorten or rotate, then it should be statically locked. If the fracture configuration is transverse, and therefore unlikely to rotate or shorten, it can be dynamically locked.

Flexible nails

Flexible nails are small-diameter solid metal nails. They predate modern intramedullary nails. The most common of these are the Enders and Rush nails, but they are not commonly used in the UK. The use of Enders nails in trochanteric fractures of the femur remains relatively common in Eastern Europe. They are not easy to use to gain good stability and they cannot be interlocked.

External fixation

External fixation is where pins, screws or wires are inserted into or through the bone, then linked to an external frame which allows both reduction and stabilization of the fracture. External fixators may be divided into pin and bar fixators, circular fixators, or a combination of the two – a hybrid fixator.

Pin and bar fixators. In pin and bar fixators pins are inserted into or through the bone, and are then connected to a bar by some sort of clamp. They have been the most popular method of external fixation in fracture management in this country and have most commonly been employed for the management of severe open fractures of the tibia.

Pin and bar fixators can be constructed as a unilateral or bilateral frame. Other constructions, such as the delta frame, are also possible. The rigidity of the frame depends on a number of factors including the size, number and location of the pins and bars, the stability of the reduced fracture, and the conditions at the pin–bone site interface.

There are disadvantages to the use of external fixators, with pin site infection being common. Pin site infection may result in loss of stability between the pin and the bone, with loosening and subsequent loss of control of fracture alignment and consequent mal-union or non-union. Comparative studies between external, internal and conservative management of fractures are poor or non-existent, but the use of external fixation in simple closed fractures of the long bones of the lower limb is not advised – other methods of operative fixation will produce better results.

Ring fixators. In a ring fixator, wires are passed through each principal fragment and held by clamps attached to a ring which is then connected to rods. This type of fixator allows correction of bony defects, length and deformity, and even so-called bone transport 'callotasis' with bridging of segmental defects. Their use is highly technical and at present is limited to specialist centres. These devices are more widely used in reconstructive surgery for the correction of angulation in fractures which have healed with deformity (in particular loss of bone length or angulation), rather than in the primary management of fractures. Their use may become more popular in the future as the skills involved become more widely disseminated.

Combined minimal internal and external fixation

Some fractures are notoriously difficult to manage, such as multifragmentary intra-articular fractures of the proximal and distal tibia. The nature of the fracture pattern makes anatomical reduction and absolute stability desirable, but thin soft tissue cover means that attempts to achieve it with plates and screws have often resulted in disaster.

One way around this has been to use a combination of interfragmentary screws inserted percutaneously with an external fixator to buttress the construct. This avoids the insertion of bulky plates into soft tissue which may already be traumatized. As a concept it seems to be satisfactory in the metaphyseal zone, though less so in the diaphysis where the screws often fail. It is not an easy technique, but these are not easy fractures to manage.

Mobilization

Mobilization, the fourth AO principle, should begin as soon as possible. The stability of the fracture implant construct will dictate the speed at which active joint exercises can begin and how soon weight-bearing commences. If a fracture cannot be fixed in a stable enough fashion to allow early mobilization, it is probably better not to operate on it at all. The combination of immobilization and operative fixation almost invariably results in significant joint stiffness.

Just as in mobilization with non-operative treatment, a knowledgeable physiotherapist is vital. Overenthusiastic early weight-bearing may result in the fatigue failure of the implant and loss of position of the fracture. Close collaboration and good communication is essential if such disasters are to be avoided. Surgeons must understand the limits of what can be achieved – partial weight-bearing in a demented elderly patient with a multifragmentary fracture of the proximal femoral shaft, however desirable, may not be practically achievable! The patient's ability to cooperate with physiotherapy must be taken into account when considering a surgical strategy for the management of fractures.

Conclusion

Fracture management has changed out of all recognition over the past 20 years, but no doubt the greatest changes are yet to come, as the molecular biologists unlock the secrets of fracture healing. What will not change, however, is the emergency workload and people's ability to inflict trauma on themselves and others.

As the technology available for treating patients becomes ever more sophisticated we would perhaps all do well to remember the words of Sir Robert Hutchison (1871–1960), a former President of the Royal College of Surgeons:

> From inability to leave well alone;
> From too much zeal for what is new and contempt for what is old;
> From putting knowledge before wisdom, science before art, cleverness before common sense;
> From treating patients as cases; and
> From making the cure of a disease more grievous than its endurance,
> Good Lord, deliver us.

References

Charnley, J. (1961) *The Closed Treatment of Common Fractures*, 3rd edn. Churchill Livingstone.

Court-Brown, C. M., Will, E., Christie, J. and McQueen, M. M. (1996) Reamed or unreamed nailing for closed tibial fractures. *Journal of Bone and Joint Surgery*, **78B**(4), 580–583.

De Lacey, G. and Bradbrooke, S. (1979) Rationalising requests for X-ray examination of acute ankle injuries. *British Medical Journal*, **1**, 1597–1598.

Frost, H. M. (1989) The biology of fracture healing I. *Clinical Orthopaedics*, **248**, 283–293.

Haas, N., Krettek, C., Schandelmaier, P. *et al.* (1993) A new solid unreamed tibial nail for shaft fractures with severe soft tissue injury. *Injury*, **24**, 49–54.

Nicholl, E. A. (1964) Fractures of the tibial shaft: a survey of 705 cases. *Journal of Bone and Joint Surgery*, **46B**, 373–387.

RCR Working Party (1993) *Making the best use of a department of clinical radiology*. Royal College of Radiologists.

Renner, N., Regain, P., Bast, R. and Ross, R. (1993) Initial experiences with the unreamed tibial nail. *Helvetica Chirurgica Acta*, **59**, 665–668.

3

The physiological effects of trauma

Jacqueline Scott

Introduction

The complexity of the physiological response to trauma presents a challenge to those trying to maintain the patient's physiological equilibrium and regain the homeostatic norm before irreversible damage occurs.

This chapter provides an overview of the physical effects and impact of trauma on the individual. A 'systems' approach provides a structure with the focus being the importance of clinical observations and their impact on recovery. Trauma patients may have several coexisting problems with varying degrees of severity, differential diagnosis being the key to effective decision-making and treatment.

Stress response

The maintenance of the body in a healthy state depends on its ability to respond appropriately to environmental changes in a coordinated fashion. However, the body's response to trauma, planned or otherwise, can have a profound effect on all systems. The normal homeostatic mechanisms of the body may be disrupted, homeostasis being the maintenance of a constant intracellular environment.

Normal cellular function depends on the ability of cells to maintain the physical and chemical properties of their constituents, temperature, hydration, concentration of nutrients, waste products, electrolytes and hydrogen ions

(Montague *et al.*, 1996). A homeostatic mechanism is a regulatory mechanism triggered by an alteration in a particular physiological property of extracellular fluid which acts to produce a compensatory or restorative change. This action is undertaken via negative feedback to restore or preserve the norm. In order for this to be achieved, receptors, effectors and the coordinating action of an integrating mechanism are required. If homeostasis is not maintained, an adverse effect on the balance of health may ensue (Guyton, 1991); the homeostasis of the individual is disrupted following trauma.

Acute traumatic shock can be identified by a variety of clinical signs (Table 3.1). Shock is a clinical state in which cardiac output is insufficient and therefore unable to meet tissue requirements. These requirements are defined as an adequate supply of oxygen and nutrients, together with the effective removal of waste products of metabolism. Shock results in reduced tissue perfusion which leads to tissue hypoxia and the accumulation of metabolites. In the severely injured patient shock can manifest itself in several ways (Table 3.2).

The principal aim in the treatment of a severely injured or shocked patient is the control of haemorrhage and the restoration of circulating blood volume. Identification of the source of blood loss is essential and it is important to remember that bleeding can be both external and internal. The amount of blood loss must be estimated as accurately as possible.

Table 3.1 Shock: signs and symptoms (Adapted from Sheehy *et al.*, 1989)

Signs and symptoms	Physical basis
Sweating, pallor, dry mouth, indigestion, vomiting	Reduced blood volume
Nausea, vomiting, frequent diarrhoea, constipation	Decreased/increased mobility of gastrointestinal tract
Tachycardia, palpitations, increased blood pressure, headache, chest pain	Increased cardiac rate and output
Increased rate and shallow depth of breathing, tingling in fingers/hands/feet, dizziness, disorientation, dilated or unequal pupils, restlessness	Depression of central nervous system
Headache, muscle tremor, spasm, lack of co-ordination	Increased arousal of central nervous system

Table 3.2 Types of shock (Adapted from Huggins, 1990)

Haemorrhagic shock	• Sudden loss of blood or fluid from the intravascular compartment • Dehydration, vomiting, diarrhoea, diabetic ketosis, heat stroke
Anaphylactic shock	• Results from an antibody–antigen reaction causing contraction of bronchial smooth muscle and narrowing of the airways, dilatation of the micro-circulation and pooling of blood, increased capillary permeability and loss of intravascular fluid
Endotoxic/Gram-negative shock	• Responsible for the peripheral circulatory failure in septicaemia • Common organisms responsible are *Escherichia coli, Pseudomonas aeruginosa*
Cardiogenic shock	• Sudden fall in cardiac output
Psychogenic shock (vasovagal syncope)	• Sudden emotional shock can cause severe peripheral arteriolar dilatation and pooling of blood leading to a low cardiac output
Neurogenic shock	• Injury to sensitive autonomic ganglia, such as those associated with the testicles or abdomen, can lead to a temporary dysfunction in the autonomic control of blood vessels
Refractory shock	• Depending on the amount of blood loss this can be fatal, however the compensatory mechanism, aided by treatment, can gradually restore circulation to normal • In some patients shock may persist for hours, gradually progressing to a stage where there is no longer any response to vasopressor drugs, and despite blood volume being returned to normal – cardiac output remains depressed.

In haemorrhagic or traumatic shock the primary cause is blood loss. Treatment should include the early and rapid infusion of adequate amounts of compatible whole blood. Saline is of limited temporary value as it is distributed into the extracellular fluid and only 25% of the amount administered stays in the vascular system (American College of Surgeons Committee on Trauma, 1993).

Hypertonic solutions and human albumin expand the blood volume by drawing fluid out of the interstitial spaces. These fluids are invaluable in emergency management, but they do dehydrate the tissues in an already compromised patient.

The immediate aims are to restore intravascular volume, to ensure pulmonary gas exchange and to restore cardiac output. Massive blood loss presents a serious threat to survival and the aim of circulatory restoration is to maintain adequate oxygen-carrying capacity in order to produce a minimum urine output of > 30 ml/hr, a normal systolic blood pressure and pulse, with a haemoglobin > 10 g/dl.

Blood loss is not the only reason an injured person may be shocked. The recording of baseline vital signs is essential prior to the administration of intravenous fluids; careful subsequent monitoring will provide an accurate record of patient response to treatment.

Fluid and electrolye imbalance

All cellular metabolic processes depend on the maintenance of homeostasis; this can be disrupted by fluid or electrolyte disturbances. These are among the most frequently seen phenomena following trauma.

Observation, assessment and early reporting of abnormalities will prevent or lessen life-threatening complications such as:

- Dehydration – abnormal combined loss of water and sodium chloride without reduction in intracellular water and electrolytes
- Overhydration – extracellular fluid volume excess with expanded interstitial cell volume

In assessing fluid balance, clinicians must be aware of the potential for a sudden and massive fluid shift into a potential space. This may be mediated by decreased plasma proteins, increased capillary permeability or lymphatic blockage. It may occur after major trauma, when remobilization of fluid usually occurs 1 week post-insult, posing a threat in terms of rapid re-expansion of intravascular volume.

Body acidity and alkalinity is expressed in pH; this term represents the concentration of the hydrogen ions – which ordinarily range between about 1 and 10^{-14} gram equivalents per litre, into numbers between 0 and 14. This is regulated in three ways – by the blood buffers, the respiratory system, and the renal system. The renal system is responsible for the maintenance of acid base balance via excretion of acids and reabsorption of bicarbonate. When renal malfunction occurs following major trauma, the remaining blood buffer system and respiratory system are frequently incapable of compensating adequately. The resulting complications are metabolic acidosis and metabolic alkalosis.

Metabolic acidosis

This is defined as a reduction in bicarbonate concentration and an increase in hydrogen ion concentration. Neurologically the patient will be confused or in a coma. The respiratory reaction is hyperventilation, or so-called Kussmaul respiration. The gastrointestinal reaction

is nausea and vomiting.

Normal values: Plasma pH < 7.35
P_{CO_2} normal 36-46 mmHg
H_{CO_3} < 22 mEq/l

Metabolic acidosis: P_{CO_2} < 36 mmHg

Metabolic alkalosis

This is an increase in bicarbonate concentration and a reduction in hydrogen ion concentration. Neuromuscular changes include muscle cramps, tetany and fits. The respiratory response is hypoventilation and hypoxia. The gastro-intestinal reaction is of an ileus and gastric retention.

Normal values: Plasma pH > 7.45
H_{CO_3} > 26 mEq/l
P_{CO_2} normal 36-46 mmHg

Metabolic alkalosis: P_{CO_2} > 46 mmHg

Neurological system

Head injury is the leading cause of death in road traffic accidents (RTAs). In 1990, 2390 out of 4898 deaths in England and Wales were due to head injury (OPCS, 1991).

Assessment is critical and regular monitoring of vital signs mandatory. The physical impact of head injury is indicated by fluctuations in the level of consciousness. It is essential to establish a baseline level – the sooner that this is established after the accident the better.

Hypoxia and hypotension may present as a result of neurological impairment following trauma. Therefore regular monitoring of blood oxygen saturation and blood pressure is essential.

The Glasgow Coma Scale (GCS) provides an objective neurological assessment of the head-injured patient – however, the scale is only effective if there is consistency in the assessment. The GCS (Table 3.3) consists of quantifying the level of responsiveness, identifying the motor function in each extremity, together with the observation of pupil reaction (Teasdale and Jennett, 1974).

Table 3.3 The Glasgow Coma Scale

Eye opening	Spontaneous	4
	To voice	3
	To pain	2
	None	1
Verbal response	Orientated	5
	Confused	4
	Inappropriate words	3
	Incomprehensible sounds	2
	None	1
Motor response	Obeys commands	6
	Localizes pain	5
	Withdraws (pain)	4
	Flexion (pain)	3
	Extension (pain)	2
	None	1

In using the GCS, points are allocated for each response on the scale, starting from zero for no response, up to 4, 5 or 6 for the maximum response. The scores for each part of the scale are added together to produce a total. It is important to stress that the assessment should be based on the patient's best response in each category, while remembering that factors such as intubation, periorbital swelling or paralysis can invalidate all or part of the assessment. The three categories evaluated are eye opening, verbal response and motor response, as explained in Table 3.4.

Pupil size and response are critical parts of the assessment and should be undertaken with a bright, reliable torch and the assessment carried out on both eyes. Unequal pupil sizes in conjunction with a reduced level of consciousness may be indicative of raised intracranial pressure (ICP) – albeit a late sign (Table 3.5).

It is equally important to examine a patient thoroughly 12–24 h post-injury in order to identify any additional signs of injury around the head, including bruising around the ears. Contusion over the mastoid indicates a basal skull fracture (this is known as Battle's Sign). Unilateral deafness of acute onset, or leakage of cerebrospinal fluid (CSF) from the ear (otorrhoea) or nose (rhinorrhoea), should be further investigated. To test for CSF, place a drop of fluid onto blotting paper: a dense red area will appear surrounded by a lighter pink/red area – this is known as the ring sign. The ear affected should be covered with a sterile dressing and specialist advice obtained. Periorbital ecchymosis (bruising), otherwise known as 'panda eyes',

Table 3.4 The Glasgow Coma Scale – assessment specifics

Eye opening

Score 4	Appropriate level of wakefulness
Score 3	Patient may be lethargic due to fatigue, analgesics, post-ictal state, early signs of raised intracranial pressure or hypoxia.
Score 2	Consistent use of nail bed pressure eliciting no response or little response indicates a definite decrease in level of consciousness (pinching the skin and puncturing the skin with pins is not an acceptable method of providing a painful stimulus)
Score 1	It is essential to rule out previous neurological disorder, otherwise indicative of profound decrease in level of consciousness and an alteration in cerebral perfusion and cerebral metabolism

Verbal response

Score 5	Communicates appropriately
Score 4	Disorientated, but able to converse. Questions such as 'What is your name?' 'Where do you live?' 'What year is it?' should be asked regularly – minimal dysfunction in frontal lobe, ? hypoxia
Score 3	Incomplete words and phrases – dysfunction in primary speech, ? oedema
Score 2	Unintelligible sounds – severe dysfunction in speech
Score 1	No verbal response – increasingly severe dysfunction in speech centre

Motor response

Score 6	Appropriate level of wakefulness
Score 5	Patient lethargic – evidence of impaired neurological dysfunction
Score 4	Evidence of alteration in level of consciousness due to a neurological dysfunction
Score 3	Flexion response to pain – indicates severe alteration in level of consciousness and disruption of motor pathway at the pontine level in the brainstem
Score 2	Extension response to pain – severe alteration in level of consciousness and disruption of motor pathway at medullary level in the brainstem
Score 1	No response to pain – indicates complete blockage at lower brainstem – profound coma

may be indicative of an orbital fracture or a basal skull fracture.

Table 3.5   Neurological assessment of the eye

Direct pupillary reflex	Pupils equal in size – it is important to chart the reaction as brisk, sluggish or non-reactive, and the numerical/pictorial size of the pupil should be recorded
	Cranial nerve III is affected if one pupil is fixed, dilated and non-reactive
	Bilateral dilated and fixed pupils which are unreactive to light indicate mid-brain lesion and major neurological dysfunction
Extraocular movements	Ability to move the globe of the eye in all directions. A disruption indicates problems with cranial nerves III, IV and VI
Visual field integrity	If the visual field is affected in either eye this is indicative of optic nerve involvement

Changes in the rate and volume of respiratory effort are key indicators of trauma to the respiratory centre. Damage to the hypothalamus, the temperature regulating centre, can lead to hyperpyrexia (core temperature over 40°C) or conversely hypothermia (core temperature under 35°C). The measurement of blood pressure is also critical in the overall picture. Raised ICP may be indicated by a gradual rise in blood pressure. This is caused by the heartbeat becoming stronger as the blood is forced into the brain in order to counteract capillary resistance (Nelson, 1989). The baroreceptors in the carotid arteries respond by acting on the cardiac centre in the brain to slow the heart rate, leading to a slow pulse and an increasingly high blood pressure. The same baroreceptor action takes place in reverse when a patient is in shock: the pulse increases rapidly and the blood pressure falls.

In the multiply-injured patient a complete neurological assessment must be undertaken with assessment of muscle tone and power, reflexes and sensation, together with cranial nerve function.

Reflexes and muscle groups are conveniently matched to myotomes, as described in Figure 3.1.

The spinal cord can go into spinal shock and mimic full spinal physiological disturbance. Spinal shock can be reversed by time and rest.

Respiratory system

The basis of successful management in thoracic trauma is effective cardiopulmonary resuscitation followed by the early detection and correction of life-threatening injuries. These may include intrathoracic visceral injuries such as pneumothorax, cardiac tamponade, and laceration of the heart or aorta which may follow a deceleration injury. Hypoxia and acidosis may occur secondary to major airway obstruction haemopneumothorax or pulmonary contusion. The patient is frequently tachypnoeic and distressed. Treatment includes maintenance of the airway, oxygen via mask, pulse oximetry and arterial blood gas and pH estimation.

Major trauma or damage to the respiratory system may result in adult respiratory distress syndrome (ARDS), which is a complex, poorly understood syndrome. There is diffuse damage to the alveolar–capillary membrane. It is known by other names such as pulmonary oedema or shock lung and is characterized by alveolar pulmonary oedema which results from increased permeability of the pulmonary microvasculature. Physical signs and symptoms in ARDS include restlessness, tachypnoea, hyperventilation and progressive dyspnoea, fine diffuse crackles in the lungs on auscultation, and a deterioration in level of consciousness. Moderate to severe changes in $Pa\,o_2$ ($<$ 50 mmHg) are seen even when the inspired oxygen concentration is greater than 60%, and there may be hypercardia with the $Pa\,co_2$ being $>$ 50 mmHg. The potential complications include respiratory arrest, respiratory failure, pulmonary fibrosis and disseminated intravascular coagulation (DIC) – a complex, acquired haematological disorder characterized by a combination of both coagulation and haemorrhage (Doughty and Murphy, 1997). Precipitating factors for DIC are shock, sepsis, severe hypoxia, trauma, burns, lengthy surgery or other types of tissue injury. Signs in DIC may be petechial haemorrhage, purpura, ecchymosis, rash or epistaxis. Tachypnoea, haematemesis, melaena, haematuria and seizures may also be observed.

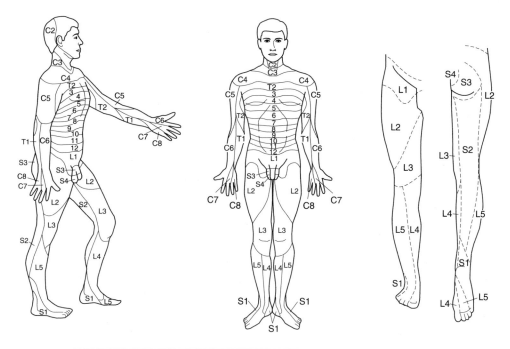

Muscle group	Reflex (nerve supply)
Diaphragm	C3, C4, C5
Shoulder abductors	C5
Elbow flexors	C5
Supinators/pronators	C6
Wrist extensors	C6
Wrist flexors	C7
Elbow extensors/fingers	C7
Finger flexors	C8
Intrinsic hand muscles	T1
Hip flexors	L1, L2
Hip abductors	L2, L3
Knee extensors	L3, L4
Ankle dorsiflexors	L4, L5
Toe extensors	L5
Knee flexors	L4, L5, S1
Ankle plantar flexors	S1, S2
Toe flexors	S1, S2
Anal sphincter	S2, S3, S4

Figure 3.1   Spinal dermatomes (From Grundy *et al.*, 1986)

Digestive system

Most abdominal trauma can be identified as either penetrating (impaling or stabbing) or blunt (e.g. crush injuries, direct blows, or as a result of deceleration in road traffic accidents). Resuscitation remains a high priority, hypovolaemia being a major threat to life. It is vital to ascertain the mechanism of injury if possible.

However, the principle of look, listen and feel can provide valuable clinical information during the course of a rapid initial assessment.

External evidence of abdominal trauma, such as bruising or wounds, entry and exit sites and possible impressions of tyres or seat belts ('witness marks') can provide valuable information. Signs of peritoneal irritation following a rupture of the viscera may be slow to develop

Table 3.6 Abdominal trauma: signs and symptoms

Signs and symptoms	Possible causes
Abdominal rigidity	Visceral injury, peritonitis, ruptured spleen
Evidence of blood at the urethral meatus (men)	Bladder trauma or ruptured urethra
Loin tenderness, loss of loin contour	Renal trauma
Retention of urine	Fracture of the pubis
Haematuria	Genitourinary injury and renal damage
Vaginal bleeding (excluding menses)	Gynaecological trauma
Bruising/swelling around perineum and lower abdomen	Pelvic fracture
Blood loss – hypovolaemic shock	Pelvic fracture, femoral fracture, visceral injury
Pain on rectal examination	Major pelvic fracture
Spinal deformity or paravertebral haematoma	Retro-peritoneal injury
Relaxed rectal tone	Spinal cord injury
Absence of bowel sounds	Development of paralytic ileus

and it is therefore essential to reassess on a regular basis. Table 3.6 illustrates some of the clinical signs and symptoms.

Major fractures of the pelvis, together with disruption of the pelvic ring, can cause extensive blood loss, and in excess of 30 units of blood may be required to regain haemostasis. Injuries of this severity are life-threatening and immediate stabilization via external fixation may be required in order to stem blood loss. The bladder is unlikely to be damaged unless it is full at the time of injury. Ruptures of the rectum or sigmoid colon may accompany fractures of the blade of the ilium. Complications following pelvic fractures include neurological lesions, persistent low back pain and, for some men (depending on fracture pattern), impotence may become a problem.

Musculoskeletal system

Musculoskeletal injuries are inevitable in multiply-injured patients. However, the management of fractures and dislocations of the appendicular skeleton do not take precedence over the resuscitation of the patient – maintenance of the airway, breathing and circulation must be the first priority (Maull *et al.*, 1993). Tenderness, swelling, deformity, laceration, bruising, abnormal alignment, pain, loss of sensation, and colour are all signs indicative of possible injury. The amount of blood which can be lost following an apparently minor injury is remarkable – the quadriceps muscles can accommodate 1 litre of extravasated blood with an increase in thigh diameter of only 1 cm.

Patients with multiple injuries and reduced tissue perfusion and oxygenation are at a high risk of developing compartment syndrome. There are 46 compartments in the human body and 38 of these are found within the lower extremities (Gamron, 1988). A compartment is made up from a group of muscles surrounded by fascia. These compartments are large enough to contain entry and exit points for nerves, tendons and arteries.

Acute compartment syndrome may develop following fractures of the tibia, femur or forearm following gluteal muscle injury or simply by immobilization (Maher *et al.*, 1994). The fascial compartments do not expand and increasing swelling will result in tissue contusion and haemorrhage, which can lead to infarction of the compartment muscle. The signs and symptoms of compartment syndrome can, in some instances, develop within 2 h of the initial trauma (Ross, 1988), yet in others up to 6 days post-injury (Maher *et al.*, 1994). It is important to note that irreversible damage and deformity can occur within only 6 h (Callaghan, 1985). Immediate action should be taken by elevating the limb to reduce swelling and relieve any additional pressure caused by restrictive dressings such as bandages, splints or casts. In many instances surgical decompression is required as an emergency procedure, where fasciotomies are performed to re-establish arterial blood supply. Regular observation of the limb is of paramount importance. Mourad and Prouste (1988) suggest that colour, sensation, movement and warmth are critical factors (Table 3.7).

Table 3.7 Compartment syndrome: signs and symptoms

Pain – deep, unrelenting, poorly localized, unrelieved by elevation and analgesia, experienced on passive movement

Weak active movement of digits

Compartment tense and warm on palpation

Colour and temperature – normal

Capillary filling and pulses frequently normal

Risk of severe, irreversible tissue damage

(After Gamron, 1988; Proehl, 1988; Ross, 1991; Slye, 1991 and Gluchacki, 1991)

The importance of maintaining regular and accurate records of the neurovascular status of injured limbs, noting and reporting any changes in circulation, motor function and sensation cannot be overemphasized (Table 3.8).

Table 3.8 Neurovascular assessment (Adapted from Mourad and Prouste, 1988)

Check limb peripheries for:

Colour – should be pinkish, not pale or blanched

Temperature – should be warm; injured tissue is cooler than well perfused tissue

Capillary refill of nails – should refill in 2–4 s; if this slows to 4–6 s it should be reported

Oedema – its presence indicates venous stasis; injured tissues are noticeably more swollen

Movement – injured tissues have decreased mobility

Sensory function – complaints of pins and needles, tingling and numbness suggest damage

Pain – increased or unexpected pain suggests pressure or trauma to tissues

Eden-Kilgour and Miller (1993) suggest using the five 'P's to inform assessment:

Pain	Which may account for oedema, nerve injury, deep vein thrombosis (DVT), or the first signs of muscle ischaemia
Pallor	Lack of blood supply
Paraesthesia	Nerve compression disrupting nerve function
Paralysis	As for paraesthesia, but secondary to increasing oedema (would be considered to be a late sign)
Pulse	Anomalies may be suggestive of arterial blood flow disruption.

Evidence of neurological or nerve injury may be difficult to obtain initially, but absence of any pain or feeling may imply severe oedema and neurological impairment such as neurapraxia. There is evidence that neurological damage following dislocation is far greater than with fractures. Disturbance of nerve function can be classified by severity (Table 3.9).

Table 3.9 Classification of peripheral nerve damage

Neurapraxia	A temporary physiological nerve dysfunction – in the absence of structural damage recovery invariably occurs
Axonotmesis	Nerve fibre damage, however recovery should be complete, or very nearly so
Neurotmesis	Nerve injury in which all essential structures have been divided – suturing is required

Conclusion

The aim of this chapter has been to emphasize the importance of the initial assessment of the multiply-injured patient and to identify some of the complex physiological responses to trauma. The use of a systems approach within the context of a single chapter can only provide an overview of such an extensive subject. However, it aims to give some insight into the demands made on clinicians whose diagnostic skills are frequently tested in circumstances where speed and efficiency may well determine whether a patient lives or dies.

References

American College of Surgeons Committee on Trauma (1993) *Advanced Trauma Life Support*. American College of Surgeons.

Callaghan, J. (1985) Compartment syndrome. *Orthopaedic Nursing*, **4**(4), 11–14.

Doughty, H. A. and Murphy, M. F. (1997) Haematological emergencies, blood products and transfusions. In *Cambridge Textbook of Accident and Emergency Medicine* (D. Skinner, A. Swain, R. Peyton and C. Robertson, eds). Cambridge University Press.

Eden-Kilgour, S. and Miller, B. (1993) Understanding neurovascular assessment. *Nursing*, **23**(8), 56–58.

Gamron, R. B. (1988) Taking the pressure out of compartment syndrome. *American Journal of Nursing*, **8**(7), 1076–1080.

Gluchacki, B. (1991) Recognising compartment syndrome. *Nursing*, **21**(10), 33.

Grundy, D., Russell, J. and Swain, A. (1986) *ABC of Spinal Cord Injury*. Cambridge: Cambridge University Press.

Guyton, A. C. (1991) The nervous system motor and integrative neurophysiology. In *Textbook of Medical Physiology*. W. B. Saunders.

Huggins, B. (1990) Trauma physiology. *Nursing Clinics of North America*, **25**(1), 1–10.

Maher, A. B., Salmond, S. W. and Pellino, T. A. (1994) *Orthopaedic Nursing*. W. B. Saunders.

Maull, K. I., Enderson, B. L. and Frame, S. B. (1993) Comprehensive management of the trauma patient. In *Current Practice Surgery* (B. Levine *et al.*, eds). Churchill Livingstone.

Montague, S., Herbert, R. and Watson, R. (1996) *Physiology for Nursing Practice*. Baillière Tindall.

Mourad, L. A. and Prouste, M. M. (1988) *The Nursing Process in the Care of Adults with Orthopaedic Conditions.* Wiley.

Nelson, P. (1989) Head and neck pain. In *Accident and Emergency Medicine* (W. Rutherford *et al.*, eds). Churchill Livingstone.

OPCS (1991) *Mortality Statistics, England and Wales.* Government Statistical Service.

Proehl, J. (1988) Compartment syndrome. *Journal of Emergency Nursing*, **14**(5), 283–290.

Ross, D. (1988) Compartment syndrome: applying nursing diagnosis to adult critical illness. In *Manual of Critical Care*. Mosby.

Sheehy, B. S., Marvin, J. A. and Jimmerson, C. L. (1989) *Manual of Clinical Trauma Care*, Mosby.

Slye, D. (1991) Orthopaedic complications. *Nursing Clinics of North America*, **26**(1), 113–134.

Teasdale, G. and Jennett, B. (1974) Assessment of coma and impaired consciousness. *Lancet*, **2**, 81–84.

4

The psychological effects of trauma

Sarah Banner

Introduction

This chapter explores the psychological impact of trauma and discusses the associated implications for healthcare professionals. Examples from practice will be used to highlight points for discussion. By developing an understanding of how the emotional impact of trauma affects the individual, healthcare professionals can utilize their skills to help such victims cope with their experiences, and support them through a period of adjustment.

The concept of trauma as a crisis will be discussed, illustrating how individual interpretations of crisis can lead to a stress response. The stress response needs to be considered, as differences in the degree of stress, and the individual's way of dealing with it, are linked to one's psychological wellbeing and coping behaviours (Kleber and Brom, 1992). There are many influences on coping behaviour. The mechanisms with which this chapter is concerned relate specifically to coping with the emotional consequences of trauma. Trauma can be described as the severe mental and emotional disruption that can follow the experience of certain events, including those where no physical injury is present (Buck, 1991). Trauma as a bereavement process is illustrated, and effective coping mechanisms which lead to the correct balance between empowerment and the need for social support is analysed.

Crisis

Experiencing traumatic injury has emotional consequences – it is a crisis. Crisis is defined as a crucial point or situation in the course of anything (Murgatroyd and Woolfe, 1982). It is often unexpected and beyond our control, bringing sudden change, worry and both physical and psychological instability. One's routine and sense of security are disrupted and vulnerability is induced. Buck (1991) describes trauma as a crisis because it causes severe mental and emotional disturbance to an individual's wellbeing. The concept of crisis to an individual is subject to continual fluctuation and is influenced by a variety of foreseen threats. The management of trauma care as part of a continuum requires healthcare professionals to be aware of the victim's perception of crisis and how this perception may vary throughout the recovery phase.

This example shows how trauma creates a whole spectrum of crises throughout the total experience. The way in which these crises are perceived by the individual directly affects the stress response and is a major influence on coping behaviour.

Example

Robert, a 19-year-old teenager, was knocked off his motorbike by a lorry and rushed into A&E for assessment of his injuries. The accident was initially interpreted by Robert as a crisis as it had ruined his new motorbike. Following x-rays of his injuries Robert was told that he had fractured his pelvis and would require surgery, as a result of which he would be immobile and in hospital for at least 6 weeks. A new crisis

---

then emerged for Robert as he realized he would be unable to walk for some time; his usual routine and any short-term plans he had made would now need to be changed. Compared to his physical condition, the impact of losing his motorbike was now not such a crisis. Robert made a good recovery and finally returned home, walking with the aid of crutches. It was then that the reality of the seriousness of the accident hit him and another crisis came to the fore – his thoughts turned to how easily he could have been killed. Other problems he was now experiencing included a change in self-image, together with the permanent scarring he was left with as a result of his injuries and the subsequent surgery.

Stress response

A wide variety of nursing, psychological and sociological literature recognizes that the experience of crisis is a most obvious form of stress (Atkinson *et al.*, 1993). Benner and Wrubel (1989) define stress as a disruption of meanings, understandings and smooth functioning so that harm, loss or challenge is experienced, and sorrow, interpretation or new skill acquisition is required. This proposes that stress interferes with an individual's stable wellbeing, and some sort of change of behaviour is needed in order to overcome this disruption. Clarke (1984) characterizes stress as an interaction between the individual and his or her environment. In comparing these definitions, Clarke does not indicate that any action or coping behaviour is required to manage the situation, hence it is of little assistance in relating to coping mechanisms. Murgatroyd and Woolfe (1982) define stress not as the traumatic event, but the process in which the person experiences the event and their ability to develop coping strategies to deal with it. It is the result of the interaction between the environment and the person perceiving the experience (Bailey and Clarke, 1989).

Following a crisis such as traumatic injury a certain amount of stress is inevitable. The resulting sudden change from a normal lifestyle can have a profound effect on the individual (Horavitz, 1986). All of a sudden the security of daily existence has been destroyed and victims are confronted with their own vulnerability,

mortality and the ultimate threat of their own annihilation (Lenehan, 1986). However, we all react to stressful situations differently (Lazarus, 1976). Some people may take longer than others to recover from stress in terms of time and emotional intensity (Castledine, 1993). Differences in the intensity of stress created by a given situation, and the individual's unique way of dealing with this stress, lead to variations in coping behaviours (Kleber and Brom, 1992). For example, the victim of a house fire who has suffered minor burns may perceive the whole experience as greatly stressful, having an enormous emotional impact on their wellbeing. However, another individual in similar circumstances may simply brush the experience off as part of life, accepting that these things happen.

The role of the healthcare professional is to find out the patient's perception of the stressful encounter. Pearson *et al.* (1991) suggest that this should be done during assessment, together with an attempt to discover how this stress has affected their usual pattern of living in addition to the individual's ability to cope with previous stressors. This history will inform planned interventions in order to strengthen the patient's defence or assist in adaptation. However, such interviews must be handled sensitively as trust, respect and intimacy may not yet have been established with the individual, and this is essential for the sharing of information (Muetzel, 1988). The interviewer must also have the necessary skills and experience to undertake such assessment. At this stage the patient may also not understand fully what the experience means to them, as they may well be distracted by other crises such as their physical injuries, the hospital environment and a change of role. This latter point introduces the concept of the different stages of grief reaction such as denial, as mentioned by Kubler-Ross (1984), and will be examined, together with coping strategies, later in the chapter.

The psychological and physical reactions commonly experienced following trauma can in most situations be described as normal, but nevertheless distressing, reactions to an abnormal experience (Bamber, 1994). The majority of individuals experiencing trauma are eventually able to regain a quality of life equivalent to that which they enjoyed pre-injury (Taylor, 1983; Castledine, 1993). The coping mechanisms and behaviours explored in this chapter are based on the 'normal' reaction to crisis.

However, not everyone fully readjusts to the experience (Taylor, 1983) and one must be aware that in some cases of trauma the impact upon the individual's wellbeing is so severe, intense and stressful that a psychiatric disorder can result (Buck, 1991), commonly referred to as post-traumatic stress disorder. Why exposure to trauma should lead to this response in some but not in others is uncertain, but an important factor may be the severity of stress both in terms of scale and violence (Buck, 1991). This then provides a link between the degree of stress and associated coping. When relating this to practice, it implies that an individual who slips while ice-skating and sustains an ankle fracture will cope with the experience better than the individual who survives a road traffic accident having suffered multiple injuries. The rationale is that the threat of mortality and the severity of injury is greater for the latter. While in one respect this may seem common sense, it must be noted that this is only one influence affecting coping behaviour, and other mechanisms yet to be discussed are similarly influential.

The experience of trauma is perceived as stressful because victims are removed from the security of normal life, wrestling with turbulent emotions and unanswered questions as to what might have been if only. . . . A similar experience can create differing levels of stress according to the individual. The impact of stress influences individual coping mechanisms and behaviours. Additional theories and influences on coping with trauma will now be considered.

Coping mechanisms

Coping is a multifactorial concept. It is the process through which the individual manages the demands of the person–environment relationship that is perceived to be stressful and how the emotions thus generated are managed (Lazarus and Folkman, 1984). The individual manages these demands (such as coping with morbidity) by calling upon coping mechanisms that have proved favourable in the past, or by initiating new ones (White, 1995). This concept allows for the individual differences which are characteristic to human beings (Clarke, 1984). For instance, one individual could perceive a situation as demanding, whereas another individual would not. Similarly, action seen by

one person as a satisfactory coping mechanism might fail with someone else.

Coping does not necessarily terminate the experience, but is the effort made by the individual to overcome the stressful situation in an attempt to recover self-esteem and tolerance (White, 1995). Coping can never remove the individual from the experience of the traumatic event, nor its physical and emotional effects; however, it can provide light at the end of the tunnel and aid in the development of strategies to overcome the source of the problem (McHaffie, 1992).

There are many influences which determine the way in which an individual copes with the psychological impact of trauma. As already mentioned, an individual may cope with a situation by applying previous coping strategies which were successful in the past. This may be intentional or even subconscious coping behaviour. Alternatively, one may be forced to acquire additional coping mechanisms to deal with the stressful encounter.

The concept of coping with stressful life events was traditionally viewed as a trait (Lazarus and Folkman, 1984). It is a direct result of the individual's personality according to Bailey and Clarke (1989) and Hagstrom (1995). For example, individuals may be repressors, conformists, challengers, etc., and their reaction to the trauma experience will be influenced by this. Kelly (1985) shows that pretraumatic personality has an effect on response to crisis, as does the individual's motivation, which can also be described as part of their personality. Welch (1995) notes that those with a positive personality cope well under stress. Numerous studies have supported the trait and personality concept of coping, such as that of Kobasa (1979). However, the validity of this is questioned as it is very difficult to assess, measure and compare coping behaviours.

Coping cannot be purely the direct result of a trait or personality, as it does not consider the environment of the individual. Coping as a trait is seen as unidimensional (Lazarus and Folkman, 1984). Moos and Tsu (1977) offer empirical evidence in support of the fact that patients coping with physical injury must deal with many sources of stress, including pain, the hospital environment and the demands imposed by professional staff. The patient must also preserve an emotional balance, a satisfactory self-image and a successful relationship with his or her family and friends (Moos and Tsu, 1977). These are multiple tasks that require an array of coping strategies. Personality can only be considered in so far as it enables different responses to change to be identified and understood (Burns, 1993).

Appraisal theory and the significance of the experience to the individual

Lazarus and Folkman (1984) have studied the effectiveness of different coping strategies through observation of those experiencing stressful life events, and suggest that in order to understand variations among individual coping behaviours in comparable conditions, the cognitive processes that intervene between the encounter and the reaction must be taken into account. This suggests that the mind is not distinct from the external world (Benner and Wrubel, 1989).

A phenomenological interpretation emphasizes that coping mechanisms and emotional reactions are influenced by the way a person appraises the traumatic event. Appraisal is a judgement about the personal meaning or significance of a situation (McHaffie, 1992). Coping can be considered as an attempt to find meaning in what has happened (Kleber and Brom, 1992) and to make sense of this (McHaffie, 1992). For example, was the experience harmful and threatening, or was it favourable and enhancing? The appraisal will differ as the experience is evaluated in the light of an individual's emotions, belief systems, cognitive styles, past experiences and personal disposition (McHaffie, 1992). Situations that the individual has previously experienced as harmful, such as past traumatic injury, will now also be appraised as threatening and stressful. Lazarus (1976) and Bailey and Clarke (1989) both illustrate that the appraisal of a situation as threatening leads to a greater degree of stress and greater difficulties in coping when compared to appraisal being considered a challenge, where positive adaptation is expected. This is of relevance in trauma as it suggests that the more serious the injury and experience of danger, the greater the degree of stress and coping difficulties, and the increased likelihood of pathological outcomes such as post-traumatic stress disorder. Hagstrom's (1995) empirical evidence

from victims of a serious train crash in Gothenburg in 1987 revealed that 24% of the victims felt that their lives had been threatened. These people experienced more problems than the remaining 76% who did not perceive the event as life-threatening. This evidence can be viewed as valid and reliable as it is research based and undertaken by scientific investigation (Hockey, 1991), the hypothesis being supported by research findings. How representative this study is can be open to question, as it is difficult to make comparisons with other sources due to lack of research-based evidence on the psychological effects of the trauma experience (Kleber and Brom, 1992).

Atkinson *et al.* (1993) propose that appraisal is affected by the controllability and the predictability of the trauma. The more uncontrollable the event, the more likely it will be appraised as a threat (Atkinson *et al.*, 1993). Likewise, being able to predict the occurrence of a stressful event usually decreases the severity of the stress, altering the meaning of the experience, as the individual may have been able to initiate some sort of preparatory process to lessen the threat (Atkinson *et al.*, 1993). McHaffie (1992) criticizes this view, arguing that perceiving an event to be controllable or predictable does not necessarily reduce stress or lead to a positive outcome. One cannot comment on the validity of these opinions for trauma, as none of the studies of actual patients' experiences of coping with traumatic events revealed such qualitative or quantitative results.

Grief and bereavement

Coping is not static, but changes with the person–environment relationship (Murgatroyd and Woolfe, 1982; Lazarus and Folkman, 1984). It varies in intensity as the individual searches, sifts through and evaluates the cues within a situation (McHaffie, 1992). The coping strategies utilized to deal with the stressful encounter continually adapt in response to the relevant stage of the coping process. Examples of this are illustrated in the studies of loss, adjustment and grieving, with different coping mechanisms being applied at each stage. The body of knowledge on coping with loss and adjustment of Kubler-Ross (1984) and Parkes

(1986) suggests that a grief reaction may occur in order to cope with loss or adjustment. Whatever the physical implications resulting from the experience, the individual will always have to adjust to the fact that the event has happened and may also need to adjust to temporary environmental changes and a subsequent loss of control and autonomy (Welch, 1995). This will consequently lead to grief. The coping mechanisms of the individual will be influenced by his or her reaction to loss and grief. These will be transitional and change according to the stage of the grief reaction. Parkes (1986) suggests that this grief reaction can be displayed by numbness, denial, yearning, pining and despair. Kubler-Ross (1984) further identifies anger, isolation and bargaining as consequent grief reactions. These emotions are experienced before acceptance and recovery are achieved. Coping behaviour will be influenced according to the grief stage and the intensity of this reaction. This in itself may well explain the variations in coping mechanisms following the experience of trauma.

Attribution theory and blame

Attribution theory suggests that one of the major strategies for coping with serious life events is affording meaning to the experience (Taylor, 1983). Davis (1987) finds that those who are unable to arrive at some meaningful explanation of the experience may have more difficulty in coping during convalescence. The individual may make causal attributions in an attempt to understand why something happened and what impact it has had (Taylor, 1983). This is similar to appraisal as mentioned by Lazarus (1976). Attributions are either accounted for externally, viewed perhaps as 'bad luck' (Miller and Porter, 1983), or internally, with the individual believing that they themselves are responsible for the event (Taylor, 1983). Reutter and Northcott (1995) view assigning responsibility or blame to oneself as a functional way in which to cope with the encounter. Miller and Porter (1983) cite empirical evidence which describes the degree of self-blame evidenced by victims of negative life events as positively correlating with subsequent coping. Hence such individuals cope more functionally than those with external attributions.

> *Example*
>
> Josie, a 37-year-old mother of two teenage children, after a stressful day at work was hurriedly driving to meet her children from school. She failed to notice the traffic slowing on the dual carriageway and drove into the back of a lorry. She sustained severe bruising to her chest and a whiplash injury to her neck. She required 48 hours' observation in hospital to ensure no other injuries were present, then was discharged home with painkillers and advice.
> Josie felt intensely angry about this accident, could find no explanation for it within herself, so blamed others. This anger was unresolved and led to social isolation and depression. Josie's behaviour was causing problems within the family, so in desperation the family sought help from their general practitioner.
> Eventually Josie agreed to see a psychologist and, with the support of her family and friends, she was helped to come to terms with the situation, regaining control, restoring her social networks and readjusting to normal life.

Bullman and Wortman (1977) found similar results from interviews of paralysed accident victims who blamed themselves for their accidents. Such studies are valuable, representative and reliable as they are research based. Various explanations for the theory of blame have been proposed. Individuals who blame themselves for an event cope more favourably than those blaming external causes, because they perceive themselves as having control over the situation (Miller and Porter, 1983; Bullman and Wortman, 1977). The concept of control enables individuals to be confident about their future, even if it means accepting responsibility for misfortunes in the past. This research is comparable with findings of Atkinson *et al.* (1993) that stress is increased with the uncontrollability of unfavourable events. Control and confidence in one's environment are a vital influence in coping (Atkinson *et al.*, 1993) and are reflected by Bailey and Clarke (1989) characterizing coping as the individual's attempt to reach goals of personal control. Taylor (1983) notes that the perception of gaining control over the event and one's life leads to a theme of mastery and adjustment which Lazarus (1976) acknowledges as a positive outcome of coping mechanisms. Other explanations of self-blame are concerned with how it preserves the belief that the world is a just place where bad things do not happen merely by chance (Lenehan, 1986). This is easier to accept than the possibility that life is capricious and unfair, and also gives meaning to otherwise incomprehensible events (Miller and Porter, 1983).

There are critics to the self-blame approach, such as Reutter and Northcott (1995), who mention that external blaming protects one's self-esteem, which likewise is a relevant and influential factor in coping. Taylor (1983) also found that self-blame was associated with poor coping in rape victims. This, however, is an exceptional trauma experience with unique and complex coping mechanisms, incomparable to other traumas such as traffic accidents, burns and falls.

Lenehan (1986) claims that self-blame provokes feelings of guilt. Such guilt should not be discouraged, and patients should be allowed to explore the circumstances and events surrounding the situation in order finally to move on (Lenehan, 1986).

Other influences on coping mechanisms

Hagstrom (1995) proposes the age of the individual as a variant in coping behaviour. He reveals quantitative results that older victims experience more difficulty in coping, having persistent thoughts and feelings about the experience. This could be a question of ageing and facing the end of life. Welch (1995) found a high incidence of prolonged depression in older sufferers despite a reduced severity of injury, lack of disfigurement and the fact that many were active participants in religion. Like Hagstrom (1995), she believed this to be due to the multiple impact of dealing with situational stress and the effects of ageing.

However, Welch (1995) found that younger victims described intense depression due to boredom associated with the sick role following injury. Sigmon (1984) notes that victims of trauma are predominantly young adults who may already be struggling with the demands of studies, relationships and employment. Unforeseen injury and hospitalization can complicate these demands and make coping more difficult. However, this literature is purely opinion based

and there is no empirical evidence to support this view. It would not be possible to rank the coping strategies of varying age groups in order of who copes best, but one can accept in broad terms that age does influence the coping mechanisms of the trauma patient.

The cultural background of the individual must also be considered when determining coping behaviour. Different cultures display different values and beliefs when interpreting the significance and meaning of an experience (McHaffie, 1992). They also have different family structures and communities.

Penson (1993) believes that culture determines the patterns and responses of individuals to life events such as trauma. Albon (1986) illustrates this, comparing how the Samoan culture coped with the traumatic experience of a serious fire in their community in 1970 with a similar traumatic fire that affected a community of Americans in 1942. This narrative source of literature indicated, from the results of interviewing representatives from the two cultures, great differences in their coping behaviours. The Samoans, who appeared to accept the experience, were unemotional and quickly readjusted to their normal pattern of living. The Americans showed aggression, fear and hysteria as a result of the trauma, and required significant psychiatric input before adjusting to it. Albon (1986) proposes that these differences in coping mechanisms were due to the different values, attitudes and beliefs of the two cultures which were passed down from generation to generation. The Samoans had a high tolerance of stressful situations, withstood injury and pain and believed that life should go on, whereas the Americans believed that life had been ruined as a result of their experience. The Samoans had strong religious beliefs, putting their experience down to God's will. The Americans did not show such attribution to religion. Also, in the case of the Samoans, the strong family and community support network facilitated coping. Reliability in comparing the studies is limited as the research is dated, there were 15 years between the two fires, and different methodologies were used. Also, the article is narrative which, although broadening the reader's understanding of the topic, risks being subjective (Benton and Cormack, 1991). However, despite these factors, the studies do indicate that coping is influenced by culture.

Social support

The social network of the individual experiencing trauma is a coping resource and can be very influential, as the way people cope largely depends on the resources available to them (McHaffie, 1992). An individual with a limited social support network will cope differently from someone who can draw on the help of a strong social network of friends.

Hagstrom (1995) also found significant differences in coping mechanisms, purely due to different forms of social support. Numerous authors acknowledge that strong and stable social relationships with others are positive components in recovering and coping with the experience of trauma (Braulin *et al.*, 1982; Hagstrom, 1995; Welch, 1995). A strong network of support allows the individual to express fears, worries, feelings and emotions related to the trauma and to receive advice from those who care during these difficult times (Argyle and Henderson, 1985). This is a valuable form of amateur psychotherapy, as a problem shared is a problem halved.

Atkinson *et al.* (1993) also note that strong social support increases an individual's self-esteem and confidence due to companionship and feelings of being loved and cared for. This in turn facilitates recovery. Typically, individuals do not seek professional help when dealing with personal problems as they initially use their social network and individual resources (Taylor, 1983). However, there are some drawbacks to consider which could hinder the coping process. For instance, individuals may find it difficult to discuss with close family and friends their feelings of anger, guilt or frustration as a result of a traumatic experience (Murgatroyd and Woolfe, 1982). Healthcare professionals need to be readily available to offer support to those without a support network and those finding it difficult to express intense feelings to family and friends.

The effect trauma has on the family is a complex subject in itself and has not been explored in any depth. Information about support agencies and self-help groups should be offered. Buck (1991) suggests that this may enable individuals to come to terms with events. It may benefit recovery, as individuals are able to compare feelings and emotions which Burns (1993) notes is an important way to improve the emotional, social and physical health of those who are stressed.

Conclusion

The experience of trauma inevitably creates stress. An abundance of literature supports this, suggesting that such an experience may induce morbidity, vulnerability and annihilation. It is such feelings that an individual must cope with and which are unique to everyone. The perception of threat from the experience and the intensity of stress both influence coping mechanisms. Additional influences, such as attribution and appraisal theory, age, cultural beliefs and social support will all in some way determine outcomes for the individual.

It is the responsibility of all healthcare professionals associated with the provision of treatment and care to those who have suffered trauma to be aware of the complexity of the psychological response. It is only through knowledge, skill and understanding that the recovery of such individuals can be facilitated.

References

Albon, J. (1986) Reactions of Samoan burn patients and families to severe burns. In *Concepts of Health and Disease: a Comparative Perspective* (C. Currer and M. Stacey, eds). Berg.

Argyle, M. and Henderson, M. (1985) *The Anatomy of Relationships and the Rules and Skills to Manage them Successfully*. Heinemann Nursing.

Atkinson, R., Smith, E. and Ben, D. (1993) *Introduction to Psychology*. Harcourt Brace Jovanovich.

Bailey, R. and Clarke, M. (1989) *Stress and Coping in Nursing*. Chapman and Hall.

Bamber, M. (1994) Providing support for emergency service staff. *Nursing Times*, **90**(22), 32–33.

Benner, P. and Wrubel, J. (1989) *The Primacy of Caring, Stress and Coping in Health and Illness*. Addison-Wesley.

Benton, D. and Cormack, D. (1991) Reviewing and evaluating literature. In *The Research Process in Nursing* (D. Cormack, ed.) Blackwell Science.

Braulin, J., Rock, J. and Sill, G. (1982) Families in crisis: the impact of trauma. *Critical Care Quarterly*, Dec., 38-45.

Buck, C. (1991) Treating the individual. *Nursing*, **4**(22), 24–28.

Bullman, R. and Wortman, C. (1977) Attributions of blame and coping in the real world: severe accident victims reactions to their lot. *Journal of Personality and Social Psychology*, **35**, 351–363.

Burns, R. (1993) *Managing People in Changing Times*. Allen and Unwin.

Castledine, G. (1993) First-aid management of psychological emergencies: 2. *British Journal of Nursing*, **2**(21), 1078–1082.

Clarke, M. (1984) Stress and coping: constructs for nursing. *Journal of Advanced Nursing*, **9**, 3-13.

Davis, L. (1987) Convalescence and implications for nursing research. *IMAGE: Journal of Nursing Scholarship*, **19**(3), 117–120.

Hagstrom, R. (1995) The acute psychological impact on survivors following a train accident. *Journal of Traumatic Stress*, **1**(3), 391–402.

Hockey, L. (1991) The nature and purpose of research. In *The Research Process in Nursing* (D. Cormack, ed.). Blackwells Scientific Publications.

Horavitz, M. (1986) Stress-response syndrome: a review of patients and adjustment disorders. *Hospital and Community Psychiatry*, **37**(3), 241–249.

Kelly, M. (1985) Loss and grief reactions as responses to surgery. *Journal of Advanced Nursing*, **10**, 517–525.

Kleber, R. and Brom, D. (1992) *Coping with Trauma: Theory, Prevention and Treatment*. Swets and Zeitlinger.

Kobasa, C. (1979) Stressful life events, personality and health: an inquiry into hardiness. *Journal of Personality and Social Psychology*, **37**, 1–11.

Kubler-Ross, E. (1984). *On Death and Dying*. Routledge.

Lazarus, R. (1976) *Patterns of Adjustment*. McGraw-Hill Book Company.

Lazarus, R. and Folkman, S. (1984) *Stress, Appraisal and Coping*. Springer.

Lenehan, G. (1986) Emotional impact of trauma. *Nursing Clinics in North America*, **21**(4), 729–740.

McHaffie, H. (1992) Coping: an essential element of nursing. *Journal of Advanced Nursing*, **17**, 933–940.

Miller, D. and Porter, C. (1983) Self blame in victims of violence. *Journal of Social Issues*, **39**(2), 139–152.

Moos, R. and Tsu, V. (1977) The crisis of physical illness: an overall view. In *Coping with Physical Illness* (R. Moos, ed.). Plenum.

Muetzel, P. (1988) Therapeutic nursing. In *Primary Nursing: Nursing in the Burford and Oxford Development Units* (A. Pearson, ed). Croom Helm.

Murgatroyd, S. and Woolfe, R. (1982) *Coping with Crisis: Understanding and Helping People in Need*. Harper and Row.

Parkes, C. (1986) *Bereavement*. Penguin.

Pearson, A., Vaughan, B. and Fitzgerald, M. (1991) *Nursing Models for Nursing Practice*. Butterworth-Heinemann.

Penson, J. (1993) *Bereavement: A Guide for Nurses*. Chapman and Hall.

Reutter, L. and Northcott, H. (1995) Managing occupational HIV exposures: a Canadian study. *International Journal of Nursing Studies*, **5**, 493–505.

Sigmon, H. (1984) Helping your long term trauma patient travel the road to recovery. *Nursing*, **14**(1), 58-64.

Taylor, S. (1983) Adjustment to threatening events: a theory of cognitive adaptation. *American Psychologist*, **38**(11), 1161–1173.

Welch, M. (1995) Clients' experiences of depression during recovery from traumatic injury. *Clinical Nurse Specialist*, **9**(2), 92–97.

White, K. (1995). The transition from victim to victor: application of the theory of mastery. *Journal of Psychosocial Nursing*, **33**(8), 41–44.

5

The causes and effects of trauma – the child

Marie-Noelle Orzel

Introduction

Trauma remains one of the major causes of death and disability for children under the age of 16 years. Caring for children and their families presents unique challenges. It must be remembered that children are not small adults; they differ anatomically and physiologically, and have different emotional needs. These differences vary as a child progresses through the stages of maturity from infant to adolescent. A child is dependent on its family for the fundamental needs of comfort and security. For this reason they cannot be cared for in isolation from their family. It is important that practitioners have an appreciation of both the emotional needs and the developmental stages of growth and maturity; each will influence a child's ability to respond physically and psychologically to traumatic injury. In order to provide optimal care for the child, the health-care team must have an understanding of the normal changes occurring within each of these stages. This will enable them to adapt their assessment techniques whilst facilitating the planning and delivery of care appropriate to the developmental level of the child. The aims of this chapter are to:

- Outline the anatomical, physiological and psychosocial developments that occur between the ages of 0 and 16 years.
- Identify how these developments influence the child's ability to understand and cope with a traumatic event.

- Highlight some of the implications to those caring for paediatric trauma patients in order to ensure the child's physical and emotional needs are met.
- Consider the pertinent legal issues in relation to consent.
- Briefly review the issue of child abuse in relation to trauma.

Anatomical and physiological differences

Anatomical and physiological differences occur throughout a child's growth and development. Practitioners should be aware of the physical changes that occur during these periods, as these will affect not only assessment and management, but also the type and size of equipment utilized in the delivery of care. Such changes are not necessarily incremental and, within the developmental continuum, periods of growth and change may occur at different times. For this reason a child's weight is usually used as a basis for the calculation of normal parameters in relation to both equipment size and, most importantly, drug dosages. In an emergency situation it may not be possible to weigh a child accurately, but it is important that as accurate an assessment of the weight as possible is made. This may be done using simple formulae (Table 5.1) or charts which are useful as *aides-mémoire* (Table 5.2). The most accurate method for rapid assessment is the use of a 'paediatric resuscitation measuring tape' such as the Broselow tape. These are designed to relate the weight of a child to its length. Using this information, the tape then calculates the correct drug dosages while recommending the appropriate size of equipment required and the expected normal parameters for a child's clinical observations.

Table 5.1 Simple formulae to aid rapid assessment of the sick child

Weight in kg	=	2 + (age×4)
Blood volume	=	80 ml/kg
Fluid replacement	=	20 ml/kg (crystalloid)
Urine output	=	2 ml/h (<1 year)
		1 ml/h (>1 year)
Blood pressure	=	80 + (age in years×2)

Table 5.2 Paediatric clinical observations

	Pulse rate (beats/min)	Respiration rate (breaths/min)	Systolic blood pressure (mmHg)
Infant	110–160	30–40	70–90
Toddler	95–140	24–40	80–100
Pre-school	80–120	20–30	80–100
School-age	60–100	15–20	90–110
Adolescent	60–100	12–16	100–120

As assessment of the injured child follows the same principles as that of an adult; the anatomical and physiological differences will be considered following the ABCDE assessment process, as described in the subsections below.

Airway

The young child's tongue is larger in relation to the mouth than that of an adult. This means that the airway may easily be obstructed and it is important to ensure patency. The chin-lift jaw-thrust manoeuvres help displace the tongue from the back of the airway, but caution must be taken in positioning fingers, as the floor of the mouth is easily compressible. If an oropharyngeal airway is required, it should be measured in the same way as that for an adult. However, it should be put in position with the aid of a tongue depressor and inserted directly into the mouth rather than rotated, as is the case with an adult, in order to prevent trauma to the child's upper palate. A child's airways are much smaller than those of an adult, making them more prone to obstruction from swelling, mucus, secretions or foreign bodies. In addition, the cartilage of the larynx is much softer, more cephalad and anterior in position. If the neck is hyperextended or flexed this will cause airway obstruction. The cricoid cartilage is the narrowest portion of the larynx and provides a natural seal for an endotracheal tube. For this reason, cuffed endotracheal tubes are not ordinarily used in children under the age of eight (Figure 5.1).

Breathing

At birth an infant's lungs are immature, with a relatively small total surface area for gaseous exchange. Under the age of 4 weeks a baby is an obligate nasal breather. It is therefore vital that nasal passages are kept clear of mucus or secretions. As a child has a faster metabolic rate (about twice that of an adult) the requirement for oxygen is much greater (6–8 ml/kg/min compared with 3–4 ml/kg/min in the adult (Kitt *et al.*, 1995). This means that if a child's respirations are inadequate for any reason, the

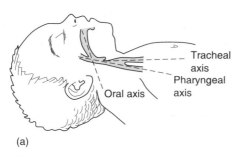

(a)

Tracheal axis
Pharyngeal axis
Oral axis

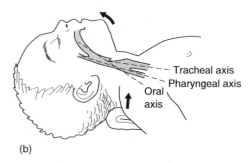

(b)

Tracheal axis
Pharyngeal axis
Oral axis

Figure 5.1 Positioning the child before intubation. Note the relationships among the oral, tracheal and pharyngeal axes (a) before and (b) after placing the child in neutral position. Intubation is easier to accomplish when the axes are in close relationship with each other. (Eichelberger *et al.* 1992)

child is more susceptible to hypoxaemia. A child has a thin chest wall and the sternum and ribs are cartilaginous. As a result the chest is pliable and energy forces are easily transmitted to the underlying structures. Following trauma to the chest wall it is possible to damage underlying structures without fracturing the ribs. If rib fractures are evident, they often indicate the presence of a severe chest or abdominal injury.

The respiratory rate of the very young child is faster than that of an older child or adult (see Table 5.2). However, they have less respiratory reserve than adults, as the intercostal muscles are poorly developed and the ribs lie more horizontally. Infants rely mainly on diaphragmatic breathing to assist the intercostal muscles. Using the diaphragm is less efficient and more likely to result in fatigue. When ill or injured, the child's respiratory effort is increased, which may predispose to respiratory distress or failure. Injury or a full stomach may impede resulting diaphragmatic excursion in hypoventilation and possibly respiratory failure.

Circulation

A child's total blood volume is less than that of an adult (80 ml/kg). However, it is larger on a ml/kg basis than an adult (70–80% of a newborn's body weight is water, compared with 50–60% of an adult's). Therefore even small amounts of blood loss can compromise perfusion and reduce the circulating blood volume. A child normally has a faster heart rate and lower blood pressure than an adult (see Table 5.2). This means that the assessment of shock in the very young can be difficult. It is important that the child's clinical observations are recorded on a frequent basis and compared with the normal parameters for the same age range (see Table 5.1). Tachycardia is the first response to decreased oxygen delivery and will occur with a blood loss of as little as 10–15%. It is not until a blood loss of 20–25% occurs that hypotension develops. This means that hypotension and bradycardia are late signs of circulatory failure.

Hypovolaemia is the commonest cause of shock in the child (Advanced Life Support Group, 1994). The abdomen of a child is susceptible to blunt injury for various reasons. The abdominal wall is thin and the weak abdominal muscles offer little protection to

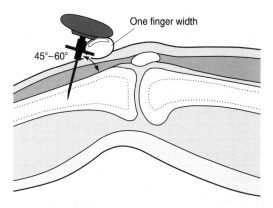

Figure 5.2 Site for intraosseous infusion (American College of Surgeons, 1993)

the relatively large abdominal organs. These organs lie in close proximity to each other because of the child's compact size, making the likelihood of multiple injuries more common than in an adult. The spleen and liver are more vulnerable as they lie in a lower position because of the horizontal diaphragm. Furthermore, the bladder is intra-abdominal rather than within the pelvic cavity, making it more prone to injury. As bruising is not always present, it is important that clinical staff suspect potential abdominal injury based on the mechanism of injury alone; for example, a high-impact injury, or hitting the handlebars when falling off a bike. Establishing intravenous access in a sick child can present a great challenge to clinical staff. Preferred sites include the dorsum of the hand, antecubital fossa and the saphenous vein of the ankle. However, in the critically injured child whose tiny veins are inaccessible, it may be necessary to use an intraosseous needle which is inserted 2–3 cm below the tibial tuberosity on the anterior surface (Advanced Life Support Group, 1994). As the insertion technique is relatively easy, it enables clinical staff to gain rapid circulatory access through which all resuscitation medications and fluids can be administered (Figure 5.2).

Disability and neurological assessment

The child has an increased head–body size ratio in comparison with an adult (in the infant the head is approximately 18% of the total body size in comparison with 9% in the adult). They also have weaker neck muscles and this may lead to a greater incidence of head injury. Head injury is the single most common cause of death in children aged 1–15 years and accounts for 25% of deaths in the 5–15-year age group (Advanced Life Support Group, 1994). The younger the child, the more prominent the occiput, which causes slight flexing of the neck when the child is placed in the supine position. In a child who has a suspected cervical or spinal injury it is necessary to raise the shoulders and chest using a small pad in order to achieve a safe supine cervical position. In addition, the infant's skull is more malleable, and the sutures and fontanelles remain open until around the age of 16 months. One of the signs of increased intracranial pressure may include a bulging or tense fontanelle when palpated. Conversely, a dehydrated infant may present with a sunken fontanelle.

When performing a neurological assessment on a child it is important to acknowledge how the child's age and development will affect the neurological responses. For this reason it is necessary to use a modified Glasgow Coma Scale for continuous neurological assessment (Table 5.3). Generally the child's level of consciousness is determined by whether the child is alert or awake. An alert infant should maintain eye contact and be wary of strangers. If any child under the age of 5 years responds indifferently to his strange environment or fails to recognize their parents, this is suggestive of an altered level of consciousness. A child who has developed verbal skills should be able to say their name, identify where they are and say what has happened to them. If unsure, it is useful to ask the parents how they would normally expect their child to respond. Generally, in any child who appears unconcerned or uninterested by what is happening, then hypovolaemia, hypoxia or head injury should be suspected. Other pertinent signs include irritability, vomiting or aggression alternating with lethargy.

Exposure

In comparison with an adult, the child has a larger body surface area to weight ratio and a lesser amount of fat. The very young child also has an immature temperature-regulating system. One cause of heat loss is a child's higher circulating blood flow, especially to the head. As a result the child is extremely susceptible to heat loss and when exposed, especially during resuscitation, can lose critical body heat rapidly. Compared to an adult, a child requires up to three times as many calories for basic homeostasis. Whereas a young child has the ability to shiver to maintain body temperature, infants do not. Instead, thermogenesis takes place and involves the breakdown of brown fat (Kitt *et al.*, 1995). This physiological mechanism increases oxygen consumption and further compromises the child. To minimize heat loss and potential hypothermia the child should not be exposed unnecessarily. If possible the room temperature should be increased. Where exposure of the child is unavoidable, for example during the resuscitation period, then adjuncts such as overhead heaters should be used, particularly for very young infants. For the older child, the use of warming blankets and simple measures such as covering the head will help minimize heat loss.

Within this section it is appropriate to discuss one further anatomical feature that is particular to the musculoskeletal system of the child – the presence of epiphyseal plates (growth plates). Growth plates are located between the epiphysis and metaphysis at the distal and proximal ends of long bones and do not ossify until puberty. They are responsible for longitudinal bone growth. Injury at the site of the epiphyseal plate may affect bone growth and deformity may result. Periosteum in children is stronger, thicker and more osteogenic than in adults. This allows bone to bend rather than break (Kitt *et al.*, 1995). It also means that rapid callus formation occurs and fractures take less time to heal.

Communication

Children are difficult to assess in comparison with adults for several reasons. A child's response to an injury is dependent on their stage of development. Communication can be difficult because of limited vocabulary and understanding. For this reason a child may or may not be able to identify what is hurting or how they are feeling. Interaction with the sick child requires patience and the ability to interpret subtle assessment clues. When caring

Table 5.3 Modified Glasgow Coma Scale (Adapted from Semonin-Houeran, 1991)

Eyes opening

Score	> 1 year	< 1 year
4	Spontaneously	Spontaneously
3	To verbal command	To shout
2	To pain	To pain
1	No response	No response

Best motor response

Score	> 1 year	< 1 year
6	Obeys	Spontaneous movement
5	Localizes to pain	Localizes to pain
4	Flexion withdrawal	Flexion withdrawal
3	Flexion abnormal	Flexion abnormal
2	Extension	Extension
1	No response	No response

Best verbal response

Score	> 5 years	2–5 years	0–24 months
5	Orientated and converses	Appropriate words and phrases	Smiles, coos appropriately
4	Disorientated and converses	Inappropriate words and phrases	Cries appropriately
3	Inappropriate words	Cries and/or screams	Persistent inappropriate crying and/or screams
2	Incomprehensible sounds	Grunts	Grunts
1	No response	No response	No response

for a child, communication should be considered as a three-way process between the practitioner, the child and the family. As part of this process the practitioner acquires information through direct observation of the child's verbal and non-verbal responses. In addition, the child's family are more than likely to be able to understand and interpret the child's verbal responses, also distinguishing between what is normal or abnormal behaviour. Wherever possible the parents should be encouraged to remain with the child, to be active participants in their care. The following are general principles for communicating with any child:

- avoid sudden advances towards the child or removing the child from the parent
- give the child time to become acquainted with the practitioner
- get down to the child's level, preferably eye level
- speak clearly using simple terms – discussing something personal such as a toy will help establish a rapport
- talk directly to the child, but try to include the parent or another sibling, especially if the child is particularly shy
- be honest at all times
- take time and wait for replies.

Psychosocial development and practical implications

In addition to the anatomical and physiological changes that occur through childhood, it is important to develop an understanding of both the cognitive and psychosocial developments that occur during maturation. Depending on the stage of cognitive development, a child's perception of a situation may be radically different from that of an adult. They have a 'mental picture' of their body image that may influence their understanding of what they are experiencing. At different developmental stages the child will also demonstrate different coping behaviours to experiences such as pain, anxiety or fear. A knowledge and understanding of all these factors will enable the practitioner to develop an appreciation of a child's understanding of their injury. It will also help them to provide age-appropriate explanations while recognizing and responding to the distressed child. Generally speaking, these stages of development are described as:

- infant   0–12 months
- toddler   1–3 years
- pre-school child   3–5 years
- school-age child   5–12 years
- adolescent   12–18 years

Infant

The primary psychosocial development during infancy is the development of trust (Erikson, 1968). Babies are thought to learn mainly through their senses and their activity within their environment by crying, kicking, smiling and sucking. Their motor abilities progress from rolling over to sitting upright, crawling and standing. If unsupervised, these actions may cause injury as a result of falls from a bed or a couch. During the first year of life a child explores the world by grabbing and placing objects in their mouth. This means that they are at risk from ingesting foreign bodies and choking, or grabbing dangerous objects that may cause harm, for example hot drinks. The infant's actions generate responses from people around them and trust develops when needs are consistently recognized and met, primarily by a parent. By the age of 3 months a baby is able to recognize and respond to familiar routines and people. Encouraging the parents to remain with the infant and wherever possible to feed, hold, rock and care for their child, maintains both comfort and security. This is particularly important as the infant gets older. By the age of 7 months, infants start to demonstrate stranger-anxiety, especially if approached abruptly, so it is important to spend time allowing the infant to get used to their surroundings and new people. This can be achieved using a quiet soothing voice, together with play prior to any clinical interventions. Ensuring that one's hands and equipment are warm during procedures further promotes comfort and trust.

Cognitively, infants are unable to understand cause and effect. While they are able to have feelings associated with pleasure and discomfort, they will not understand the reasons for this. However, they are able to sense their parent's distress, and this may cause them to become more fretful. For this reason it is vital that parental trust is also promoted, through the provision of careful explanation and emotional support. Distressed infants use self-comforting measures as a coping strategy; these include sucking on a thumb or a dummy. It is thought that sucking provides the infant with comfort by blocking out noxious stimuli (Porter, 1989). If a baby likes to suck a thumb then, where possible, any intravenous cannulation should be avoided in that hand or arm.

Toddler

As children progress from infancy into the toddler stage they begin to experience a sense of autonomy (Erikson, 1968). Through their increasing motor and language abilities toddlers demonstrate an increasing ability to help themselves and make their desires known. They are extremely inquisitive, but have no concept of right or wrong or danger. Their increased mobility can lead them into dangerous situations where they may inadvertently fall from heights or into water. As with the infant, they tend to grab objects without thinking, and this age group is particularly at risk from kettle scalds and drinks being pulled from kitchen counters. Many toddlers may have experienced some separation from their family, either through day nurseries or when cared for by childminders. However, their autonomy is dependent on the maintenance of security that is associated with their normal routine. Exposing the toddler to an environment or experience that is strange and unfamiliar is likely to threaten their security and cause a great deal of anxiety. Although stranger-anxiety decreases by the age of 18 months, emotionally toddlers are still very dependent on adults. Ideally, the presence of parents will in most cases help reduce any anxiety. This may not always be possible, so a further strategy is to provide objects that the toddler is familiar with. It is at this age that many children have a 'comforter' such as a favourite blanket or toy that should be kept with them at all times.

Cognitively, toddlers' language abilities are increasing. They are able to identify certain external parts of their bodies, though they have limited understanding of their bodily functions. It is important to note that a child of this age is able to understand more than they can verbalize. When providing age-appropriate explanations it is helpful to use familiar words. Many families have their own words for urinating, bowel movement and sometimes pain. The toddler's thought processes often appear illogical to the adult. At this age children perceive their body's boundaries as indefinite and if their arm is placed in a cast or bandage it may take careful explanation to convince the child that the limb is still there (Kitt *et al.*, 1995). A toddler's memory and attention span is usually quite short and their understanding of time is quite poor. To avoid any undue anxiety, practitioners, when planning clinical interventions, should ensure that any explanation is done immediately prior to the intervention.

Toddlers use verbal activities such as crying and screaming as part of their coping mechanisms. They may also express their anxiety through kicking and hitting out at those near them. While it may be important to restrain their physical activity for some clinical procedures, the toddler should be allowed to cry and scream as this will help them to cope with the experience. Following such an experience, rewards such as badges and certificates are a good method of promoting the child's sense of control and self-worth.

Pre-school child

Pre-school children are beginning to develop a sense of initiative (Erikson, 1968). It is at this stage that they try their best to please and demonstrate pride in their accomplishments. They like to help and are able to complete activities such as undressing themselves. Their verbal skills are developing and they should know most of their external body parts and some internal organs. The child is able to follow simple instructions and it is important to reward the child for any cooperation which they have demonstrated with procedures. In their daily activities they may blur fantasy and reality, believing they can fly in the same way as their favourite cartoon heroes and this may lead to injury. At this age children are developing better coordination skills, but still have a poor sense of direction and undeveloped peripheral vision, making them vulnerable in busy environments such as roads and crowds. They often have imaginations that are vivid and they may engage in 'magical thinking' (Carter and Dearmun, 1995). When carrying out clinical procedures it is useful to make up stories about the techniques and instruments being used, even going so far as to give them names and identities such as 'Freddy' the forcep, or 'Gertie' the gauze. Some children of this age perceive their injury or illness to be the result of a real or imaginary wrong doing and the child will begin to fear both pain and the idea of body mutilation. Using simple concrete language to explain procedures will help gain the child's trust and help them to understand what is happening.

Children of this age should be encouraged to verbalize their feelings and be reassured that they are allowed to feel afraid. If something is going to hurt, it is useful to allow the child to scream 'ouch!' as loud as they can, as this will give them some control over the situation and help them to cope. Holding a parent's hand and squeezing as tightly as possible is another strategy that may be used to encourage the child to maintain control.

School-age child

The school-age child works hard to gain approval for tasks they have completed and if they do not achieve they may develop a sense of inferiority (Erikson, 1968). They will have developed a sense of independence and self-control. Through their social contacts they will also have developed strong relationships with their peer group. It is during this period that children become more involved in sporting activities such as riding bicycles. The child gains confidence and begins to understand the concept of competitiveness. However, they may not have acquired the cognitive and motor abilities to master successfully all that they attempt, putting them at risk on roads or, for example, when climbing trees. Despite their increased independence, the child's family is still extremely important during this period and these children should be given a choice about having their parent present during procedures and examinations. A child's body image plays a bigger part at this age and children may fear being exposed or the thought of disfigurement. Therefore their modesty should be respected at all times.

The school-age child has a large vocabulary, though may still be confused about some bodily functions. Their appreciation of time is more developed. Generally, the school-age child understands simple scientific explanations, as their level of understanding and reasoning abilities are becoming more refined. Obtaining information is one coping strategy that school-age children use (Kitt *et al.*, 1995). For this reason, practitioners should encourage the child to ask questions and participate in their care. It enables the practitioner to explain the purpose of different equipment and procedures, while using such opportunities to teach the child about bodily functions.

Adolescent

Adolescence is a period of great change, due to the rapidly occurring hormonal, physical and psychosocial changes that are taking place. It is a time when people establish their own identities (Erikson, 1968) through increasing independence. It is also a time when an individual develops strong ties with their peers and worry about acceptance within a social group. Part of this process is an increase in 'risk-taking' behaviour. The adolescent is able to make choices based on logical and abstract thought processes, and should be able to understand the consequences of their actions. Despite this, they often partake in risky behaviour based on the belief that bad things will not happen to them. While they should be respected and treated in the same way as adults, it is also important to have their families nearby to provide emotional support as needed. The adolescent should have a basic knowledge of anatomy and physiology and practitioners should use appropriate terminology to explain any findings during clinical procedures. During this changing period the adolescent's body image may be in a state of turmoil. It is vital that privacy and confidentiality are maintained.

To enable adolescents to cope, it is important that they are allowed to feel in control of their situation. They should be encouraged to ask questions and be given choices when discussing treatment plans.

Legal considerations in caring for children

Health professionals responsible for the care of children must be aware of the rights of children and to what extent children should be involved in decision-making. The younger the child, the more reliant they are on their parents or carers to make appropriate decisions for them. Occasionally, other adults may be invested with the power to consent on a child's behalf, a typical example being schoolteachers. They are responsible for children during certain periods of the day, and are thus able to provide proxy consents for any child involved in an accident while at school. As such, adults are legally recognized as capable of consenting to medical and nursing procedures on behalf of children (Royal College of Nursing, 1998). However,

under the Family Law Reform Act 1969, a child over the age of 16 years is able to give valid consent on their own behalf as though they were an adult. In addition, following the decision in the House of Lords in Gillick v West Norfolk and Wisbech AHA (1985), a child under the age of 16 years is able to consent to medical treatment if they are able to understand fully the nature and consequence of the treatment. The outcome of the Gillick case has been replicated in the Children Act 1989, which implies that parents and carers should listen to children, provide them with appropriate information and take account of their wishes and feelings. To facilitate this, practitioners must ensure that they have an adequate understanding of individual children's development levels and the necessary communication skills.

Child abuse

Child abuse refers to non-accidental harm that is inflicted on children by their parents or other adults. Abuse can either be active or passive and can occur in the form of neglect or physical, emotional or sexual abuse (Home Office *et al.*, 1991). Nationally the true incidence of child abuse is not known, but estimates indicate that at least 1 million children a week are at risk of being harmed (National Commission of Inquiry into the Prevention of Child Abuse, 1996). The role of the healthcare professional in child protection lies within the framework of legislation and government guidelines for inter-agency working (Powell and Perriment, 1998).

Within the acute setting the nurse may be the first person to identify children who are either at risk or who have suffered actual harm. For this reason all healthcare professionals caring for children should be knowledgeable about the possible indicators of abuse and neglect (Table 5.4). They should also have an understanding of their responsibilities and the importance of collegiate relationships with agencies (police, social services) and multi-professional teams (paediatric teams, community liaison teams) who share responsibility for child protection (Department of Health, 1997). If child abuse is suspected, for whatever reason, the information must be passed on to a specialist paediatric team who can then involve other inter-agency teams as necessary. It is vital that any information is carefully and factually documented for future use should it be required either for case conferences or, if necessary, subsequent court action.

Table 5.4 Classic indicators of child abuse or neglect

Delay in seeking medical help for the injury

History of accident is vague and lacks detail

Conflicting and varying history of events from carers and child

History given by accompanying adults that does not fit the presenting injuries

Other unexplained injuries are present such as lacerations, burns, bite marks

Parents' interaction with the child is abnormal, e.g. lack of concern, more preoccupied with own problems than condition of the child

Parents' behaviour may give cause for concern, e.g. hostile for no apparent reason or unwilling to wait for treatment

Child's interactions with the parent or other carers may be abnormal

Child's appearance may be sad, withdrawn or displaying fearful body language

There may be obvious evidence of failure to thrive with no pathological cause

Child may openly disclose being a victim of abuse

Conclusion

Within the constraints of this chapter it has only been possible to provide a broad overview of the factors that should be considered when caring for children. As mentioned at the beginning of the chapter, children are not small adults. They have special needs that arise from the fact that they are continually changing as they grow and develop. For these reasons children should be cared for by practitioners with the required specialist training (DHSS, 1976), in an environment that meets their needs (Department of Health, 1991, 1993). Despite these recommendations there are still areas where such facilities and staffing are not available due to organizational constraints. It is the responsibility of all nurses to safeguard the wellbeing and interests of their patients,

while recognizing their own abilities and limitations (UKCC, 1992). This chapter has outlined the key principles for all practitioners responsible for the care of children and has provided a basis for the further exploration of their unique needs.

References

Advanced Life Support Group (1994) Advanced paediatric life support: the practical approach. *British Medical Journal*.

American College of Surgeons (1993) *Advanced Trauma Life Support – Programme for Physicians*. American College of Surgeons.

Carter, B. and Dearmun, A. (1995) *Child Healthcare Nursing: Concepts Theory and Practice*. Oxford Blackwell Science.

Department of Health (1991) *The Welfare of Children and Young People in Hospital*. London: HMSO.

Department of Health (1993) *Audit Commission: Children First – a Study of Hospital Services*. London: HMSO.

Department of Health (1997) *Child Protection: Guidance for Senior Nurses, Health Visitors and Midwives*. London: HMSO.

DHSS (1976) *Fit for the Future: Report for the Committee on Child Health Services*. (Court Report). London: HMSO.

Eichelberger, M., Pratsch, G. and Runion, E. (1992) *Paediatric Emergencies*. Prentice Hall.

Erikson, E. (1968) *Identity: Youth and Crisis*. Norton.

Home Office, Department of Health, Welsh office *et al.* (1991) *Working Together Under the Children Act 1989: A Guide to Arrangements for Inter-agency Co-operation for the Protection of Children from Abuse*. London: HMSO.

Kitt, S., Selfridge-Thomas, J., Proehl, J. and Kaiser, J. (1995) *Emergency Nursing: A Physiological and Clinical Perspective*. Saunders.

National Commission of Inquiry into the Prevention of Child Abuse (1996) *Childhood Matters*. London: HMSO.

Porter, F. (1989) Pain in the newborn. *Clinics in Perinatology*, **16**, 549–564.

Powell, C. and Perriment, D. (1998) Child protection in paediatric ambulatory care settings. In *Innovations in Paediatric Ambulatory Care: A Nursing Perspective* (E. Glasper and S. Lowson, eds.) Macmillan.

Royal College of Nursing (1998) *Nursing Children in the Accident and Emergency Department*. RCN.

Semonin-Houerin, R. (1991) Paediatric trauma patients, differences and implications for emergency nurses. *Journal of Emergency Nursing*, **17**(1), 24–31.

UKCC (1992) *The Code of Professional Practice*. United Kingdom Central Council for Nursing, Midwifery and Health Visiting.

6

The causes and effects of trauma – the young adult

Kerri Rance

Introduction

In 1996 the car industry celebrated its one hundredth anniversary; during this time over 0.5 million people have died on the roads. Pedestrians make up half that number and the drivers responsible are frequently in their early twenties (Hamer, 1996). It is widely recognized that trauma is the leading cause of death in the under 44-year age group (Haddon, 1980; Emergency Nurses Association, 1995) (Figure 6.1).

Trauma accounts for 63% of all deaths in the 15–24-year age group (Haddon, 1980; Hamilton, 1991), with the overall death rate due to trauma being twice that for males than females. For every person killed there are 400 non-fatal injuries serious enough to require medical attention (Hamilton, 1991).

In Oxford city the 15–29-year age group makes up 30.4% of the population (Figure 6.2), whereas in England and Wales as a whole this age group makes up 21.3% of the population (Office for National Statistics, 1996). This

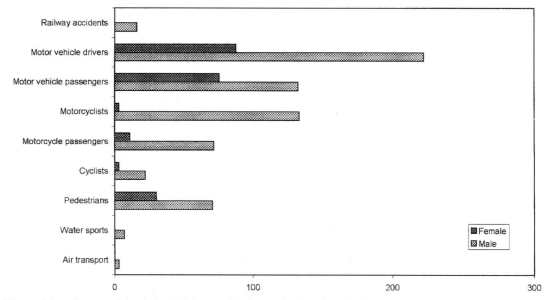

Figure 6.1   Causes of death in 15–24-year-olds in England and Wales in 1994 (From the Office of National Statistics, 1993–1994)

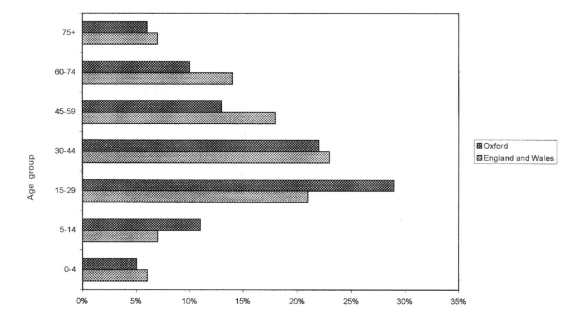

Figure 6.2 Age range as a percentage of the population

therefore can be seen as a contributory factor to Oxfordshire's higher than average national death rate in this age group (Figure 6.3).

The incidence of fractures in younger males peaks in 15–24 year olds (Donaldson *et al.*, 1990; Court-Brown *et al.*, 1998). Fractures of the shafts of the tibia, fibula and femur are common injuries among young men, frequently due to contact sports and road accidents, especially motorcycle accidents. There are many factors which affect accident death rates, including the ingestion of alcohol and the use of illegal substances, both of which warrant further discussion.

Risk-taking

Linked with any traumatic injury is an element of risk-taking, whether it be taking part in sports, driving, the use of drugs and alcohol, or of being subjected to peer pressure (Denscombe, 1993). **There is growing evidence that intentional and unintentional injuries are closely related to risk-taking behaviours** (Redeker *et al.*, 1995).

It has been found that certain individuals repeatedly present at hospitals with new injuries. Kaufmann *et al.* (1998) found in a study

undertaken in the USA that these individuals were generally in the 20–24-year age group, with males 1.5 times more likely than females to be regular attenders. It has been shown that repeated hospital attendance is linked to alcohol abuse and that individuals who are intoxicated at the time of the initial injury are more likely to return than those who were not (Rivara *et al.*, 1993; Schwarz *et al.*, 1994).

Redeker *et al.* (1995) have put forward the theory that risk-taking behaviours are linked to the following:

- developmental characteristics
- environmental characteristics
- social network
- psychological factors

They suggest that these are the antecedents to risk-taking behaviours which in turn increase the likelihood of trauma occurring.

Developmental characteristics

These include poor judgement about the negative outcome of their behaviour, an unrealistic sense of competence, control, optimism and sense of invulnerability (Irwin and Millstein, 1988; Denscombe, 1993).

It has been found that young men are

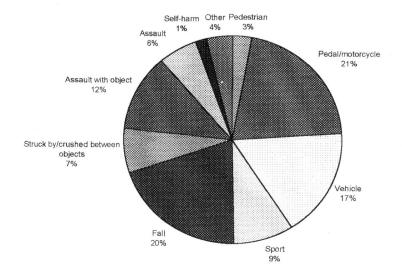

Figure 6.3 Injuries received by 15–24-year-olds in the Oxford area, 1996–1997

particularly vulnerable to the excitement and macho status of driving fast cars. Inexperience on roads and peer pressure are a lethal combination (Shapiro *et al.*, 1998).

Case study

John, 18, was involved in a minor collision with the central reservation on a dual carriageway. He was unhurt in this incident and got out of the car. However, he was then hit by a car travelling at 70 mph. The injuries he received were as follows:

- closed head injury – intracerebral bleeds and brainstem haemorrhage
- unstable fracture of the second cervical vertebra
- closed fracture of the right femur
- closed fracture of the right tibia
- open fracture of the left femur
- open fracture of the left tibia
- open fracture of the right forefoot
- closed fracture of the left humerus

John was transferred to ICU from a District General Hospital 8 days post-injury.

Days post Treatment received
injury

2	Above-knee amputation of the left leg
	External fixator to the right tibia
7	External fixator to the left humerus
	External fixator to the right femur
	Intramedullary nail to the left femur
9	C2/3 fusion
11	Intramedullary nail to the right femur
	'K' wires to the 1st–5th metatarsals of the right foot
	Internal fixation of the right talus
	Wound debridement over the right tibia
	Intramedullary nail to the left humerus
14	Split skin grafting to wounds on the left arm
	Split skin grafting to wounds over the left tibia
15	Formation of tracheostomy
28	Insertion of percutaneous endoscopic gastrostomy (PEG) tube

Following a lengthy recovery period John was eventually transferred to a rehabilitation centre 2½ months post-injury. By this time he had had his tracheostomy tube removed and could feed himself with one hand and wash his face. Nine months from the accident he was discharged home to the care of his parents, able to independently propel his wheelchair and practising with his artificial limb. John still suffers from memory problems as a result of his head injury and still has further to go in order to fulfil his potential.

Environmental characteristics

1. Poverty, availability of weapons and increased exposure to risk-taking behaviours (Hammond and Yung, 1993).
2. Violent behaviour which is on the increase within inner cities where the risk of becoming a victim is high (Singer, 1986).
3. Unemployment and living in an urban area associated with drug-taking increases the likelihood of engaging in risk-taking behaviours (Redeker and Smeltzer, 1995).

Williams *et al.* (1996) suggest that children from low family affluence are more likely to be involved in fighting, and as a result to sustain head and facial injuries. The incidence of this increases when alcohol is involved.

Risk-taking is part of youth culture. It has been suggested that having friends who engage in dangerous activities and choosing to undertake dangerous activities is more common among adolescents whose parents are generally not in employment (Williams *et al.*, 1996).

It has also been suggested that children from poorer households are at higher risk of traffic-related injuries (Williams *et al.*, 1996; DiGallo *et al.*, 1997).

Social network

Failure in school, unemployment, lack of job skills and underdeveloped social skills often isolate adolescents and young adults from the positive influences associated with education (Eccles *et al.*, 1993).

Joy-riding and the theft of motor vehicles is a contributory factor in the severity of injuries received by an unrestrained driver travelling at speed. In addition to the intrinsic amusement factor, it is likely that little effort is made to avoid a crash just because of the presence of the police. It may also be that the intention is to drive recklessly in order to initiate a police chase (Livingstone *et al.*, 1998). It was shown in one UK city that car crime accounted for 20% of road traffic accident (RTA) deaths in hospital, and 13% of RTA admissions to ICU (Marshall *et al.*, 1996). This study showed that, except for one death, the joy-riders sustained less severe injuries than the innocent individuals also involved. Where pedestrians are involved, the injuries sustained are invariably severe (Marshall *et al.*, 1996).

Psychological factors

It has been suggested that one of the main motivators for engaging in or avoiding risk-laden behaviour has been the anticipated reward which results from that behaviour (Heimer, 1988).

Within a group situation there is a tendency for risky decisions to be considered as acceptable (Denscombe, 1993). This may be because the group exerts pressure to conform (Dion *et al.*, 1970).

The traditional view on risk-taking behaviours casts males within this role and tends to exclude females. Shapiro *et al.* (1998) challenged this view, suggesting that females are engaging in more risk-taking behaviour at higher rates than before in areas such as drug use, smoking and drinking. **It has also been shown that the number of women who drink above the recommended level of alcohol is on the increase** (Central Statistical Office 1996).

Risk-taking and the use of bicycle and motorcycle helmets

Research undertaken by Oxford Brookes University showed that teenage cyclists were influenced by friends in relation to the use of helmets, even to the extent that some left home wearing a helmet but removed it prior to arriving at school (The Health of Oxfordshire, 1993–94). Many people do not like wearing helmets as they are seen as cumbersome (Clayton, 1998); one way to encourage their use is to change their image.

Cycle helmets reduce the risk of head injury (Thompson *et al.*, 1989; Thomas *et al.*, 1994) by as much as 85% (Discala, 1991). It has also been found that the wearing of a cycle helmet has some limited protection against facial injury (Bjornstig *et al.*, 1992; Thompson *et al.*, 1996). Harrison and Shepherd (1997) have found that in cycling accidents the face is most likely to impact with the surface (e.g. car, road, windscreen) and this alone can result in head injury. It has been suggested that child accident rates and the wearing of helmets are associated with social class (McCarthy, 1996) and that deaths are 15 times more frequent in areas of greatest deprivation (Sharples *et al.*, 1990). It is worth mentioning that British Standard cycle helmets only afford protection when the rider falls to the ground, not when any other vehicle is involved

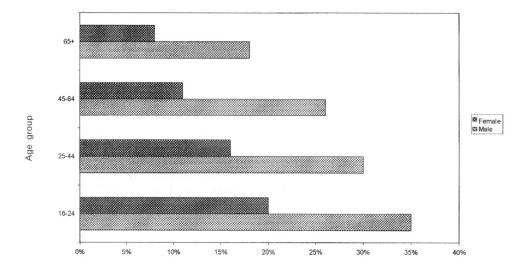

Figure 6.4 Consumption of alcohol above sensible levels: by gender and age, 1994–95

(British Standards Institution, 1990). Many cyclists feel that enforcing the use of helmets is taking away their freedom and that heavy-duty motorcycle helmets would be needed in order to offer protection when in collision with motor vehicles (Clayton, 1998). However, some form of head protection is better than none, even in the most severe situations.

Wagle *et al.* (1993) suggest that if an individual is wearing a motorcycle helmet it has a significant effect on the outcome of an accident and the likelihood of death is greatly reduced. The use of a motorcycle helmet also reduces the likelihood of facial fractures (Bachulis *et al.*, 1988; Johnson *et al.*, 1995).

Alcohol and trauma

Risk-taking is directly linked to alcohol consumption. Alcohol alters one's perception and one's abilities, both cognitive and physical. According to large numbers of authors, alcohol is a major factor in adult trauma (Henderson, 1987; Shepherd et al., 1988; Denscombe, 1993; Spain et al., 1997), contributing to the frequency, severity, mortality and disability from injury in a variety of causes (Meyer, 1998). It has also been found that alcohol consumption may adversely affect decision-making in other areas of road safety such as the wearing of seat belts and motorcycle helmets. It is unlikely that

individuals willing to risk arrest for drink driving would be overly concerned with the chance of getting caught not wearing a seat belt (Foss *et al.*, 1994; Spain *et al.*, 1997).

The rapid consumption of excessive amounts of alcohol produces a deterioration in brain function, with changes in behaviour progressing through slurred speech and unsteady gait to unconsciousness (Trounce, 1990; Walsh, 1996). Alcohol is a depressant, not a stimulant, as is commonly thought (Figure 6.4).

Alcohol is absorbed from the stomach and intestines, although more from the latter (Paton, 1994). The rate of absorption is variable, but more rapid when on an empty stomach and when the concentration of alcohol in the drink is 20–30% (e.g. sherry or vermouth).

In the West Midlands, Clayton *et al.* (1977) found that 25% of all fatally injured pedestrians had a blood alcohol level above the legal limit for driving. At blood alcohol levels 2½ times the legal driving limit (approximately 5 pints of beer) the chances of being killed were 23 times greater than the control group. Drinking is a well-known pastime among students. In 1992 a study showed that 87% of college students drank alcohol in the previous year; 40% consumed 5 or more drinks on a single occasion – more than the non-college attendees of the same age (Kivalian *et al.*, 1989; Hingson *et al.*, 1992). In the 18–24-year age group over a third of men and a fifth of women drank more than the recommended sensible level of alcohol (see Figure 6.4). According to the Central Statistical Office (1996) the proportion of men drinking above the recommended sensible level has remained virtually unchanged between 1986 and 1995, while the corresponding proportion of women increased from 11% to 13%. Drinking among students occurs often as a result of peer pressure due to the need to relax within a social situation (Collins and Marlatt, 1981) (Table 6.1).

Table 6.1 Blood alcohol concentration and its effect (Adapted from Trounce, 1990)

Blood level	Effect
20 mg/100 ml	Relaxed
30 mg/100 ml	Talkative
50 mg/100 ml	A little uncoordinated (knock over glass)
80 mg/100 ml	Legal driving limit
100 mg/100 ml	Fall about, vomiting
300 mg/100 ml	Stupor

Spain *et al.* (1997) found that alcohol had been consumed in 40% of all traffic fatalities. Meyer (1998) showed that alcohol is associated with a higher incidence of death from crashes, with damage to the vehicle also being more severe. It has also been noted that intoxicated individuals who survive an RTA are 5–10 times more likely to suffer serious injuries and a higher incidence of post-injury complications (Gentitello *et al.*, 1993; Spain *et al.*, 1997). Alcohol makes the performance of drivers more erratic and causes them to experience difficulty staying 'on task' (Synder and Ladu, 1985). Intoxicated drivers feel excessively confident, causing them to take more risks than if they were sober (Synder and Ladu, 1985; Paton, 1994). Although their average performance may seem acceptable, the many minor deviations and errors they make, then correct (or over-correct), increase their vulnerability to accidents. This same pattern is typical of many new drivers who have not yet mastered the skill of operating a car and so tend to be insecure. Many make errors; therefore drinking by inexperienced drivers is particularly risky (Synder and Ladu, 1985; Hingson *et al.*, 1992). This association between inexperience and fatal crash involvement has been studied by Mayhew *et al.* (1986), who also showed that each alcoholic drink consumed before driving increases the fatal crash risk for drivers in this category.

Alcohol intoxication has long been associated with aggression (Shepherd *et al.*, 1990; Wright and Kariya, 1997). Yates *et al.* (1987), who performed studies in Manchester, found that 60% of assault victims had positive blood alcohol readings. This same figure is corroborated in research undertaken in Strathclyde (Wright and Kariya, 1997). Shepherd *et al.* (1988) undertook research within an inner city accident and emergency (A&E) department to find out whether there was a link between alcohol intake and assault. They discovered that patients who reported abstinence from alcohol tended to have injuries which were relatively minor, whereas individuals who had consumed in excess of 10 units of alcohol tended to have more severe injuries. The authors suggest that the link between alcohol and the severity of the injuries received may have arisen because alcohol-induced aggression and loss of judgement in the victims prolongs violence, or simply because such victims are less able to avoid blows during assault. Wright and Kariya (1997) found that 41% of assault victims who presented in A&E had suffered previous assaults.

Illegal substances and trauma

The cause and effect of alcohol in relation to accidental and non-accidental injury is well documented; not so the use of illegal substances. Very few studies have been undertaken which look at the number of individuals involved in road traffic accidents who have been using illegal substances. The majority of studies are American, but they can still provide useful indicators from which to draw conclusions in the UK.

In Great Britain in 1993/1994 there were thought to be 21 000 people with a drug problem, of whom 34% were aged between 15 and 24 years (Central Statistical Office, 1996). These figures increase to 42% of 16–19-year-olds and 44% of 20–24-year-olds within inner cities, of whom one-third were male and one fifth female. Within the inner city population of 16–25-year-olds it has been suggested that 1%

have misused crack-cocaine, 2% heroin and 4% cocaine. These figures do not include those who have used marijuana. In two government papers it found that 18% of people aged 16–19 and 14% aged 20–24 reported misuse of marijuana in the previous year (Home Office, 1995). It is acknowledged that marijuana is the most widely misused illegal drug (Keene, 1997). A great contributor to the misuse of drugs in the 1990s has been the integration of LSD and Ecstasy into mass youth culture. Among 16–19-year-olds 11% have tried amphetamines, 9% Ecstasy and 8% LSD (Keene, 1997).

Between 1988 and 1991 a number of studies looked at the use of cocaine and marijuana in trauma patients and found that between 26.1% and 37% had used marijuana (Sonderstrom *et al.*, 1988; Sloane *et al.*, 1989; Rivara *et al.*, 1989) and 9% to 34% had used cocaine (Sloane *et al.*, 1989; Rivara *et al.*, 1989; Dischinger, 1991). Lindenbaum *et al.* (1989) found the figure for cocaine use and trauma patients to be as high as 54.4%. Rivara *et al.* (1989) also found that between 0.5% and 2% of those fatally injured in road traffic accidents had used opiates.

A random study undertaken in America found that from a group of cocaine users studied in the A&E department, 52.1% had accidental injuries and 47.9% had injuries relating to violent crime. Of this number, 80.5% were male and 19.5% female (Lindenbaum *et al.*, 1989). Of those involved in violent crime and those who had received accidental injures, 80.3% and 69.3% respectively tested positive for alcohol and drugs. At present in the UK, individuals are not routinely tested for illegal substances when they present in A&E.

According to Braun *et al.* (1998) marijuana is the most commonly used illicit substance in the USA. Of fatally injured males in the 15–34 age group 37% tested positive for marijuana, and of these 81% also tested positive for alcohol. In this study it was found that 42.6% of male college graduates and 44.3% of female graduates used marijuana, though the study found that there was no relationship between the use of marijuana and accidents.

Marijuana acts as a depressant on the central nervous system – it lowers the sensory threshold and causes euphoria, relief of anxiety and disorientation in time and space (Mckenry and Salerno, 1989; Foster, 1996). It is therefore surprising that despite it being proven that the use of marijuana causes cognitive impairment, this cannot be shown to be associated with injury, as supported by Braun *et al.* (1998). However, other authors have found that it degrades driving skills (Smart and Feyer 1976; Moskowitz, 1985; Gieringer, 1988) by affecting the individual's attention span and reaction time (Weil *et al.*, 1968; Reeve *et al.*, 1983; Pope and Yurgelun-Todd, 1996). Screening for marijuana is problematic as the active ingredient, delta-9-tetrahydrocannabinol, is taken in and stored by fatty tissue. Long-term users may continue to test positive for more than 48 h following abstinence (Sonderstrom *et al.*, 1988). This therefore indicates that despite having marijuana present in the body, its effects may have passed, making it difficult to cite as a factor in the causation of accidents.

Case study

Lee, a 19-year-old, was an unrestrained back seat passenger in a car involved in a collision with the wall. The car's impact with the wall occurred across the length of the driver's side. All three occupants had consumed large quantities of alcohol and marijuana. The driver was killed instantly, the front seat passenger, who was restrained, suffered a whiplash injury and Lee, who had managed to get himself out of the car, suffered a displaced fracture of his right hemi-pelvis, a fractured left medial malleolus, a fractured right femur and tibia, myocardial contusions and a ruptured spleen. He was admitted to A&E in the early hours of the morning and underwent a laparotomy and splenectomy, intramedullary nailing of his femur and tibia, the application of an external fixator to his pelvis and internal fixation of his ankle. Lee spent four days in ICU and 19 days post-injury he discharged himself (against medical advice). Lee was non-compliant with treatment and physiotherapy while in hospital and at home. Due to his illiteracy he found it difficult to find work. Prior to his accident he had been a labourer. He has now become increasingly depressed.

Sports injuries

Most sports injuries occur as either an acute traumatic episode or as the result of overuse, where repetitive forces cause injury over a period of time (Holt Paletta, 1997). Certain injuries are often associated with particular sporting activities (Table 6.2).

Table 6.2 Injuries commonly associated with specific sports

Injury Associated sports

Head and wrist
(Regan *et al.*, 1991; Barton, 1997) Gymnastics, skating, football, climbing, horse-riding
Head injury
(Strong *et al.*, 1978) Rugby, horse-riding, football
Ankle injuries
(Ekeland, 1997; Dawson *et al.*, 1998) Parachuting (civilian sport and military)
Pelvic injuries
(Chitnavis *et al.*, 1996; O'Farrell *et al.*, 1997) Horse-riding
Knee and lower leg
(Crisp, 1995) Football, rugby
Spinal injuries
(Wetzler *et al.*, 1998) Rugby

Cox *et al.* (1989) suggest that most musculoskeletal injuries sustained during sporting activities are avoidable. They feel that the problem lies with poor training in preparation for participation in competitive sport. Some individuals are influenced by their family and peers and many athletes will continue to compete despite pain and injury.

Horse-riding

It has been estimated that over 3 million people ride horses in the UK (Silver and Lloyd Parry, 1991; Chitnavis *et al.*, 1996) for either work or leisure. It has been found that young females are particularly at risk (Chitnavis *et al.*, 1996; Temes *et al.*, 1997).

The suggestion that riding is one of the most dangerous sports in the country (Firth, 1985; Silver and Lloyd Parry, 1991) is due in the main to the following factors: **horses can weigh up to 500 kg; are capable of speeds of 40 mph and can kick with a force of up to 1 ton** (Silver and Lloyd Parry, 1991; Kriss and Kriss, 1997). Horse-riding is also the only sport in which the two partners are members of different species (Hamilton and Tranmer, 1993). Whether as a competitive sport or as a leisure activity, horse-riding has been found to be 20 times as dangerous as motorcycling (Firth, 1985), lar-

gely due to the unpredictability of the horse! (Table 6.3).

Table 6.3 Causes of injury in horse-riding

Falls from the horse
Crushing against stationary objects
Entrapment in reins/stirrups
Kicks or being stamped on
Bites

While most horse-related injuries are of moderate severity, some accidents can also result in major life-threatening injuries, most notably head injuries and pelvic injuries (Nelson and Bixby-Hammet, 1992; Robertson and Redmond, 1994). Spinal injuries may result from horse-riding accidents, but these make up a very small percentage.

Football

Football is the most popular team sport, with 21 million regular players (Crisp, 1997) with an average age of 23 years. The highest rates of injury lie in the 15–24 year age group (Shaw *et al.*, 1997). Crisp (1995) found that in one sports centre 74% of football injuries occurred to the lower limbs, with injuries to the knee and fractures of the tibia the most commonly encountered.

Goalkeepers sustain 33% of footballing hand injuries (Barton, 1997). Lawson *et al.* (1995) showed that 54% of distal radial fractures caused by football occurred on synthetic pitches due to the force involved in a direct fall.

Rugby

Rugby is a skilled but collision-orientated sport requiring a combination of muscular strength, stamina and endurance (Gibbs, 1993). Players in forward positions generally receive more injuries than backs due to more physical contact (Gibbs, 1993; Stephenson *et al.*, 1996). It has also been shown that the ball carrier is most likely to receive an injury (Gissane *et al.*, 1997). Approximately 46% of rugby players are aged between 16 and 24 years and they sustain 55% of all injuries (Scher, 1991; Garraway and Macleod, 1995).

The most common types of injury received

are dislocations, strains and sprains of the knee (Garraway and Macleod, 1995). However, research undertaken by Gissane *et al.* (1998) found that in the winter season the majority of injuries were to the head and neck. Wetzler *et al.* (1998) found that 58% of spinal injuries occur during a scrum and, despite changes in the rules to try to reduce the incidence, this number remains fairly constant (Hodgson Phillips, 1998).

Factors affecting outcome

It has been suggested that the length of time an individual takes to recover from an accident depends on their lifestyle prior to the event (Breslau *et al.*, 1995). It has also been suggested that greater age, level of education and income prior to the accident will result in improved outcomes (Morrison *et al.*, 1991; Michaels *et al.*, 1998). However, Van der Sluis *et al.* (1998) disagree in part, and do not feel that level of education is a significant factor.

Fatigue can also be a major factor affecting outcome, especially following head injury (Ponsford *et al.*, 1995). Persistent pain can be a contributory factor in chronic fatigue (Van der Sluis *et al.*, 1998) which in turn can cause low self-esteem (Hancock, 1998) leading to withdrawal from social activities (Gilbert, 1996).

Conclusion

It is hard to know how best to appeal to the youth of today, and indeed tomorrow, in order to reduce accidents and injuries. Despite the best efforts of those engaged in accident prevention, health promotion and safety in sport, the rogue and delinquent element will continue to contribute to accident statistics and in many instances will also involve the innocent bystander. Taking risks is part of youth culture and, sadly, wisdom seems to come only with age and experience.

References

Bachulis, L. B. Sangster, W. and Gorrell, G. W. (1988) Patterns of injury in helmeted and non helmeted motorcyclists. *American Journal of Surgery*, **155**, 708–711.

Barton, N. (1997) Sports injuries of the hand and wrist. *British Journal of Sports Medicine*, **31**(3), 191–196.

Bjornstig, U., Ostrom, M. and Eriksson, A. (1992) Head and face injuries in bicyclists – with special reference to possible effects of helmet use. *Journal of Trauma*, **33**, 887.

Braun, B. L., Tekawa, I. S., Gerberich, S. G. and Sidney, S. (1998) Marijuana use and medically attended injury events. *Annals of Emergency Medicine*, **32**(3) 353–360.

Breslau, N., Davies, G. C. and Andreski, P. (1995) Risk factors for PTSD related traumatic events: a prospective analysis. *American Journal of Psychiatry*, **152**, 529.

British Standards Institution (1990) *Catalogue*. London: BSI.

Central Statistical Office (1996) *Social Trends*. London: HMSO.

Chitnavis, J. P., Gibbons, C. C. M. H., Hirigoyen, M. *et al.* (1996) Accidents with horses: what has changed in 20 years? *Injury*, **27**(2), 103–105.

Clayton, B., Booth, A. C. and McCarthy, P. E. (1977) *A Controlled Study of the Role of Alcohol in Fatal Adult Pedestrian Accidents.* Transport and Road Research Laboratory.

Clayton, M. (1998). Encouraging children to use cycle helmets. *Paediatric Nursing*, **10**(3), 14–17.

Collins, R. L. and Marlatt, G. A. (1981) Social modelling as a determinant of drinking behaviour: implications for prevention and treatment. *Addictive Behaviours*, **6**, 233–240; cited in Taylor, S. T. (1991) *Health Psychology*. McGraw-Hill Inc.

Court-Brown, C. M., Rimmer, S., Prakash, U. and McQueen, M. M. (1998) The epidemiology of open long bone fractures. *Injury*, **29**(7) 529–534.

Cox, M., Miles, D. and Bomz, J. (1989) Physical fitness and its relation to orthopaedics and sports medicine. In *Orthopaedics in Sports Medicine for Nurses* (S. Gates and P. Mooar, eds). Williams and Wilkins.

Crisp, T. (1995) Football injuries: tackling the damage. *The Practitioner*, **239**(1577), 703–709.

Crisp, T. (1997) Football injuries: a new season begins. *The Practitioner*, **241**, 440–444.

Dawson, M., Asghar, M., Pryke, S. and Slater, N. (1998) Civilian parachute injuries; 10 years on and no lessons learned. *Injury*, **29**(8), 573–575.

Denscombe, M. (1993) Personal health and the social psychology of risk-taking. *Health Education Research*, **8**(4) 505–517.

DiGallo, A., Barton, J. and Parry-Jones, W. L (1997) Road traffic accidents: early psychological consequences in children and adolescents. *British Journal of Psychiatry*, **170**, 358–363.

Dion, K., Baron, R. and Miller, N. (1970) Why do groups make riskier decisions than individuals? *Advances in Experimental Social Psychology*, **5**, 305–377; cited in Denscombe, M. (1993) Personal health and the social psychology of risk-taking. *Health Education Research*, **8**(4), 505–517.

Discala (1991) Children with traumatic head injury: morbidity and post-acute treatment. *Archive of Physical Medical Rehabilitation*, **72**, 662–666.

Dischinger, P. C. (1991) *The Shock Trauma Patients Toxicology Database*. Baltimore: National Study Centre for Trauma and Emergency Medicine Systems; cited in Sonderstrom, C. A., Daily, J. T. and Kerbs, T. J (1994) Alcohol and other drugs: an assessment of testing and clinical practices in US trauma centres. *Journal of Trauma*, **36**(1), 68–71.

Donaldson, L. J., Cook, A. and Thomson, R. G. (1990) Incidence of fractures in a geographically defined population. *Journal of Epidemiology and Community Health*, **44**, 243–245.

Eccles, J. S., Midgely, C., Wigfield, A. *et al.* (1993) Development during adolescence: the impact of stage-environment fit on young adolescents: experience in schools and in families. *American Psychology*, **48**(2), 90–101.

Ekeland, A. (1997). Injuries in military parachuting: a prospective study of 4499 jumps. *Injury*, **28**(3), 219–222.

Emergency Nurses Association (1995) *Nursing Core Course Manual*. Chicago: Emergency Nurses Association.

Firth, J. (1985) Equestrian Injuries. In *Sports Injuries, Mechanisms, Prevention and Treatment* (R. C. Schneider, J. C. Kennedy and M. L. Plant, eds). Wilkins.

Foss, R. D, Beirness, D. J. and Sprattler, K. (1994) Seatbelt use among drinking drivers in Minnesota. *American Journal of Public Health*, **84**, 1732.

Foster, R. W. (1996) *Basic Pharmacology*. Butterworth-Heinemann.

Garraway, M. and Macleod, D. (1995) Epidemiology of rugby football injuries. *The Lancet*, **345**, 1485–1487.

Gentitello, L., Cobean, R. A., Walker, A. P. *et al.* (1993) Acute ethanol intoxication increases the risk of infection following penetrating abdominal trauma. *Journal of Trauma*, **34**, 669–674.

Gibbs, N. (1993) Injuries in professional rugby league: a three year prospective study of the South Sydney professional rugby league football club. *American Journal of Sports Medicine*, **21**(5), 696–700.

Gieringer, D. M. (1988) Marijuana, driving and accident safety. *Journal of Psychoactive Drugs*, **20**, 93–101; cited in Brookoff, D. (1998). Marijuana and injury: is there a connection? *Annals of Emergency Medicine*, **32**(3), 361–363.

Gilbert, S. E. A. (1996) Implications of severe trauma to the hand. *Professional Nurse*, **11**(5) 358–370.

Gissane, C., Jennings, D. C. and Cumine, A. J. (1997) Differences in the incidence of injury between rugby league forwards and backs. *Australian Journal of Sport Medicine*, **21**, 91–94.

Gissane, C., Jennings, D. C. and Cumine, A. J. (1998) Injury in summer rugby league football: the experiences of one club. *British Journal of Sports Medicine*, **32**(3) 149–152.

Haddon, W. H. (1980) Advances in epidemiology of injuries as a basis for public policy. *Public Health Report*, **95**, 411.

Hamer, M. (1996) A hundred years of carnage. *New Scientist*, Aug., 14–15.

Hamilton, M. G. and Tranmer, B. I. (1993) Nervous system injuries in horseback-riding accidents. *Journal of Trauma*, **34**(2), 227–232.

Hamilton, S. M. (1991) Coalition on trauma – trauma prevention and trauma care: Presidential Address, Trauma Association of Canada. *Journal of Trauma*, **31**(7), 951–957.

Hammond, W. R. and Yung, B. (1993) Psychology's role in the public health response of assaultive violence among young African-American men. *American Journal of Psychology*, **48**(2), 142–154.

Hancock, B. (1998). Paraplegia. *Professional Nurse*, **14**(3), 181–184.

Harrison, M. and Shepherd, J. P. (1997) Facial protection conferred by cycle safety helmets: use of digitized image processing to develop a new nondestructive test. *Journal of Trauma*, **43**(1), 78–82.

Heimer, C. A. (1988) Social structure, psychology and the estimation of risk. *Annual Review of Sociology*, **14**, 491–519.

Henderson, M. (1987) *Living with Risk. The British Medical Association Guide*. Wiley.

Hingson, R., Berson J. and Dowley, K. (1992) Interventions to reduce college student drinking and related health and social problems. In *Alcohol, Minimising the Harm* (M. Plant, E. Single and T. Stockwell, eds). Free Association Books.

Hodgson Phillips, L., Standen, P. J. and Batt, M. E. (1998) Effects of seasonal change in rugby league on the incidence of injury. *British Journal of Sports Medicine*, **32**(3), 144–148.

Holt Paletta, J. (1997) Nursing care of sports-related injuries. *Orthopaedic Nursing*, **16**(6), 43–46.

Home Office (1995) *Tackling Drugs Together: A Strategy for England 1995–1998*. London: HMSO.

Irwin, C. E. and Millstein, S. G. (1986) Biopsychosocial correlates of risk-taking behaviours during adolescence. *Journal of Adolescent Health Care*, **7**, 82–96.

Johnson, R. M., McCarthy, M. C. and Miller, S. F. (1995) Craniofacial trauma in injured motorcyclists: the impact of helmet usage. *Journal of Trauma*, **38**, 876–878.

Kaufmann, C. R., Branas, C. C. and Brawley, M. L. (1998) A population-based study of trauma recidivism. *Journal of Trauma*, **45**(2), 325–332.

Keene, J. (1997) *Drug Misuse: Prevention, Harm Minimisation and Treatment*. Chapman and Hall.

Kivalian, D. R., Coppel, D. B., Fromme, K. *et al.* (1989) Secondary prevention of alcohol related problems in young adults at risk. In *Biobehavioural perspectives* (K. D. Craig and S. M. Weiss, eds). Springer.

Kriss, T. C. and Kriss, V. M. (1997) Equine-related neurosurgical trauma: a prospective series of 30 patients. *Journal of Trauma*, **43**(1), 97–99.

Lawson, G. M., Hajducka, C. and McQueen, M. M. (1995) Sports fractures of the distal radius – epidemiology and outcome. *Injury*, **26**, 33.

Lindenbaum, G. A., Carroll, S. F., Daskal, I. and Kaposnick, R. (1989) Patterns of alcohol and drug abuse in an urban trauma centre: the increasing role of cocaine abuse. *Journal of Trauma*, **29**, 12.

Livingstone, D. H., Merritt, S., Callori, S. and Vanek, S. (1998) Auto theft related trauma. *Journal of Trauma*,

45(5), 780–784.

Marshall, C., Boyd, K. T. and Moran, C. G. (1996) Injuries related to car crime: the joy-riding epidemic. *Injury*, **27**(2), 79–80.

Mayhew, D. R., Donelson, A. C., Bierress, D. J. and Simpson, H. M. (1986) Youth alcohol and relative risk of crash involvement. *Accident Analysis and Prevention*, **18**, 273–287.

McCarthy, M. (1996) Controversy: cycle helmets – the case against. *Child Care, Health and Development*, **22**(2), 105–111.

Mckenry, L. M. and Salerno, E. (1989) *Pharmacology in Nursing*. C. V. Mosby.

Meyer, A. A. (1998) Death and disability from injury: a global challenge. *Journal of Trauma*, **44**(1), 1–12.

Michaels, A. J., Michaels, C. E., Moon, C. H. *et al.* (1998) Psychological factors limit outcomes after trauma. *Journal of Trauma*, **44**(4) 644–648.

Morrison, J. A., Sanchez, A. A. and Bass, S. M. (1991) Trauma patients return to productivity. *Journal of Trauma*, **31**, 827.

Moskowitz, H. (1985) Marijuana and driving. *Accident Analysis Preview 2*, 105–120; cited in Brookoff, D. (1998). Marijuana and injury: is there a connection? *Annals of Emergency Medicine*, **32**(3), 361–363.

Nelson, D. E. and Bixby-Hammet, D. (1992) Equestrian injuries in children and young adults. *American Journal of Diseases of Children*, **146**, 611–614.

O'Farrell, D. A., Irshad, F., Thorns, B. S. and McElwain, J. P. (1997) Major pelvic injuries in equestrian sports. *British Journal of Sports Medicine*, **31**(3), 249–251.

Office for National Statistics (1993–94). *Mortality Statistics Injury and Poisoning*. London: Office for National Statistics.

Office for National Statistics (1996) *Key Population Vital Statistics for Local and Health Authority Areas*. London: Office for National Statistics.

Paton, A. (1994). *ABC of Alcohol*. BMJ Publishing.

Ponsford, J. L., Oliver, J. H. and Curran, C. (1995) A profile of outcome 2 years after traumatic brain injury. *Brain Injury*, **275**, 521–527.

Pope, H. G. and Yurgelun-Todd, D. (1996). The residual cognitive effects of heavy marijuana use in college students. *Journal of the American Medical Association*, **275**, 521–527.

Redeker, N. S., Smeltzer, S. C., Kirkpatrick, J. and Parchment, S. (1995) Risk factors of adolescent and young adult trauma victims. *American Journal of Critical Care*, **4**(5), 370–378.

Reeve, V. G., Robertson, W. B., Grant, J. *et al.* (1983) Hemolyzed blood and serum levels of delta-9-THC: effects on the performance of roadside sobriety tests. *Journal of Forensic Science*, **28**, 963–971; cited in Brookoff, D. (1998) Marijuana and injury: is there a connection? *Annals of Emergency Medicine*, **32**(3), 361–363.

Regan, P. J., Roberts, O., Feldberg, L. and Roberts, A. H. N. (1991) Hand injuries from leading horses. *Injury*, **22**(2), 124–126.

Rivara, F. P., Koepsell, T. D., Jurkovich, G. *et al.* (1993).

The effect of alcohol abuse on readmission for trauma. *Journal of the American Medical Association*, **279**, 1962–1964.

Rivara, F. P., Muellar, B. A., Fligner, C. L. *et al.* (1989) Drug use in trauma victims. *Journal of Trauma*, **29**, 462–470.

Robertson, C. and Redmond, A. (1994) The management of major trauma. In *Oxford Handbooks in Emergency Medicine*. Oxford University Press.

Scher, A. T. (1991) Spinal cord concussion in rugby players. *American Journal of Sports Medicine*, **19**(5), 485–488.

Schwarz, D. F., Grisso, J. A., Giles, C. G. *et al.* (1994) A longitudinal study of injury morbidity in an African–American population. *Journal of the American Medical Association*, **271**, 755–760.

Shapiro, R., Siegel, A. W., Scovill, L. C. and Hays, J. (1998) Risk-taking patterns of female adolescents: what they do and why. *Journal of Adolescence*, **12**, 143–159.

Sharples, P. M., Storey, A., Ansby-Green, A. and Eyre, J. A. (1990) Causes of fatal childhood accidents involving head injury in a Northern region 1979–1986. *British Medical Journal*, **301**, 1193–1197.

Shaw, A. D., Gustillo, T. and Court-Brown, C. M. (1997) Epidemiology and outcome of tibial diaphyseal fractures in footballers. *Injury*, **28**(5), 365–367.

Shepherd, J., Irish, M. and Scully, C. (1988) Alcohol intoxication and severity of injury in victims of assault. *British Medical Journal*, **296**, 1299.

Shepherd, J. P., Robinson, L. and Levers, B. G. H. (1990) The routes of urban violence. *Injury*, **21**, 139.

Silver, J. R. and Lloyd Parry, J. M. (1991) Hazards of horse-riding as a popular sport. *British Journal of Sports Medicine*, **25**(2), 105–110.

Singer, S. I. (1986) Victims of serious violence and their criminal behaviour: subcultural theory and beyond. *Violence Victims*, **191**, 51–70; cited in Redeker, N. S., Smeltzer, S. C., Kirkpatrick, J. and Parchment, S. (1995) Risk factors of adolescent and young adult trauma victims. *American Journal of Critical Care*, **4**(5), 370–378.

Sloane, E. P., Zalenski, R. J., Smith, R. F. *et al.* (1989) Toxicology screening in urban trauma patients: drug prevalence and its relationship to trauma severity and management. *Journal of Trauma*, **29**(12), 1647–1653.

Smart, R. and Feyer, D. (1976) Drug use and driving risk among high school students. *Accident Analysis Preview 8*, 33–38; cited in Brookoff, D. (1998). Marijuana and injury: is there a connection? *Annals of Emergency Medicine*, **32**(3), 361–363.

Sonderstrom, C. A., Triffilis, A. L., Shanker, B. S. *et al.* (1988) Marijuana and alcohol abuse among 1023 trauma patients. *Archives of Surgery*, **123**, 733–737.

Spain, D. A., Boaz, P. W., Davidson, D. J. *et al.* (1997) Risk-taking behaviours among adolescent trauma patients. *Journal of Trauma*, **43**(3), 423–426.

Stephenson, S., Gissane, C. and Jennings, D. (1996) Injury in rugby league: a four year prospective survey. *British Journal of Sports Medicine*, **30**, 331–334.

Strong, I., MacMillan, R. and Jennett, B. (1978) Head injuries in accident and emergency departments at

Scottish hospitals. *Injury*, **10**, 154–159.

Synder, S. H. and Ladu, M. H. (1985) *Alcohol: Teenage Drinking*. Burke.

Temes, R. T., White, J. H., Ketai, L. H. *et al.* (1997) Head, face and neck trauma from large animal injury in New Mexico. *Journal of Trauma*, **43**(3), 492–495.

The Health of Oxfordshire (1993–94) *Report of the Director*. Oxfordshire Department of Public Health and Health Policy.

Thomas, S., Acton, C. and Nixon, J. (1994) Effectiveness of bicycle helmets in preventing head injury in children: case control study. *British Medical Journal*, **308**, 173.

Thompson, R., Rivara, F. and Thompson, D. (1989) A case control study of the effectiveness of bicycle safety helmets. *New England Journal of Medicine*, **320**, 1361.

Thompson, C. Rivara, P. and Thompson, R. (1996) Effectiveness of bicycle safety helmets in reducing head injuries. *Journal of the American Medical Association*, **276**, 1968.

Trounce, J. (1990) *Pharmacology for Nurses*. Churchill Livingstone.

Van der Sluis, C. K., Eisma, W. H., Grouthoff, J. W. and Ten Duis, H. J. (1998) Long-term physical, psychological and social consequences of severe injury. *Injury*, **29**(4), 281–285.

Wagle, V. G., Perkins, C. and Vallera, A. (1993) Is helmet use beneficial to motorcyclists? *Journal of Trauma*, **34**(1), 120–122.

Walsh, N. (1996) *Accident and Emergency Nursing: a New Approach*. Butterworth-Heinemann.

Weil, A. T., Zinberg, N. E. and Nelsen, J. M. (1968) Clinical and psychological effects of marijuana in man. *Science*, **162**, 1234–1242; cited in Braun, B. L., Tekawa, I. S., Gerberich, S. G., Sidney, S. (1998) Marijuana use and medically attended injury events. *Annals of Emergency Medicine*, **32**(3), 353–360.

Wetzler, M. J., Akpatra, T., Laughlin, W. and Levy, A. S. (1998) Occurrence of cervical spine injuries during the rugby scrum. *American Journal of Sports Medicine*, **26**(2), 177–180.

Williams, J. M., Currie, C. E., Wright, P. *et al.* (1996) Socioeconomic status and adolescent injuries. *Social Science and Medicine*, **44**(12), 1881–1891.

Wright, J. and Kariya, A. (1997) Aetiology of assault with respect to alcohol, unemployment and social deprivation: a Scottish accident and emergency department case control study. *Injury*, **28**(5), 369–371.

Yates, D. *et al.* (1987) Alcohol consumption of patients attending two A&E departments in north-west England. *Journal of Royal Society of Medicine*, **80**, 486–489.

7

The causes and effects of trauma in mid-life

Rachel Steel

Introduction

It has often been said that in the middle years people are in the prime of their life. It is during this time that decisions such as choice of partner, further study and the establishment of a career assume a high profile. Much energy is required in order to deal effectively with such life choices. Individuals at this phase in their lives are better equipped, both physically and emotionally, to meet these challenges than at any other age (Groenman *et al.*, 1992).

In our society, work is at the heart of our way of life during the middle years. Employment not only provides status among contemporaries but is also essential in order to achieve financial security. Furthermore, for many people work makes up a central part of their lives, providing social contacts and leading to self-actualization through the attainment of personal goals and achievements. In addition to work, it is generally expected that during this period individuals realize their need for human contact by entering into a relationship with a partner and perhaps starting a family. Financial stability, accommodation and establishing a role within the family unit are fundamental components of life at this time. In view of this, the impact of trauma to someone in their middle years may have significant consequences for their lifestyle, leaving both the individual and their family in a state of financial and emotional crisis.

To ease discussion, this chapter focuses on two separate aspects of trauma. First, the causes of trauma and the associated risk-taking behaviours of this age group. Secondly, the impact of trauma on individuals' lifestyles and the way in which their needs should be met. This section also includes the emotive area of domestic violence. To augment the discussion, relevant case studies observed in practice are described.

The causes of trauma

The mere nature of an individual's life at this age incorporates a variety of latent causes of trauma which are summarized in Table 7.1.

Table 7.1 Causes of trauma

Sports injuries
Work-related injuries
Stress from social change, e.g. unemployment or bereavement – leading to suicide or risk-taking behaviours, e.g. alcohol or substance abuse
Road traffic accidents
Domestic violence
Pregnancy

Work-related injuries

For the majority of people of this age, work takes up a large part of their daily routine. It is therefore not surprising that a significant number of accidents take place at work (Martella *et al.*, 1992). In 1995/96 about 1.06 million employed people suffered a workplace injury in Great Britain (Health and Safety Executive, 1997). Of these, 403 000 injuries led to more than 3 days' absence from work

(Health and Safety Executive, 1997). Obviously the type and prevalence of injuries sustained in the workplace is largely dependent on occupation. For example, manual and factory workers may be exposed to hot materials, poisonous substances or lifting of heavy objects. In this type of environment accidents may well result in burns, back injuries and fractures.

Suicide and risk-taking behaviours

The onset of stressful situations arising from the workplace or some other source, such as unemployment, bereavement or social change, has been directly linked with incidents of attempted suicide and increased uptake of risk-taking behaviours such as alcohol or substance abuse and violence (Redeker *et al.*, 1995). With reference to attempted suicide Wright (1993) states: 'There are a number of people who experience some sudden change to which they could adapt if they gave themselves time. Instead they resort to suicide on impulse, being overwhelmed by the disorganisation and disruption.'

The types of injuries resulting from attempted suicide and other risk-taking behaviours range from multiple fractures of the limbs and spinal column to head injuries (mild to severe) or, in the worst cases, a combination of both.

Road traffic accidents

In 1997, 154 700 British people in this age group were involved in an accident either as a pedestrian, cyclist or car user (DETR, 1997); of these, 20 323 were killed or seriously injured (DETR, 1997). The incidence of road traffic accidents is higher in the middle years than in any other age group, accounting for approximately half of all road traffic accidents (DETR, 1997). This may not be surprising as individuals in this age group are all above the legal age required to possess any type of vehicle licence, and increasing numbers of people are vehicle owners (DETR, 1997). The types of injuries these individuals present with range from simple isolated limb fractures to multiple fractures, head injuries, limb amputations and spinal cord injuries.

Domestic violence

This is the leading cause of injury to women in their middle years, causing more injuries than muggings, rapes and car accidents combined (Dunn, 1995). Although there is an increasing awareness that men can also be abused in a relationship, the extent to which findings about battered women can be applied to men who are abused, or the under-recognized problem of violence within gay and lesbian relationships, is not known. Victims face the ongoing, debilitating experience of physical, psychological and/or sexual abuse, associated with increased isolation from the outside world (Wright, 1993). Although some women are able to escape a violent relationship after the first assault, most abuse is recurrent and escalates in both frequency and severity (Dunn, 1995).

Sports injuries

Individuals in this phase of life are often active and enjoy taking part in some kind of sport or leisure activity outside work. It is therefore not surprising that a significant number of injuries in this age group arise as a result of sporting activities. With the increase in availability of more dangerous leisure pursuits, such as parachuting and bungee jumping, the number of accidents in this area continues to rise. However, injuries resulting from such accidents often involve isolated limb fractures, and a quick recovery is not uncommon.

Pregnancy

The physical changes experienced in pregnancy frequently lead to a decline in a woman's ease of mobility and independence. In later pregnancy this can give rise to circumstances in which the pregnant woman is prone to injury. This is exemplified in the following case study.

Case study

Louise, a 26-year-old, was 5 months pregnant when she experienced the abrupt onset of vaginal bleeding and abdominal pain. In a state of panic her partner Daniel assisted her into his car in order to drive Louise to the nearest hospital. Whilst driving, Louise's abdominal pain worsened to a point where she cried out suddenly – this made Daniel briefly lose control of the vehicle resulting in a head-on collision with another car. Although Daniel was not injured, Louise suffered a fractured left pubic ramus and humerus.

The impact of trauma and meeting individual needs

Traumatic injury sustained by individuals during this phase of life will often involve the unravelling of decisions made earlier in life in order to enable either short- or long-term adjustments. The aftermath of personal injury, whether it is the need to be non-weight-bearing on a limb for a period of time, or coping with the loss of a limb, obviously involves a psychosocial transition and adaptation. For those with a severe disability there may be major difficulties in coming to terms with a change in body image, and the disruption of life plans at this stage in life may be particularly devastating. Not only are there physical losses, but life plans and goals in key areas such as marriage, children and career may have to be questioned. Whatever the circumstances, it is essential that both the individuals and their families are included in setting and working towards shared goals (Wright, 1993).

The impact of trauma on an individual's lifestyle is dependent on a number of factors, which include the nature of the injury, the individual's lifestyle and their socioeconomic environment. The four most commonly encountered areas of need are identified in Table 7.2, but it is of paramount importance to remember that people's needs vary. These needs are often interrelated, impacting on each other, and each must be assessed on an individual basis. The impact of domestic violence on relationships within the home environment is obviously quite unique and will therefore be discussed separately.

Table 7.2 Impact of trauma

Loss of independence in mobility or daily needs
Change in body image
Loss of employment
Alterations in relationships with family or friends, e.g. following domestic violence

Loss of independence in relation to mobility and daily needs

The degree to which an individual experiences a decline in independence with mobility and other daily needs, such as washing, dressing, eating and shopping, will depend on the severity of the injury sustained. For example, in the event of a complex fracture of the tibia, the application of an external fixator for some months is unlikely to have a significant effect on mobility or daily needs, since individuals at this age are usually able to mobilize effectively with crutches. In contrast, the loss of a limb, or severe spinal cord injury resulting in paraplegia, will impose restrictions and permanent adaptations, such as the fitting of an artificial limb or adjustments to the home environment for wheelchair access.

The severity of impact on an individual's lifestyle is mediated by a range of psychological and social factors (Taylor and Field, 1993). What health professionals tell patients about the severity of their condition and its likely consequences is crucial in shaping their expectations of what is possible. Similarly, the reactions of others play an important part in shaping the interpretation of the psychological needs of the individual (Taylor and Field, 1993; Livneh and Antonak, 1994). This is discussed below, in the subsection entitled 'Change in body image'.

An important role of the nurse is in coordinating the multidisciplinary team (Wright, 1993). In terms of mobility and daily needs, a number of health professionals, including physiotherapists, occupational therapists, social workers and dieticians, should be involved in planning short- and long-term goals and in psychologically preparing the individual for discharge. If the individual has suffered a permanent disability for which significant home and care arrangements are a prerequisite for discharge, it is imperative to involve both the social worker and the individual's family in discharge planning. Early referral to all key health professionals is of paramount importance.

Change in body image

Body image means much more than what we think we look like. It includes the way we perceive our strengths and weaknesses and even how we perceive our sexuality (Wright, 1993). Any change in appearance or function of a part of our body threatens our body image (Groenman *et al.*, 1992). Whether it is the need to wear a halo jacket following spinal fracture or the

Table 7.3 Change in body image: key points for healthcare professionals (Adapted from Wright, 1993)

The external changes will be the ones which the patient finds most distressing and it is important to focus on these first

Internal changes, although less distressing, can concern organs of special significance, especially those associated with sexuality, role and reproduction

The loss of self-esteem, role and strong sexual identity may induce feelings of fear as to how a relationship will be resumed

Anticipatory guidance preoperatively may prevent a crisis response, especially if it takes the form of exploring the process of grief and other expected responses

The healthcare professional should remember that the individual has inner resources and strengths which need to be exploited

It is helpful to touch the affected parts and encourage the individual to do this

Involve the individual's partner and close family. Encourage discussion of loss with the partner, and also the expressions of feeling which the loss brings about

It is important to work at the individual's pace. As well as coming to terms with psychological adjustment, the individual is coping with the after-effects of surgery and resuming their activities of living

---

need for a colostomy due to an injury to the large bowel following a pelvic fracture, a change in body image is likely to occur. Some individuals experience terrible embarrassment because they have to wear a bandage or plaster of Paris, as it focuses attention on the body highlighting areas they would prefer remained unnoticed.

Clinicians and researchers have posited several theoretical models to account for the nature, structure and ordering of the observed reaction to physical impairment or disability. Reviews of research concerning psychosocial adjustment most often single out the reactions of shock, anxiety, denial, depression, internalized anger, hostility and final adjustment (Livneh and Antonak, 1994; Wright, 1993). Wright (1993) identified a number of important issues that healthcare professionals must consider in caring for individuals facing physical change, and these are shown in Table 7.3.

Although the reaction of some individuals to physical changes will involve denial, not all denial has psychological origins. In the case of phantom limb pain there is a physiological explanation. When an individual has had a recent limb amputation they may experience pain or itching. Such sensations are a consequence of severed nerve endings which continue to send impulses that appear to come from the limb. A warning to the patient that this is likely to happen is necessary to provide reassurance that this is a normal reaction (Wright, 1993).

Case study

John, a 46-year-old, had his arm torn off in a baling machine while working on a farm. Following admission an above-elbow amputation and the necessary skin grafts were performed. For approximately 2 weeks John experienced severe pain in his absent limb, which he found both distressing and confusing. Initially it was essential to explain the physiological reasoning behind the phenomenon in terms that John could understand, and to reassure him that this experience was quite normal following the loss of a limb. It was also important to carry out pain assessment and management in the aftermath of surgery and to inform John that phantom pain might occur intermittently for months or even years following the accident.

Loss of employment

The period of leave from work which an individual takes following an accident depends on the type of injury, the length of recovery period and the individual's occupation. Some individuals will have access to statutory sick pay and their position will be held open by their employer until they are able to recommence work. For those who are self-employed, loss of income commences the moment they suffer an injury severe enough to prevent them working. Others, whose injuries are very severe, may have to face the prospect of permanent unemployment. Loss of employment, whether on a temporary or permanent basis, is likely to affect an individual in a number of ways. First, unemployment will have a profound effect on the financial stability of a family. Douthwaite (1994) claims that unemployment entails relative, if not absolute, poverty for many of those affected by it. In Ireland, Whelan *et al.* (1991) reported that while roughly 7.7% people in employment fall below the poverty line, this is true of almost 40% of the unemployed. It is therefore essential to involve both the social worker and the occupational therapist when loss of employment is foreseen, so that the financial implications and the availability of benefits can be discussed with the individual and their family as soon as is appropriate.

Unemployment has also been found to cause a psychological deterioration in the relationship between the injured person and their spouse, inducing feelings of personal disappointment, lack of self-worth and depression (Warr and Jackson, 1985; Morris *et al.*, 1994). Men who are married with children are the worst affected by unemployment due to the pressure imposed by society in viewing the man as the 'breadwinner' (Douthwaite, 1994). However, the impact of loss of employment for any length of time on all individuals should not be underestimated. In such circumstances it is important for the healthcare professional to give the individual time to talk about their loss of job and earning capacity. It is also necessary to examine the individual's situation in terms of their perceptions of the role of work, the role of leisure and outside interests, the implications of being without work and the psychological consequences (Likeman, 1997). It may be that the individual's physical condition permits part-time employment as an alternative, or that a career change is necessary in order to find more suitable work, in which case a career adviser may need to be involved at the appropriate time. Finally, Likeman (1997) suggests that writing a daily journal helps the individual reflect on a day-to-day basis and enables them to look ahead.

Alterations in relationships

The imbalance introduced by injury can unhook relationships that have become rigidly bound over time, or it may stretch families beyond tolerable limits (Altschuler, 1997). For a partner, guilt or embarrassment about their own well-being, and frustration and even anger about restrictions in their lives, can make it difficult to share concerns, limiting access to support and the right to needs of their own. Groenman *et al.* (1992) believe that 'the traumatic effects on the family should not be underestimated'.

The impact of trauma on the family may take several forms. Immediately after the accident members of the injured person's family may experience feelings similar to those of the grief reaction. It is essential for the healthcare professional to include the family in care planning, and to provide them with reassurance, counselling and support. Furthermore, Altschuler (1997) believes that delay in adjusting to the long-term implications can occur when there is failure to acknowledge the seriousness of the injury. In view of this, it is imperative that healthcare professionals work at the family's own pace when helping them to cope with change. Families who have given up trying because it seems hopeless need encouragement. In contrast, a family that holds onto hope by denying the seriousness of an injury needs to have this explained, or reiterated, and may need help in mourning the loss of well-being.

Case study

David, a 35-year-old father of two children aged 9 and 13 years, was involved in a road traffic accident in which he sustained a complex fracture of his tibia and fibula. He required surgical fixation and muscle grafting. David's ability to regain full mobility and range of movement in the long term was unclear as his rehabilitation programme depended on the degree of bone unification attained. While talking to David on one occasion he became very upset and said 'My eldest son asked me today when I would be able to go home and play football with him. I don't think my wife or children understand that I will not even be able to walk properly for a long time'.

This incident highlighted the family's lack of understanding, or perhaps acceptance, of the long-term implications of David's injury and the need for further information, support and time to discuss their concerns and feelings.

For individuals confronted with long-term rehabilitation, loss of independence or permanent disability, the impact on family relationships is likely to involve a number of difficult questions and decisions. It is important to work closely with both the individual and their family and to encourage them to ask questions and to talk openly about the concerns they may be experiencing so that they can provide support for each other. High levels of social support, particularly in the community, have been found in research studies to have a beneficial effect on patterns of recovery (Taylor and Field, 1993; Gronwall *et al.*, 1991). The aftermath of some injuries means that individuals may take longer to recover or require assistance with simple tasks such as eating and drinking. This may limit the lives of people around them by restricting their activities and requiring the reorganization of their previous routines, roles and ways of viewing life. On a short-term basis such disruption may be acceptable and perhaps even welcomed. However, in the long term it is likely to be disruptive and to cause difficulties for 'lay carers' and others closely associated with the person (Taylor and Field, 1993). For these families it is important that the social worker is closely involved with the family should further support be deemed necessary.

Finally, individuals who suffer injuries that result in physical changes, such as skin discoloration from muscle grafts, loss of a limb, or facial injuries, may be prone to stigmatization (Wright, 1993). Stigmatization is based upon oversimplified ideas about people known as stereotypical thinking (Taylor and Field, 1993) and is likely to have an adverse effect on an individual's self-perception, identity and ability to manage their social interactions. As a result of having a central role in the care of such people, the healthcare professional is in a key position to shape their experiences through the way in which they respond to the physical change, and through the help and support they provide both to the individual and their family (Altschuler, 1997). It is also important to assist the individual to gain insight into their injury through self-help organizations and informal contact with other sufferers.

In the case of domestic violence, if a victim discloses the reasons for their injury and expresses the desire to leave their home environment, this will obviously have a profound effect on the relationships with their partner, children and other family members. The nature of the change will depend on who has inflicted the abuse, but is likely to involve the permanent breakdown of a family, perhaps leading to divorce, or decisions regarding the long-term care of children. Often the consequences of violence go unrecognized by colleagues, friends and family members as denial and rationalization are powerful coping mechanisms (Dunn, 1995). It may be that this hospital admission is the first encounter with a healthcare provider and it may be the only opportunity to intervene before the violence escalates. It is also important to remember that the victim can exhibit a range of responses, such as appearing frightened or embarrassed, and may be unwilling to talk about their abuse (Dunn, 1995). In the healthcare setting, domestic violence must be treated sensitively and the healthcare professional must ensure confidentiality and safety for the individual involved. Questions need to be asked in an appropriate manner in order for safe discharge to be planned. In these circumstances it is important to offer support if advising the individual that they should not return to their home environment and, if appropriate, offer them the opportunity to take legal action. The social worker must be involved and early referral is vital. Finally, all individuals should be offered information about self-help organizations and given an emergency contact number before leaving hospital.

Conclusion

This chapter has raised a number of issues relating to trauma in the middle years of an individual's life, the time in which responsibilities are frequently focused on achieving financial security and raising children. Causes of trauma have been identified which relate to individuals' lifestyles, including work-related injuries, domestic violence and sports injuries. Traumatic events are unexpected, and coming to terms with long-term disability is undoubtedly painful for both individuals and their families. Outcomes such as loss of independence, altered body image or a change in relationships are all too common. Within this chapter a number of practical recommendations have been suggested for healthcare professionals. However, it is important to recognize and respond to the particular needs of the injured person given the significance of many individuals' responsibilities within the context of family and relationships in this mid-life stage.

References

Altschuler, J. (1997) *Working with Chronic Illness.* Macmillan Press.

DETR (1997) *Road Accidents in Great Britain – The Casualty Report.* London: Department of the Environment, Transport and Regions.

Douthwaite, J. (1994) Unemployment: a challenge to occupational therapy. *British Journal of Occupational Therapy*, **57**(11), 432-436.

Dunn, K. (1995) Domestic violence. *Nursing News*, **45**(4), 1, 6-7.

Groenman, N. H., Slevin, O. D. A. and Buckenham, M. A. (1992) *Social and Behavioural Sciences for Nurses.* Campion Press.

Gronwall, D., Wrightson, P. and Waddell, P. (1991) *Head Injury – the Facts: A Guide for Families and Care Givers.* Oxford University Press.

Health and Safety Executive (1997) *Annual Abstract of Statistics.* London: Government Statistical Service/Office of National Statistics.

Likeman, J. (1997) Coping with redundancy. *Nursing Management*, **4**(7), 24-25.

Livneh, H. and Antonak, R. F. (1994) Psychosocial reactions to disability: a review and critique of the literature. *Critical Reviews in Physical and Rehabilitation Medicine*, **6**(1), 1–70.

Martella, R. C., Marchand-Martella, N. E. and Agran, M. (1992) Work-related accident causes: a neglected transitional area. *Canadian Journal of Rehabilitation*, **6**(2), 117–122.

Morris, J. K., Cook, D. G. and Shaper, A. G. (1994) Loss of employment and mortality. *British Medical Journal*, **308,** 1135–1139.

Redeker, N. S., Smeltzer, S. C., Kirkpatrick, J. *et al.* (1995) Risk factors of adolescent and young adult trauma victims. *American Journal of Critical Care*, **4**(5), 370-378.

Taylor, S. and Field, D. (1993) *Sociology of Health and Health Care: An Introduction for Nurses.* Blackwell Scientific.

Warr, P. and Jackson, P. (1985) Factors influencing the psychological impact of prolonged unemployment and re-employment. *Psychological Medicine*, **15,** 795–807.

Whelan, C. T., Hannan, D. F. and Creighton, S. (1991) *Unemployment, poverty and psychological distress.* General research paper no. 150. Economic and Social Research Institute.

Wright, B. (1993). *Caring in Crisis. A Handbook of Intervention Skills.* Churchill Livingstone.

8

The causes and effects of trauma – the older person

Sharon Christie

Introduction

The needs and care of the older trauma patient are many and varied. This chapter aims to introduce some concepts of ageing and other relevant gerontological issues. Causes of trauma are examined and a subjective evaluation of attitudes and care is explored. The management and care of the older patient is outlined and suggestions are made which could improve their care.

Demography

Over the last 100 years the number of people of pensionable age in Britain has increased from 2 million to over 10 million. In addition to the numerical increase, the proportion of older people has also risen from 5% to 18.3% of the population (Bond *et al.*, 1993).

Current figures and projections show that the older population is growing, and is expected to do so until 2050 (Warnes, 1992). This does not simply mean an increase in the numbers of older people, but also a change in the proportion of older people to younger, economically active people.

These trends are based on projections, and assumptions are made about future trends in mortality, migration and fertility which may prove to be inaccurate. However, projections regarding numbers of older people have proved accurate (Phillips Report, 1954, cited in Victor, 1994) but it has been acknowledged that it is more difficult to predict health and mortality rates which are subject to many variables (Craig, 1983; Fennell, 1988; Bond *et al.*, 1993).

The OPCS Disability Survey (1988) census of disability showed an exponential relationship between age and the prevalence of disability. Tallis (1992) lists the major causes of disability as:

- stroke
- Alzheimer's disease
- Parkinson's disease
- osteoarthritis
- fractured neck of femur.

The incidence of these increases with age. As half of the UK's hospital beds are occupied by people aged 65 years and over (Coni *et al.*, 1993), any increase in this section of the population is likely to lead to increasing numbers of older people requiring hospital admission.

The ageing process

Ageing can be defined as the progressive loss of an individual's adaptability, or the impairment of homeostasis. The physiological processes which keep our organs and systems balanced and functioning effectively become less sensitive, less accurate, slow and less well sustained. When we meet a challenge to which we can no longer respond effectively, we die (Grimley-Evans, 1994).

The process of ageing is a combination of intrinsic (genetic) and extrinsic (environment and lifestyle) factors.

It is recognized that much difficulty exists in separating pathology from physiology in old age (Rudd and Millard, 1988; Fairweather, 1991). Disease is sporadic, affecting only certain individuals. However, many diseases are age-related and, whilst ageing itself is universal, it affects different people at different rates.

Key issues affecting the older trauma patient

Osteoarthritis

Osteoarthritis could be said to be part of the ageing process, as it is characterized by a number of degenerative changes in the joints. However, although ageing is accepted as an important contributor, there are other causes such as traumatic injuries involving articular surfaces, internal joint derangement due to injury or disease and possibly metabolic abnormalities (Goldie, 1986).

To be attributed to ageing, osteoarthritis must be universal and, although Felson (1988) reported evidence of osteoarthritis in the majority of people aged 65 and in 80% of people over 75, the disease does not affect everyone. It is progressive though, and in an earlier study he found that radiographically there was an increase in osteoarthritis with age. Extrinsic factors such as diet, obesity and mobility also contribute to the occurrence of this disease.

Confusion

Confusion is not an inevitable consequence of ageing, although the older person may be more vulnerable to it as a result of the effects of the ageing process diminishing the reserves required to deal with physical and psychological crises. For example, changes in respiratory function and homeostatic control leading to hypoxia and electrolyte imbalance may cause confusion.

There is some debate as to whether Alzheimer's disease is part of the ageing process, because the increase in characteristic plaque deposits are found to a lesser extent in the brains of non-sufferers. However, it is argued that if we lived to our maximum life span we would all develop the disease and that what we see at present is a manifestation of those who exhibit the signs of ageing earlier than others – similar to the way some people develop wrinkles earlier than others (Randall, 1991).

Confusion is a presenting symptom of illness and not a diagnosis in itself; many health professionals still fail to differentiate between confusion and dementia (Walsh and Ford, 1994). The label of 'dementia' has sometimes been applied, when investigation into the cause of a patient's confusion would be a more appropriate course of action. Acute confusion can last from a few minutes to 3 months, the main features being disorientation in time and place, labile mood, poor memory, drowsiness, hallucinations and delusions (Bennett, 1994). Possible causes are infection, myocardial infarction, stroke, diarrhoea and vomiting, diabetes, drugs, electrolyte imbalance and post-anaesthesia. Moving house, admission to hospital and failing sight or hearing can also cause confusion. It is critical to identify and treat the cause as confusion is reversible.

If confusion persists for longer than 3 months it is considered to be chronic, but still reversible. Possible causes can be hypothyroidism, anaemia, depression, head injury, brain tumour, Parkinson's disease and alcoholism. All these conditions are treatable, or can be managed in such a way so as to reduce the associated confusional state.

Dementia is progressive and irreversible. In addition to the aforementioned manifestations, the person may display personality changes, difficulties in communicating, loss of judgement, loss of practical skills and changes in behaviour (Sugden and Saxby, 1985).

As healthcare professionals we come into contact with many older people suffering from dementia and it is easy to assume that the disease affects a significant number. In fact only 10–15% of 65–75-year-olds and 20–25% of the over-80s suffer from it (Department of Health, 1996). Interestingly though, one study did find that one-third of older patients admitted with a fractured neck of femur also had dementia (Campbell, 1976).

Causes of trauma

The causes of trauma which apply to all age groups can apply equally to the older person –

falls, road traffic accidents, accidents in the home and garden, violence and sports injuries. However, the difference lies in the amount of force required to cause significant injury, and the types of injury sustained.

One overall effect of ageing is a slowing down and decline in certain functions, which may leave the older person less adaptable and less able to respond to crises.

The decline in sensory functions may contribute to falls and accidents. Poor sight and hearing or confusion can lead to reduced awareness of potential hazards, and the slower reactions of the nervous system mean a reduced ability to avert a fall or injury.

Changes in cardiovascular and respiratory function can lead to diminished physical ability. The increased incidence of cardiovascular disease in the older person may lead to falls and accidents as a result of the blood supply to the heart or brain being interrupted.

The effects of ageing on the kidneys and bladder may contribute to falls by increasing the urgency with which an older person must get to the toilet, together with nocturia resulting in attempting to mobilize hurriedly or when half asleep.

All these changes are factors in the causes of trauma in the older person, but changes in the musculoskeletal system are the most significant. In particular, the marked decline in musculoskeletal strength puts the older person at risk of sustaining injury, especially fractures. Osteoporotic changes make the bones of the older person fracture more readily (Pennig, 1992). Interestingly, there has been an increase in the number of older people who sustain fractures and Pennig (1992) suggests this may be due to the increase in levels of activity of older people nowadays compared to previous generations.

Society's perception of all older people as isolated, inactive and frail is inaccurate and the author has experience of caring for older people following skiing and horse-riding accidents, injuries sustained on the dance floor and on boating trips. However, these are exceptions rather than the rule and falls are still one of the most common causes of trauma leading to hospital admission in this age group.

Falls

In the over 75 age group 82% of injuries resulting in hospital treatment are caused by falls (ROSPA, 1994). In the 64–74 group the figure is 51%. In addition to this, it is estimated that 40% of falls are not reported (Livesley, 1988).

Falls can be distinguished as trips or turns (Roberts, 1989). Trips are due to extrinsic factors such as the home environment, lighting, steep stairs and loose carpets; turns come from within the person. The characteristics of ageing which are important in relation to falls are decreased muscle strength, decreased flexibility of joints, reduced coordination of movement, decreased light penetration to the retina and diminished efficiency of proprioception (Williamson, 1990). These lead to changes in balance and gait and decreased visual capacity (intrinsic factors), together with any concomitant medical problems such as heart block, postural hypotension, Parkinson's disease and dementia.

The effect of medications – potency or side effects – is another major factor (Brocklehurst, 1989; Roberts, 1989; Williamson, 1990; Williams and Nolan, 1993). Stevens and Mulrow (1989) found that increased incidence of hip fracture paralleled the rate of prescription of drugs which affected overall stability.

The tendency to fall does increase with age (Stevens, 1992) and the interaction between the fall, bone strength and protective responses may determine the type of injury sustained (Dias, 1992).

Osteoporotic changes, essentially loss of bone mass, are significant in that isolated injuries commonly sustained by the older person, i.e. fractures of the neck of femur, distal radius and proximal humerus (Pennig, 1992), occur at the sites most commonly affected by the disease.

A fall onto an outstretched hand or directly onto the shoulder may cause fracture of the proximal humerus, the incidence of which increases from the age of 50 due not only to the inability to check a fall, but also to osteoporosis (Stableforth, 1992). Fracture of the distal radius is also a very common injury resulting from a fall onto an outstretched hand. Interestingly, in men the incidence shows no change with age, but in women there is a rise between the ages of 45–60 (Alffram and Bauer, 1962). However, from age 65 onwards there is no general upward trend (Winner *et al.*, 1989).

The pattern in older people of an increased risk of femoral neck fracture but a constant rate

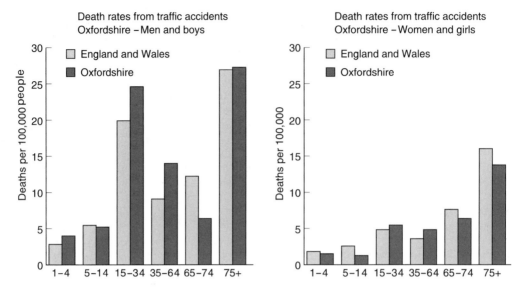

Fig 8.1 Deaths from road accidents in Oxfordshire – by age and gender (From The Health of Oxfordshire (1993–1994))

of wrist fracture may suggest that with age a person is less likely to throw out their arm in time to break a fall, in consequence a hip fracture becomes more likely (Grimley-Evans, 1990).

The increasing number of older patients being admitted with femoral neck fractures has been acknowledged nationwide and has been said to be reaching epidemic proportions (Royal College of Physicians, 1989; Wallace 1983). The fracture rate for femoral neck fractures doubles in each decade of life over 50 (Gallagher *et al.*, 1980), women being affected more than men.

However, the increase cannot be accounted for purely by growth in the ageing population. Zetterberg *et al.* (1984) found that the incidence of femoral neck fractures had increased by 109% from 1965 to 1983 and yet the increase in the older population was only 20%. Attempts to discover the reason for such an increase have merely been able to confirm that decreasing bone density and a lack of mobility predispose to hip fracture, but fail to find a link to the increasing incidence (Wallace, 1983; Elliot *et al.*, 1992; Keene *et al.*, 1993).

Falls cause nine out of ten femoral neck fractures (Audit Commission, 1995) and 70% of these fractures sustained by older people are caused by falls indoors (Aitken, 1984), which may suggest that those most affected are less active.

Some studies have shown that increases in the incidence of femoral neck fractures did not occur in rural populations (Larrson *et al.*, 1989; Harnlo *et al.*, 1989). Finsen and Benum (1987) suggest that this may be due to the more physically active lifestyle of those living in such areas. People who are more physically active are less likely to sustain a fractured neck of femur (Boyce and Veasey, 1988; Astrom *et al.*, 1987).

Road traffic accidents

On the roads, older drivers are involved in many more accidents per distance travelled than younger drivers (Gatherer, 1994). Impaired vision, slower reaction times and loss of hearing may all be contributory factors. Surprisingly, the number of deaths from road accidents nationwide is highest not in the young adult as may be expected, but in the over 75 age group for both sexes (Figure 8.1). One factor is that older people today tend to be more active compared with previous generations. For example, in 1976 less than 60% of men aged over 60 held a driving licence, but by 2000 this figure will have risen to 80% (Friedel, 1985). The over 65 age group accounts for 50% of all pedestrians killed in road traffic accidents (Friedel, 1985) and the increase in death rate from injuries to pedestrians aged over 70 is fivefold compared with people in their 20s. The majority of older multiple trauma victims are pedestrians knocked down by motor vehicles (Friedel, 1985; Haeske-Seeberg, 1988). In multiple trauma involving an older person, the injuries are likely to be similar to those of a younger person. However, whether driver, passenger or pedestrian, the older person has a higher risk of injury.

Attitudes towards the older trauma patient

The older trauma patient is often viewed in a negative light. In the Accident and Emergency (A&E) Department the older person may often be referred to as 'a fall – another neck of femur' and scant notice taken regarding the circumstances of that fall. The hurried clerking of such patients may allude to 'a fall' with no further details. This is in contrast to the detailed documentation regarding injuries sustained by younger people. Ward staff may perpetuate this behaviour by completing assessment forms by simply writing 'fall' rather than 'tripped on kerb while out shopping' or 'transferring from bed to commode and slipped to floor'.

Similarly, admission details show all older people as 'retired', with no further thought as to whether they may still be working, or indeed what their previous occupation may have been. This illustrates the stereotypical image that some professionals have of older people, thereby denying the individuality of the person.

The author observes that often nurses will know all about the activities and interests of their younger patients through conversations conducted while delivering care, but know very little about their older patients other than their immediate health problems. There seems to be an ignorance of how interesting the lives and life experiences of the elderly can be – a lumping together of the 'old' as one, not recognizing that each person is an individual.

As well as a lack of recognition of the individuality of the older patient, there is a tendency to see the presenting problems of the older patient as a consequence of age, rather than ill-health. Symptoms, particularly incontinence and confusion, are attributed to age and become diagnoses, denying the older patient

proper assessment and investigation.

There is also the risk within an acute service that the focus of treatment will be the injury, and other aspects contributing to the overall condition of the patient may be afforded secondary consideration. A perfectly fixed fracture is of limited value if the person has multiple medical problems which are not addressed concurrently.

This approach and the attitudes displayed all have their roots in ageism, which is defined as discrimination on the basis of age alone.

Ageism in society

Ageist attitudes abound in society. We live in a youth-centred culture (Sontag, 1972) where growing old is feared (Harris, 1975) and seen as a negative experience strongly associated with frailty and dependence (Day, 1986; Bond *et al.*, 1993). Mandatory retirement takes away a major role in a person's life (Cowgill and Holmes, 1972) and may leave them feeling they no longer have a contribution to make to society or indeed are a burden on that society.

The 'aged' or the 'old' are used as collective nouns to encompass a hugely diverse group of people. There are references to the aged and the rest of society as if they are a separate element. The 'old' are made up of individuals, each with their own experiences, hopes and aspirations; we do not suddenly become 'old' and lose our individual characteristics.

Psychology of ageing

In defining old age it could be said that you are old when you feel old (Hazan, 1994). Ward (1984) found that health problems, retirement, physical and mental deterioration and changes in social contact were all factors which led to a person identifying themselves as old. Midwinter (1987) defined four stages in life – the third and fourth relating to life after paid work. It is the onset of illness or frailty that heralds the fourth age, the point at which a person becomes dependent.

The psychological aspects of ageing itself present challenges to the individual in coping with concepts of loss (of job, income, status, spouse, friends), low self-esteem due to lack of role or worth to the family or society, guilt associated with being a burden and a resignation that declining health is inevitable. It is difficult to separate whether these feelings come purely from inside the individual or whether they exist because of the attitudes of society towards ageing.

Much of the literature suggests that the key to 'successful ageing' is flexibility and adaptability (Solomon and Peterson, 1994; Lundh and Nolan, 1996). As a person grows old they are forced to adjust to a different role in life. Finding a meaningful one is considered a major step towards successful ageing. In addition, being connected to family and friends and having control over one's life are important factors. Adaptability involves the efficient use of one's physical and emotional resources, expending energy on activity that is meaningful (Solomon and Peterson, 1994).

Brandstadter *et al.* (1993) suggested that older people successfully adapt to ageing and the degenerative changes associated with it by maintaining a 'sense of self'. Being in hospital, particularly as a result of a fall, reinforces the physical demise of the older person and the attitudes encountered may reinforce a loss of control and change in role. To adapt to the challenge of recovery may be difficult when faced with professionals and family who make assumptions about older people as a whole rather than as individuals.

Hazan (1994) suggests that some older people happily adopt the sick role, perhaps because of the attention they receive, but it may be because they are playing the role society creates for them – that of the frail, dependent old person.

Ageism in healthcare

The ageist attitudes that exist in society and the media are bound to exist in health professionals as well; they are ingrained in us (Weber, 1980). Studies have shown that nurses prefer to care for patients other than the elderly, mainly due to difficulties in communication, anti-social behaviour and their slowness to accomplish tasks (Weber, 1980; Fielding, 1986).

Hazan (1994) puts forward the view that we have turned the phenomenon of ageing into a pathology by looking no further than age as the cause of many symptoms. There is a tendency to attribute problems we cannot account for to old age, perhaps to eliminate the need for further investigation or simply to hide the clinician's inability to explain the cause.

'Of course, we're all geriatricians now' is the popular cry from doctors in all specialities (Newman, 1992). This comment shows a sadly ignorant and somewhat arrogant view that simply by coming into contact with older patients within their own specialities, these doctors consider themselves also to be gerontologists. This attitude not only devalues the gerontologists' expertise, but more importantly is detrimental to the care of the older person, denied access to specialist input.

Management and nusing care of the older trauma patient

In many respects the care of the trauma patient is the same regardless of age. Priorities of care should be maintenance of airway and oxygen saturation, maintenance of cardiovascular stability, pain control and the prevention of complications arising either as a result of the injury itself or as a consequence of reduced mobility. Many trauma patients require surgical treatment. Ongoing care consists of working towards independent mobility and discharge home. Psychological support throughout the hospital admission is also a very important aspect of care. The differences in the physical care required by an older patient, as opposed to a younger patient relate to needs linked specifically to the effects of ageing. The ageing process renders the older person more vulnerable, less adaptable and with fewer reserves to respond to a crisis.

On admission, a comprehensive assessment of the respiratory and cardiac system is important, particularly if surgery is required. An electrocardiograph is essential to identify any problems, particularly as a myocardial infarction in older people can occur without chest pain (Pathy, 1967). Although expedient surgical intervention is preferable, if reversible symptoms are present it is better to delay surgery and improve the patient's medical condition prior to anaesthetic (Eastwood, 1991; Stevens, 1992). This would include treatment for atrial fibrillation, heart block, cardiac failure, hypertension, anaemia, dehydration or chest infection.

General anaesthesia and major surgery will present higher risks in relation to postoperative hypoxia and confusion for an older person than would be experienced by a younger individual.

A decrease in efficient renal function and

homeostatic control means that the older person is more prone to dehydration, particularly when stressed by illness or fluid deprivation (Bagnall, 1992). If dehydration is not corrected it can lead to hypotension, an imbalance of electrolytes and confusion. Therefore intravenous hydration is paramount, but care must be taken to avoid circulatory overload leading to pulmonary oedema.

Administration of oxygen therapy, monitoring of vital signs including pulse oximetry and accurate recording of fluid balance are necessary.

Adequate pain control is essential to enable movement to relieve pressure points and to allow early mobilization. It should be remembered that older patients may have increased sensitivity to opiates, resulting in reduced respiratory function and confusion. It is good practice to administer low doses initially and thereafter to titrate the dose, allowing a balance between pain control and the level of sedation.

Regular oral analgesia is essential to allow mobilization, and a sound knowledge of pain management is required by the nurse as some older people may deny pain or refuse analgesia when it is required.

Changes brought about by the ageing process put older patients at higher risk of developing pressure sores, chest infection, urinary tract infection, deep vein thrombosis and pulmonary embolus. Thus, early mobilization is a priority in the care of the older trauma patient in order to minimize these risks which are all associated with immobility. Patients need to commence mobilizing before muscle bulk and strength diminish, which occurs at a loss of 3% per day (Payton and Poland, 1983).

Pressure sore prevention should start in A&E, with the time spent on trolleys kept to a minimum. Assessment of pressure areas on admission and the use of pressure sore prediction scores facilitate the appropriate use of pressure-relieving mattresses, greatly reducing the risk of pressure sores. However, the use of pressure-relieving aids does not eliminate the need to assist patients to change position and allow the observation of pressure areas.

Catheterization may be appropriate as a short-term measure to allow accurate monitoring of output, as well as minimizing the pain and discomfort caused by using bedpans and decreasing the risk of pressure sores if the patient is incontinent. As soon as mobilization is commenced, the catheter should be removed to allow a return to normal bladder function.

Wound care in the older patient requires special consideration as the skin may be thin and friable. Adequate nutrition is essential for skin care, wound and bone healing, maintaining electrolyte balance and preventing constipation. Hospital menus often fail to cater for the older person's tastes, and lack of access to snacks between mealtimes hinders attempts to encourage dietary intake 'little and often'. A major issue raised in the HAS 2000 report was the inflexibility of ward catering and failure to assist patients with eating and drinking. Encouraging diet, fluids and feeding, where necessary, requires skill and patience. Taking time to assist with nutrition has to be a recognised priority as it is a fundamental need.

Management of confusion

The care of confused patients is challenging and time consuming; there are no easy answers.

As discussed earlier, confusion is a symptom and the cause must be investigated. It is often the nurse who assesses the level of confusion and has to instigate the investigative process. Involving the family in assessing confusion can be useful, but seeing a confused relative is distressing, so giving explanation and reassurance to the family is an important role.

In dealing with a confused patient, the first priority is to maintain safety. This may involve the removal of potentially harmful objects from the patient's reach, and the use of cotsides on the bed. Despite the controversy surrounding their use, the author believes cotsides are necessary in an acutely busy area in order to prevent falls out of bed. Cotsides are also recommended as a safety measure by the manufacturers of some pressure-relieving support surfaces which are used in conjunction with standard hospital mattresses. If a patient is constantly trying to get out of bed, the nurse needs first to establish if there is a reason for this. It is interesting to observe how many times some nurses will tell a patient to get back into bed or put them back into bed without actually exploring why they are trying to get up.

Taking time to talk with confused or demented patients can be most helpful. A calm, relaxed approach may help to reassure the person. Reorientation in time and place is important and sometimes the use of notebooks recording past or anticipated visits by friends and family can useful.

A key point when dealing with very confused and agitated patients is to appreciate that what the person is thinking and feeling is totally real to them – they do believe you are holding them prisoner, trying to kill them or stopping them from going home to their family. However strange the behaviour or the words that are spoken, there are strong feelings beneath: 'I want to go home' or 'I want my mother' show fear and anxiety. By choosing your language carefully you can acknowledge these feelings without collusion or dispute. You may be able to reassure the person, but if your presence causes them to become more distressed or agitated, simply leave them and go back later.

If a patient is agitated and fighting against nursing intervention, then flexibility is needed to balance the importance of the intervention against the amount of distress caused. Persisting in attempting to carry out care in this situation is poor use of nursing time and often leads to an unsatisfactory outcome.

Managing a confused patient does take time and patience. It is easy to become stressed and frustrated, but controlling such feelings and taking a calm approach is paramount. The value of good quality nursing care for the older person cannot be underestimated, but the key is the way in which that care is given.

A different generation – dignity and respect

The initial meeting with a patient is important and it is good practice to address them by title and surname to show respect. Many older people address even their own friends using the titles 'Mr' or 'Mrs' and to use a first name without first being given permission is impolite. Asking a patient how they wish to be addressed can make them feel obliged to volunteer their first name. They may then feel uncomfortable when addressed this way by staff much younger than themselves. It is best to use the surname until the patient invites you to do otherwise.

Giving patients and their families clear information and an understanding of how the ward operates is essential. The culture of healthcare has changed greatly over the years

and previous hospital experiences may have been very different. Establishing the expectations of both patients and staff will help to build therapeutic relationships, enabling both parties to work towards shared goals.

Rutter (1996), on talking to discharged patients following hip fracture, found that what older patients valued most was the support and encouragement of nurses and being given time. The HAS 2000 report highlights that older people want professionals to listen to them, allow them to have control over their own lives and choices, which in turn provides motivation.

The motivation to overcome a significant injury and its consequences can be a problem for many older people. It will depend on how the older person has coped with the psychological aspects of ageing and their ability to adapt to new challenges. The amount of effort required to recover may outweigh the perceived positive outcomes, especially if the person feels that the quantity or quality of life remaining will be low.

The level of nursing assistance required by the older trauma patient will initially be high and reinforce their perception of being dependent and helpless. Nurses can use the time spent giving care to get to know the person, their life experiences, feelings and hopes. If the patient can see your interest in them as a person, rather than a patient with problems, it may well help their motivation. In a busy ward it can be easy to do things for a patient because it is quicker, whereas enabling patients to do things for themselves is much more beneficial. The climate of the ward needs to remain focused on the individual rather than the system.

Positive images of old age, such as poems on display, can help to promote an anti-ageist atmosphere. Negative attitudes towards older patients must be checked, through education and good practice. The rewards are there. Listening to the life experiences of an older person can provide staff with privileged insight into some of the most significant historical events and personalities of the twentieth century. The author recalls particularly caring for a 1936 Olympic rowing medallist, and an escapee from Nazi-occupied Poland who went on to became a fighter pilot. Even the more personal aspects of life, such as attitudes towards relationships, marriage and children, can be of fascination to later generations.

Case study

I remember helping to care for Dr Gray (pseudonym), a 98-year-old lady who had sustained a femoral neck fracture. Her diminutive stature and frailty gave no hint of the catalogue of achievements that she had accomplished throughout her life: qualifying as a doctor, when this was considered by many to be an unsuitable job for a woman; gaining an international reputation for research/work with children in developing countries; surviving as a prisoner of war in the Far East. The needs of children had formed a huge part of her working life.

Postoperatively Dr Gray became very ill and recovery was deemed unlikely. She was listless, breathless and at times confused. One day her primary nurse noticed that another patient was being visited by a family proudly showing everyone their new baby. The nurse asked if she could show the baby to Dr Gray, explaining how much she loved children and, with the permission of Dr Gray's family, a little of her background. They were happy to agree. The nurse handed the baby to Dr Gray whose expression changed from one of sadness to one of joy. She talked coherently and with authority about the contrast in life expectations that this child would have in comparison to some of the children she had known. She seemed to enjoy the experience of having been recognized as someone who had a special affinity with children. Her family were also very moved by the spontaneous action of the nurse. She had responded to 'the person' not the patient.

Dr Gray died peacefully soon after.

Surgery to fix a fractured neck of femur is the third most common surgical procedure carried out on the over 65s; it cannot be seen simply as an injury and procedure. The care of older patients requires special skills because of high morbidity rates, different patterns of disease presentation, multiple symptoms, slower response to treatment and the combination of underlying frailty and illness. Indeed, Newman (1992) suggests that individuals in their 70s and 80s require a level of expertise comparable to that provided for a neonate.

The role of gerontologists in rehabilitation following hip fracture is well recognized (BMJ Editorial, 1978; Harries and Eastwood, 1991; Coni *et al.*, 1993) and essential to postoperative rehabilitation. However, there is still more scope to improve collaboration with gerontologists preoperatively, with more attention being given as to why patients have fallen. All staff must be exhorted to recognise older people as individuals, ensuring that ageism, whether by an individual or the system, is not permitted.

Summary

- Older patients will continue to make up a large proportion of trauma patients.
- Knowledge of research into ageing and the effects of the ageing process enhance practice.
- Recognize the special needs of the older person and utilize that expertise to enhance practice.
- Communication and teamwork are essential.
- Time and support must be given to older patients.
- Value the life experiences of a patient – they are unique to that individual.
- Adopt a 'people' first, 'patient' second and 'age' last approach.

References

Aitken, J. (1984) Relevance of osteoporosis in women with fractures of the femoral neck; cited in Newman, R. (1992) *Orthogeriatrics: Comprehensive Orthopaedic Care for the Elderly Patient*. Butterworth-Heinemann.

Alffram, P. and Bauer, G. (1962) Epidemiology of fractures of the forearm; cited in Newman, R. (1992) *Orthogeriatrics: Comprehensive Orthopaedic Care for the Elderly Patient*. Butterworth-Heinemann.

Astrom, J., Ahnqvist, S., Beertema, E. and Johnson, B. (1987) Physical activity in women in sustaining fracture of the neck of femur; cited in Newman, R. (1992) *Orthogeriatrics: Comprehensive Orthopaedic Care for the Elderly Patient*. Butterworth-Heinemann.

Audit Commission (1995) *United We Stand: Co-ordinating Care for Elderly People with Hip Fracture*. London: HMSO.

Bagnall, W. (1992) General medical problems of the elderly patient; cited in Newman, R. (1992) *Orthogeriatrics: Comprehensive Orthopaedic Care for the Elderly Patient*. Butterworth-Heinemann.

Bennett, G. (1994) *Alzheimer's Disease and other Dementias*. Vermillion.

BMJ Editorial (1978) Falls and fractures, *British Medical Journal*, **2**(61361), 552.

Bond, J., Coleman, P. and Peace, S. (1993) *Ageing in Society*. Sage Publications.

Boyce, W. and Veasey, M. (1988) Habitual physical inertia and other factors in relation to risk of fractures of the proximal femur; cited in Newman, R. (1992) *Orthogeriatrics: Comprehensive Orthopaedic Care for the Elderly Patient.* Butterworth-Heinemann.

Brandstadter, J., Wentura, D. and Greve, W. (1993) Adoptive resources of the ageing self: outlines of an emergent prospective; cited in Lundh, U. and Nolan, M. (1996) Ageing and quality of life 1: Towards a better understanding. *British Journal of Nursing*, **5**(20), 1248–1251.

Brocklehurst, J. (1989) After the fall. *Nursing the Elderly*, Sept. 16–17

Campbell, A. (1976) Femoral neck fractures in elderly women: a prospective study. *Age and Ageing*, **5**, 102–109.

Coni, N., Davidson, W. and Wester, S. (1993) *Lecture Notes on Geriatrics.* Blackwell Scientific.

Cowgill, D. and Holmes, L. (1972) Ageing and modernisation. In *An Ageing Population* (V. Carver and P. Liddiard, eds). Hodder and Stoughton/Open University Press.

Craig, J. (1983) *The Growth of the Elderly Population.* OPCS 32. London: OPCS.

Day, E. (1986) Time to value the golden age. *Nursing Times*, **82**(42), 67–69.

Department of Health (1996) Mental illness, mental health and older people. In *The Health of the Nation*. London: HMSO.

Dias, J. (1992) Wrist fractures; cited in Newman, R. (1992) *Orthogeriatrics: Comprehensive Orthopaedic Care for the Elderly Patient.* Butterworth-Heinemann.

Eastwood, H. (1991) The social consequences of surgical complications for patients with proximal femoral fractures. *Age and Ageing*, **22**, 360–364.

Elliot, J., Hanger, H., Gilchrist, N. *et al.* (1992). A comparison of elderly patients with proximal femoral fractures and a normal elderly population: a case control study. *New Zealand Medical Journal*, **105**, 420–422.

Fairweather, S. (1991) Ageing as a biological phenomenon. *Reviews in Clinical Gerontology*, **1**(3), 16.

Felson, D. (1988). Epidemiology of hip and knee osteoarthritis; cited in Neman, R. (1992) *Orthogeriatrics: Comprehensive Orthopaedic Care for the Elderly Patient.* Butterworth-Heinemann.

Fennell, G., Phillipson, C. and Evers, H. (1988) *The Sociology of Old Age.* Open University Press.

Fielding, P. (1986) *Attitudes Revisited: An Examination of Student Nurses' Attitudes Towards Older People in Hospital.* RCN.

Finsen, V. and Benum, P. (1987) Changing incidence of hip fractures in rural and urban areas of central Norway; cited in Newman, R. (1992) *Orthogeriatrics: Comprehensive Orthopaedic Care for the Elderly Patient.* Butterworth-Heinemann.

Friedel, B. (1985); cited in Newman, R. (1992) *Orthogeriatrics: Comprehensive Orthopaedic Care for the Elderly Patient.* Butterworth-Heinemann.

Gallagher, J., Melton, L., Riggs, B. and Bergstrath, E. (1980) Epidemiology of the proximal femur in Rochester, Minnesota; cited in Newman, R. (1992) *Orthogeriatrics:*

Comprehensive Orthopaedic Care for the Elderly Patient. Butterworth-Heinemann.

Goldie, I. (1986) Failed joint replacement; cited in Newman, R. (1992) *Orthogeriatrics: Comprehensive Orthopaedic Care for the Elderly Patient.* Butterworth-Heinemann.

Grimley-Evans, J. (1990) The significance of osteoporosis; cited in Newman, R. (1992) *Orthogeriatrics: Comprehensive Orthopaedic Care for the Elderly Patient.* Butterworth-Heinemann.

Grimley-Evans, J. (1994) Can we live to be a healthy hundred? *MRC News.* Autumn, 18–21.

Haeske-Seeberg, H. (1988); cited in Newman, R. (1992) *Orthogeriatrics: Comprehensive Orthopaedic Care for the Elderly Patient.* Butterworth-Heinemann.

Harnlo, G., Jakobsson, B., Ceder, L. and Throngren, K. (1989) Hip fracture incidence in Lund, Sweden; cited in Newman, R. (1992) *Orthogeriatrics: Comprehensive Orthopaedic Care for the Elderly Patient.* Butterworth-Heinemann.

Harries, D. and Eastwood, H. (1991) Proximal fractures in the elderly: does operative delay for medical reasons affect short-term outcome? *Age and Ageing*, **20**, 41–44.

Harris, L. (1975) The myth and reality of ageing in America; cited in Hendricks, J. and Hendricks, C. (1977) Ageism and common stereotypes. In *An Ageing Population* (V. Carver and P. Lidiard, eds). Hodder and Stoughton/Open University Press.

HAS (2000) *HAS 2000 Report – review of care older people receive in acute sector.* Commissioned by Frank Dobson, 1996.

Hazan, H. (1994) *Old Age: Constructions and Deconstructions.* Cambridge University Press.

Keene, G., Parker, M. and Pryor, G. (1993) Mortality and morbidity after hip fractures. *British Medical Journal*, November, **307**, 1248–1250.

Larrson, S., Eliasson, P. and Hansson, L. (1989) Hip fractures in northern Sweden; cited in Newman, R. (1992) *Orthogeriatrics: Comprehensive Orthopaedic Care for the Elderly Patient.* Butterworth-Heinemann.

Livesley, B. (1988) Safety in the home in old age. *Health Visitor*, **61**(9), 284–286.

Lundh, U. and Nolan, M. (1996) Ageing and quality of Life 1: towards a better understanding. *British Journal of Nursing*, **5**(20), 1248–1251.

Midwinter, E. (1987) Ageing is opportunity: education and older people; cited in Hazan, H. (1994) *Old Age: Constructions and Deconstructions.* Cambridge University Press.

Newman, R. (1992) *Orthogeriatrics: Comprehensive Orthopaedic Care for the Elderly Patient.* Butterworth-Heinemann.

OPCS Disability Survey (1988) Cited in Coni, N., Davidson, W. and Wester, S. (1992) *Ageing, the Facts.* Oxford University Press.

Pathy, M. (1967) Clinical presentation of myocardial infarction in the elderly. *British Heart Journal*, **29**(2), 190–199.

Payton, O. and Poland, J. (1983) Ageing process: implications for clinical practice. *Physical Therapy*, **63**(1), 41–48.

Pennig, D. (1992) Principles of fracture management in elderly patients; cited in Newman, R. (1992) *Orthogeriatrics: Comprehensive Orthopaedic Care for the Elderly Patient*. Butterworth-Heinemann.

Phillips Report (1954) Cited in Victor, C. (1994) *Old Age in Modern Society*. Chapman and Hall.

Randall, T. (1991) Is it 'Old Timer's Disease' or just growing old? *Journal of the American Medical Association*, **265**(3) 310–311.

Roberts, A. (1989) Systems of life (no. 176). Senior systems. *Nursing Times*, **85**(41), 45–48.

ROSPA (1994), cited in Gatherer, A. *The Health of Oxfordshire 93–94*. Report of the Director of Public Health, Oxford Dept of Public Health Policy. Seacourt Press Ltd.

Royal College of Physicians (1989) Report on fractured neck of femur: prevention and management, *Journal of the Royal College of Physicians* **23**(8), 8–12.

Rudd, A. and Millard, P. (1988) What is ageing? *Baillières Clinical Obstetrics and Gynaecology*, **2**(2), 241–259.

Rutter, D. (1996) *'I don't want to bother people.' Patients' and Carers' Experience and Views of Care, Treatment and Rehabilitation Following Fracture of the Neck of Femur*. Audit Commission/College of Health.

Solomon, R. and Peterson, M. (1994) Successful ageing: how to help your patients cope with change. *Geriatrics*, **49**(4), 41–47.

Sontag, S. (1972) The double standard of ageing. In *An Ageing Population* (V. Carver and P. Liddiard, eds). Hodder and Stoughton/Open University Press.

Stableforth, P. (1992) Shoulder injuries in the elderly; cited in Newman, R. (1992) *Orthogeriatrics: Comprehensive Orthopaedic Care for the Elderly Patient*. Butterworth-Heinemann.

Stevens, A. and Mulrow, C. (1989) Drugs affecting postural stability and other risk factors in the hip fracture epidemic; cited in Newman, R. (1992) *Orthogeriatrics: Comprehensive Orthopaedic Care for the Elderly Patient*. Butterworth-Heinemann.

Stevens, J. (1992) Fractures of the femoral neck; cited in Newman, R. (1992) *Orthogeriatrics: Comprehensive Orthopaedic Care for the Elderly Patient*. Butterworth-Heinemann.

Sugden, J. and Saxby, P. (1985) The confused elderly patient. *Nursing*, **2**, 1022–1025.

Tallis, R. (1992) Rehabilitation of the elderly in the 21st century. The F. E. Williams Lecture, 1992.

The Health of Oxfordshire (1993–4) *Report of the Director*. Oxford: Oxfordshire Department of Public Health and Health Policy.

Wallace, W. (1983) The increasing incidence of fractures of the proximal femur: an orthopaedic epidemic. *Lancet*, **1**, 1413–1414.

Walsh, P. and Ford, M. (1994) *New Rituals for Old*. Butterworth-Heinemann.

Ward, R. (1984) The ageing experience; cited in Victor, C. (1994) *Old Age in Modern Society*. Chapman and Hall.

Warnes, A. (1992) Demographic processes and health forecasts; cited in Newman, R. (1992) *Orthogeriatrics: Comprehensive Orthopaedic Care for the Elderly Patient*. Butterworth-Heinemann.

Weber, H. (1980) *Nursing Care of the Elderly*. Reston.

Williams, M. and Nolan, M. (1993) Prevention of falls among older people at home. *British Journal of Nursing*, **2**(12), 609–13.

Williamson, J. (1990) *Falls – Whose Concern?* Age Concern.

Winner, S., Morgan, C. and Grimley-Evans, J. (1989) Perimenopausal risk of falling and incidence of distal forearm fracture; cited in Newman, R. (1992) *Orthogeriatrics: Comprehensive Orthopaedic Care for the Elderly Patient*. Butterworth-Heinemann.

Zetterberg, C., Elmerson, S. and Anderson, G. (1984). Epidemiology of hip fractures in Goteborg, Sweden; cited in Newman, R. (1992) *Orthogeriatrics: Comprehensive Orthopaedic Care for the Elderly Patient*. Butterworth-Heinemann.

Part II

The continuum of trauma care

9

The Injury Minimization Programme for Schools

Lynn Pilgrim

Introduction

There is definitely a need for accident prevention teaching to start earlier in life. If we want to create a society in which individuals become more caring and capable in times of emergency, the value of educating the present generation of adults may be limited (Morgan *et al.*, 1996). A far better option is to educate our children. Children absorb and retain knowledge easily and can also exert considerable influence on their parents to change attitudes and behaviour. Frederick and Orzel (1999) found that following an Injury Minimization Programme for Schools (IMPS) there was an increase in safety awareness in children.

IMPS is an accident prevention programme delivered to children between the ages of 10 and 11 years. The programme was developed in 1994 by a multi-professional group based at the John Radcliffe Hospital Oxford. The objective of the IMPS programme is to reduce disability and death as a result of accidents.

The need for IMPS

Government White Papers (Health of the Nation, 1986; and Our Healthier Nation, 1997) show that accidents are recognized as a serious public health problem – not only because of physical injury and possible disability, but also because of the huge financial cost to the NHS.

- Accidents are the leading cause of death among children between the ages of 1 and 15 (Constantinides, 1987).
- The majority of accidents are avoidable. However, for those who survive, injury may result in disability, ill-health and an inability to work (British Orthopaedic Association, 1992).
- Road traffic accidents account for almost twice as many lost years of life nationally than any other single cause (Towner *et al.*, 1996).
- The UK child pedestrian death rate is one of the highest in Europe, with mortality from childhood injuries in Sweden half that of the UK (Schelp, 1987).
- Each year approximately 700 children die as a result of accidents, and approximately 10 000 become permanently disabled (Carter and Jones, 1993).
- The cost to the NHS has been estimated at £100 million per annum (Child Accident Prevention Trust, 1992).
- Childhood injuries account for 14% of all general practitioner consultations; 1 in 4 children attend a casualty department every year (2 million attendances) and use 1 in 6 paediatric beds (Child Accident Prevention Trust, 1989).
- Young people aged 15–24 exhibit a high level of risk-taking behaviour which, combined with inexperience, leads to accident and injury (Barker and Power, 1993)

The National Curriculum Council (1992)

suggests that the national curriculum should incorporate first aid principles and procedures for all children, as accidents often occur in their presence. This is supported by the European Resuscitation Council (1992) who suggest that all European Schools should incorporate basic life support into their curriculum.

Staff from the Accident and Emergency (A&E) Department at the John Radcliffe Hospital were increasingly being asked to visit schools to teach first aid treatment in support of curricular requirements. This situation was becoming unsustainable due to the number of schools requesting visits, leading to staff providing this training in their own time.

As a result, the IMPS programme was set up. The programme was devised by a trauma consultant, A&E lecturer practitioner, and a liaison health visitor with a special interest in accident prevention.

Target group

IMPS targets children who are in year 6 at school (10- and 11-years-old). At this age children are capable of understanding formal reasoning and hypothetico-deductive thinking (Piaget, 1983). Children of this age also have the mature physical and cognitive skills needed to gain maximum benefit from the programme content. The IMPS programme is delivered as part of the National Curriculum, meeting Key Stage 2 attainment targets.

Road traffic accident death statistics show that children between the ages of 11 and 15 are at greatest risk. Therefore the IMPS programme targets children before this most vulnerable period.

Children are encouraged to increase their knowledge and skills through experiential learning, and to explore their own environment in relation to safety issues.

IMPS is a unique multi-agency health education initiative, originally delivered by a multi-professional team based in the Oxford Radcliffe Trust, now operating at a national level. IMPS aims to provide a better understanding of accidents and injuries, and to develop a generation of children who, as adult citizens, have a different attitude to injury prevention and the immediate care of their neighbour.

The IMPS concept is one of linking accident prevention knowledge to the core curriculum and then giving it credibility by experiential learning within a hospital environment. This completes the education loop – the link between education and healthcare services – ensuring all teaching is delivered by appropriate professionals.

The IMPS programme is free to schools.

Programme structure

The programme is delivered to year 6 children in two sections, with most of the teaching occurring at school with the class teacher. During the term when the majority of IMPS teaching occurs, the class visit a hospital for further skills training.

School environment learning

The IMPS 'Resource Pack' is provided by the programme and used by the teachers within the school classroom setting. It is provided free on a long-term loan while the school is enrolled on the IMPS programme. Drawing from the children's own experiences, the extensive teaching materials explore all aspects of accidents, injury minimization and environmental risk factors.

The resource pack is multi-curricular and emphasizes Key Stage targets outlined in the National Curriculum. The programme links to a topic web that incorporates safety skills into all the curricular requirements (Figure 9.1).

Safety skills covered by the resource pack include:

- road safety
- sport and leisure safety
- pedestrian safety
- water safety
- home safety

These safety skills are linked to the curricular subject, as indicated below.

English

The children are asked to write a letter to their parish council about safety conditions at their local playground, suggesting strategies that may be implemented to improve the environment.

Science

Children learn about the concept of electricity,

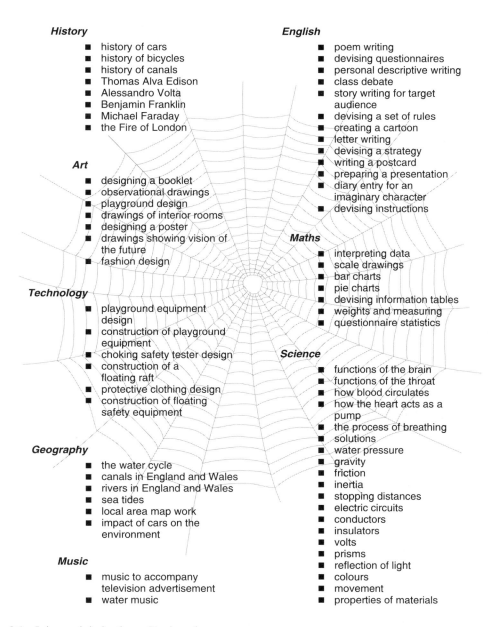

History
- history of cars
- history of bicycles
- history of canals
- Thomas Alva Edison
- Alessandro Volta
- Benjamin Franklin
- Michael Faraday
- the Fire of London

Art
- designing a booklet
- observational drawings
- playground design
- drawings of interior rooms
- designing a poster
- drawings showing vision of the future
- fashion design

Technology
- playground equipment design
- construction of playground equipment
- choking safety tester design
- construction of a floating raft
- protective clothing design
- construction of floating safety equipment

Geography
- the water cycle
- canals in England and Wales
- rivers in England and Wales
- sea tides
- local area map work
- impact of cars on the environment

Music
- music to accompany television advertisement
- water music

English
- poem writing
- devising questionnaires
- personal descriptive writing
- class debate
- story writing for target audience
- devising a set of rules
- creating a cartoon
- letter writing
- devising a strategy
- writing a postcard
- preparing a presentation
- diary entry for an imaginary character
- devising instructions

Maths
- interpreting data
- scale drawings
- bar charts
- pie charts
- devising information tables
- weights and measuring
- questionnaire statistics

Science
- functions of the brain
- functions of the throat
- how blood circulates
- how the heart acts as a pump
- the process of breathing
- solutions
- water pressure
- gravity
- friction
- inertia
- stopping distances
- electric circuits
- conductors
- insulators
- volts
- prisms
- reflection of light
- colours
- movement
- properties of materials

Figure 9.1 Injury minimization – Topic web

and about the anatomy and physiology relating to the body's circulatory system.

Mathematics

Children may explore issues relating to the number of road accidents that occur locally. Using data from the county council they are taught to create pie charts, bar graphs and tables.

The lessons and work cards (Figure 9.2) are pre-prepared and include a resource list for the teacher. The resource pack was written by a Key Stage 2 teacher.

The school programme aims to develop a number of skills and attitudes. These include:

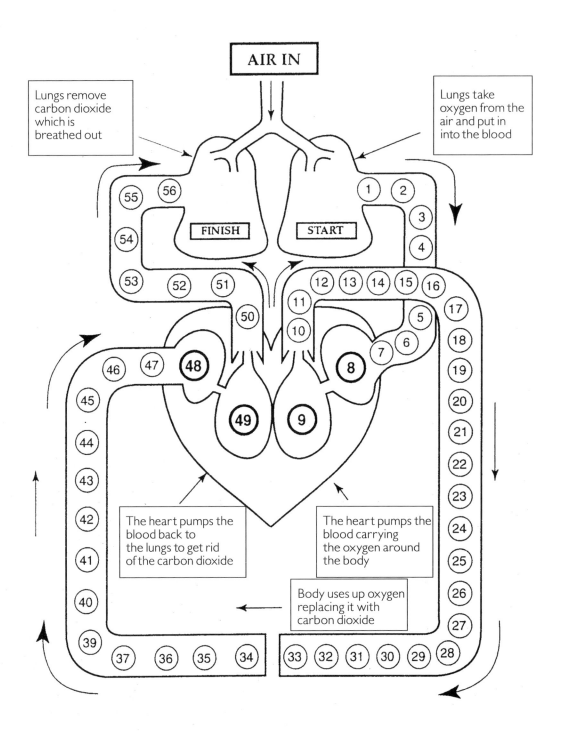

Figure 9.2   Example of a pupil's work card

- critical thinking and decision-making
- responsibility
- empathy
- assertiveness
- independence
- the ability to link action with outcome
- effective communication/concentration and cooperation with peers.

The class use the resource pack during the school term of the hospital visit. It is important that the children learn the basic core elements prior to the visit – these include resuscitation sciences (anatomy and physiology of breathing, the circulation of blood) and how to keep themselves safe.

The hospital visit

This consists of three elements (Figure 9.3):

1. Basic life support training (BLS).
2. First aid training using an interactive video.
3. Tour of the A&E department.

Basic life support training

The principles of basic life support are taught following the European Resuscitation Council (1997) guidelines. The approach has been adopted in line with their recommendations. The children are taught basic life support skills using individual manikins, role play and scenarios.

The aim of each session is for all children to learn and practise 123 ABC resuscitation and the recovery position during group work:

1. **Keep yourself safe.**
2. **Approach.**
3. **Call for help.**

A. **Airway.**
B. **Breathing.**
C. **Circulation.**

As the resuscitation session only lasts 75 minutes, it is unrealistic to expect each child to become proficient at resuscitation during this time; therefore the objectives of this session are:

- **for all children to be aware of dangers and ensure their own safety**

- **for all children to know the importance of calling for help and phoning for an ambulance.**

Experiential learning is encouraged and all the children, teachers and adult helpers practise the techniques using individual manikins (Figure 9.4). Adult single rescuer basic life support is taught, and children are reminded never to practise resuscitation on each other.

First aid training using an interactive video

The children watch a short video containing five first aid scenarios:

- burns and scalds
- cuts and bleeding
- falls and fractures
- electrocution
- choking (infant).

After watching a 'snapshot' of these accidents the children are asked:

- What has happened?
- Why has it happened?
- How it could have been prevented?
- What action could be taken to minimize injury?

The video then resumes, reinforcing the correct course of action.

During this session the IMPS trainers discuss the importance of wearing cycle helmets, asking the children questions such as 'Who owns a bicycle?', 'Who owns a cycle helmet?', 'Who always wears their helmet every time they go for a ride?', 'Why do you wear your cycle helmet?'

The function of the brain is discussed. An analogy of a skull and brain is used, likening it to an egg with its protective shell and soft delicate centre. A helmet that has been damaged in an accident is shown. With these facts, the children are then in a position to make an informed decision to change their attitudes and behaviour.

The treatment for a choking adult is explained and the abdominal thrust manoeuvre demonstrated and discussed.

Children are reminded never to practise making 999 calls or to perform the abdominal thrust manoeuvre unnecessarily.

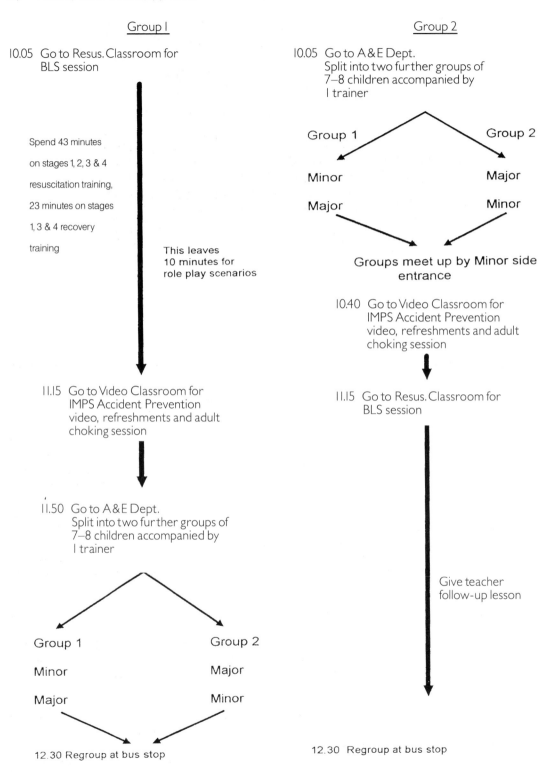

Figure 9.3 Flow chart of hospital visit (BLS, basic life support training; IMPS, Injury Minimization Programme for schools)

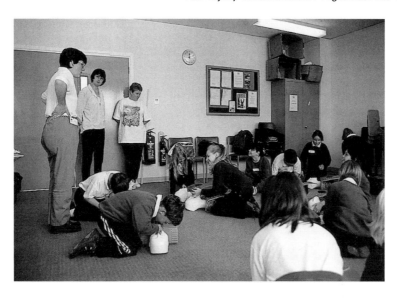

Figure 9.4 An IMPS class

Tour of the A&E department

The aims of the tour are:

- to familiarize children with the A&E department, reducing their fear of the unknown in the event of an accident or ill health
- to relate the core skills of 123 ABC taught in the classroom to the real world of the A&E department.

The A&E tour gives further opportunities for experiential learning, providing real experience of a working hospital. This lends credibility to and consolidates all that has been learnt before in the school and classroom environment.

Small groups of approximately 7 children are guided around the department by IMPS trainers. The areas visited include:

Triage nurse area. This reinforces the importance of assessment of injured people and links to principle number 2 'assess'.

Resuscitation room. This focuses on the ABC aspect of basic life support. The children are able to see equipment, e.g. cardiac monitors, defibrillators, Guedel airways, and link these to the skills learnt in the classroom.

X-ray room. Within this area the uses and

dangers of radiation and X-rays are explored, linking principle number 1 'keep yourself safe'. The treatment of fractures is discussed using a series of X-ray pictures.

Plaster room. The children have plaster of Paris applied to a finger and the principles of chemical reaction are demonstrated. This element is considered great fun by the pupils!

Major incident cupboard. This area will reinforce the importance of principle number 1 'keep yourself safe', as the children are shown the protective clothing worn by healthcare workers when they go out on a major incident call.

Theatre. The treatment of lacerations is discussed, in addition to the safe disposal of syringes and needles found in the environment. Information relating to safe disposal of sharps is given to the class teacher.

Potential blood donors are encouraged by showing the children a unit of blood and discussing the importance of donation.

The tour of A&E is modified each time to fit in with the changing demands on the department and could not take place without the full support and cooperation of all the staff. The children do not come into contact with distres-

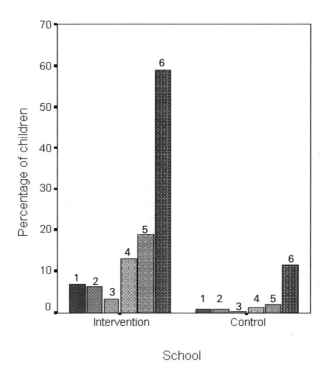

Figure 9.5 Percentage of children in intervention and control schools undertaking key cardiopulmonary resuscitation skills (1, recovery position – call for help; 2, recovery position – physically get help; 3, good compressions; 4, good mouth to mouth; 5, good overall; 6, inappropriate sequence)

sing or frightening sights.

The teacher is provided with follow-up lessons to complete in the classroom; these are designed to consolidate the IMPS visit. Many classes will make a presentation to a whole school assembly, thus demonstrating and sharing their new skills. Teachers have stated that some children have initiated safety changes at school following their IMPS training (Frederick and Orzel, 1999).

The children are provided with a pocket-sized leaflet that includes all the first aid and basic life support information taught during the hospital visit.

Structure of the IMPS programme

IMPS is a health education initiative working as a charitable fund linking education and health agencies.

A programme coordinator liaises between the schools and the hospital to ensure smooth delivery of the programme. The IMPS trainers are recruited from within the hospital and are paid on a sessional basis. In the main they are healthcare professionals who have both an interest in health education and experience with well children. All trainers are monitored to ensure that a standard approach is maintained.

Funding

IMPS is part of the hospital charitable fund and has charity status. Funding is secured by a combination of grant applications and business donations. Fund-raising activities are organized throughout the year and schools are asked to make a financial donation. The co-ordinator role includes fund raising. IMPS is only able to function with the full support of many hospital departments.

Research

IMPS has completed a two-year multi-method non-randomized controlled study to evaluate its effectiveness (Frederick and Orzel, 1999). The objective was to examine the learning that took place in children who had been exposed to the IMPS programme, comparing it with those who had not. The study was conducted over the course of one academic school year (September 1997–July 1998), in Oxfordshire's primary and middle schools. It included children's quizzes, parent and teacher questionnaires and basic life support testing.

A total of 1200 year 6 children took part in the study; 600 in the intervention group and 600 in the control group.

Changes in knowledge, skills, attitudes and behaviour in relation to accident prevention and injury minimization were measured involving the use of the 'Draw and Write' investigative tool (Noreen Wetton, Southampton University Health Education Unit).

The results were highly encouraging for the provision of effective injury prevention and demonstrated the positive outcomes of the combination of academic and experiential learning used in the IMPS programme. This teaching strategy has resulted in a significant increase in children's knowledge and skills (Figure 9.5), together with changes in their attitudes and behaviour towards their own safety, the safety of others and their awareness of their environment (Frederick and Orzel, 1999).

Children in the intervention schools were more likely to initiate 'good life-saving procedures'. Both groups of children performed basic life support in an inappropriate sequence. This was due to failure to assess the circulation prior to commencing cardiac massage. As a result, the 'four-stage approach' of BLS training has been adopted by the IMPS programme.

Conclusion

The research has conclusively proved that the IMPS programme can play a significant role in the objective to provide children with the knowledge and skills that will influence their attitude and behaviour in relation to injury minimization. The short-term aim is to provide children with the skills to enable them to act promptly to save life, prevent disability and to help others appropriately. The long-term aim is to reduce injury numbers.

The future

The future looks promising – the IMPS programme is expanding to three further centres nationwide, and ultimately the aim is for IMPS to be included in the National Curriculum for Schools.

References

Barker, M., and Power, C. (1993) Disability in young adults: the role of injuries. *Epidemiology and Community Health*, **47**, 349–354.

British Orthopaedic Association (1992) BOA. *The Management of Skeletal Trauma in the United Kingdom*.

Carter, Y. H. and Jones, P. W. (1993) Effectiveness of the BBC's 999 training roadshows on cardiopulmonary resuscitation: video performance of cohort of unforewarned participants at home six months afterwards. *British Medical Journal*, **43**, 463–465.

Child Accident Prevention Trust (1989). Basic Principles of Child Accident Prevention. CAPT.

Child Accident Prevention Trust (1992) *The NHS and Social Costs of Children's Accidents: a Pilot Study*. CAPT.

Constantinides, P. (1987) *The Management Response to Childhood Accidents: Primary Healthcare Group*. London: King's Fund Centre.

European Resuscitation Council (1992). Guidelines for Basic Life Support, **24**, 1033–1110.

Frederick, K., Bixby, E., Orzel, M. N. *et al.* (2000) An evaluation of the effectiveness of the Injury Minimization Programme for Schools (IMPS). *Injury Prevention* (in press).

Health of the Nation (1986) *The Strategy for Health in England*. London: HMSO.

Morgan, C. *et al.* (1996) General practitioners' beliefs about their role in the prevention or treatment of accidents involving children. *British Medical Journal*, **313**, 912–915.

National Curriculum Council (1992) *Physical Education Non Statutory Guidance*, section G, paragraph 1.14, G4.

Our Healthier Nation (1998). London: HMSO.

Piaget (1987), cited in Gregory, R. L. (1987). *The Oxford Companion to the Mind.* Oxford University Press.

Schelp, L. (1987) Community intervention and changes in accident patterns in a rural municipality. *Health Promotion*, **2**(2) 109.

Towner, E., Dowsell, T., Simpson, G. *et al.* (1996) *Health Promotion in Childhood and Young Adolescence for the Prevention of Unintentional Injury.* London: London Health Education Authority.

10

Pre-hospital assessment and treatment

Duncan Moore, Steve Double and Tracey Wright

Introduction

Pre-hospital assessment and treatment cover a wide range of accident situations and injury severity – from the individual who suffers a seemingly minor injury, to a major disaster requiring multi-agency involvement. This chapter aims to give some insight into the decision-making processes which pre-hospital providers utilize when responding to emergencies in the field. It also includes the perspective of another perhaps little-recognized service provider, that of the vehicle recovery operator. Her observations make interesting reading and identify yet another avenue down which the injured person and those close to them may experience.

Pre-hospital care

Teamwork in pre-hospital care is crucial. The necessity of working to predetermined protocols and procedures is of paramount importance, as the scene, the nature of injuries sustained, and other members of the team will be ever-changing factors – from one extreme, the single vehicle road traffic accident (RTA) with bystanders constituting part of the team, to the other where prolonged entrapment of the victims involves the participation of other agencies such as the fire service, police and on-site medical staff.

The practice of pre-hospital skills also has a team focus. The use of a skill deemed appropriate in hospital may be inappropriate in the

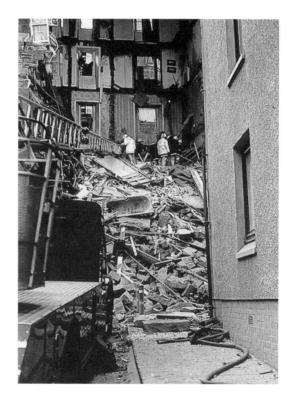

Figure 10.1 The accident

field, as any delay in transportation caused by performing the skill may be more detrimental to the patient's overall condition than the clinical benefit gained from the intervention. Remember the 'golden hour' (Cowley, 1976).

Hospital-based staff need to be aware of the

problems faced by those providing care and treatment in the field. Following arrival at the scene, during the initial 15 seconds a primary survey is carried out, and information is gathered and passed on to other members of the team. This 15-second period affords a unique opportunity to establish a baseline from which the whole team can potentially base its assessment and actions. A rapid but confident assessment will win patient confidence and alleviate anxiety, it may identify life-threatening injuries, and will begin the monitoring of any improvement or deterioration in the patient's overall condition – essential information for the receiving hospital. A multiply-injured patient will rarely, if ever, be presented to the receiving facility having had a full secondary survey completed, as rapid transportation to hospital is imperative.

To the bystander, the pre-hospital provider's immediate input may appear to consist merely of walking up to a patient, holding his hand and talking to him. However, while approaching the patient the accident scene is assessed. The hand on the wrist feels for a pulse, checking rate, rhythm and volume (which may indicate a fall in blood pressure) and an appraisal of the skin – temperature, texture and colour – may indicate shock. The 'Hello, can you hear me?' is a stimulus delivered as part of the visual and auditory appraisal of the patient's reaction and level of consciousness.

The scene is set.

The purpose of pre-hospital care

The purpose of pre-hospital care is to deliver effective and appropriate treatment to patients prior to their transportation to a definitive care facility.

How do we achieve this?

All training in the preservation of life is based around airway, breathing and circulation – ABC. The delivery of care by all disciplines in the field must follow the same principles. To this end staff both in the field and within the receiving hospital must be trained and familiar with the relevant protocols for care (American College of Surgeons, 1997).

The scene

On arrival at the scene (Fig 10.2) a primary survey is carried out following the criteria in Table 10.1. Other factors to be considered are detailed in Table 10.2.

Communication

From the moment you arrive on scene, communicate your intentions and actions to your patient, colleagues in the field and, as soon as possible, the receiving hospital:

'To sing from the same song sheet we must first all know the tune.'

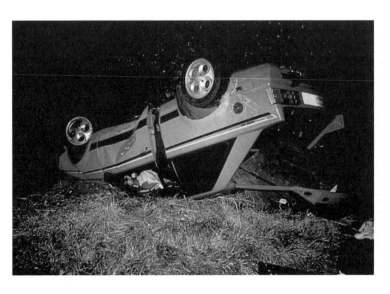

Figure 10.2 The car at an RTA

Table 10.1 Primary survey at the accident scene

Global overview	Is the scene safe to you, the patient, any bystanders? Is the patient conscious? Note patient's colour, position and mechanism of injury Obtain brief history, look for clues regarding current illness or injury
Airway	Check airway is clear Clear and maintain airway If cervical spine injury possible, then apply in-line immobilization
Breathing	Is patient breathing adequately?
Circulation	Are adequate carotid and radial pulses present? Is there severe haemorrhage – external/internal?
Disability	Assess level of consciousness using the AVPU scale – alert/responds to voice/responds to pain/unresponsive
Expose	Expose the patient's body surfaces to look for indications of life threatening conditions or trauma e.g. medic alert tags, pacemakers, large wounds, fractures of long bones, rigid abdomen

Table 10.2 Decision-making at the accident scene

Time critical	Stay and stabilize
• Immobilize • Extricate • Immediate transport	• Baseline observations – respiratory rate, pulse, blood pressure, level of consciousness
During transportation: • Gain intravenous access • Treat other injuries if appropriate or possible • Monitor respiratory rate, pulse, blood pressure, blood oxygen saturation, level of consciousness	• Secondary survey • Treat priority injuries • Extricate • Treat other injuries • Transport and monitor

A simple methodical approach is best, working to a story-line with four key elements:

1. Mechanism of injury.
2. Injuries found.
3. Signs and symptoms.
4. Treatment already given.

This will provide the receiving team with the information required to inform treatment decisions. The story can always be retold at a later stage, at which time more information can be given, e.g. the social and family history.

The following two scenarios provide examples of assessment and treatment in the field.

The handover should be comprehensive, yet concise; time may be of the essence (Figure 10.3). Rapid transportation is of no benefit if the handover is lengthy and delays the patient's treatment.

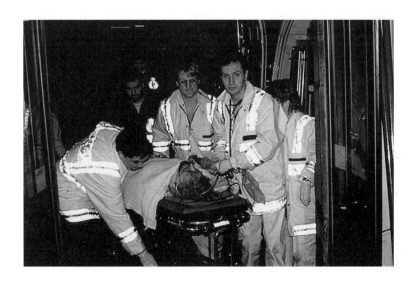

Figure 10.3 Arrival at hospital of paramedics and patient

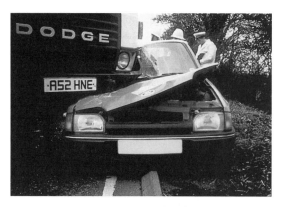

Figure 10.4 Road traffic accident involving a car and a heavy goods vehicle

Scenario 1 (Figure 10.4)

A 30-year-old male, side impacted by HGV, impact speed 45 mph, severe side intrusion, right-sided chest injury, flail chest, open fracture right femur, respiratory and heart rate raised, paradoxical movement right side of chest, alert and orientated.

Global overview:

- Scene safe.
- Side impacted by HGV, severe vehicle intrusion.
- Restrained driver in stationary car – impact speed 45 mph.

Primary survey:

- Airway patent.
- Potential cervical spine injury.
- Breathing – rate raised and shallow.
- Circulation – radial pulse present, tachycardic.
- Disability – alert.
- Expose – chest, paradoxical movement right side, right leg deformed with external haemorrhage.

Decision

- Time critical

Treatment

- Oxygen via face mask.
- Intravenous access.
- Pain relief administered.
- Immobilized on spinal board.
- Right leg immobilized and traction applied.

Then:

- Rapid transportation
- Concise handover

Scenario 2 (Figure 10.5)

A 55-year-old male, thrown from vintage aircraft on crash landing at air show, high-speed impact, severe head injury, obstructed airway, hypoxic, respiratory rate 6, bradycardic, pupils dilated, unresponsive.

Global overview:

- Scene safe.
- Aircraft crashed on landing at air show.
- Thrown from aircraft following high-speed impact.

Primary survey:

- Airway – partial obstruction potential.
- Cervical spine injury.
- Breathing – deep and laboured.
- Circulation – radial pulse present, bradycardic.
- Disability – unresponsive.
- Expose – helmet lost on impact.

Decision:

- Time critical.

Treatment:

- Intubated.
- Ventilated.
- Oxygen administered.
- Immobilized on spinal board.

Then:

- Rapid transportation
- Concise handover

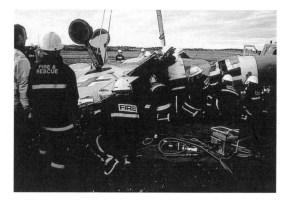

Figure 10.5 Aircraft crash

The role of the recovery operator

All car drivers or passengers will have considered at one time or another the possibility of being involved in a road traffic accident. For thousands of people each year this thought becomes reality.

The call to recover accident damaged vehicles from an RTA can happen at any time, day or night. Brief details of the accident will be given, for example the number of vehicles involved, makes and models of the vehicles, the damage and position of the vehicles (on the road, upside down), and of course the location. However, despite this information you never really know what to expect until you arrive at the scene of the accident itself.

RTAs vary – from the minor accident shown in Figure 10.6 where a 55-year-old female driver drove into her garage too fast and ploughed right through the garage wall, sustaining only minor injuries (incidentally, seconds after pulling her and her car out, the whole garage collapsed!); to the serious road traffic accident

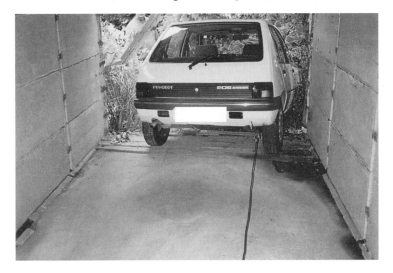

Figure 10.6   Car through garage wall

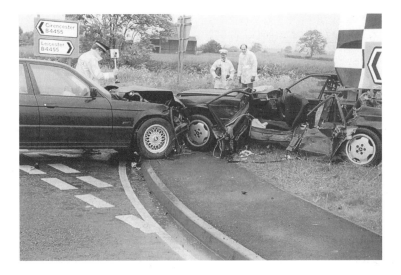

Figure 10.7   The scene following a high-speed head-on collision

shown in Figure 10.7 where two drivers were involved in a high-speed head-on collision, both sustaining multiple injuries; to the fatal accident shown in Figure 10.8 where the young driver of this vehicle lost control at high speed, hit a wall and was killed instantly.

On approaching the accident scene you are met by flashing lights, piercing sirens and people wandering about everywhere – both emergency personnel and bystanders.

RTAs and vehicle recovery hold a fascination for the public and the media. Figure 10.9 shows

just such an accident – the recovery was watched by dozens of bystanders plus the customers in the restaurant.

No two RTAs are the same, nor is the vehicle recovery. However, the following principles always apply:

- **The safety of the recovery crew is paramount**, so it is important to wear fluorescent coats, hard hats and steel toe-capped shoes, along with strong waterproof gloves as there are invariably traces of human flesh and blood

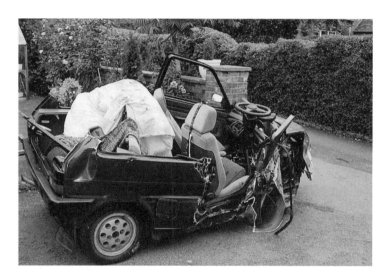

Figure 10.8   The scene of a fatal RTA

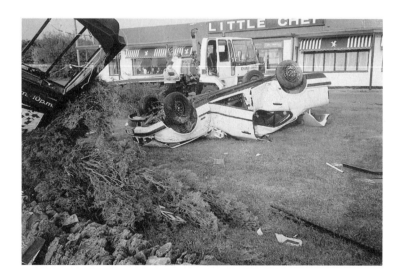

Figure 10.9   Vehicle recovery scene

in the vehicle. All recovery personnel are advised to be vaccinated against hepatitis B.

- **The correct hydraulic lifting equipment applicable to the damage must be employed.** For example, following a typical head-on collision such as that shown in Figure 10.7, a lift and suspended tow would be used, or following the accident in Figure 10.9 total lift equipment would be necessary.
- **The safety of the vehicles and other road users while recovery is taking place must be considered.** Recovery of the vehicles in

Figure 10.10 involved closing the road, as a hi-ab crane was required to lift the vehicles apart.

- **The journey back to the garage takes place when the car is loaded and secured,** and in the event of a fatal accident the front of the car is covered as a measure of discretion and respect.
- **On arrival at the garage, the car is unloaded from the recovery vehicle, stored in a secure compound and all property is logged, bagged up by two personnel and made secure.**

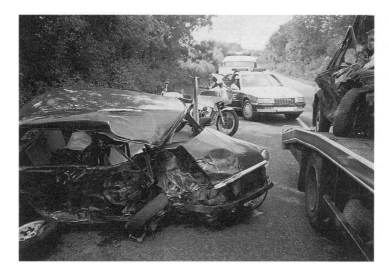

Figure 10.10 Road closure during vehicle recovery

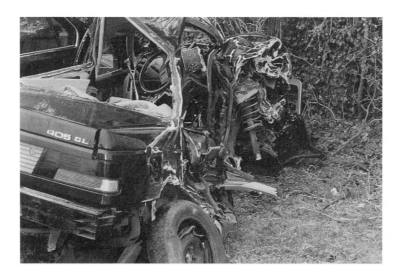

Figure 10.11 Badly smashed vehicle involved in an RTA

Over the years the author has lost count of the number of times the main priority on discharge from hospital for the victim of an RTA is to see their car and collect their possessions, rather than go home and rest. For example, the driver of the car in Figure 10.11 was discharged after a 6-week stay in hospital and arrived at our garage, in a wheelchair, 1 hour later!

On reflection, at times some drivers seem more interested in their cars than themselves. Perhaps this is not so surprising when, for many, a car is the second most expensive possession after their home.

For those whose vehicles have been recovered, reactions have been varied – anger, shouting, crying, shock. People have been witnessed dancing around their cars, some who have sat silently in their cars and others who just cry. These are different coping mechanisms following a trauma which for some may have been the worst experience of their life.

Although the role of the recovery operator may seem exciting and interesting, it is a dangerous, dirty job, done in all weathers, day or night, with the risk of battery acid, petrol and diesel all over the road, not to mention broken glass, jagged edges and human blood and flesh. This is what the injured person remembers – they hear it, see it, smell it and were probably the cause of it.

Reference

American College of Surgeons Committee on Trauma (1997) *Advanced Life Support Student Course Manual.* ACSCT.

Cowley, R. A. (1976) The resuscitation and stabilisation of major multiple trauma patients in a trauma care environment. *Clinical Medicine*, **83**, 14.

11

The 'golden hour'

Lisa Hadfield-Law

A 48-year-old beautician, Ann, was running late on her way to do some Christmas shopping when she rounded a corner to be faced by another car on the wrong side of the road. She swerved, but was unable to avoid a head-on collision at a combined speed of around 60 mph. Her car had about 23 inches of deformation on the front bumper and she was trapped in it. The driver of the other car was killed. It took 55 minutes from the crash before Ann could be extricated from the car. There was then a 35-minute transport time to the hospital.

On arrival at the hospital Ann was agitated and in pain. She had severe facial injuries which were bleeding and swelling. She was complaining of chest pain and difficulty in breathing and was asserting, loudly, that if something was not done quickly she would die. Her observations were:

Blood pressure (B/P) 90/50
Pulse   140
Respiratory rate   38

The police were present and sent a message to her husband about the crash.

Ann is the patient referred to in this chapter, where appropriate.

Introduction

Major injuries can result in death within seconds. Those who do survive, can suffer long-term problems both physically and emotionally. The first couple of hours following injury are critical, as the patient is at her most vulnerable. This critical time period is often referred to as the 'golden hour' (Cowley, 1976). Some, or even all, of this time may be spent in the pre-hospital setting. Usually a significant proportion is spent in the Accident and Emergency (A&E) Department.

During the golden hour the patient requires rapid assessment to identify injuries, both actual and potential, together with timely resuscitation. A systematic approach will ensure that no injury is missed, minimizing the risks to this vulnerable group. Advanced Trauma Life Support (ATLS) principles have now been adopted in many countries as standard practice, and will be used to underpin this chapter (American College of Surgeons, 1997).

The Advanced Trauma Life Support programme

In the UK the ATLS programme is the standard approach to managing trauma (American College of Surgeons, 1997). This programme of training is based upon a sequence of priorities of care with the aim of minimizing death and morbidity.

ATLS is underpinned by an assessment which comprises:

1. Preparation.
2. Primary Survey (ABCDEs).
3. Resuscitation.
4. Secondary survey (head-to-toe evaluation and history).
5. Continuous monitoring and evaluation.

6. Definitive care.

During the management of trauma patients many of these activities occur concurrently, as there are usually a number of staff involved. The primary and secondary surveys should be repeated to monitor any change in the patient's condition.

Although the physiological aspects of trauma resuscitation take priority within the ATLS programme, it is often the emotional damage that lasts longer for the patient. While this aspect of care has traditionally fallen into the realms of nursing, psychosocial care should be considered by all team members. Evidence has started to emerge which seriously questions the wisdom of advocating the one-off interventions post-trauma which have become popular over the last decade (Bisson *et al.*, 1997). This should stimulate research into more effective initiatives which may be started in A&E.

Pre-hospital care

In the past, hospital clinicians have made the mistake of considering the golden hour as starting from the moment the patient arrives in A&E rather than from the moment trauma occurs. This has, at times, resulted in errors of judgement when making decisions about management. By training paramedics (McSwain *et al.*, 1994) and even the general public, we can at least minimize some of the damage suffered by patients at the beginning of the golden hour.

It is important to consider the conditions from which trauma patients have been dying. Some of these conditions are not difficult to identify or complicated to deal with. Some are as simple as lack of oxygen, inappropriate volume replacement and delays in suitable treatments. Paramedics are in an excellent position to take appropriate action early. By developing professional collaboration between pre-hospital and in-hospital care providers, the patient will benefit from an unbroken chain of care (Hadfield-Law, 1999).

Community cardiac resuscitation programmes around the world have proved very successful and by building on these principles we can make sure that members of the general public can also make a contribution to improve trauma outcomes.

Preparation

A&E staff will usually be alerted to the impending arrival of a trauma patient by pre-hospital staff. This provides a window of opportunity in which to prepare facilities and people. Although there will be a wide variation between the numbers of people and levels of skill available in each hospital, the best level of human resource can, at least, be rallied. The principles of effective trauma management will not vary. Each person should have a clear role which matches their skills (Hadfield-Law *et al.*, 2000).

This window of opportunity can also be used to prepare the environment and equipment. With everything ready, the team can focus on the patient as soon as she enters the resuscitation room. Universal precautions are essential. Nobody should come into contact with the body fluids of others before putting on suitable protective clothing. As a minimum this should include goggles, gloves and plastic aprons to protect staff against contamination, and vulnerable patients from nosocomial infection and death due to sepsis (American College of Surgeons, 1997). There is a period of time, weeks or months following injury, when the patient may be at risk of morbidity or mortality, as a result of infection. By wearing suitably weighted and effective lead aprons, trauma teams can remain with the patient during assessment while X-rays are taken without having to worry about exposure to dangerous levels of radiation.

Trauma teams

Cudmore (1996) identified that one of the main problems associated with trauma management is related to inadequate numbers of suitably trained staff and poor skill mix on certain shifts in A&E.

A large number of people make a contribution to patient care in A&E. This may be an informal group of individuals or a more formal resuscitation team, as identified by Driscoll and Vincent (1992a). Although there are the more obvious members of the team, including nursing and medical staff, there are a number of others who may have less direct, but equally important roles, e.g. clerical, portering and domestic staff, pharmacists, laboratory technicians, radiographers, chaplains, learners, witnesses to the incident and, most importantly, the patient and relatives.

Good trauma care relies heavily on a multi-disciplinary approach (Hadfield-Law *et al.*, 2000). However, large numbers of people may attend a trauma resuscitation who are either there to provide a particular service, or to learn. It can be tempting to send some away, which may discourage collaboration at a later date, and will prevent learners from experiencing irreplaceable opportunities. Either situation will jeopardize optimal patient care in the future. Team leaders should consider these eventualities beforehand and decide on a strategy. Groups of people who are unsure of their roles can cause confusion and chaos. However, roles can be outlined and then delegated to make full use of human resources, resulting in good trauma care, reduced overall assessment time and fulfilment of the needs of individual team members (Driscoll and Brook, 1993). These roles may include responsibility for the airway or liaison with relatives. Certainly the way team members are organized and trained affects how well the trauma team functions (Driscoll and Vincent, 1992b; Lomas and Goodall, 1994).

To establish crowd control make sure that anyone not involved in treating the patient to assess, treat or support them, remains at least 2 metres away from the patient trolley, behind a line painted on the floor. By organizing the area in this way you can avoid having to ask members of staff to leave. If possible, anyone who can make a contribution to patient care or who might learn from the situation and be able to perform better at another trauma resuscitation, should be able to stay.

Primary survey

The initial physical examination of the patient identifies potentially life-threatening injuries. A quick evaluation will help the team to set priorities by using the ABCDE system:

A Airway maintenance with cervical spine control.
B Breathing and ventilation.
C Circulation with haemorrhage control.
D Disability: assessment of neurological status.
E Exposure/environmental control: completely undress patient but prevent hypothermia.

During the primary survey life-threatening injuries are identified and treated as soon as they are identified. Therefore primary survey and resuscitative measures are taken together.

Airway maintenance with cervical spine control

Anyone who approaches the patient initially should take immediate measures to protect her cervical spine. It is important to enter the patient's field of vision before she is spoken to, to prevent her moving her head and risking further injury. While the team are making sure that adequate cervical spine precautions are in place, you should ask the patient a question which requires a simple response, such as 'Hello, what's your name?' or 'How are you, Ann?' If the patient is adequately oxygenated and her brain perfused, she should respond appropriately. The team can be satisfied that the airway is clear and the patient's brain is adequately perfused with blood. Such questions, as well as helping to assess the airway, will help to start a supportive relationship with the patient. It is very helpful if one person is responsible for talking to her and keeping her informed of what is happening, whether the patient is conscious or not (Hadfield-Law, 1999).

Even if the airway appears clear, it is important to look carefully to check for any potential problems. Damage to the teeth, soft tissues, facial bones or neck may indicate impending problems with the airway. By taking measures to secure a safe airway at this point you can prevent unexpected problems later; for example swelling from facial injuries can occur quickly and prove dangerous if it compromises the airway. By intervening early, an adequate airway can be secured under controlled circumstances, thereby avoiding having to respond to a crisis (American College of Surgeons, 1997).

Simultaneous cervical spine precautions must be taken from the time of injury (Tippett, 1993). All multiply-injured patients, particularly those who have injuries above the clavicle or a change in level of consciousness, should be treated as though they have a cervical spine injury, until this has been ruled out. Manual immobilization of head and neck should be followed as soon as possible by the application of a semi-rigid cervical collar and head immobilizers specifically designed to protect the spine.

Sometimes patients are unable to remain still. They may be agitated, confused or in pain.

These patients should have a semi-rigid collar in place until they are calm enough to tolerate full spinal precautions. By trying to restrain a thrashing patient, we are more likely to endanger the patient's spine. The team should strive to identify the reason for the patient's agitation or confusion as soon as possible.

When the patient does not respond appropriately to a question, immediate measures should be taken to secure an airway. Often the obstruction is due to the partial or complete occlusion of the oropharynx by the tongue. A simple chin lift or jaw thrust will often pull the collapsed soft tissues out of the airway. There may be saliva, vomit, blood, teeth or other foreign bodies which will need to be removed. Suction through an adequately bored rigid sucker with wide-bore tubing should be used. Flexible suction catheters and even a tonsil-tip sucker can easily be blocked by large pieces of vomit or other foreign matter.

Trauma patients can vomit or regurgitate profusely and unexpectedly. Under such circumstances airway and cervical spine control can become difficult. The head end of the patient trolley should be dropped 20 degrees, so that the patient is tipped head downwards, and with the use of suction apparatus her airway may be cleared (Hadfield-Law, 1999). This initiative should be taken *immediately* in order to reduce the risk of aspiration of gastric contents. Every second counts and the team must be absolutely sure that equipment is fully functional and available without delay.

Once a chin lift or jaw thrust has been done, the patient's airway will need to be made more secure. A nasopharyngeal airway can be very useful in patients who still have a gag reflex. It is particularly useful for patients whose level of consciousness fluctuates. For those who have no gag reflex, an oropharangeal (Guedal) airway must be used (American College of Surgeons, 1997). To provide adequate security these airways must be of a suitable size for the individual patient. Nasal airways are of a standard length, but the diameter should match the diameter of the patient's smallest finger. Oral airways should be measured from the middle of the lips to the angle of the jaw.

For some trauma patients such basic measures are not adequate to maintain an effective airway and these patients require endotracheal (ET) intubation. Patients with severe head injuries and an altered level of consciousness or a Glasgow Coma Scale score of less than 8 usually need intubation. (Driscoll and Skinner, 1998). There are a number of serious risks involved in intubation and it should be carried out by an appropriately skilled team member. Such intubation must often be performed under stressful circumstances with no knowledge of the patient's past medical history. There can be damage to the airway and the complication of a full stomach. This is not the time for those with limited experience to practise their skills.

Very occasionally ET intubation fails. Nobody should persist for more than 60 s without stopping and reventilating the patient with a bag-valve mask device and high-flow oxygen (American College of Surgeons, 1997). Patients like Ann, with facial fractures, can be very difficult to manage, and the team should be prepared to perform an emergency surgical airway. Prolonged periods of apnoea resulting from repeated failures to intubate can lead to potentially fatal hypoxia. While setting up the equipment needed to perform a surgical airway, a needle cricothyroidotomy will allow a delay of 30–45 min before a full cricothyroidotomy or a tracheostomy are required.

Breathing and ventilation

Once the patient's airway has been safely secured, the assessor can assess the adequacy of breathing. Following exposure of her chest, the team can look for any obvious injury and listen and feel for adequate breathing. By watching the patient's chest wall rising and falling the rate, depth and symmetry of breathing can be ascertained. The team can listen for breath sounds and feel for exhaled breath (American College of Surgeons, 1997).

If the patient's breathing is inadequate or absent, then high flow oxygen and mechanical ventilation through a bag-valve mask system should begin immediately. It is difficult to deliver specific percentages of oxygen using this technique, but by turning the oxygen flowmeter up to 12–15 litres of oxygen, a high enough flow should be delivered. Two team members should assume this role together, so that one can ensure a complete seal around the patient's mouth while the other squeezes the bag to the right depth at the right pace. The patency of airway should continually be rechecked, and the efficacy of breathing be established by noting:

1. Rate and depth of breathing.
2. Cyanosis – central or peripheral.
3. Use of accessory muscles.
4. Tracheal shift from the midline.
5. Engorged neck veins.
6. Any sucking chest wounds.

All these signs indicate an impending or actual problem with breathing, although perhaps the most important, and one of the first, is a change in conscious level, which may be very subtle indeed. Pulse oximetry can be used to monitor oxygenation. However, misleading information can be generated when sensors are placed distal to a blood pressure cuff or the patient is peripherally shut down.

All trauma patients without exception should receive high flow oxygen (American College of Surgeons, 1997). By attaching a reservoir bag to the oxygen mask running at 15 litres of oxygen per minute, a concentration of approximately 85% can be achieved.

If a life-threatening condition is identified during the assessment of breathing it must be corrected immediately. Such conditions include:

- tension pneumothorax
- flail chest with pulmonary contusion
- massive haemothorax
- open pneumothorax.

Sucking chest wounds should be covered. To avoid a resultant tension pneumothorax, a needle thoracentesis should be performed immediately.

If a tension pneumothorax is identified this should be relieved immediately with a needle thoracentesis. A 16 g cannula is inserted into the second intercostal space in the mid-clavicular line. The release of air relieves the pressure within the chest, allowing time for a chest drain to be inserted to reinflate the lung.

In the event of massive haemothorax or pneumothorax, a chest drain should be inserted into the 4th–5th intercostal space just anterior to the mid-axillary line to drain the haemothorax. It is worth ensuring that venous access is secured at the same time. A haemothorax can be defined as massive if it is over 1.5 litres or collects at greater that 20 ml/h over a 4-hour period (American College of Surgeons, 1997).

Once any manoeuvre is performed which will affect ventilation, breathing should always be rechecked.

Circulation with haemorrhage control

Blood loss is the main cause of preventable death due to trauma. The most important vital signs indicating the state of the patient's circulation are the level of consciousness, skin colour and pulse (Hadfield-Law, 1999).

The brain does not compensate well and needs a constant supply of oxygen. In an attempt to increase oxygen to the brain, vasodilatation occurs; vasodilatation results in raised intracranial pressure. Therefore the first sign of shock may be a change in level of consciousness. This can vary from a slight sense of unease through to agitation, drowsiness and eventually loss of consciousness (Conley, 1998).

A grey face and white body is very suggestive of hypovolaemia. It is surprising how such an accessible and quickly measured vital sign can be missed when sophisticated equipment is now available.

A rise in pulse is another early compensatory mechanism. Most people will not suffer a drop in blood pressure until a rise in pulse and vasoconstriction have failed to adequately compensate. This will often not occur until at least 30% of the circulating blood is lost (American College of Surgeons, 1997).

If a pulse is absent, cardiac massage should begin. Equipment should be available for pericardiocentesis if cardiac tamponade has occurred and/or open or needle thoracentesis in cases of tension pneumothorax.

Any sources of external bleeding should be located as early as possible and stemmed. Although it may be tempting to attempt delicate procedures to stop bleeding, the application of direct pressure is quick and effective. In the resuscitation room, tourniquets tend only to be used when an affected limb is deemed unsalvageable, as tissue hypoxia resulting from their use can cause irreversible damage after only a very short time (Driscoll and Skinner, 1998).

Sources of internal bleeding should also be considered. Pelvic and long-bone fractures can result in irreversible hypovolaemic shock surprisingly quickly. Be aware of complications associated with the very fit, patients on beta blockers or with pacemakers, those under the age of 12 and over 70, and those in pain or hypothermic or who may mask signs of hypovolaemic shock.

By assuming all trauma patients have hypovolaemic shock, the trauma team can err on the side of caution and minimize morbidity and mortality. Some question the wisdom of giving large quantities of fluids to patients who may become overloaded; however, many more patients die of hypovolaemia as opposed to fluid overload (Anderson *et al.*, 1988).

By inserting two short wide-bore venous cannulae of at least 14–16 gauge, an initial fluid bolus of at least 2 litres may be given. For the hypovolaemic patient a blood transfusion is the best method of fluid replacement. Failing that, crystalloid solution such as Hartmann's, warmed to a temperature of 39°C will suffice. By administering this through a blood giving-set the infusion may be changed to a blood transfusion, with the minimum of delay, once blood is available. The rate of infusion is determined by the internal diameter of the cannula and not the size of the vein, and the rate slows as the cannula lengthens.

Two peripheral intravenous lines should be commenced in uninjured extremities, preferably upper limb. If insertion proves difficult, venous cutdown should be performed. The aim of fluid resuscitation is to restore adequate circulating blood volume and oxygen-carrying capacity.

A great deal of debate surrounds the issue of fluid replacement. Crystalloids, e.g. normal saline and Hartmann's solution, are cheaper than colloids such as Haemaccel and Gelofusin. Crystalloids are also considered more effective in restoring intravascular volume (Schierhout and Roberts, 1998). As indicated earlier, the most effective fluid of choice is blood, with its oxygen-carrying capacity.

Once the initial fluid bolus has been administered, if there is no response, a rapid blood transfusion should begin. Ideally, blood should be grouped and cross-matched. However, group-specific blood is adequate in the event of any delay, as the risk of reaction for the patient is relatively low. If the patient is seriously hypovolaemic, a transfusion of O negative blood should be given. A small supply of O negative blood stored in A&E will save valuable minutes for the most critically injured patients. The risks associated with such transfusions, of reactions and later difficulties with grouping and cross-matching, should be balanced against the risks of continued hypovolaemia.

While the circulatory status is being assessed and intravenous access established, a blood sample should be taken for the grouping and cross-matching of at least 6 units, a full blood count, a urea and electrolyte baseline and pregnancy test (in females of childbearing years). An arterial sample will also need to be taken for blood gas and pH analysis. However, this can wait until resuscitation is complete at the end of the primary survey.

By attaching the patient to a cardiac monitor, dysrhythmias may be identified which may indicate cardiac damage or hypothermia (American College of Surgeons, 1997). Electromechanical dissociation may be the result of cardiac tamponade, tension pneumothorax or hypovolaemia.

A urinary catheter should be inserted and attached to a urometer to provide accurate monitoring of urine output. This should only be done once contraindications have been considered:

- blood at the external urinary meatus
- scrotal haematoma (in men)
- perineal bruising.

all of which may indicate urethral damage. If damage is a possibility, a suprapubic catheter may be used. By maintaining a urinary output of 0.5 ml/kg/h the patient would be considered to be responding well to resuscitation (American College of Surgeons, 1997).

Vomiting and regurgitation is a serious risk to the patient and a nasogastric tube should be inserted to decompress the stomach. Blood-stained gastric contents may indicate damage. The passage of a tube carries some risk as it can induce vomiting, so insertion should be conducted carefully. Large particulate matter may be vomited around the tube. If a fracture of the cribriform plate is suspected, as in the case of Ann, any tube should be passed orally. A tube entering the nose under these circumstances may accidentally be passed into the cranium and should be avoided (American College of Surgeons, 1997).

Disability: assessment of neurological status

A rapid neurological assessment can be carried out by using the AVPU method to describe the level of consciousness. The patient should be asked to put her tongue out, wriggle her toes and to squeeze the assessor's fingers. A judgement can then be made about whether she is:

A Alert.
V Responding to **V**erbal stimuli.
P Responding to **P**ainful stimuli.
U Unresponsive to all stimuli.

Pupil size and reactivity must also be assessed.

A full Glasgow Coma Scale score is completed at this stage. Although this score is considered by some to be a crude measure of level of consciousness, a sequence of readings will tend to show fairly subtle changes quickly (Conley, 1998). A change in level of consciousness may be a sign of reduced perfusion or oxygenation of the brain, or it may be due to head injury. Certainly, any change must be carefully evaluated by checking and rechecking through the primary survey.

Even when there is evidence of alcohol or drug use, this should be disregarded as a possible cause of change in level of consciousness at this stage: 'No patient should be considered drunk until they have a hangover the next day' (Hadfield-Law, 1999).

Exposure/environmental control

Once the primary survey is completed and all life-threatening injuries have been identified and dealt with, the patient should be undressed completely. By leaving the patient lying on her back, the team are only able to examine the front half of the body. This is often an appropriate point at which to log-roll the patient onto her side, to assess her back. Life-threatening injuries are occasionally missed when teams leave this crucial assessment until the end of the secondary survey. Some patients, particularly adolescents and some from ethnic minorities, can be particularly self-conscious when their bodies are exposed. Every effort should be made to help the patient retain as much dignity as possible under these difficult circumstances.

Four members of the team are required to turn the patient and an additional member should have their hands free to examine the patient properly, remove any debris from under her and consider performing a rectal examination.

The team member who takes control of the patient's head and neck should take control of instructing the team. Before anyone touches the patient the procedure should be explained to her, even if she does not appear fully conscious. Once all four pairs of turners' hands are appropriately placed, she can be confidently and swiftly turned on her side.

Hypothermia poses a significant threat to the trauma patient. Many of them have been exposed to the elements and are unable to move. Blood loss further contributes to a drop in core temperature. Hypothermia has been associated with increases in morbidity and mortality and should be prevented if possible and reversed quickly once it occurs.

Once the patient enters the resuscitation room the team have responsibility for keeping her as warm as possible. Patients lying exposed on trolleys will lose heat very quickly. To maintain or increase core temperature (Hadfield-Law, 1999):

- place warm, dry blankets from a warming cabinet, radiator or even a microwave over the patient
- make sure intravenous fluids, including blood and any lavage fluids, are warmed to at least 39°C
- maintain reasonably high environmental temperatures in the resuscitation area
- suspend specially designed radiation plates over the patient trolley
- apply an external warming device, e.g. Behr Hugger.

X-rays should not interfere with the progress of resuscitation. However, cervical spine, chest and pelvic films can provide useful information.

Full history

By taking a careful history of the trauma incident and the patient's past medical and social history, the team are in a better position to plan their care. The best source of information is the patient, if they are conscious and can remember what happened. If not, paramedics, witnesses to the incident and relatives can provide missing pieces of information.

To plan care appropriately, it is necessary to take an AMPLE history:

A Allergies.
M Medications.
P Past illnesses or operations and pregnancy.
L Last meal or drink – important when considering the security of the airway.

E Events preceding the injury.

By understanding what happened leading up to the incident, not only can we plan appropriate care for the patient, but we can gather valuable data for accident prevention. Other important details include tetanus status, date of last period in women, the patient's approximate height and weight and the geographical location of the incident.

By carefully noting the place, we can help to communicate clear information to relatives and police to avoid unnecessary confusion.

Details regarding the mechanism of injury can help us predict the site and seriousness of a number of injuries. This can save a great deal of time and may save the trauma patient's life. Many paramedic crews now take polaroid pictures at the scene of an incident which can then be examined by trauma teams in the hospital.

Table 11.1 summarizes the primary survey and resuscitation procedures.

Table 11.1 Key to the primary survey and resuscitation

Secure and maintain an airway
Stabilize cervical spine
Assess and treat any problems with breathing and ventilation
Assess circulatory condition
Control external haemorrhage
Insert two large-bore peripheral cannulae
Send blood sample for analysis
Assess conscious level
Establish supportive relationship
Remove all clothes
Cover and keep warm
Record observations every 5 minutes
Log-roll
Insert catheter and gastric tube

Secondary survey

Once the primary survey is completed and the patient has been successfully resuscitated the secondary survey can begin. The patient must be stable before moving on and each step of the primary survey should be repeated until stability is achieved (American College of Surgeons, 1997). Less obvious injuries are identified during the secondary survey, but such injuries

may still pose a threat to life. The entire surface of the body should have been examined by the end of the secondary survey. A full set of vital signs should be recorded at this point including a temperature. Tympanic membrane is the route of choice, which provides a swift and reasonably accurate temperature measurement (Hadfield-Law, 1994a). The trauma team can detect the early signs of shock in patients, with a raise in pulse and respiration and a fall in blood pressure. If the same team member takes vital signs every 5 minutes, subtle changes should be noted more readily.

Head

Starting at the top, the patient should be examined for any evidence of injury to the bones, soft tissues, mouth or eyes and asked about pain. Any discharge from the nose or ears should be noted, and tested to check for the presence of cerebrospinal fluid following a basal skull fracture. If the team needs to remove spinal immobilization devices to examine the patient properly, then manual in-line immobilization must be maintained.

In cases like Ann's, despite extensive facial injuries, a complete eye examination should be performed if possible, including visual acuity and pupillary response

Neck

While continuing to maintain safe spinal immobilization, the neck should be examined for injury. Such injury will alert the team to the possibility of impending airway obstruction. The patient should be checked for deviation of the trachea from the midline or distended neck veins which could indicate tension pneumothorax or cardiac tamponade (American College of Surgeons, 1997). Cervical spine injury should only be ruled out once a full set of cervical spine X-rays have been reviewed by a doctor experienced in detecting such injuries. Patients who arrive in A&E on a spine board should be transferred from the board as soon as possible to prevent the development of pressure sores (Cooke, 1998). Spine boards are designed to keep the patient immobile only until they arrive in A&E.

Any lacerations should be inspected, but should never be probed with instruments or fingers in case further damage results.

Chest

Ask the patient about pain or difficulty in breathing. Is there any obvious injury, subcutaneous emphysema, bruising or pain over the ribs? Remember that all chests have a back to them, and this should have been examined during the log-roll at the end of the primary survey (Tippett, 1993).

Listening to the chest can be difficult in a noisy resuscitation room, but can be very useful. Distant heart sounds and narrow pulse pressure can indicate cardiac tamponade. This may cause distended neck veins, which may also suggest tension pneumothorax. However, hypovolaemia can mask this sign. Tension pneumothorax may have occurred where decreased breath sounds, hyper-resonance and signs of shock are present. This requires immediate decompression (American College of Surgeons, 1997).

In addition to cardiac monitoring, a 12-lead electrocardiograph should indicate any cardiac damage. Pulmonary and cardiac contusions are potentially life-threatening and should be considered when the chest wall has received a significant direct blow. Ann is a powerful example of what happens when there is a collision between the driver's chest and a steering wheel following a road traffic accident. She sustained a fractured sternum, several fractured ribs, a fractured and displaced clavicle and a pneumothorax.

Abdomen

The most important aspect of assessing the abdomen is to determine whether the patient requires surgery or not. Does the patient have any pain, obvious injury, distension, rigidity, guarding, contusions or scars? Does she have bowel sounds? This part of the examination must be carried out very carefully as life-threatening hypovolaemia is frequently caused by intra-abdominal damage. Re-evaluation is essential, particularly in the case of blunt abdominal trauma, and changes may occur over time (American College of Surgeons, 1997).

If diagnostic peritoneal lavage (DPL) is to be performed, a gastric tube and urinary catheter must always be inserted first. This way abdominal and pelvic organs are at reduced risk of damage. DPL is a reliable and swift investigation to determine intra-abdominal bleeding. It is a valuable test when physical examination is difficult or the results are equivocal. The surgeon likely to take the patient to theatre should always be present during this procedure.

Pelvis and genitalia

Does the patient have pain, the urge to pass urine, bruising or blood at the urethral meatus, or priapism? Is there bruising or swelling and are femoral pulses present? Pelvic fractures can be devastating for patients and are too often the cause of death from hypovolaemia.

A rectal examination should have been performed when the patient was log-rolled at the end of the primary survey. The examiner should check for blood in the rectum which may indicate damage to the intestine or pelvis. High-riding prostate may be the result of urethral injury, and a loss of anal sphincter tone can indicate spinal injury. In women, a vaginal examination revealing blood and lacerations results either from direct damage or pelvic fractures. The pelvis should not be 'sprung' by applying pressure to the iliac crests as this can be extremely painful and can cause further damage and haemorrhage (American College of Surgeons, 1997).

Extremities

Each arm and leg should be examined and assessed for:

- pain
- colour
- pulse
- paraesthesia
- paralysis
- cold
- perspiration
- instability
- crepitus.

Any injury discovered should be realigned and immobilized. Each time a limb is moved it should be reassessed. Open wounds should be covered with a sterile dry dressing.

Injuries to the hands, wrists and feet are often missed in A&E. These can cause significant disability for patients in the future and should be managed carefully and correctly from the beginning.

Different team members may need to examine open fractures. By taking a polaroid photograph of the wound before it is covered, the number of times the dressing needs to be removed will be reduced, which should limit the incidence of contamination (Hadfield-Law, 1999).

Very careful attention must be paid to prevention of pressure sores. Trauma patients are particularly vulnerable and plans to protect the skin should be made as early as possible.

Analgesia

Relief of pain can be forgotten during the activity of resuscitation; however, it is an essential part of good care. Intravenous opiates are usually most effective, in titrated doses. Intramuscular routes should be avoided as muscles may well not be perfused and therefore analgesia will not be absorbed. Entonox can be very useful in the initial stages until the primary survey is complete.

If the patient's condition starts to deteriorate during the secondary survey, the team should return to the beginning of the primary survey.

Paediatrics

Trauma in children can be a frightening prospect for everyone concerned. However, the principles for managing children are exactly the same as in adults, but it is essential that paediatric specialists join the trauma team at this time. Priorities for assessment and management are exactly the same. In a child over 1 year, a urinary output of 1 ml/kg/h should be expected. We should aim for 2 ml/kg/h in children under 1 year. For those who have had limited experience with children, the main differences lie with their anatomy, physiology and emotional development (American College of Surgeons, 1997).

Due to the different size and shape of the child, mechanisms of injury tend to be different with an increased susceptibility to multiple injuries. Children's bones are much more pliable, which means they tend to bend rather than break, allowing damage to structures beneath. Hypothermia is a significant risk due to the high ratio between body surface area and volume. Psychosocial aspects of care are particularly important in children as they have not had the experience to develop emotional coping strategies. If possible, someone familiar to the child should be available to them throughout the golden hour (Reynolds and Ramenofsky, 1988).

Definitive care

Once the patient has been adequately assessed and successfully resuscitated she can be moved to the next stage of care. Such care can be delivered in a number of different areas including general wards, other specialist hospitals, the intensive care unit or the operating theatre. It is essential that the patient reaches the best possible condition before transfer either within the hospital or to another facility. Patients are particularly vulnerable during these transfers as they are more difficult to monitor and facilities are limited. Equipment should be carried by the team accompanying the patient, in case of sudden deterioration. When identifying the most appropriate personnel to accompany the patient, the team leader should anticipate the ways in which the patient might deteriorate *en route*. A team member who is able to deal with such events should do the transfer.

Copies of all documentation should be maintained for the patient and should accompany her to wherever she goes. If one member of the trauma team assumes responsibility for recording all data, gaps in information will be avoided. Preprinted trauma sheets can be useful to save time and to act as an *aidé mémoir*. Good documentation is an essential part of patient safety, effective communication, risk management and retrospective audit (Harrahill, 1997).

Family and friends

Friends and family should be kept carefully informed of events. If staff with resuscitation skills are required in the resuscitation room, other members of the hospital team can be called for assistance such as the chaplain or social worker. If staff who are likely to be caring for the patient later on in their hospital stay are available, a valuable and supportive relationship can be started in A&E, either with the patient herself or her family.

Friends and relatives are an important source of information and their inclusion in trauma team efforts will be beneficial to both the patient and their loved ones. There is good evidence to suggest that the bereavement process is eased if a partner or relative witnesses the resuscitation (Mitchell and Lynch, 1997). Relatives could be offered the opportunity to witness resuscitation if staff training and the establishment is geared towards their presence in these circumstances (Barratt and Wallis, 1998).

Conclusion

It is during the golden hour that trauma patients who have survived the initial minutes following an event can be particularly at risk. The patient needs rapid assessment to identify injuries, both actual and potential, and timely resuscitation. A systematic approach will ensure that no injury is missed, minimizing the risks to this vulnerable group.

In the past, multiply-injured patients have died from reasonably easily treated problems such as lack of oxygen and circulating blood volume. The last decade has seen a raising of awareness among those concerned with this group of patients. We know what needs to be done, we know how to reduce morbidity and mortality, but trauma teams need to be available and appropriately trained.

Some centres have developed new roles in an attempt to continue to improve trauma systems cost-effectively (Holmquist *et al.*, 1996). However, these initiatives have still to be evaluated.

Lack of appropriately trained staff remains a problem when trying to plan the expert care required for multiply-injured patients attending A&E departments. Training is available, but not accessible to all those involved in trauma care, due to limitations of funding (Hadfield-Law, 1994b).

The price of trauma is high, not just in terms of money, but in terms of human suffering. Investment in training to prepare for the golden hour is not a luxury, but a necessity. A great deal of progress has been made in the field of trauma in recent years, particularly concerning the golden hour. However, 'even if you are on the right track, you will get run over if you just sit there'.

Postcript

Six months after the crash, Ann is doing very well physically. She had multiple facial fractures with extensive soft tissue injury. These have all healed well, and although she does not look quite the same as before the accident, she remains as physically attractive, with no visible scars. She has recovered fully from her chest injuries. Her fractured clavicle has been internally fixed, and is functional and comfortable.

Ann has suffered from debilitating headaches since the accident and finds it difficult to leave the house unaccompanied without suffering from panic attacks. It is the panic attacks which have prevented her from returning to work and to her normal lifestyle. She is seeing a behavioural psychologist to try to speed up her recovery.

References

American College of Surgeons Committee on Trauma (1997) ATLS. *Student Course Manual.* ACSCT.

Anderson, I. D., Woodford, M., de Dombal, F. T. and Miles Irving (1988) Retrospective study of 100 trauma deaths from injury in England and Wales. *British Medical Journal*, **296**, 1305–1308.

Barratt, F. and Wallis, D. N. (1998) Relatives in the resuscitation room: their point of view. *Journal of Accident and Emergency Medicine*, **15**, 109–111.

Bisson, J. I., Jenkins, P. L., Alexander, J., and Bannister, C. (1997) Randomised controlled trial of psychological debriefing for victims of acute burn trauma. *British Journal of Psychiatry*, **171**, 78–81.

Conley, R. L. (1998) Head Injury. In *The Comprehensive Curriculum for Trauma Nursing.* Emergency Nurses Association.

Cooke, M. W. (1998) Use of the spinal board within the accident and emergency department. *Journal of Accident and Emergency Medicine*, **15**, 108–109.

Cowley, R. A. (1976) The resuscitation and stabilisation of major multiple trauma patients in a trauma care environment. *Clinical Medicine*, **83**, 14.

Cudmore, J. E. (1996) Trauma nursing: the team approach. *British Journal of Nursing*, **5**(12), 736–753.

Driscoll, P. A. and Brook, S. (1993) Resuscitation and stabilisation of the severely injured patient. In *Trauma Resuscitation: The Team Approach.* McMillan.

Driscoll, P. and Skinner, D. (1998) *Trauma Care – Beyond the Resuscitation Room.* BMJ Books.

Driscoll, P. A. and Vincent, C. A. (1992a) Organising an efficient trauma team. *Injury*, **23**(2), 107–110.

Driscoll, P. A. and Vincent, C. A. (1992b) Variation in trauma resuscitation and it's effect on patient outcome.

Injury, **23**(2), 111–119.

Hadfield-Law, L. V. (1994a) Review of tympanic membrane thermometry. *Accident & Emergency Nursing*, **2**, 57–58.

Hadfield-Law, L. V. (1994b) The development of trauma education for A&E nurses in the UK. In *Issues in Accident and Emergency Nursing* (L. Sbaih, ed.). Chapman and Hall.

Hadfield-Law, L. V. (1999) *Advanced Trauma Nursing Course Manual*. Oxford ATNC Committee.

Hadfield-Law, L. V., Kent, A. and McNulty, L. (2000) The role of the trauma nurse. In Skinner D., Driscoll, P. and Earlam, R. *ABC of Major Trauma. British Medical Journal*.

Harrahill, M. (1997) Strategies for improving trauma documentation. *Journal of Emergency Nursing*, **23**(2), 187–188.

Holmquist, P. J, Yamamoto, L., Didonna, D. and Sise, M. J. (1996) Nursing role innovations: improved outcomes in a trauma centre. *Nursing Economics*. **14**(6), 357–365.

Lomas, G. A. and Goodall, O. (1994) Trauma teams versus non-trauma teams. *Accident and Emergency Nursing*, **2**, 205–210.

McSwain, N. E. Jr, Paturas, J. L. and Wertz, E. (1994) *Prehospital Trauma Life Support – Advanced*. Mosby Yearbook.

Mitchell, M. H. and Lynch, M. B. (1997) Should relatives be allowed in the resuscitation room? *Journal of Accident and Emergency Medicine*, **14**, 366–369.

Reynolds, E. A. and Ramenofsky, M. L. (1988) The emotional impact of trauma on toddlers. *Maternal, Child, Nurse*, **13**, 106–109.

Schierhout, G. and Roberts, I. (1998) Fluid resuscitation with colloid or crystalloid solutions in critically ill patients: a systematic review of randomised trials. *British Medical Journal*, **316**, 961–964.

Tippett, J. (1993) Spinal immobilisation of the multiply injured patient. *Accident and Emergency Nursing*, **1**(1), 25–33.

12

Principles of trauma care in intensive care

Maureen Coombs and Ann Dillon

Background

The trauma patient admitted into the intensive care unit (ICU) is at risk of developing complications as a direct result of their primary injuries. These complications, as a result of infection and multisystem organ failure, contribute to the deaths occurring within the third phase of the trimodal distribution of mortality following trauma (Trunkey, 1983).

Eighty per cent of all trauma fatalities will have occurred at the scene of the incident or in the accident and emergency department (Neff and Kidd, 1993). The remaining fatalities occur approximately 3–4 weeks post-injury. The goal for the healthcare practitioner therefore is to provide an organized approach to care with preventative and supportive measures to minimize complications and ultimately reduce the risk of mortality. Maximal support for the patient, family and loved ones during this stressful time can be optimized when goals are based on agreed and coordinated treatment protocols delivered within a focused and collaborative team approach.

The aim of this chapter is to focus on the needs of the adult trauma patient while they are in the intensive care environment. To help apply theory to practice, brief illustrations from practice will be presented and discussion of care will be explored within the main text of this chapter. The broader issues of resourcing, healthcare costs and ethical dilemmas arising from instigation of trauma care will be highlighted and the challenge for practitioners explored as issues arise during the chapter.

Introduction

The nature of intensive care is to provide 'one-to-one nursing' 24 hours a day (National Health Service Executive, 1996); this environment allows intensive monitoring of the respiratory and cardiovascular systems of the trauma patient. To inform this care, communication between the intensive care team and the emergency personnel regarding primary assessment, resuscitation and retrieval are vital to the management of ongoing problems and the anticipation of potential problems.

Proactive care planning can be optimized through an understanding of:

- how the injuries were sustained (e.g. road traffic accident, assault, gunshot)
- the type of energy released (e.g. kinetic, thermal, chemical)
- the force involved (e.g. speed at impact, height of fall, head-on, lateral)
- the use of any protective devices (e.g. seatbelts, airbags, helmets)

Case study

Mr Turner is admitted to ICU following a high-speed road traffic accident (RTA). He was the driver of the car and was wearing his seatbelt. What specific injuries will this patient be at risk of?

Discussion. Mr Turner's assessment should include a thorough review, with anticipation of

---

> pelvic injury from lap restraint and cervical fracture from shoulder restraint. An unrestrained driver would risk patella, head, facial and larynx fractures. Such information can form an outline of the potential problems Mr Turner may sustain.

High-impact forces such as the following lead to more severe injuries (Neff and Kidd, 1993):

- falls over 6 m
- high road speeds (cars > 40 miles per hour (mph), motorcycles > 20 mph, pedestrians > 5 mph
- space intrusion above 30 cm
- rollover or ejection from vehicle.

Throughout all stages of care accurate communication and documentation should be maintained. The increasing use of computerized patient information management systems, especially when linked between departments, may improve the process of care (Gross, 1995). Handover between all team members needs to be precise and needs to cover all pertinent issues (Table 12.1).

Table 12.1 Important handover details

Name, age and home address

Any pre-existing medical conditions or allergies

Nature and mechanism of injury and details of other casualties

Time of accident and length of extrication

Concern regarding intoxicants or drugs involved

Time of last meal (if known)

Significant events, e.g. period of respiratory or cardiac arrest

Status of spinal clearance and time on backboard if spine uncleared

Details of injuries, procedures performed and instructions for positioning

Access lines and drains present

Fluid status (crystalloid/colloid/output) and blood status

Update on vital signs

Tetanus immunization status

Location of property

Details and location of family

Police details, if involved

Information regarding the need for special equipment, such as spinal beds, should be discussed early with the emergency staff. If possible, this should be prior to transfer to the ICU in order to allow any necessary arrangements to be made. To maintain continuity of care and to prevent the loss of vital baseline information, handover of the patient between accident and emergency staff to ICU staff must be thorough. A trauma chart (Figure 12.1), allowing documentation and charting of all patient injuries, is helpful in subsequent patient handovers and a useful adjunct to planning future care needs.

Equally important in the handover of the patient is information regarding the care of relatives and friends. The move from the emergency room to the ICU can cause further distress for the relatives. Introduction of the intensive care nurse and team by the emergency nurse may help towards establishing and building a relationship of trust. This is important to help the relatives feel supported and respected during their loved one's time in the ICU.

The recent demand on intensive care beds has exceeded supply, receiving a wide coverage in the national press (Craven, 1999). Additionally, a shortage in specially educated intensive care nurses has led in some units to the closure of intensive care beds. These events also occur against a backdrop of increased pressure on ward staff to manage higher dependency patients while striving to meet government waiting list targets. The use of independent agencies, such as the Emergency Bed Service, to locate the nearest intensive care bed if one is not locally available has meant that the process of care may not run as smoothly and therapeutically as described above. It is into this political arena that many healthcare professions must consider entering if such resourcing issues are ever to be resolved.

However, once the patient is settled into an intensive care bed, it is important that a comprehensive treatment plan is formulated to continue the process of care delivery. Current emergency room practice advocates the use of the Advanced Trauma Life Support as a framework for patient assessment. This provides a useful framework for initial assessment and planning within the ICU environment and this chapter will therefore outline the care required based around this framework.

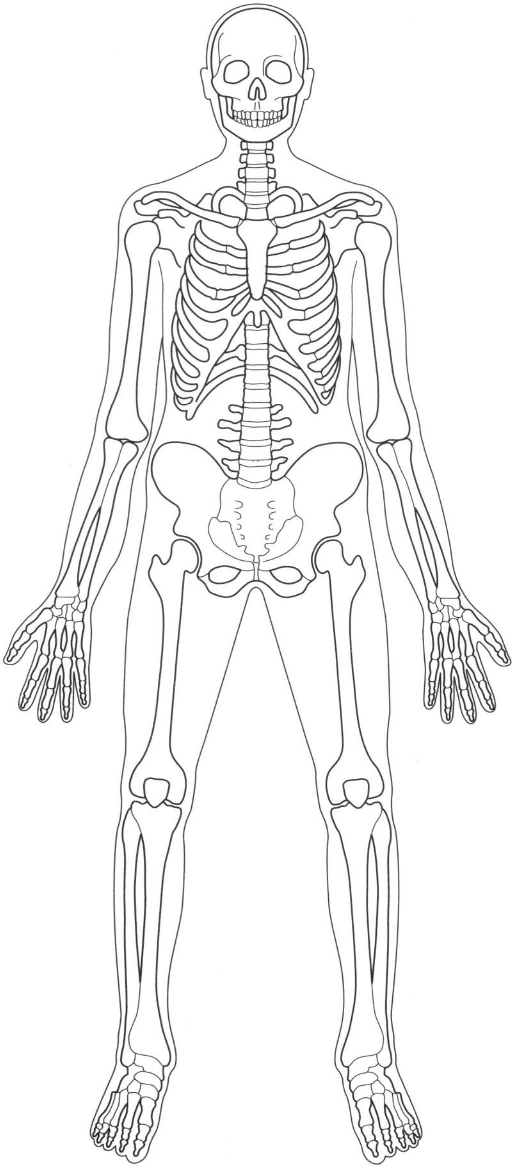

Patient
Name: ....

Date of Admission: ....

Time of Admission: .... hrs

Admitted from:

☐ A&E

☐ Theatres

☐ Other (specify)

Type of Accident:

Motor Vehicle: Motor Cycle:

Pedal Cycle: Pedestrian:

Burns: Sports:

Other:

GCS

☐ At Scene

☐ In A&E

History of Accident:

Spinal Clearance

	Yes/No	Method	Date
Cervical			
Thoraco			
Lumbar			

Fractured bones should be
shaded – specify left or right

Figure 12.1   Bone injuries trauma chart

Management of airway and spine

As outlined earlier, admission to the ICU usually indicates that airway management has been, or remains, a problem. The majority of patients admitted to intensive care will have been orally or nasally intubated. Patients with major facial trauma or oedema with respiratory failure will require nasal intubation or, in extreme cases, a tracheostomy. Patients with suspected basal skull fractures must not be nasally intubated and must only have an orogastric tube placed.

In addition to routine airway management procedures, further precautions must be taken with the trauma patient with an uncleared cervical spine. The cervical area is the most vulnerable part of the spine due to the relative heaviness and mobility of the head which is supported by weak muscles. Accidents involving hyperflexion from head-on collisions and lateral flexion from lateral impacts can cause more serious damage than hyperextension. For patients with radiologically uncleared spines, intubation must be undertaken with in-line mobilization either manually or with the use of a collar or sandbags.

Further details regarding airway management and spinal clearance are covered in the chapters on the emergency department. Spinal clearance in unconscious and intubated patients is difficult and criteria will vary throughout units. X-rays that can be undertaken to reveal the lower cervical spine include:

- cross-table lateral cervical spine
- normal lateral
- normal anterior posterior
- transoral odontoid
- computerized tomography scan.

Practitioners are referred to local unit policy regarding this issue to ensure safe practice is delivered.

Management of breathing and ventilation

Respiratory management of the trauma patient in the ICU can range from the self-ventilating patient recovering from emergency trauma surgery to the patient requiring a high level of mechanical support and ventilation. Patients may require long-term ventilation as a result of the following (Bradley, 1987):

- underlying respiratory disease
- severe aspiration during the accident
- severe pneumonia
- adult respiratory distress syndrome (ARDS) due to severe lung contusion
- fat embolism
- blood transfusion
- sepsis

Direct trauma to the lungs can lead to difficult and protracted ventilation. Multiple rib fractures can lead to flail chest with a high risk of sputum retention and atelectasis. In the absence of spinal damage or coagulopathy, an epidural can promote good respiratory function and provide analgesia, thereby minimizing the risk of intubation.

Case study

Sally was a motorcycle rider involved in an RTA. She was in collision with a car, thrown off her bike and onto the car's bonnet. Among other injuries she sustained fractured ribs on the left 1–6. She was self-ventilating on 80% oxygen. Two hours following admission she became tachypnoeic, anxious and complained of shortness of breath. On auscultation there was no bronchospasm, but no breath sounds could be heard on the left lung. What potential problems and actions should be considered?

Discussion. Twenty per cent of all rib fractures are associated with a haemothorax and 25% with a pneumothorax. A haemothorax of less than 250 ml does not cause problems for the patient, but a haemothorax greater than 1500 ml will cause tracheal deviation with ventilatory management problems (White and Kenner, 1992). This requires draining through a chest drain. Sally should be positioned upright and if arterial blood gases demonstrate a drop in oxygenation, increased oxygen should be administered and medical assistance sought. Respiratory distress is very frightening both to experience and to see, and Sally should be comforted, kept calm and informed. This may necessitate one person sitting with her while another informs the doctor and prepares for possible chest x-ray or chest drain insertion.

Modern mechanical ventilators now provide a wide range of ventilatory support that include sophisticated weaning modes. Where severe lung injury is present, prone positioning has been demonstrated to improve oxygenation (Richardson, 1997); however, the need for safety and team coordination in this manoeuvre is paramount. The input of the physiotherapist to help clear secretions and reinflate collapsed lung areas is essential in this aspect of care. It is important that the nurse and physiotherapist work in close collaboration to coordinate care. Regular sputum specimens must be taken to detect any new bacterial growth to ensure appropriate antibiotics are prescribed. Prolonged intubation (greater than 7 days) may require tracheostomy to reduce respiratory effort and increase patient comfort. This procedure can, for the majority of patients, be performed on the ICU using a percutaneous approach and prevents transfer of the patient to theatre.

Patients with severe lung injury who are unable to tolerate physiotherapy with posturing may benefit from the use of special kinetic therapy beds, which allow posturing without incurring cardiovascular instability. A range of special beds for patients with or without spinal injury are now commercially available. It is important that if these beds are used regularly, costing is built into the non-pay budget.

Patients are often transferred to the ward when their cardiovascular and respiratory systems have been stabilized. The next stage in the recovery process is to the high-dependency unit, if this facility is available. This allows a gradual adjustment to a less critical environment to be made, while still being closely observed. During this time both the patient and relatives can adapt to a different environment. However, transfer to a ward may be the only option. Only with careful planning and communication with the patient and family will the ward nursing staff feel informed and equipped to manage. The development of high-dependency units (HDUs) and the use of intensive care beds remains a resource issue in the National Health Service (Edbrooke, 1996). While HDUs are more expensive in terms of nurse staffing in comparison with ward areas, these units provide both a 'step down' unit from the ICU and a 'step up' unit from the wards, potentially averting a readmission to ICU. The financial investment required to create and sustain these units remains a topic for debate.

Cardiovascular and temperature management

Management of cardiovascular instability requires timely and accurate assessment by all members of the healthcare team. This data is obtained both from technology and monitoring, as well as from the use of touch and sight in patient assessment. Changes in capillary refill and warmth of peripheries may indicate poor fluid resuscitation or ongoing fluid loss.

Blood loss in trauma is often underestimated. A loss of up to 4.5 litres following pelvic fracture is not uncommon, frequently accumulating in the retroperitoneal space. One to two litres can be lost following humeral or femoral fractures. This is compounded by the fact that hypotension may not be noted until 20–30% of the circulating volume is lost (Ihde *et al.*, 1987). Adequate central and peripheral access with large-bore cannulae is important and has often been established in the emergency department. Some clinical points to consider during fluid replacement are outlined in Table 12.2. If aggressive fluid management is required, insertion of a pulmonary artery catheter may be considered to measure left-sided cardiac function and filling pressures.

Table 12.2 Pointers for fluid replacement

Avoid the use of Ringer's lactate with blood as this precipitates out the ionized calcium in the blood – normal saline 0.9% is the fluid of choice

Stored blood has a high potassium level with decreased ionized calcium stores and may affect the electrolyte balance

If emergency blood is required, O negative blood is stored in most emergency departments

Consider the use of autotransfusion, which will reduce the risks of coagulopathy and disseminated intravascular coagulation associated with massive blood transfusion

Use the patient's haemoglobin and haematocrit to guide colloid and crystalloid in fluid resuscitation

Trauma can lead to vascular and peripheral nerve damage resulting, for example, from an open fracture. Neurovascular assessment is

Case study

Mary was a front seat passenger involved in a head-on, high-speed RTA. On admission to the unit vital signs were monitored and she was noted to have multifocal ventricular ectopics greater than 6 per minute. Her serum potassium was 4.5 mmol/l. On closer examination she had marked bruising across her chest from the seat belt. What should be considered in Mary's care plan?

Discussion. Direct cardiac injury can result from trauma. In blunt acceleration/deceleration injury the heart muscle is injured by compression of the heart between the sternum and the vertebra, and bruising of the tissue or cardiac rupture occurs as a result of raised intracardiac and abdominal pressures. Cardiac contusion

can also occur in head-on trauma or from the impact of the steering wheel. Sudden or new onset angina post-injury, precordial bruising, sternal fracture or dysrhythmias should be regarded with a high degree of suspicion as they usually indicate cardiac injury. A repeat 12-lead electrocardiogram should be carried out, blood pressure readings should be taken in both arms (suspicion of aortic dissection) and close cardiovascular observation for cardiac rupture or tamponade is necessary. Urgent discussions with the medical staff will ascertain whether further referral or advice from the cardiac specialists is required.

important, including checks on the circulation, sensation and motor power. Local skin trauma and soft tissue assessment should be made for the five Ps:

1. Pain.
2. Pulselessness.
3. Pallor.
4. Paraesthesia.
5. Paralysis.

These assessments must be documented and any deterioration reported immediately to the medical team.

Patients who have experienced a prolonged extraction from their vehicle or a prolonged resuscitation are often hypothermic on admission to the ICU. While hypothermia may offer some protection from tissue and cellular da-

mage, it can cause cardiac rhythm disturbances and shivering, thereby increasing tissue oxygen demands. Cautious warming should be achieved through use of space or warming blankets and warming of intravenous fluids.

Patients may become pyrexial as a result of an inflammatory reaction to injury, surgery, or blood transfusion. Pyrexia with raised white cell count indicates infection. A full sepsis screen should be undertaken and surgical intervention or administration of appropriate antibiotics may be required.

The incidence of nosocomial infection rises with the increasing severity of injury in conjunction with the number of clinical procedures. If the patient has been in hospital for more than 5 days, the incidence of a hospital-acquired infection is high. The signs of infection, together with the cellular sequelae of cellular and tissue hypoxia, may precipitate the development of systemic inflammatory response syndrome (SIRS) and sepsis syndrome. This can necessitate intensive monitoring and inotropic support.

Minimizing neurological damage

Neurological problems can result from trauma due to direct injury to the cranium or brain structures, e.g. intracranial haematoma (Table 12.3) and secondarily due to changes in the brain structure as a result of cerebral oedema.

Table 12.3 Types of intracranial haematoma

Extradural haematoma resulting from a temporal linear fracture lacerating the middle meningeal artery

Subdural haematoma resulting from a (usually) venous bleed between the dura and arachnoid. The older patient is particularly at risk due to a decrease in brain size with an increase in the dura – skull space

Subarachnoid haematoma seen over the convexities of the brain

Intracerebral haematoma seen as small, localized or generalized punctuate bleeds

In severe brain damage brainstem death may result. The patient will subsequently undergo a series of brainstem tests which indicate irreversable brain damage. The issue of organ donation will then be raised with the next of kin prior to the withdrawal of ventilatory support. This is a very sensitive aspect of care, requiring support from local transplant coordinators (Franklin *et al.*, 1996). The care and support required by all during this time is crucial.

The skull is a rigid container affording limited capacity for changes in volume as measured by increased intracranial pressure (ICP). ICP can be directly monitored through use of an ICP bolt or fibreoptic catheter (normal value < 10 mmHg) and indirectly monitored through frequent neurological observations using the Glasgow Coma Scale (Smith, 1994). Cerebral perfusion pressure (CPP) (derived from ICP, mean arterial and central venous pressures) can then be calculated and used in directing patient treatment. In some centres, jugular venous oximetry (normal value is 54–75%) is undertaken via a catheter placed in the jugular venous bulb, just below the base of the skull. This is perceived as a more accurate means of assessing cerebral perfusion and requires specialist equipment and specific actions in the care of the patient. Jugular venous oximetry below 54% and CPP below 55 mmHg suggest hypoperfusion, and requires increased perfusion pressure through titrating a noradrenaline infusion once the patient is normovolaemic.

Neurosurgical treatment options can resolve surgically recoverable problems. Medical treatment options, offered as standard in intensive care, include the administration of up to 1 g/kg mannitol to reduce brain tissue volume, and effective patient assessment includes the use of sedation scoring systems for pain, anxiety and fear, together with the effective use of analgesics, sedatives and muscle relaxants. If these options do not reduce a high ICP, then a barbiturate coma can be commenced (Eisenberg *et al.*, 1988). Previously, the standard practice was towards hyperventilation in the head-injured patient. However, more recent work indicates that this may result in a further reduction in cerebral blood flow where intracranial hypertension is not the result of cerebral vasodilatation. Ventilation should therefore be guided by local unit policy. Hypothermia has been shown to confer some protection from cerebral ischaemic damage, although as yet this is not part of standard intensive care therapy.

The presence of rhinorrhoea and otorrhoea must be reported as these indicate dural tears as a consequence of possible basal skull fractures. A simple dry dressing can be used to cover the area. Similarly, periorbital bruising or 'panda eyes' may indicate anterior fossa injury. Such signs therefore indicate specific injuries which need closer assessment.

Case study

John was involved in an RTA while riding a motorbike and sustained a severe head injury. He was intubated, ventilated and fully sedated. A subdural bolt was inserted to manage his intracranial pressure more effectively. His ICP had been steady at 12 mmHg, but 10 minutes after tracheal suctioning his ICP remained at 21 mmHg. What actions should be taken?

Discussion. After any care it is important that the ICP returns to baseline within 5 minutes. Immediate checks should include assessment of the patient's level of sedation, with increase in sedation if required. Neurological observations should be repeated to ensure that in John's case the elevation is not a reflection of ongoing raised ICP requiring mannitol or further interventions. The patient's head should be checked to ensure it is in neutral position and the head of the bed should be elevated to 30 degrees (Feldman *et al.*, 1992). Any obstruction around the neck area, e.g. endotracheal tube ties or cervical collar, should be appropriately loosened and further tracheal suctioning should be limited to two suction catheters only (10 seconds in each 60 seconds), allowing 60 seconds of 100% oxygen after each suction attempt (Mitchell *et al.*, 1992). These events should then be incorporated into the patient's care plan and documented.

Renal and nutrition management

Renal management in intensive care is focused on the injuries resulting directly from renal trauma and those resulting from low cardiac output due to ineffective fluid resuscitation or comorbidity of cardiac disease. Structurally, the kidneys are well protected and blunt renal trauma is often due to compression of the kidney against the lumbar spine by the twelfth rib. Hollow organs (e.g. stomach and bladder) are compressible when force is applied, so are less likely to rupture. Bladder injury is therefore more likely when it is distended, i.e. after excessive drinking or after the fourth month of pregnancy when the bladder rises above the umbilicus and is less protected.

Renal assessment not only includes the quantity of urine produced against input and observation of renal chemistry (urea and creatinine and potassium), but also the colour and appearance of the urine produced. Signs of haematuria need early discussion with the medical team regarding subsequent management. Clinical tests may include abdominal CT scan and intravenous pyelogram. Myoglobinuria, associated with severe crush injuries, may also cause haematuria. Confirmation of this is through laboratory electrophoresis of a urine specimen. Treatment is then directed towards forced diuresis with volume loading, diuretics and possible alkalinization of the urine. In the ICU most patients have urinary catheterization for close monitoring of renal function and output. It should be noted that in suspected urethral damage, suprapubic catheterization should occur.

In a hypercatabolic state, post-injury, the commencement of a feeding regimen is recommended as early as possible. However, injury may hinder enteral feeding. Within the abdominal cavity, the spleen (particularly vulnerable to lower left rib fractures), liver (lower right rib fractures) and colon are closest to the abdominal wall and are therefore at a higher risk of injury (Thal *et al.*, 1985). Liver trauma can be especially problematic, leading to coagulopathy, intra-abdominal abscess, biliary leak, late haemorrhage and the release of potent digestive enzymes and virulent bacterial contents into the vascular and peritoneal spaces. These can be potent initiators of the systemic inflammatory response cascade, resulting in sepsis.

If gut integrity is impaired and enteral feeding (with or without gut motility agents) is unachievable, then intravenous feeding must be established to provide sufficient energy sources for healing to occur. Stress ulcer protection with sucralfate or ranitidine should also be considered. Monitoring of blood glucose levels, with possible insulin infusion, is important to detect any stress-induced diabetes or to control a pre-existing diabetic state.

It is important to obtain advice from dietary and pharmacy services in order that gut protection is maintained, together with sufficient calorific intake to enable tissue and cellular regrowth while in the ICU. This provides a sound base for continued healing to occur, thereby facilitating maximum rehabilitation.

Managing hygiene

This aspect of care can sometimes present a challenge to the intensive care nurse. The nurse must be able to comprehend the patient's total needs. These include assessing the degree of mobility that the patient's injuries will allow and maintaining cardiovascular and respiratory stability while dealing with the hygiene needs.

Patients with uncleared or confirmed spinal injuries will need to be strictly log-rolled as per local unit protocol. If there is actual or potential spinal damage, then dynamic pressure relieving mattresses must not be used. An appropriately sized collar should be applied, and headblocks or sandbags used if necessary. At least four staff will be required to log roll the intubated patient. This has resourcing issues with regard to staffing and the frequency of turning that can be offered. It also places responsibility both on individual staff and unit managers to ensure that manual handling education and resources are available to reduce the incidence of back strain within the health service (Royal College of Nursing, 1996).

Most centres now advocate early internal fixation of long bone fractures to reduce the incidence of fat embolism and to assist in patient hygiene and early mobility (Burgess and Brunback, 1987). Specific instructions from the trauma team regarding mobility and fracture stability should be built into the care plan. Elevation of limbs to reduce swelling, use of traction and plaster of Paris splints all require specific actions and observations from the intensive care nurse. Close working relationships with trauma ward nurses, physiotherapists and plaster technicians are paramount. Optimum use of skills will maximize early rehabilitation and minimize pressure sore incidence, the total costs of which were estimated to be in the region of £400–£1000 million per annum (Moody, 1997). Effective passive limb movements reduce the risk of deep vein thrombosis, together with the use of prophylactic subcutaneous heparin. Joint stiffness is also minimized.

Following admission to the ICU a full body inspection is important, not only to ascertain skin integrity, but also to check for any additional signs of penetrating injury or bruising. The skin is elastic and entry sites can be deceptive, not revealing the full extent or direction of injuries. In missile injuries the ballistics of certain missiles produce injury beyond the missile's tract, causing tissue damage related to energy dissipation from gaseous combustion and explosive agents. Missiles do not always travel in a straight line and contamination can result from unsterile air or fragments and tissue which are sucked in during the missile's trajectory. All entry and exit wounds must be visualized, documented and appropriate action taken.

In turning a patient, knowledge of the injuries sustained will enable safe patient posturing and care. Inspection of the urine for haematuria is important in trauma victims with a fractured pelvis, as 15% will also present with urinary tract injuries. The pelvis is a 'vascular sink' and any pelvic injury has a high incidence of bleeding and soft tissue damage. For example, a fractured ilium can tear the internal iliac vein, leading to an extensive retroperitoneal haematoma. Any laceration of the perineum, groin or buttocks must be assumed to be caused by compound open pelvic fractures until proved otherwise.

Hygiene observations must include monitoring for the development of compartment syndrome, defined as elevated interstitial pressures in a space defined and limited by a fascial envelope (Burgess and Brunback, 1987). This is usually associated with fracture of the tibia and fibula (especially transverse and comminuted fractures) and can also occur following haematoma, vascular and crush injury, as well as arterial/vascular obstruction. The increased venous pressures, decreased local arteriovenous gradient, diminished local blood flow and decreased tissue oxygenation lead to temporary or permanent ischaemia and soft tissue damage. Observations must include inspection of at risk extremity sites for swelling and reduced capillary refill. The medical team must be alerted so that emergency fasciotomies can be performed if the risk of ischaemia is increasing.

As has been outlined, care of the trauma patient can be complex. However, there are some essential aspects of care, e.g. mouth and eye care, which, with support, the family can become involved in. This can be one area which can empower the family during an otherwise stressful and traumatic time. This will be covered in the next section.

Emotional support of the patient, family and healthcare team

An essential part of care delivery, even for the unconscious patient, is the reorientation, appropriate reassurance and information-giving that must accompany any procedure or event. Most emotional problems as a result of intensive care do not emerge until transfer to the ward. However, patients in intensive care may suffer from the 'ICU syndrome' usually occurring on the third to fourth conscious day in intensive care.

The ICU syndrome may be suffered by 30% of all patients in intensive care. Impaired memory, confusion, disorientation, hallucination and personality and emotional changes, more pronounced at night and early morning, are characteristic of this problem (Campbell, 1995). While tranquillizers (e.g. haloperidol) can be used, the manner in which practitioners deliver their care can offer much to alleviate the distress caused. Caring for the patient in a truly humanistic way, minimizing competing or distracting stimuli and using strategies to promote rapid eye movement sleep can be of use. The use of clocks, calendars and familiar objects may also help to orientate. Glasses and hearing aids should be worn by the patient if needed. The evaluation of intensive care follow-up clinics has affected intensive care practice to reduce the physical and psychological problems experienced post-ICU (Jones and Griffiths, 1998).

The care required by those suffering from post-traumatic stress is given substantive cover later in the book. It is important that even when the patient is in intensive care, the nurse can support the patient and family as they begin to make sense of what has happened and address the long-term effects of the event. In achieving this, the use of primary or primary team nursing in the intensive care environment has been held to be pivotal in providing patient centred care (Audit Commission, 1991), although extensive evaluation of these models has yet to occur (Bray, 1996). Active listening and communicating skills throughout the team, helping patients and relatives to identify actual and perceived roles in the trauma, and working through feelings of self-blame and guilt are all important aspects of care and support. Strategies for relaxation, e.g. visual imagery, focusing on one object and deep breathing, can all be used and incorporated into the patient's care, especially if anxiety is a problem (Fortinash and Holoday Worret, 1995). Intensive care nurses should familiarize themselves with the resources that are available to support the patient and family, and know how these resources can be mobilized.

Case study

Mrs Jackson comes to visit her son John (see earlier case study). She was contacted at work and has come straight in to see him. Throughout her time with her son she appears distant, with an overriding sense of anger. She is constantly blaming her son for riding on his motorbike. How can Mrs Jackson be supported during this time?

Discussion. The emotional pressures faced by Mrs Jackson, as by any family member in these circumstances, are great. With little or no time to prepare and little experience as to what to expect, relatives may experience a sense of loss of control, with possible issues of anger or guilt to deal with. In some cases previous experiences of trauma and hospitalization or intensive care may be revived. It is therefore understandable that relatives can experience and demonstrate a whole range of emotions. It is important when talking with Mrs Jackson that clear, simple, accurate and consistent information is given which can be documented to ensure that all are aware of what has been discussed. In taking time to talk with Mrs Jackson it becomes evident that her nephew had been involved in a motorbike accident and she felt that she should have been more conscientious in warning her son about the dangers. Active listening and the use of humanistic skills can enable Mrs Jackson to express her guilt and grief in a non-judgemental environment so that she feels able to be with her son, to support him and deal with the situation as it presents.

The opportunity for family and friends to ask questions is important and it can be suggested that writing questions down may help to organize their thoughts. Written sources of information regarding the unit and hospital as well as information relating to the patient's illness and any established support groups can be informative at this time. Encouraging the family to participate in care, as they feel able, can help to re-establish a sense of control and of 'doing something'. Financial support may be required by the patient or the family and a social services referral should be made at an early stage.

The demands placed on the clinical team in this environment can be great. Caring for a complex, unstable trauma patient can be physically, mentally and emotionally demanding. Previous life events experienced by healthcare staff may trigger memories, and coping mechanisms will be brought into play. While staff are dealing with their own reaction to the injuries, disfigurement and possible death, the patient, the family and other team members still have to be supported. Well-facilitated case conferences and debriefing sessions can be used to allow exploration of feelings in order to develop effective plans for the management of similar events in the future (Cudmore, 1996). It is important that strong mentorship with channels for staff support are available on the unit. Pastoral support, together with more formal psychological support off the unit, must be available for all. It must also be recognized that to use such channels should not be seen as a sign of weakness, but as a means of self-development in order to achieve effective coping mechanisms which will support future personal and patient/family mental health.

Conclusion

Trauma is now the leading cause of death in the UK in the first four decades of life, and trauma as a result of accidents formed one of the key areas of concern identified in the Health of the Nation report (Department of Health, 1991). The intensive care team know that once a patient arrives in the ICU all care is directed towards preventing and minimizing the risk of mortality and morbidity following trauma. To facilitate this, complex skills and a diverse knowledge base are required in order both to understand the nature of the injuries sustained by individual patients, as well as the potential complications that may result. This requires a team approach to care, underpinned by good communication, appreciation and a respect for the knowledge and skills of each discipline. This combination of skills will ensure that the patient and family receive appropriate and timely care.

However, care is not solely the delivery of clinical treatments. Huge developments in medical science have brought many successes and also many dilemmas in healthcare, particularly for the intensive care team (Soderberg *et al.*, 1997). The issue of appropriate resourcing continues to maintain a high profile in the national and professional press. The provision of specialized trauma centres with the necessary support services, including intensive care, remains an acutely sensitive political and community issue (Kivell and Mason, 1997). The issues faced by patients and families of those severely injured in trauma highlight discussion on the use of living wills, advance directives, and the promotion of health education issues relating to safer driving, prevention of drink driving and the use of restraints, to name but a few. The resources required for the long-term support of many trauma patients with severe disability and disfigurement raises issues regarding the long-term costs in both emotional and financial terms. Healthcare professionals, as with society at large, have a responsibility to contribute to such debates in order to reach an informed consensus on care, given the available resources. Such an approach to trauma management can help to educate and support all those involved in the care of trauma patients, their families and their friends.

References

Audit Commission (1991) *The Virtue of Patients: Making the Best Use of Ward Resources*. London: HMSO.

Bradley, B. R. (1987) ARDS. *Focus Critical Care*, **25**, 48.

Bray, K. (1996) Changing practice to primary nursing. *Nursing Critical Care*, **1**(3), 134–136.

Burgess, A. R. and Brunback, R. J. (1987) Early fracture stablization. In *Trauma Care* (R. A. Cowley and A. M. Conn Dunham, eds), Volume 1, *Surgical Management*. J. B. Lippincott.

Campbell, A. S. (1995) Recognising post traumatic distress syndrome in intensive care patients. *Intensive and Critical Care Nursing*, **11**, 60–65.

Cudmore, J. (1996) Preventing post traumatic stress disorder in accident and emergency nursing. *Nursing in Critical Care*, **1**(3), 134–136.

Craven, N. (1999). Critically ill patients facing a desperate hunt for a bed. *Daily Mail*, 4 January, p. 4.

Department of Health (1991) *The Health of the Nation*. London: HMSO.

Edbrooke, D. (1996) High dependency – so much promise – so little progress. *Care of the Critically Ill*, **12**(3), 80–81.

Eisenberg, H. M., Frankowski, R. F. and Constant, C. F. (1988) High dose barbiturate control of elevated intracranial pressure in patients with severe head injury. *Journal Neurosurgery*, **69**, 15–23.

Feldman, Z., Kanter, M. J. and Robertson, C. S. (1992) Effect of head elevation and intracranial pressure perfusion pressure and cerebral blood flow in head injury patients. *Journal of Neurosurgery*, **76**, 207–211.

Fortinash, K. M. and Holoday Worret, N. (1995) *Psychiatric Nursing Care Plans*. St. louis, MO: Mosby Year Book.

Franklin, P., Crombie, A. and Nichols, J. (1996) Organ donation – discussing the options with the family. *Care of the Critically Ill*, **12**(3), 95–96.

Gross, M. (1995) No stars in their eyes. *Health Services Journal*, January, **26**, 6–8.

Ihde, J., Jacobsen, W. and Briggs, B. (1987) *Principles of Critical Care*. W. B. Saunders.

Kivell, P. and Mason, K. (1997) Trauma centres: where to care for major injuries. *British Journal of Health Care Management*, **3**(4), 93–98.

Jones, C. and Griffiths, R. (1998) Intensive follow-up workshop. *British Journal of Intensive Care*, **8**(4), 139–140.

Mitchell Yates, R. and Kenner, C. V. (1992) Head injuries. In *Critical Care Nursing Body – Mind – Spirit*, 3rd edn (B. M. Dossey, C. E. Guzzetta and C. V. Kenner, eds). J. B. Lippincott.

Moody, M. (1997) Fighting against pressure sores and a rise in legal suits. *British Journal of Health Care Management*, **3**(1), 40–41.

National Health Service Executive (1996) *Guidelines for Admission To and Discharge From Intensive Care and High Dependency Units*. London: Department of Health.

Neff, J. A. and Kidd, P. S. (1993) *Trauma Nursing: The Art and Science*. St. Louis, MO: Mosby Year Book.

Richardson, A. (1997) Turning a patient prone with ARDS. *Nursing in Critical Care*, **2**(4), 197–199.

Royal College of Nursing (1996) *Manual Handling for Nurses ... Issues for Nurses*. Royal College of Nursing Labour Department.

Smith, S. (1994) Examination of the central nervous system in the critically ill patient. *British Journal of Intensive Care*, **4**(4), 116–121.

Soderberg, A., Gilje, F. and Norberg, A. (1997) Dignity in situations of ethical difficulty in intensive care. *Intensive and Critical Care Nursing*, **13**, 135–144.

Thal, E. R., McClelland, R. N. and Shires, G. T. (1985) Abdominal trauma. In *Principles of Trauma Care* (G. T. Shires, ed.). McGraw-Hill.

Trunkey, D. D. (1983) Trauma. *Scientific American*, **249**, 28–35.

White, K. and Kenner, C. (1992) Chest trauma. In *Critical Care Nursing Body – Mind – Spirit* (B. M. Dossey, C. E. Guzzetta and C. V. Kenner, eds.) J. B. Lippincott.

13

Complications of trauma

Martin McNally

Introduction

The aim of treatment for any injury to the skeleton and the component joints is a complete functional recovery. To achieve this, two fundamental and interdependent principles must be observed. These are:

- restoration of the mechanical and biological integrity of the tissues
- active prevention of complications.

Observance of one and neglect of the other courts disaster.

Increasing surgical management of fractures has led to a rise in some complications with a resultant loss of confidence in some techniques. It is important to define the indications for a surgical technique, to allow a balance between the benefits of surgery and the risk of complications.

The current debate on the development and quality of major trauma centres brings the balance of active treatment and complications into acute focus. There is no question that a well-resourced trauma unit, with a concentration of experienced surgical and nursing staff, will produce better treatment with low complication rates. In reality this is often not possible, and injured patients may be dispersed to a number of small centres. In these circumstances the surgeons involved must accept that there are situations which demand the onward transfer of trauma to a centre that has more experience, has better facilities and will offer a better outcome as a result. One good example of this is the open tibial fracture. Here the soft tissue

care is paramount and, from the outset, the involvement of a plastic surgeon together with a fracture surgeon is essential. If a plastic surgeon is not immediately available, the patient must be transferred to a unit where this team approach is routine.

In recent years the drive towards increasing surgical intervention has reduced our experience with conservative methods of fracture care – skeletal traction and prolonged immobilization in a cast are now rare. It should be remembered that these methods have their own risks and complications. Pressure necrosis of skin, nerve traction injury, joint contractures and stiffness were all common in the past. Successful conservative treatment of fractures requires great attention to their prevention. In many ways non-operative fracture care is more demanding than surgical fixation.

The prevention of complications is closely interwoven with the treatment of injury. Many useful comments are made in other chapters, and there are some important areas which are the subject of major sections (tissue viability, rehabilitation, etc.). To prevent repetition these will not be discussed in this chapter, but a list of the possible complications will serve as a useful checklist in study and for revision.

Complications of skeletal trauma

Table 13.1 lists the complications of skeletal trauma, a number of which are discussed in the following subsections of this chapter.

Table 13.1   Complications of skeletal trauma

General and systemic complications

Fat embolism
Adult respiratory distress syndrome (ARDS)
Deep venous thrombosis
Pulmonary embolism
Pneumonia
Tetanus
Septicaemia
Multi-system organ failure

Local complications

Skin	Pressure, bed and cast sores
Vascular	Direct injury
	Volkmann's ischaemic contracture
	Gangrene
Nerve	Direct injury
	Traction injury
Joint	Septic arthritis
	Instability
Bone	Osteomyelitis
	Bone loss

Late complications

Muscle	Contractures
	Myositis ossificans
Bone	Delayed, non-union
	Mal-union
	Chronic osteomyelitis
	Osteoporosis
	Stress-shielding
	Growth disturbance
	Avascular necrosis
Brain	Post-traumatic stress disorder
Joint	Stiffness
	Osteoarthritis
Multiple	Reflex muscular dystrophy

Thromboembolic disease

Venous thromboembolism remains a life-threatening complication in patients with bony injury. Fractures carrying a particularly high risk include those of the hip, pelvis, tibia and spine. Pulmonary embolism has been identified at post-mortem in 45–60% of patients dying after femoral or tibial fracture. It is the primary cause of death in the majority of cases.

In the multiply-injured patient, venous thromboembolism is difficult to diagnose and little is known of its true incidence. Two-thirds of immobilized multi-trauma patients develop asymptomatic deep vein thrombosis (Figure 13.1), with half having proximal segment involvement. There is a significant increase in the likelihood of thrombosis if the patient had lower limb fracture as part of their injury complex.

A number of risk factors have been identified including age, prolonged immobilization, paraplegia, sepsis, direct venous injury, and coagulopathy. The risk is not related to Injury Severity Score, although time from injury is important. In patients who die more than 4 days after injury, pulmonary embolism is the cause in 50%, after 28 days it is present in 90%.

The issue of prophylaxis in fracture patients is controversial. No consensus has been reached on the best prevention. The efficacy of warfarin, subcutaneous heparin and low molecular weight heparin is under investigation, but concern has been expressed over the risk of bleeding complications. Elderly patients with hip fractures and multiply-injured patients are least able to survive excessive bleeding. 'Safe' prevention, by the use of external pneumatic compression, pneumatic foot pumps and electrical calf muscle stimulation has been advocated to avoid bleeding complications. Intravenous dextran 70 or standard heparin and external pneumatic compression have been shown to decrease the incidence of pulmonary embolism following hip fracture. Initial results with the A-V impulse foot pump system in patients with hip fracture are encouraging.

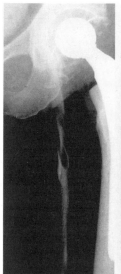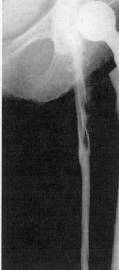

Fig 13.1 This venogram identified a deep vein thrombosis in a patient who had a hip replacement after a femoral neck fracture.

The diagnosis of post-traumatic deep vein thrombosis can be difficult. Patients with lower limb trauma will often have symptoms and signs normally associated with thrombosis, but caused by their injury or surgery. Duplex ultrasound scanning or early pulmonary scanning should be considered in these patients.

Tetanus

This disease is caused by the *Clostridium tetani* bacillus which is anaerobic and is widespread in the soil and faeces of animals. It is rarely encountered in the developed world, where wound hygiene is carefully sought in all cases. However, tetanus remains a potent cause of mortality in the developing world. Prevention takes two forms. The first, and most important, is good wound debridement and toilet. All wounds must be explored by a competent surgeon. Devitalized tissue must be removed, and if there is any doubt about tissue that is preserved then the wound must be inspected on a daily basis with the facility for further excision if necessary. Contaminated wounds should be left open and lightly dressed. Prophylactic antibiotics should be given using intravenous benzylpenicillin.

Immunization of the population is the second defence. Adsorbed tetanus toxoid is effective and safe. The antibody levels are satisfactory after a second dose and booster doses every 10 years are required. The usual course is one dose followed in 6 weeks with a second, and a third at 6 months. Booster doses should be carried out at 10-year intervals and after any penetrating injury.

In most cases the onset of tetanus is insidious. The more rapid the onset, the more severe the disease. The symptoms will intensify for the first 10 days and then tend to plateau for a similar period before settling – if the patient survives.

The disease is mediated by the neurotoxin secreted by the bacilli. The toxin travels to the spinal cord and the medulla by means of the peripheral nerves, and blocks the release of inhibitory spinal neurotransmitters. This permits the motor nerves to fire without central inhibition, producing the characteristic spasm and tetanic contractions of the disease. The disease first becomes manifest in the short motor neurons of the neck and head, followed by the longer trunk neurons and then finally in the long neurons of the limbs. The spasms merge into hypertonicity, producing the classical lockjaw and risus sardonicus. Treatment is with intravenous antibiotics and human anti-tetanus gamma globulin. The muscle spasms are controlled by sedation, relaxants, neuromuscular blockade and respiratory support. Active metabolic support is given and severe cases should be treated in an intensive care unit.

Skin pressure sores

Tissue viability as a general topic is considered in detail in Chapter 20. This section deals with the problems of skin and subcutaneous tissue viability locally in the injured limb.

Local pressure necrosis of the skin and underlying soft tissues may occur by many mechanisms in fracture patients. Bony fragments or displaced fractures may press on the skin from within, producing ischaemia and tissue death. Blistering of the skin occurs due to swelling around a fracture, causing separation of the normal skin layers. In all cases it is important to reduce fractures promptly to protect the skin and its blood supply. If the skin is oedematous, severely blistered or ischaemic, surgery must be postponed until the skin has recovered. High elevation of injured limbs is essential to allow swelling to resolve, prevent venous stasis and thrombosis, and reduce tension on the skin.

External stabilization of fractures by orthoses or external fixators places the patient at risk of injury from the fixation device. All such devices have pins or edges which can damage the skin of the injured limb or even another limb. Care must be taken to cover or pad external fixator pins on the medial side of the leg to protect the other leg. In children, psychiatric patients and adults with learning difficulties, the fixator should be completely covered.

Plaster of Paris sores (Figure 13.2) are a source of distress for the patient and embarrassment for the nurse or surgeon. They usually represent poor technique at the primary application of a cast or splint. They can also arise from inexpert repair of damage to the plaster, or can be due to an object lodged between the plaster and the skin. In all cases the patient will complain of pain which is inappropriate to the injury, and this must be investigated by removal of the cast. It is far better to take off a cast to be sure of the skin condition than to risk a pressure sore. Once tissue breakdown is identified, the cast must be modified to prevent further pressure necrosis. A 'window' may be cut in the new cast to facilitate this and to allow wound inspection and dressings.

Traction can also be a source of pressure sores, either generally due to immobility and dependence, or locally due to pressure from the traction splint or pin. If traction is used as a definitive treatment, daily inspection of vulnerable bony prominences is essential, particularly in the early days of the treatment. Although no longer practised by the Oxford Trauma Service, some centres still use skin traction in the elderly prior to surgery for femoral neck fractures. Great care must be taken to ensure that foam is placed over the ankle malleoli and that pressure is alleviated from the heel. In this group of high-risk patients, pressure necrosis will arise very rapidly over these bony prominences.

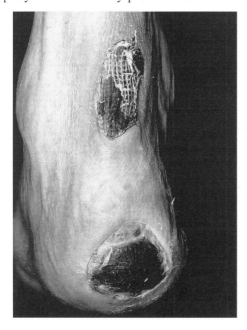

Fig 13.2 On removal of a short leg cast, this diabetic patient was found to have full thickness plaster sores over the achilles tendon (at top) and over the calceaneus. Diabetic patients may have poor sensation in the limb peripheries and are at high risk of cast sores.

Vascular complications

Every injured limb must be examined to ensure that there is adequate peripheral circulation. The examination must be repeated regularly over the first few days, as there are occasions when the arterial circulation is intact on admission but may become compromised later.

Displaced fractures may divide or occlude major vessels in a limb. Limb deformity may twist vessels, especially veins, producing ischaemia or venous congestion. When these are found at examination, the fracture should be reduced and the limb observed for a few minutes. Often the circulation will improve, but if it is not restored then angiography may be required and the patient must be taken to theatre as soon as possible for exploration of the fracture site.

When a cast has been applied to a recently traumatized or operated limb it must be split until the reactive oedema has settled. If there is any doubt about an intact cast causing peripheral vascular impairment, it should be split without question. Failure to do this will lead to the increasing spiral of vascular occlusion and swelling. Beware also the encircling bandage that has become saturated in blood or serum and is acting like a tight cast. If bandages are suspect, split them immediately. Loss of fracture reduction is a minor problem compared with loss of a limb through ischaemia.

Ischaemia due to compartment syndrome is a common and serious complication. It arises as a result of bleeding within the muscle compartments around the long bones. These compartments are surrounded by dense fascial sheets which do not allow the muscles to swell to any degree, so the pressure in the compartment rises. The condition does not only occur with fractures. It can occur in any situation where there is a soft tissue injury or where there is an accumulation of oedema. Increasing pressure leads to capillary shut-down, further muscle swelling and ischaemia, leading to outpouring of fluid, causing further pressure increase. The circle persists until the muscles are dead and grossly swollen, the nerves are ischaemic and irrecoverable, and the arteries reach their critical closing pressure, cutting off the distal circulation. The danger signs are listed in Table 13.2.

The forearm is the classical site for compartment syndrome after radius and ulnar fractures, but it is also seen in the lower limb. In many trauma units early intramedullary nailing by closed technique is the treatment of choice for displaced tibial and femoral fractures. There have been a number of reports of compartment syndrome arising in the distal limb following a closed nailing technique. Epidural anaesthesia must not be used in these patients as it will mask the early signs of increased pressure and lead to delay in diagnosis until after muscle tissue has died.

Table 13.2 Danger signs of compartment syndrome

Pain	Pain that is increasing and which seems to be inappropriate
Pallor	The skin will be white and cool to touch
Paraesthesia	The digits will be numb or tingling
Paralysis	• The distal limb may have little or no active motion
	• Passive stretching of the involved muscle groups produces severe pain
Pulselessness	In the early stages the pulse may be bounding, but it is lost in the advancing case

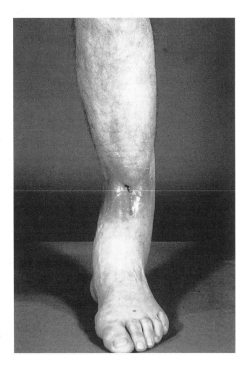

Fig 13.3 This open tibial fracture has united with some deformity and with a discharging sinus. This is a classical appearance of deep chronic osteomyelitis of the tibial shaft.

If the clinical signs are present, it is a surgical emergency to decompress the compartments. It is better to err on the side of decompression in a normal limb than to miss the opportunity of preventing disaster.

The operation of choice is a fascial decompression (fasciotomy) and it should be carried out by open incisions of the skin over the affected muscle groups. Dead muscle must be excised, and wounds should not be closed until all reactive oedema has subsided. The wound should be examined under anaesthetic 48 h after fasciotomy to ensure complete excision of all dead tissue. The limb should be splinted in the position of function, and subsequent deformity prevented by aggressive physiotherapy and orthotics.

Failure to recognize compartment syndrome early leads to joint contractures, peripheral numbness and severe loss of limb function. Less commonly, tissue death may require amputation to prevent local gangrene and systemic sepsis.

Osteomyelitis

Infection of bone is a serious complication of trauma and represents one of the commonest causes of disability worldwide. Infection after closed fractures arises from the use of open operation and internal fixation. Operative treatment in closed fractures must always be balanced against the risk of infection. The patient factors which predispose to infection include poor skin, blisters and pressure sores, diabetes, alcoholism and immunosuppression therapy or other medical diseases. Other factors include operating room environment, risks of contamination of sterile towels and equipment, level of competence of the nurses and surgeons, and the standards of postoperative care.

Prevention of bone infection begins prior to surgery with treatment of any concomitant medical conditions, particularly chest or urinary tract infection. At the time of osteosynthesis, care must be taken to handle the soft tissues gently and the wound should be liberally irrigated with saline. Drains are used to reduce the chance of a haematoma and the skin must be closed without tension. Prophylactic antibiotics are used for a period of 24 h and elevation of the limb with active physiotherapy will prevent accumulation of oedema.

If infection is suspected, the wound and any discharge from it should be swabbed and sent for culture and sensitivities. The limb must be elevated and splinted, and every effort made to correct anaemia, electrolyte imbalance or poor nutritional state. The patient should be taken to theatre and the wound opened and all infected tissue excised. Deep samples are sent for bacteriological culture. The wound should be irrigated and left open with antiseptic dressings. Broad-spectrum antibiotics (usually a cephalosporin) are given intravenously, but these can be changed to more specific agents once the microbiology is known. Serial return to theatre is essential to salvage fracture fixation and control infection. The wound is only closed when it is clean and healthy. In some cases the patient may remain on oral antibiotics as suppression therapy until fracture union is complete.

In the case of a joint being infected, a similar aggressive approach should be adopted. The joint should be explored, all debris removed and the joint space liberally irrigated. Thereafter aspiration and irrigation with a needle can be employed, provided that the infection is under control.

Occasionally infection may become established around a fracture or implant (Figure 13.3). This form of chronic osteomyelitis is a serious complication requiring complex surgery and infection control. Such patients should be referred to a specialist centre which can deal with all of the components of the disease. Treatment involves defining the extent of the infection and planned removal of all infected tissue. Reconstruction of this defect may require bone transport or other advanced techniques, together with microvascular free-tissue transfer to achieve skin cover. Nursing care and rehabilitation for these patients may extend over two or three years and is very demanding on patient and practitioner alike.

Abnormal healing of fractures

Delayed union of a fracture occurs when the signs of union fail to appear at a time that would be expected in a particular bone. Non-union is said to be present when the bone has failed to unite in a reasonable timescale and intervention is required to secure union. Until the healing of fractures can be reliably mea-sured, the clinical signs must be weighed together with the X-ray appearance and clinical experience. The clinical signs of union are stability at the fracture site, absence of pain on testing, and the presence of callus radiologically which bridges the fracture ends. These signs are highly subjective and the radiographs can be misleading, so a high index of suspicion is necessary. Even with abundant callus on X-ray the fracture may slowly deform with weight-bearing, suggesting insufficient union.

Normal fracture healing requires blood supply to the bony ends and stability to allow new bone to bridge the fracture gap. Open fractures, or high-energy fractures where there is stripping of tissue from bone, have a high risk of non-union due to loss of the blood supply around the fracture. Infection limits the blood supply, as does avascular necrosis and of course extensive periosteal stripping during internal fixation. Pathological fractures and those where soft tissues are interposed may also go on to delayed or non-union. Poor stabilization can prevent union by allowing excessive movement at the fracture site. This constantly breaks the small capillaries so vital to the process of union. There is also concern that non-steroidal anti-inflammatory drugs used for analgesia after fracture may have an adverse effect on the healing process. Anti-inflammatories should not be given to patients having treatment for established non-unions.

The management of delayed or non-union will depend on many factors: the cause of the delay; the structural needs of the bone; any complications; the response of the patient to surgery; and the local pattern of the fracture. There are, however, a number of basic principles which must be observed:

- eradication of any infection around the fracture
- stable internal or external fixation to allow bridging of new bone
- restoration of local blood supply by removal of dead bone and preservation of the viable soft tissues
- bone grafting to fill defects and to allow new bone to cross the fracture site.

In some fractures, such as displaced oblique tibial fractures or ulnar shaft fractures, the incidence of non-union or mal-union (healing in a poor position) is so high that early operative

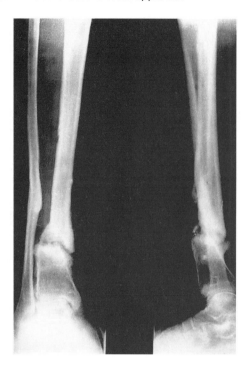

Fig 13.4 Despite prolonged immobilization in a cast, this low tibial fracture has failed to unite. It is mobile and painful on weight-bearing. It now needs surgical stabilisation to allow union to proceeed.

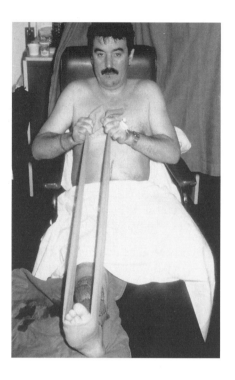

Fig 13.5 As soon as possible after fracture fixation, the patient should be actively involved in mobilizing the joints adjacent to the injured bones. Ankle dorsiflexion is often lost after tibial fractures and should be maintained with early repeated passive stretching as shown. In the unconscious patient the ankle should be splinted and passively moved by the physiotherapist.

fixation is indicated (Figure 13.4).

In the case of open fractures, the practice over the last few decades of delayed skin cover has been superseded by early plastic surgery. Early and adequate debridement and skin cover, together with bony stabilization and delayed bone grafting, has reduced the incidence of infection, and delayed and non-union. The provision of good skin cover brings new blood supply to the devitalized area of the fracture and permits new capillaries to invade the fracture site and encourage bone healing. External fixation provides excellent fixation of bone in the presence of an open wound, but more recently intramedullary nailing of open long-bone fractures has been shown to be a safe and effective treatment. This method allows much better access for plastic surgical reconstruction of the soft tissues.

Interposition of soft tissue will cause non-union. This is predominantly a problem of the fractured humerus and femur. These long bones are surrounded in muscle, and when grossly displaced at the time of fracture the ends

button-hole the muscle. Experience will indicate which fractures are at risk, but continued malposition of the fracture despite reduction and splintage suggests interposition. If interposition cannot be resolved by closed means, an open reduction will be necessary to prevent the non-union. In the femur, intramedullary nailing is now the treatment of choice, avoiding problems of interposition and non-union.

When a pathological fracture is present the tumour type must be ascertained and this will dictate the mode of therapy. Frequently the tumour will be a secondary metastatic deposit from a distant primary carcinoma. Careful internal fixation is important to provide pain relief and to re-establish skeletal function. This can be supplemented with radiotherapy. Chemotherapy may be indicated for the tumour, but it will also delay fracture healing. Both radiotherapy and chemotherapy should be

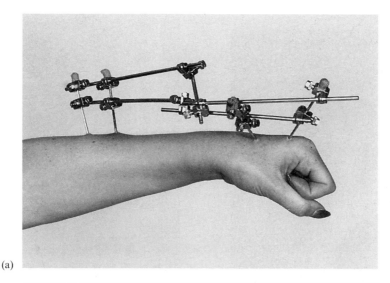

(a)

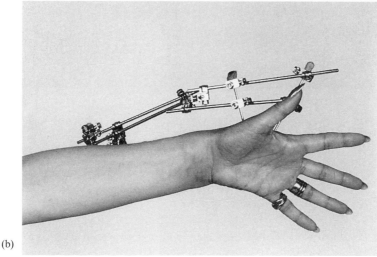

(b)

Fig 13.6 a,b External fixators and splints should be applied carefully to avoid immobilization of uninjured joints. This small fixator crosses the wrist joint

delayed until wound healing is secure.

Osteoporosis

There is a close cause-and-effect relationship between osteoporosis and fracture. Osteoporosis is a major predisposing factor in proximal femoral and vertebral collapse fractures, but it is also caused in previously normal bones by injury. It can complicate fractures managed by either conservative or operative means by two separate mechanisms.

In conservative management, there is a diffuse loss of bone density associated with disuse of the limb. This is particularly marked after tibial or foot fractures which have been immobilized for long periods in a plaster of Paris cast. Even without splintage, bone loss may be severe if the patient remains non-weight-bearing for many weeks. This may be necessary after calcaneal or talar fractures. In the upper limb, osteoporosis often complicates distal radial or scaphoid fractures in the elderly. It may occur either alone or with the other features of reflex sympathetic dystrophy. Pa-

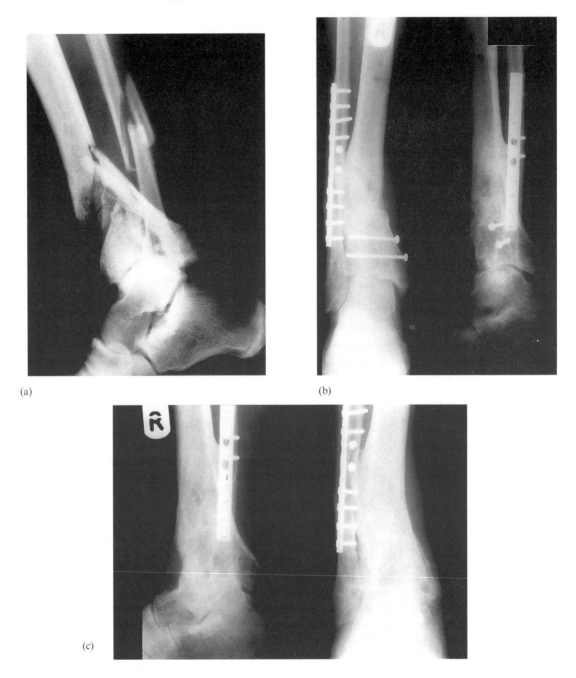

(a)

(b)

(c)

Fig 13.7 a–c   This severe open ankle fracture (a) was treated by internal fixation. Despite this, post-traumatic arthritis developed (b) and the painful, stiff ankle was fused (c) to relieve the symptoms.

tients should be warned that there is a danger of early refracture when post-traumatic osteoporosis is present.

In all cases the prevention and treatment is active mobilization of the affected limb. There is no good evidence to support the use of calcium or vitamin D supplements except in those who are grossly deficient. However, hormone replacement therapy has been shown to reduce bone loss and prevent secondary fractures in postmenopausal women.

In fractures managed by open reduction and internal fixation there is a more localized process which results in bone loss. If a fracture is rigidly fixed with a heavy plate, the normal loading of the fixed portion of bone is reduced. This is known as stress-shielding. Once the fracture has united and new bone formation has ceased, there is progressive loss of cortical bone mass adjacent to the plate. To prevent increasing local bone resorption with eventual fixation failure and fracture, plates should be removed from long bones once union is complete.

Joint stiffness

The aim of fracture treatment is a full restoration of function, and when this does not occur it is usually due to joint stiffness. There are a number of causes of stiffness which require careful differentiation. Early post-traumatic arthritis will be dealt with separately.

Stiffness may result from soft tissue damage at the time of injury. It may also arise as so-called 'fracture disease' from the method of treatment provided. Injury produces inflammatory reaction, pain, and circulatory disturbance creating disuse of the bone, muscle and joint complex. This promotes chronic oedema, soft tissue atrophy, osteoporosis and joint stiffness. In the past the great dilemma was the need to immobilize to achieve union while trying to move limbs to prevent joint stiffness. Advances in fracture fixation have permitted a resolution of this dilemma, and the aim should be to achieve stable reduction of the fracture to allow early active and pain-free motion. Movement reduces the soft tissue oedema, builds the muscle bulk, prevents disuse osteoporosis, and encourages the movement of synovial fluid in the articular cartilage.

Good-quality fracture treatment demands that the best mechanical fixation is achieved at operation so that the maximum degree of motion and weight-bearing can be achieved at the earliest opportunity. If the fixation is sound and there is some other factor preventing mobilization, there are great benefits to be gained from the continuous passive motion devices (CPM) available for both upper and lower limb. CPM has been demonstrated to improve functional outcome after knee and elbow trauma.

Joint stiffness is a particular problem in the open fracture (Figures 13.5 and 13.6a,b), where the degree of soft tissue damage is a major determinant of the loss of joint function. In the early stages after injury, joints should be splinted to prevent contractures. Once the skin cover is secure, active physiotherapy begins before weight-bearing to regain joint motion. If a major muscle group has been lost at injury, then appropriate orthoses are needed to allow function within the remaining muscles.

Post-traumatic arthritis

Progressive damage to articular surfaces may occur after injury by a number of pathways. Direct injury with fragmentation of one or both joint surfaces will predispose to early osteoarthritis (OA). This is particularly prevalent after ankle fracture, hip fracture and dislocation. Late arthritis is not uncommon after carpal or elbow fractures and fracture dislocations. Loose fragments of articular cartilage, bone or foreign material may damage the joint surface. Traumatic chondromalacia can occur without a fracture and will predispose to arthritis.

The incidence and onset of the condition is largely dependent on the initial management of the intra-articular fracture and subsequent rehabilitation, but in the large weight-bearing joints it usually begins within 1 year of injury. Residual joint deformity after initial treatment is the most potent cause of post-traumatic arthritis.

The condition is most often seen after severe ankle fractures. Radiographic OA has been reported in 15–25% of cases, depending on the degree of comminution and the presence of a talar fracture. While this joint is rarely the site of non-traumatic OA, it is a major cause of disability after injury. Arthrodesis may be required for pain relief. After central dislocation of the hip, OA may occur in 30% of cases, while in dislocations associated with a femoral neck fracture, 50–70% will have early arthritic change. Post-traumatic OA also commonly complicates fractures of the patella, calcaneus, talus (with or without avascular necrosis), scaphoid and tibial condyles.

The prevention of post-traumatic arthritis relies upon early anatomical reduction, adequate stabilization, and prompt rehabilitation of intra-articular fractures (Figures 13.7a–c).

Open reduction and internal fixation are preferred for displaced fractures. It should be remembered that intra-articular fractures are often much more comminuted than the first radiographs may suggest. In complex joint injuries the fracture should be investigated with CT or magnetic resonance scanning to define the fracture pattern. Once the fracture is fixed, motion must begin early.

Post-traumatic arthritis may also be caused by extra-articular injury. At the ankle, ligamentous injury may result in recurrent subluxation with early onset OA. This mechanism also affects the carpometacarpal joint of the thumb. Mal-union of adjacent long-bone fractures may cause abnormal loading of a normal joint, resulting in early degeneration. This is seen in unicompartment OA of the knee complicating a mal-union of the tibia.

Avascular necrosis is a cause of OA in specific joints. It is most often seen after fractures of the scaphoid, talus or neck of femur.

Reflex sympathetic dystrophy

While reflex sympathetic dystrophy, Sudeck's atrophy or causalgia is considered an uncommon disease, studies indicate that it is poorly recognized and often occurs to a mild degree. When it is not recognized in the early stages, it can develop into a major management problem well in excess of the original injury. It has been defined as a syndrome of exaggerated response to injury with the following features:

- unexpected intensity or prolongation of pain
- vasomotor disturbance

- grossly delayed functional recovery
- associated trophic changes.

The common symptoms are intense and increasing pain out of proportion to the injury, stiffness, swelling, burning sensations, and anxiety. The cause of the condition is not clear, but there are a number of features which point to autonomic over-activity.

In the upper limb there is excessive pain which tends to increase with time. The fingers become swollen and stiff very quickly, and any attempted movement is accompanied by an intense painful reaction which is genuine. If a fracture has been the precipitating cause, then check radiographs will reveal the diffuse osteoporosis that accompanies this condition.

The mainstay of treatment has been physiotherapy with good analgesia and anti-inflammatory drugs. This may be supplemented with sympathetic blockade in severe cases. The patient should have constant support and understanding, with as much analgesia as needed to reduce or abolish pain. Counselling with a clinical psychologist has been advocated for anxious patients and should be used alongside conservative measures.

FURTHER READING

Charnley, J. (1961) *The Closed Treatment of Common Fractures*, 3rd edn. Churchill Livingstone.

Pellegrini, V. D. Jr, Reid, J. S., McCollister Evarts, C. (1996) Systematic and regional complications of extremity injury. In Rockwood, C. A. and Green, D. B. (1996) *Fractures in Adults 4th edn*. Lippincott-Raven.

14

Rehabilitation

Sally Davis

Introduction

Rehabilitation can mean different things to different people. It is often thought of as something that happens in a specialized rehabilitation setting, more relevant to chronic care settings rather than acute care, whereas it should be a continuing process from admission to beyond discharge. The aim of this chapter is to explore the relationship between rehabilitation and acute trauma care by:

- defining the attributes of rehabilitation.
- exploring rehabilitation frameworks including the World Health Organisation's (WHO) International Classification of Impairments, Disabilities and Handicaps (ICIDH).
- exploring the related concepts of teamwork and goal-setting.
- discussing psychosocial aspects.
- identifying the different levels of rehabilitation from acute trauma to community.

A case study will be used to relate theory to practice and the conclusion will contain strategies for promoting rehabilitation in trauma care.

Rehabilitation

Within the literature, rehabilitation is defined in a number of ways. It is impossible to include all of the definitions here, so a variety have been chosen which reflect the general ambience of the majority.

Rehabilitation is:

- 'An active process which seeks to reduce the effects of disease (in its broadest sense) on daily life' (Ward and McIntosh in Greenwood *et al.*, 1993).
- 'The whole process of enabling and facilitating the restoration of a disabled person to regain optimal functioning (physically, socially, and psychologically) as fully as they are able or motivated to do so' (Waters, 1987).
- 'A dynamic process in which a disabled person is aided in achieving optimum physical, emotional, psychological, social or vocational potential to maintain dignity and self-respect in a life that is as independent and self-fulfilling as possible' (Hickey, 1986).
- 'Reactivation – the encouragement of patients to be active within their surroundings. Resocialisation – the encouragement of physical and/or verbal contact by patients with peers family and others. Reintegration – restoration of the patient to society and the regaining of status as a person' (Jackson, 1984).
- 'The restoration of an individual's ability to function as efficiently and normally as his condition will permit following injury, illness or accident. It involves re-education and retraining of those who have become partially or wholly incapacitated

by such conditions as blindness, deafness, heart disease, amputation, paralysis' (Blackwell, 1994).

- 'Concerned with the intrinsic worth and dignity of the individual. It is therefore committed to the restoration of the disabled to a life that is purposeful and satisfying, one that allows each individual the opportunity to function adequately as a family member and as a member of society with the capabilities to meet the responsibilities of that society' (Licht, 1968).
- 'The process by which a person works towards a former level of functioning after experiencing some type of injury or the effects of a disease. Rehabilitation is achieved by relearning skills formerly mastered and by learning new ways to do activities one no longer can accomplish with previously learned skills' (Chipps *et al.*, 1992).
- 'An educational, problem-solving process aimed at reducing disability and handicap' (Wade, 1996).

These definitions highlight the defining attributes of rehabilitation, which are process, restoration, effectiveness, enabling and facilitating, and learning and teaching, as discussed below:

Process. Rehabilitation is generally described as being a continuing process which is concerned with physical, social and psychological aspects. A process which should be active and dynamic with the client taking an active part.

Restoration. Restore or restoration is used in terms of restoring patients to regain lost elements of their life, such as physical functioning or personal and social identity. It is also used in the sense of restoring the patient to society or to a purposeful and satisfying life. To restore can imply that the emphasis of rehabilitation is on the client returning to their former life, rather than on adapting to their changed circumstances and learning new skills. The latter is the way it is meant in most of the definitions.

Effectiveness. Rehabilitation is described as promoting effectiveness or optimal functioning for the client.

Enabling and facilitating. Rather than a 'passive, doing for' process, rehabilitation is generally described as being an enabling and facilitating process which is conducive to it being dynamic rather than static.

Learning and teaching. Rehabilitation is often described as being an educational process which enables clients and carers to learn new skills.

In summary, rehabilitation can be identified as being an active, dynamic process which aims to help clients reach the maximum physical, social and psychological potential within their capabilities, through interventions which are facilitating, enabling and educational. How does this relate to trauma care? No matter where the client is in terms of their healthcare experience, the focus should be on rehabilitation. The process can still be active with client involvement, but this level of involvement will be at different levels of intensity according to the client's capabilities. This involvement must also include the family, who are a vital element in the rehabilitation process. If rehabilitation is to be successful in its aims of maximizing a person's potential, then healthcare professionals need to develop a rehabilitation 'mindset' from the onset.

Rehabilitation: a philosophy of care

One of the difficulties which healthcare professionals may find when considering rehabilitation is that by thinking of it as a process it makes it easier to think of as something that happens 'elsewhere' in a specialized setting. It would perhaps be more effective to think of rehabilitation as a philosophy of care, as well as a process which should underpin all aspects of healthcare (Preston, 1994; Royal College of Nursing, 1994). Nurses in particular are in an ideal position to adopt a philosophy of rehabilitation because of their 24 hour duty of care, whether they work in an acute or continuing care setting.

Adopting this philosophy of rehabilitation means that nurses and other healthcare professionals:

- value the client as an individual – understanding their past achievements and hopes for the future.
- identify the importance of adopting stra-

tegies which facilitate and enable the client to achieve their full potential.

- identify that although it may be necessary to put in more time to enable clients to achieve their full potential, it will be cost effective in the long term.
- though limited in being able to affect the client's level of handicap, one should certainly be thinking about how the client and their family will manage in the future and should focus the client's future quality of life.

Concepts and theoretical frameworks related to rehabilitation

Rehabilitation is a complex process with a number of related phenomena which professionals need to understand if the process is to be effective for the client and their family; for example, adaptation, stress, adjustment, independence, activities of living, self-care, motivation, illness and wellness. There are a number of theoretical frameworks or models which can help explain these phenomena.

The International Classification of Impairments, Disabilities and Handicaps (ICIDH)

This classification (World Health Organization, 1980) provides a framework consisting of three levels of illness. It enables professionals to identify goals at each of these levels which meet the client's needs in order for them to maximize their quality of life – the ultimate aim of rehabilitation. The framework is currently under review, with the suggestion that the level of disability be changed to activity, and handicap to participation. Pfeiffer (1998) identifies the need for review being due to language and perspectives which do not reflect current day thinking, but that of 20 years ago.

Within the ICIDH framework the levels identified are:

Impairment. Loss or abnormality of psychological, physiological or anatomic structure or function at organ level. The symptoms and signs are: weakness of limbs, ataxia, spasticity, dysphasia, cognitive deficits, dysphagia.

Disability (activity). The restriction or lack of ability to perform an activity in a normal manner. The functional consequences are: inability to stand, transfer, walk, wash, dress, feed, communicate, control bowel/bladder function, poor memory.

Handicap (participation). The disadvantage due to impairment or disability that limits or prevents fulfilment of a normal role. The social and societal consequences are: inability to return to role as husband/wife, parent, grandfather/grandmother, lover; inability to return to work, social life, home community; inability to resume hobbies.

It could be said that the level of handicap is loosely based on role theory which focuses on people's roles in life. Each role is a set of social norms that governs a person's behaviour in a group and determines relationships to other group members (Hoeman, 1996).

In order for rehabilitation to be effective the focus has to be on the level of handicap. This enables the professionals, the client and their family to think beyond what the client cannot do, towards what they can do. It is necessary to establish what is required to enable clients to return to their former roles in life or to establish new ones in order to achieve an acceptable quality of life. It could therefore be said that the ultimate aim of rehabilitation is to reduce the level of handicap for clients. However, this is not an aim that will necessarily be achieved in a short period of time; indeed it may take many months or years. The aim will probably not be achieved in one setting, as the client may move on through a variety of settings, e.g. acute, rehabilitation unit, community and respite care. At each stage of the journey through the rehabilitation process the client will achieve the smaller aims of rehabilitation incrementally, in order to achieve the overall goal.

The model of human occupation

Based on systems theory, this model (Keilhofner and Nichol, 1989; Kavanagh and Fares, 1995) is concerned with occupational behaviour defined as 'activity' in which individuals engage during most of their waking time. This includes activities that are playful, restful, serious and productive. Disruption caused by trauma, disease or illness will result in dysfunctional behaviour by the individual. Although this

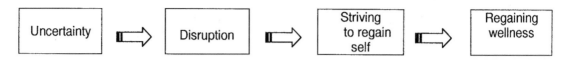

Figure 14.1   The illness experience

model is mainly an occupational therapy model, its focus on occupation makes it relevant to the concept of quality of life and therefore to all rehabilitation professionals. The model is comprehensive and enables professionals to assess clients holistically, taking into account elements such as time, the community, coping, the individual and the family. There may not be much potential for using this model within the acute area, but it does enable professionals to focus on the level of handicap and more of a wellness approach, moving away from the levels of impairment and disability which could be said to be more of a medical model approach.

The contingency model of long-term care

This model (Hymovich and Hagopian, 1992) is drawn from motivational, systems and adaptation theories and provides a comprehensive framework for clients with chronic illness and disability. Family functioning is the primary focus and the professional's role is identified as assisting individuals and their families to adapt to the condition and its effects on their daily lives. The strength of this model is that it enables professionals to assess clients holistically, taking into account elements such as time, the community, coping, the individual and the family. Elements from this model may be appropriate to incorporate into assessment at the acute stage, enabling professionals to focus more on the level of handicap.

The illness–constellation model

The focus of this model (Morse and Johnson, 1991) is on achieving wellness within the social context and it incorporates the experiences of individuals and families. Based on adaptation theory, the model identifies illness as being an experience which affects the sick person and their significant others. This illness experience is identified as a four-stage process (Figure 14.1):

The model can be seen as a process of adaptation which could be applied in the acute

area to enable professionals to identify the client and family's level of adaptation. They may be at different levels; for example the client may be at the stage of striving to regain self, where they are beginning to regain control and wanting to do things for themselves, whereas their family may be at the stage of disruption, where they are unsure of what to do and may distance themselves from the client. The stage which clients and their families have reached may determine how the team involve them in the rehabilitation process.

Orem's self-care model

This model (Knust and Quarn, 1983; Orem, 1985) is based on the theory of self-care, which explains the relationship between the kinds of day-to-day care that human beings need and their own growth, development and functioning. The major focus of this model is on self-care, dependence and independence. It enables professionals to identify the client's level of independence, so as to identify what level of intervention is required, e.g. wholly-compensatory, partially-compensatory or supporting educational needs.

One of the main concepts related to rehabilitation is the concept of teamwork, without which the aims of rehabilitation could not be achieved.

Teamwork

Rehabilitation encompasses the physical, emotional and psychological elements of care which cannot be addressed by one group of healthcare professionals, thereby highlighting the importance of effective teamwork. In order for teams to be effective, certain criteria need to be met (Table 14.1).

There are two main types of team approach identified in the literature – multidisciplinary and interdisciplinary.

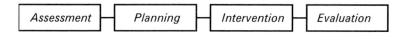

Figure 14.2 The rehabilitation experience

Multidisciplinary

This type of approach generally focuses on the level of disability, with team members conducting independent assessments, identifying independent goals and developing their own treatment plans independently of each other (McGrath and Davis, 1992; Embling, 1995; Skeil, 1995). It is the multidisciplinary approach which is mostly adopted in healthcare settings where the skill mix of professionals is uneven, e.g. one occupational therapist between a number of wards.

Table 14.1 Criteria for effective teamwork (Adapted from Dittmar, 1989; Embling, 1995)

Understanding
Respect
Regular communication
Integration of decisions and actions
Coordinated team plan
Collaboration
Coordination
Evaluation
Shared goals
Cooperation
Coordination of activities

Interdisciplinary

The interdisciplinary approach generally focuses on the level of handicap, with team members collaborating in assessment, outcomes and treatment plans (McGrath and Davis, 1992; Powell *et al.*, 1994). This type of approach lends itself more to client involvement through collaborative goal-planning. For an effective interdisciplinary approach the team needs to consist of a reasonable mix and number of professionals, which is often why this approach is only used in rehabilitation settings.

It may be appropriate for an eclectic approach to be adopted, e.g. a multidisciplinary approach with elements of the interdisciplinary approach, such as goal-setting.

Rehabilitation processes

The processes involved within rehabilitation are assessment, planning, intervention and evaluation (Figure 14.2).

Assessment

Assessment in rehabilitation needs to involve a number of instruments assessing function/self-care/mobility, cognition, emotion, vocation, perception and social circumstances. According to Hoeman (1996), information from assessment instruments can be used to:

- document the type and severity of impairments, functional limitations or disability at a given point in time
- measure clinical changes over time
- establish goals and plan treatments.

The levels of the ICIDH framework – impairment, disability and handicap – plus the level of pathology, can provide a useful framework for assessment in rehabilitation (Wade, 1996). Wade also identifies the following areas for consideration when using this as a framework:

- the focus of attention should pass from pathology through to handicap as time passes
- as the client progresses from pathology to handicap, the focus should also move from the client to the environment
- where possible, treatment should be aimed at the level of pathology
- assessments should be focused on a single level and contain only items related to that level
- losses for the client become increasingly personal and meaningful as their condition changes from impairment to handicap
- using this framework allows for the analysis of difficult problems.

Use of this framework in trauma care would

enable professionals to identify into which level the assessments they are using fit, and to identify any gaps in assessment.

Planning – client-centred goal-setting

The main element of planning in rehabilitation is goal-setting, enabling goals to be focused on the client rather than on the professional, enabling the client, carers and team to focus on the client's strengths rather than problems. Even though in the acute stage it may be appropriate for professionals to identify the goals for the clients, e.g. preventing complications, maintaining a safe environment, maintaining life, as soon as is feasible the client and relatives should be enabled to identify the goals that are meaningful for them. The team can guide the client into thinking of goals pertinent to the level of handicap, taking a more long-term view, rather than focusing solely on the level of disability. Thinking at this level needs to begin at the acute stage. Davis *et al.* (1992) developed a questionnaire to assist clients and the team in the setting of client-focused aims. The questionnaire consists of the following life areas:

- residential and domestic arrangements
- personal care
- leisure and hobbies
- work
- relationship with partner
- family life
- contacts with friends
- religion
- financial status.

Clients are asked to rate each area in relation to its level of importance to them. The questionnaire enables staff to identify what is really important to the client and to identify goals in terms of handicap. The goal-setting process consists of aims, objectives and targets. Aims can be described in terms of handicap and social role, with objectives being the steps to achieve the aims (Davis *et al.*, 1992). Objectives are interdisciplinary, being achieved by more than one member of the team, with targets being the steps each professional needs to take in order to achieve the objectives.

Example

Aim. For Bill to return to live independently at home with his family

Objective. For Bill to be able to transfer himself independently. The objective would be one of many identified to achieve the aim. In the objective chosen, a number of professionals may be involved in its achievement, e.g. nurse, physiotherapist, occupational therapist. Each professional will then identify targets to help Bill meet the objective. For example a nursing target might be:

Target. Transfer Bill from bed to chair and chair to bed using the technique identified by the physiotherapists, reporting back to them any difficulties

---

Although the aim could be identified at the handicap level in the acute area, it may not be achieved until the client is in a rehabilitation setting or in the community. However, the team in the acute area can begin to identify objectives which would work towards the client's aim, as the above example illustrates.

Interventions

Rehabilitation interventions can be conceptually divided into treatments which may be at the level of pathology, impairment, disability or handicap (Wade, 1996). When thinking of rehabilitation interventions, these should begin from the day following the client's accident and continue to beyond discharge. It is useful to relate to the four stages shown in the following example.

Example

Stage 1 At the initial critical stage where the client is in a coma, the goal of rehabilitation will be to maintain life.

- Preventing complications, including those of immobility: passive exercises, positioning.
- Providing verbal and tactile stimulation: music, touching, massage, communication.
- Supporting relatives: informing them of what is happening, giving them the opportunity to be involved in providing stimulation, giving

them written information, referring them to support groups.

Stage 2 The client is out of the coma, fully responsive and beginning to regain some function. The goals of rehabilitation will depend on the client's needs. One goal may be 'to maintain a safe, comfortable environment'. For example, clients following head injury often become aggressive and agitated at this stage and may be in post-traumatic amnesia. If possible, the process of enabling clients to use the function they have should begin now.

- Managing aggressive behaviour: assessing the client's behaviour in order to establish a baseline from which to build a behaviour modification programme which should include:
  - reinforcing acceptable behaviour and ignoring unacceptable behaviour
  - ensuring that a consistent team approach is used
  - the provision of a safe environment
  - the avoidance of overstimulation
- Often, overstimulation can be identified as the reason for aggression.
- Assessing the client's functional and cognitive ability: enabling them to do as much for themselves as they can, e.g. moving limbs, bridging and turning in bed, assisting with transfers, washing, dressing, feeding themselves.
- Beginning to establish normal activities: eating while sitting at a table, sitting out of bed, using the toilet rather than the commode.
- Giving clients choices, even if they are limited: choice of diet, choice of clothes.
- Establishing alternative forms of communication if appropriate.
- Supporting and involving relatives in these strategies so that they are also using an enabling approach.

Stage 3 This is the stage where a more active programme of rehabilitation is required and may occur in a rehabilitation ward or centre. The goals of rehabilitation are more specifically focused on the level of handicap.

- Facilitating and enabling clients to achieve their maximum potential in washing, dressing, feeding, communication and mobility.
- Ensuring that there is continuity of therapy programmes between the different disciplines, e.g. washing and dressing programmes, mobility programmes, speech exercises, cognitive programmes.

- Establishing continence programmes if appropriate.
- Empowering clients by giving them informed choice and by involving them in the setting of rehabilitation goals.
- Providing psychological support to the client and family.
- Assessing the client's needs in relation to sexuality; identifying an appropriate plan of care which may involve additional referrals.
- Acting as a coordinator between the client, relatives and the rest of the team.
- Providing a supportive, structured environment for the client and family.
- Health promotion, e.g. facilitating empowerment, incorporating health education activities.

Stage 4 At this stage the client will have reached their full potential and the focus is now on living with the disabilities they have and maintaining quality of life in relation to work, hobbies and social life. At this stage the client will either be at home or in an alternative placement. They may attend a young disabled unit for respite care or other day facilities where the role of the team and the nurse is to help them maintain their quality of life.

Reassessment

Reassessment is concerned with the evaluation of the planning and intervention stages (Wade, 1996). It is important that this evaluation occurs so that the rehabilitation programme can be renegotiated if it is not achieving the client's aims. Also, the client's overall aim may change; for example the aim may originally have been to return to work, but as the rehabilitation programme progresses the client themselves may be able to identify that this is no longer realistic. It is difficult to evaluate whether or not rehabilitation has been successful for an individual client. Outcome measures cover three main areas (Jeffrey, 1993):

1. Function – where the focus is on mobility and self-care.
2. Specific areas for people with mental health problems – such as task orientation, social interaction, role functioning.
3. Comprehensive measures which focus on the holistic approach to client care and on the client's perceptions of their recovery.

The goal planning process lends itself to an

evaluation of the effectiveness of rehabilitation for the individual client by comparing outcomes with the identified aims. It also enables professionals to focus on evaluation of the quality of life for that client.

Rehabilitation – psychosocial effects

Clients undergoing rehabilitation have often gone through some sudden major change brought about by illness or trauma, resulting in disabilities which will have major implications for the future. These changes can create enormous psychological stress, which can be defined as being a particular relationship between the individual and the environment that exceeds the individual's resources to cope, thereby endangering their well-being. This stress may also be experienced by the client's family. Examples of stressors are listed in Table 14.2.

Table 14.2 Stressors (Adapted from Hoeman, 1996)

Loss and change
Health status
Daily hassles
Environment
The rehabilitation itself
Lack of knowledge
Uncertainty factors
Individual and family characteristics
Self-esteem, hardiness and vulnerability
Sociocultural influences and perceptions of quality of life

A number of reactions to stress are identified within the literature, for example shock, anxiety, denial, depression, internalized anger, externalized hostility, acknowledgement and adjustment. It is important for professionals to identify how the client and family are reacting to the situation. Nichols (1984) identifies four main principles of psychological care which can help professionals identify the level at which they should be operating:

- *Emotional care.* Providing a relationship and environment which helps to address emotional processes. Professionals need to relate to the client and family in a manner which communicates permission, acceptance and safety. It is important that the client and family do not feel the need to suppress emotion, or feel ashamed or feel that they are a nuisance.
- *Informational care.* Identifying what the client and their family know and identifying the gaps in that knowledge. Ensuring that the relevant information is available and that it is understood by the client and family.
- *Counselling.* Healthcare professionals should have the basic skills of counselling which include listening, probing, reflecting, empathizing and challenging.
- *Monitoring of psychological state and referring on.* It is important that professionals can recognize when there is a need to refer the client and possibly members of their family on to other professionals for more formal therapy.

Keeping the family informed and giving them the opportunity to discuss their fears may be a major role of the team in the acute stage of a client's rehabilitation journey.

Case study

This case study attempts to bring together aspects discussed previously, highlighting the different levels of intervention and the environments in which they occur.

Linda, a 41-year-old woman, was admitted to the accident and emergency (A&E) department following a road traffic accident. On admission to A&E:

Pathology: Severe head injury.
Impairments: Dense right hemiparesis; unable to swallow, complete expressive aphasia; husband, Peter, very stressed.
Disabilities: Unable to stand, transfer, walk, drink unthickened fluids; unable to communicate; unable to use right arm and hand for any activities; unable to wash and dress without maximum assistance.
Handicaps: Unable to fulfil her role as a wife and mother of two children; unable to return to her part-time job as a shop assistant.

Level 1
On admission to A&E Linda had recovered consciousness but was unable to communicate

and unable to move unaided. Rehabilitation at this stage, both in A&E and on the acute ward, was concerned with recording observations to ensure that her condition remained stable, commencing passive exercises, positioning her limbs appropriately and talking to her in order to explain what was happening. Nutritional needs were met by feeding her thickened fluids and a soft diet. Peter was very stressed at this stage and needed a lot of support from the nurses and the rest of the team. They were able to give him written information about the consequences of head injury and put him in contact with Headway (a head injury support group). The aim at this stage was to prevent complications and maintain stability. Linda began to make slow progress over the next few weeks.

Level 2
Linda was now fully alert and beginning to regain some independence. The team assessed her functional and cognitive ability and agreed, following discussion with Linda and Peter, the aims of rehabilitation at this stage. These included promoting independence by encouraging Linda to bridge and turn in bed, to wash herself and carry out personal care and to wheel herself in a wheelchair. At this stage, due to the density of her hemiplegia, Linda was being transferred using a hoist on the ward, but in physiotherapy sessions she was learning how to take weight through her unaffected side and to transfer with one physiotherapist. Following a speech therapy assessment a communication board was introduced which was used by the team. Peter was involved in Linda's programme at this stage, being taught how to use the communication board and how to encourage Linda in physical activities. He also attended Linda's physiotherapy sessions with her. As Peter needed a lot of reassurance and support, Anne, Linda's primary nurse, made sure that she saw him regularly to feedback Linda's progress and to pick up on his anxieties.

Level 3
Linda was transferred to a rehabilitation unit 2 months after her head injury. The first 2 weeks of Linda's stay involved the team undertaking a full physical and cognitive assessment. As well as communication difficulties, it was discovered that Linda had poor short-term memory. She was now able to drink ordinary fluids and feed herself and identified her main aim as being to return home to look after her children. In order to achieve this she needed to be independent in washing, dressing and personal care. She

needed to maximize her physical mobility, to communicate and be able to remember to do things. At the goal-planning meeting the team identified the objectives that needed to be met in order for Linda to achieve her aim. These were discussed with Linda and Peter. The main objectives were aimed at social interaction and activities of daily living and mobility. While at the unit Linda was able to practise social skills such as shopping and communicating with different agencies. She also learnt how to use a diary to compensate for her poor short-term memory. Peter voiced his concerns regarding Linda's ability to look after the children and expressed his desire that she should not return home. His mother was very protective of him and the children and supported Peter in his view.

Level 4
Six months after admission to the unit Linda was discharged home with the assistance of a carer who could make telephone calls, monitor her correspondence and help her with heavier household tasks. On discharge into the community Linda's residual difficulties were as follows:

Impairments: Mild language impairment affecting high-level reading skills and understanding of complex sentences; no functional speech; limited short-term memory; ability to write single words only; inability to make skilled movements with accuracy; no active movements in right upper limb and right ankle and reduced active movements of right hip and knee.

Activities: Ability to walk independently with a stick and manage stairs; ability to feed herself; independence in simple domestic tasks with one-handed equipment; ability to order a taxi and 'shop mobility'; ability to go around the shops in town in a powered chair; ability to shop in the supermarket on her own if set up and planned; needs assistance in unfamiliar situations.

Participation: Ability to live in her house without adaptations; has resumed her role as mother, with the help of her mother-in-law; beginning to re-establish friendships again and becoming more confident in the community; unable to return to employment – other options not yet explored; needs support in the community regarding domestic and community matters; needs to work on community reintegration; Peter still having problems coming to terms with Linda's disabilities.

> The main focus of Linda's rehabilitation at home is on her reintegration into the community and the fulfilment of her role as mother and wife. This involves Linda attending various groups at the local community hospital and receiving counselling with Peter.

Conclusion

Rehabilitation needs to be thought of as a philosophy and a process which begins immediately following an acute incident, continuing through into the community. Rehabilitation is not often seen in that way, rather more as something that happens 'elsewhere'. The explanation for this could be due to lack of knowledge in relation to what rehabilitation means and how it fits into acute trauma care. The aims of this chapter have been to relate rehabilitation to trauma care by exploring the meaning and levels of rehabilitation, together with related concepts such as teamwork and goal-setting. The following are strategies which professionals could use in order to promote rehabilitation in trauma care:

- use the ICIDH classification as a framework for client's notes to ensure that the focus is not solely on impairment and disability
- think of rehabilitation as a philosophy as well as a process
- identify how you operate as a team – which approach do you use, what communication strategies do you use?
- reflect on your own practice – are you using enabling facilitating strategies which promote client choice and independence?

References

Blackwell (1994) *Blackwell's Dictionary of Nursing.* Blackwell Scientific.

Chipps E., Clanin, N. and Campbell, V. (1992) *Neurological Disorders.* Mosby Year Book.

Davis, A. M., Davis, S., Moss, N. *et al* (1992) First steps towards an interdisciplinary approach to rehabilitation. *Clinical Rehabilitation*, **6**, 237–244.

Dittmar, S. (1989) *Rehabilitation Nursing.* Mosby.

Embling, S. (1995) Exploring multidisciplinary teamwork. *British Journal of Therapy and Rehabilitation*, **2**(3), 142–144.

Greenwood, R., Barnes, M. P., McMillan, T. M. and Ward, C. D. (1993) *Neurological Rehabilitation.* Churchill Livingstone.

Hickey, J. V. (1986) *The Clinical Practice of Neurological and Neurosurgical Nursing.* J. P. Lippincott.

Hoeman, S. (1996) *Rehabilitation Nursing: Process and Application.* Mosby.

Hymovich, D. P. and Hagopian, G. A. (1992) *Chronic Illness in Children and Adults: A Psychological Approach.* W. B. Saunders.

Jackson, M. F. (1984) Geriatric rehabilitation on an acute care medical unit. *Journal of Advanced Nursing*, **9**, 441–448.

Jeffrey, L. I. H. (1993). Aspects of selecting outcome measures to demonstrate the effectiveness of comprehensive rehabilitation. *British Journal of Occupational Therapy*, **56**(11) 394–400.

Kavanagh, J. and Fares, J. (1995) Using the model of human occupation with homeless mentally ill clients. *British Journal of Occupational Therapy*, October, **58**(10) 419–422.

Keilhofner, G. and Nichol, M. (1989) The role of the nurse in the rehabilitation of acute stroke patients: towards a unified theory. *Advances in Nursing Science*, **19**(4) 55–64.

Knust, S. J. and Quarn, J. M. (1983) Integration of self-care theory into rehabilitation nursing. *Rehabilitation Nursing*, **8**(4), 26–28.

Licht, S. (1968) *Rehabilitation Medicine.* Waverly Press.

McGrath, J. and Davis, A. (1992) Rehabilitation: where are we going and how do we get there? *Clinical Rehabilitation*, **6**, 225–235.

Morse, D. I. M. and Johnson, J. U. L. (1991) *The Illness Experience: Dimensions of Suffering.* Sage.

Nichols, K. A. (1984) *Psychological Care in Physical Illness.* Croom Helm.

Orem, D. M. (1985) A concept of self-care for the rehabilitation client. *Rehabilitation Nursing*, **10**, 33–36.

Pfeiffer, D. (1998) The ICIDH and the need for its revision. *Disability & Society*, **13**(4) 503–523.

Powell, T., Partridge, T., Nicholls, T. *et al.* (1994) An interdisciplinary approach to the rehabilitation of people with brain injury. *British Journal of Therapy and Rehabilitation*, **1**(1), 8–13.

Preston, K. (1994) Rehabilitation nursing: a client-centred philosophy. *American Journal Nursing*, February, 66–70.

Royal College Nursing (1994) *Standards of Care for Rehabilitation Nursing.* Scutari Press.

Skeil, D. (1995) Individual and staff professional development in a multidisciplinary team: some needs and solutions. *Clinical Rehabilitation*, **9**, 28–33.

Wade, D. T. (1996) Designing district disability services – the Oxford experience. *Clinical Rehabilitation*, **4**, 147–158.

Waters, K. (1987) The role of the nurse in rehabilitation. *CARE – Science and Practice*, **5**(3), 17–21.

World Health Organisation (1980) *International Classification of Impairments, Disabilities and Handicaps.* WHO.

15

Trauma and mental health

Mike Hobbs

Introduction

Physical trauma is always associated with stress which, if severe, may generate a range of psychological and psychiatric reactions. Stress most obviously affects the person who is injured, but may also have a dramatic impact on those who are exposed to a traumatic event, but not injured. Those around the primary victim are often affected too, including the professional staff whose work involves the rescue, resuscitation and treatment of those who are injured.

Some degree of emotional distress is quite natural after a traumatic experience, and may persist or recur for several weeks. The psychological reaction would be regarded as abnormal and of psychiatric significance, however, if the person's usual emotional, social or occupational functioning was undermined to a significant degree; though this may be less easy to judge when normal functioning is impaired by physical injury.

A range of early and later psychiatric reactions to trauma are recognized, including post-traumatic stress disorder (PTSD). Related post-traumatic syndromes, anxiety disorders and depression are more common than PTSD, however. This chapter will examine these disorders, addressing their origins, clinical features and treatment. Particular emphasis will be given to their recognition and management in the setting of accident department, trauma ward or rehabilitation unit. Reference will be made also to the impact on health staff of working with people who have been traumatized.

The psychology of trauma

Stress

The psychological impact of trauma is mediated by stress, which in this context is termed 'traumatic stress'. Stress is the psychophysiological response to challenge or threat, and is both natural and adaptive. In the face of adversity, stress is generated by the person's perception of a discrepancy between available and required resources. Stress galvanizes the psychophysiological arousal which is essential for effective response to danger, both physical action (e.g. to escape from danger) and psychological adaptation, or coping. The absence of stress indicates that there is no recognition of, or reaction to, a challenge. Increasing arousal mobilizes established coping resources, and then new resourcefulness. Excessive arousal, however, is associated with diminishing effectiveness and ultimately the breakdown of functioning.

Traumatic events cause sudden, severe and sometimes incapacitating stress, i.e. traumatic stress. The perceived threat of pain, injury or death creates intense fear or terror. Very high levels of arousal are generated, habitual coping resources are overwhelmed and the person's usual resourcefulness may evaporate. This state of perceived powerlessness and ineffectiveness, which may completely negate the person's previous view of themselves, is the basis for the post-traumatic stress syndromes.

Traumatic stress

In psychiatric terms, a traumatizing event is one

in which the person

1. **Experiences, witnesses, or otherwise encounters an event which involves death, the threat of death or serious injury, or a threat to the physical integrity (e.g. rape) of self or others;**

and

2. **Experiences intense fear, helplessness or horror** (American Psychiatric Association, 1994).

Not everyone who is exposed to such experiences develops post-traumatic psychiatric problems, however, and the factors which influence risk will be further examined.

Traumatic events may be categorized usefully according to the complexity of the psychological reactions to which they may give rise (Terr, 1991). Type I traumas are single incidents, typically sudden, unexpected and short-lived (e.g. road accident), and, if pathogenic, they tend to give rise to clear-cut post-traumatic disorders such as phobic anxiety or PTSD. Type II traumas often comprise prolonged, repeated, and thereby anticipated, terrifying experiences (e.g. torture, or sexual abuse in childhood); these give rise to more complex, and often more enduring, post-traumatic disorders. 'Crossover' conditions occur when a type I trauma gives rise to a prolonged traumatic ordeal, as for example when the victim of a brutal physical assault is intimidated into silence by threats of further violence.

Causes of traumatic stress

Experiences which are psychologically traumatizing may or may not be associated with physical injury. Events which cause physical injury will usually have the potential to cause traumatic stress and its related psychiatric disorders.

Traumatic events, particularly when large-scale, are sometimes differentiated as natural ('acts of God') or perpetrated by humans ('man-made'). This distinction is not absolute, but does draw attention to the fact that many so-called 'accidents' are avoidable, the result of human error, carelessness or antisocial action. Traumatic events which are perceived to be the result of human failing or malice are often associated with more lasting psychiatric problems.

Traumatic events sometimes occur in combi-

nation, of course. Such combinations may be particularly traumagenic, as for example when a loved person is killed in the same accident in which the individual is injured and permanently disabled.

Some causes of traumatic stress are listed in Table 15.1.

Table 15.1   Traumatic stressors

Physical assault
Sexual assault – including childhood sexual abuse and rape
Accident – on road, in the workplace or home
Fire – in the home, workplace, or elsewhere
Traumatic bereavement by sudden, unexpected death (e.g. accident, suicide, homicide)
Hostage experience, with threats of death
Torture
Threatened or actual criminal/terrorist shooting, bombing
Disaster (large-scale destructive events) • natural – flood, hurricane, earthquake • man-made – transportation disasters (road, rail, sea, air), crowd disasters (sports stadium, nightclub), massacres
War combat
Genocidal violence

Psychological victims of trauma

A destructive event may traumatize not just those who are directly exposed to danger – the primary victims – but also people who are in some other way connected to it (Table 15.2). These include those who are emotionally close to the primary victims, amongst them the bereaved; people who witness or in some other way feel associated with the event, including those who might easily have been primary victims, for example the person who missed the flight which crashed ('victims by proxy'); and those whose jobs involve response to the incident or caring for its victims.

The traumatic impact of a destructive event has a ripple effect, spreading from its epicentre to involve people at progressively greater geographical, temporal and psychological distances. Because of this, it has been suggested that traumatic stress is 'contagious'. The numbers of people affected by large-scale traumatic incidents, particularly mass disaster, may be enormous.

Table 15.2 Psychological victims of traumatic incidents

Primary victims – those directly exposed to perceived danger

Family, friends, work or school mates of the primary victims, including the bereaved

Witnesses – people who see the incident, or the deaths, injury or suffering of those involved

Victims by proxy – those who might have been there

Emergency services, rescue and body-handling personnel

Media personnel who cover the incident

Front-line hospital staff in a number of areas – accident department, intensive care unit, trauma ward; also staff such as telephonists, porters, mortuary staff

Voluntary and professional support workers, counsellors and therapists who work with trauma victims

Psychological models of trauma

Traumatic experiences are those which pierce the psychological defences by which we can usually protect ourselves from awareness of danger, fear and pain (Garland, 1991). Nurses in the accident department, for example, could not work efficiently if they were always in tune with their patients' fear and pain. There may be something so dreadful about a particular patient's death, injuries or experience, however, that the horror cuts through the nurse's defences to leave him or her feeling traumatized.

When gripped by intense fear, people are no longer able to process and resolve the emotional and cognitive aspects of their experience. Their feelings (including horror or terror) remain raw, and their most basic assumptions about themselves and the world are shattered (Janoff-Bulman, 1992). People who have been traumatized frequently lose the sense of safety, invulnerability and future that most of us take for granted (Table 15.3). Some, particularly those who have been traumatized by sexual assault or torture, may lose all sense of self-worth.

Traumatic experiences frequently have a destructive psychosocial impact. People who have been seriously traumatized may lose their sense of relatedness to others and behave in a very detached manner, even with their closest family and friends. This, in conjunction with the avoidance and irritability which are symptomatic of PTSD, puts a severe strain on relationships. Broken relationships, alienation and antisocial actions are characteristic of the destructive changes in personality which may result from complex traumas such as torture or certain prolonged combat experiences.

Another result of traumatization is that memories of previous traumas and losses may be rekindled. A road accident, for example, may stir up recollections and feelings associated with a previous accident, a past bereavement or sexual abuse in childhood. It can be very puzzling for hospital staff when a patient is more distressed than their experience seems to warrant, or is more upset about a past experience than the event which led to their hospitalization.

Table 15.3 Impact of trauma on basic assumptions

Loss of basic sense of:

Orderliness and predictability of the world
Justice and fairness of life
Benevolence of others
Safety, invulnerability and immortality of oneself
Future for oneself and loved ones
Self-worth
Emotional relatedness of oneself to others

Risk factors

It is evident that people's reactions to traumatic incidents are not all the same, even when objectively their experiences are very similar. Some individuals are vulnerable to the development of psychiatric problems, while others prove more resilient. Traumatization is the product of interaction between the event, the attributes of the person experiencing it, and his or her social context. A number of risk factors have been identified and may be classified along these three dimensions.

The event

The traumatic impact will be influenced by the nature, duration and seriousness of the event. Take road accidents as an example. A few people are traumatized psychologically by road accidents in which nobody is injured, let alone killed, and material damage is minor. Many more people will be traumatized by multiple accidents in which others are killed and severely injured, even if they escape serious injury themselves. This is particularly likely if they witness the death or suffering of others, especially of people they know.

Again, the victim of a road accident is more likely to be traumatized if, rather than freeing himself from the car immediately, he is trapped in pain and terrified of the prospect of fire for a long period before being extricated by emergency service workers.

There is another issue which seems to influence risk, and which represents an interplay between the dimensions of event and person. This is the subjective meaning the incident has for the individual experiencing it (Garland, 1991).

Example: personal meaning of traumatic event

Mrs Andrews had prided herself in being strong and capable. Since childhood she had protected her psychologically vulnerable mother who was often depressed, and always kept her own feelings hidden. She supported her mother emotionally and coped with all the practical arrangements when her father and maternal grandmother died within a few weeks of each other, but did not grieve herself.

Then, when pregnant with her second child, Mrs Andrews was involved in a car accident. Nobody was injured, but Mrs Andrews was highly distressed and, over the ensuing weeks, became seriously depressed. She was preoccupied both with her helplessness at not having been able to do anything to avert the accident, and with the possibility that she and her children could have died. She saw danger everywhere, could no longer drive and would not allow her children out of her sight. When she talked with her family doctor about the accident Mrs Andrews recognized that it was the first time in her life that she had felt vulnerable and had confronted her own mortality. The accident changed Mrs Andrews' view of herself and the world and triggered delayed grieving for all that she had lost. As she came gradually to recognize the full personal meaning of the incident, her depression lifted and she resumed driving – albeit with extreme cautiousness. It was a long time, however, before she came to terms with her new self-image.

The person

The psychological impact of a threatening event is influenced by the personal attributes of the individual exposed to it, as well as its physical effects (Table 15.4).

Table 15.4 Risk factors for psychological traumatization

Persisting physical problems or disability
Disfigurement
Socioeconomic loss – job, financial security, status
Previous or concurrent psychiatric illness
Personality factors
Subjective perception of life threat
Negative cognitive appraisal of experience
Dissociation

Injury, disability, disfigurement

Research studies after destructive events have produced conflicting findings for the relationship between physical injury and psychiatric complications (Blanchard *et al.*, 1995; Ehlers *et al.*, 1998). **There is no evidence for a simple direct relationship between injury severity and the presence or severity of subsequent psychiatric problems**. People who suffer no physical injury may suffer severe psychological traumatization and develop a disabling psychiatric disorder (Mayou and Bryant, 1994). Some who sustain serious injury display no significant psychiatric complication. There is a tendency for those who suffer multiple injuries to develop psychiatric illness, however, but this may be more a product of their lasting physical problems.

There is evidence that persisting physical problems, lasting physical disability and disfigurement (perhaps particularly facial disfigurement) are associated with increased risk of psychiatric difficulties (Mayou *et al.*, 1993). In some cases the physical disability may lead to socioeconomic factors such as loss of job, career prospects and financial security, which compound the psychological impact of the trauma.

Personality, coping and psychiatric history

The individual's personality and previous coping resources are significant factors in how they cope with destructive incidents, as are previous or concurrent psychiatric disorders (Breslau and Davis, 1992; O'Brien, 1998).

Those with 'anxious' personalities, who are prone to worry and cope maladaptively with any challenge, are vulnerable to stress and likely to develop psychiatric problems in the face of intense threats to their precarious psychological adjustment. In some people their vulnerable personalities are the result of earlier adversities, including childhood abuse (physical, sexual, emotional), bereavement and other losses, psychiatric illness, or previous psychological trauma.

People who have suffered previous psychiatric disorders of any kind (including anxiety states, depressive illness, psychosis, substance misuse or even PTSD), or who are psychiatrically unwell at the time of the incident, are vulnerable to relapses or exacerbations of those disorders and to the development of specific post-traumatic disorders. Some psychiatric disorders are associated with increased risk of involvement in traumatic incidents, either as a direct consequence of the illness or as an adverse effect of the psychotropic medication with which they are treated (McDonald and Davey, 1996). For example, those who abuse alcohol or drugs are at greater risk of experiencing, and causing, accidents or assaults (Cherpitel, 1993). Depressed people are at greater risk of accidents because of impaired concentration and reaction time, and those who attempt or achieve suicide represent an enhanced risk to their relatives and friends. A small minority of psychotic patients are at increased risk of assault or accident because of their delusional beliefs, for example when they accuse others of persecuting them.

Subjective perception of danger

Another risk factor, which may be related to factors identified above, is the person's *perception* of danger. A number of studies have confirmed that the risk of developing psychiatric problems is correlated with subjective perception of danger rather than with the objective risk of injury or death (Malt and Olafsen, 1992; Blanchard *et al.*, 1995).

Reaction to traumatic event

The person's immediate reaction to the traumatic event also influences the risk of post-traumatic psychiatric problems. One significant aspect of the reaction is cognitive appraisal, that is the thoughts that occur during and after the traumatic experience. Studies of women who have been sexually or physically assaulted (Dunmore *et al.*, 1997) show they are at greater risk of post-traumatic stress disorder if:

- they 'give up' mentally during the assault, as opposed to thinking of ways to escape or protect themselves
- they subsequently blame themselves for the way they behaved during the assault
- they perceive the reactions of others to be unsympathetic and unsupportive
- their perceptions of themselves and their lives are adversely affected

Another significant aspect of the person's immediate reaction to the event is the degree to which they dissociate emotionally from it. **A minor degree of dissociation, commonly manifest as emotional numbing, is normal in the immediate aftermath of exposure to frightening events.** Numbing may be regarded as an adaptive early response, in that it confers some protection from the overwhelming fear which otherwise might compromise the victim's physical reactions, including escape from the danger. Furthermore, short-lived emotional numbing may enable the person to come to terms gradually with the seriousness of the threat to which they have been exposed, by pacing their psychological response.

More severe dissociation, however, is strongly associated with the risk of post-traumatic psychiatric problems (Koopman *et al.*, 1995; Murray, 1997). Problematic degrees of dissociation may be manifest by persisting emotional detachment, reduced awareness of the surroundings, depersonalization and derealization (feeling as if oneself or one's surroundings respectively are unreal), or a dissociative amnesia. These form part of acute stress disorder (see next section). The pathogenic effect of marked dissociation may result from its obstruction and distortion of psychological adaptation to the traumatic experience.

Social context

Psychosocial factors have a significant influence on the person's adaptation to traumatic experiences.

The first influential factor is the social environment in which the traumatized individual recovers from the ordeal, the so-called 'recovery environment'. It is apparent, clinically, that **the provision of a secure and emotionally supportive environment is essential for re-establishment of the victim's sense of security, without which the risk of psychiatric complications is enhanced**. Clinical experience is supported by empirical evidence for the protective value of social support (Joseph *et al.*, 1997; O'Brien, 1998). The interpersonal aspects of the post-trauma environment are crucial for limiting traumatic damage to the victim's sense of relatedness or attachment to others, which is the basis for his or her personal security and capacity for psychological adaptation.

Family and friends can play a significant role in the victim's recovery, particularly if they can remain sympathetic and supportive even in the face of the individual's continuing distress, which might sometimes include anger or rejection and repeated harrowing accounts of their ordeal. The social network faces a particularly great challenge when another member is killed in the incident, for grief may then compromise their emotional availability to those who survived, as well as compounding the survivor's traumatization.

Social isolation enhances the risk of developing post-traumatic psychiatric problems. For those patients who are hospitalized with physical injuries after trauma, nursing and other professional staff can make a significant contribution to the creation of an optimal recovery environment.

Other social factors which influence outcome include the restrictions resulting from: physical injury and disability; the financial problems resulting from loss of income, loss of material possessions (e.g. car, home) and loss of job or career; and the social consequences of disfigurement, particularly facial disfigurement, which sometimes lead to severe social anxiety and avoidance.

Of related concern is the adverse impact of other events which result from or follow the initial destructive incident and which serve as continuing, unwelcome reminders of the trauma. The former include the loss of home, or even community, which may occur in mass disasters such as floods, hurricanes or warfare. The latter category includes the legal process, on a wider scale involving the coroner's inquest and any formal inquiry or criminal proceedings which are initiated. On a personal scale, the individual may be reminded repeatedly of the

trauma by compensation or other legal procedures, particularly because these may drag on for years.

Psychiatric effects of trauma

Psychiatric effects

The majority of people who are exposed to traumatic events experience fear and distress, but with the care of their family and friends make a full recovery. For some, the experience leads to revised views of themselves and of life: stronger, wiser, more resourceful, but also more cautious, careful and caring. A sizeable minority, however, suffer significant and sometimes lasting psychiatric effects. These are summarised in Table 15.5.

Table 15.5 Psychiatric disorders associated with trauma

Acute stress reaction
Acute stress disorder
Post-traumatic stress disorder (PTSD)
Abnormal grief reactions
Depression
Phobic anxiety
Substance misuse
Post-concussional disorder; psychiatric effects of head injury
Enduring personality change

Normal emotional reactions

A minority of people who survive life-threatening incidents display no great emotional reaction. The majority do have an emotional reaction, however, and in most survivors this can be regarded as normal and will resolve gradually over the weeks after the incident. It is important to differentiate normal from abnormal reactions because the latter require active management.

Normal reactions to traumatic incidents vary greatly. Initial emotional numbness and disbelief is common, and may last for minutes or hours. It is sometimes followed by euphoric relief at having survived. Usually this gives way rapidly to distress, fear, and even anger as the person takes stock of what happened. At this stage anxiety may be prominent, and both sleep and concentration impaired.

In these early days and weeks survivors may recall their ordeal vividly and repeatedly, with appropriate distress. Some may be vulnerable emotionally, displaying a need for comfort and reassurance, but others may appear remote and reject sympathy. Some may be desperate to talk about their ordeal, perhaps in detail and repeatedly, whereas others may shun communication altogether, avoiding reminders or discussion of the traumatic experience. The implications of these different patterns for professional staff are considered later.

Normal reactions diminish progressively, so that the survivor is largely asymptomatic by 1 month after the traumatic incident. Recollections and distress are reactivated by reminders of the experience, however, as when the location or situation of the traumatic event is again encountered or at the time of any court hearing, inquest or memorial service; and anniversary reactions are common, particularly when bereavement was part of the trauma.

Unless acute stress disorder or another acute state develops, there may be no clear distinction between normal and abnormal reactions in the early stages; but, if the patient remains symptomatic and dysfunctional at 1 month, a post-traumatic disorder may be diagnosed.

Psychiatric disorder induced by traumatic stress

The major diagnostic classifications of psychiatric disorders, ICD-10 (World Health Organisation, 1992) and DSM-IV (American Psychiatric Association, 1992) are complex and, despite some common categories, contrasting. A pragmatic approach is adopted here, drawing from both classifications for the sake of clarity and comprehensiveness. The selection of specific diagnoses is determined by symptom profile and the time relationship to the traumatic event. The diagnosis of specific post-traumatic disorders (acute stress reaction or disorder, post-traumatic stress disorder, enduring personality change following catastrophe) requires that the person has been exposed to an extreme and exceptional stressor as described in Table 15.1.

Acute stress reaction (ICD-10)

This diagnosis is made when the onset of symptoms follows a traumatic experience immediately or within minutes. It describes a transient disorder lasting no longer than 2–3 days, and is characterized by initial 'daze' (dissociation) and then a mixed and changing picture of anxiety, depression, anger, despair, withdrawal or excited overactivity. In a small number of cases, including but not confined to those with a previous history of psychotic illness, delusional ideas or hallucinations may emerge (stress-induced psychosis).

Acute stress disorder (DSM-IV)

Acute stress disorder (ASD) can be diagnosed only when abnormal symptoms last for more than 2 days and up to 4 weeks (when a diagnosis of PTSD would be made), and if the symptoms cause clinically significant distress and/or significant impairment in communication, social, occupational or other functions.

Four symptom clusters are described, including the re-experiencing, avoidance and arousal symptoms characteristic of PTSD. The fourth cluster, which defines ASD, comprises the following dissociative symptoms:

1. Emotional numbing or detachment.
2. Reduction in awareness of surroundings ('daze').
3. Derealization or depersonalization (surroundings or self, respectively, feel unreal).
4. Dissociative amnesia (inability to recall important aspects of the traumatic experience in the absence of organic amnesia resulting from head injury).

Recent studies have confirmed that **early but persistent dissociative symptoms are associated with a higher later incidence of PTSD** (Koopman *et al.*, 1995; Murray, 1997), so ASD may require active treatment.

Post-traumatic stress disorder (ICD-10 and DSM-IV)

The diagnosis of PTSD requires the presence, for longer than 4 weeks, of symptoms in each of three clusters (Table 15.6), along with associated distress and/or impairment of social, occupational or other functioning (American Psychiatric Association, 1994).

Formal DSM-IV diagnosis of PTSD requires a minimum of one re-experiencing symptom, three avoidance symptoms and two arousal symptoms. However, partial post-traumatic

Table 15.6 Symptoms of PTSD (DSM-IV)

Re-experiencing	Avoidance (Persistent avoidance or numbing of general responsiveness)	Hyper-arousal (Persistent symptoms of heightened arousal)
Recurrent, intrusive recollections (images, thoughts, perceptions) of the event	Efforts to avoid thoughts, feelings or conversations about the incident	Sleep disturbance
Recurrent distressing dreams or nightmares of the event	Efforts to avoid situations or people who arouse recollections of the trauma	Irritability, angry outbursts
Feeling or acting as if the traumatic event were recurring, including dissociative 'flashbacks' in which the intensity of the recollection is such that the person experiences themselves as re-living the ordeal	Inability to recall important aspects of the event (dissociative amnesia)	Impairment of concentration
Intense distress or physiological reactivity when exposed to actual or symbolic reminders of the event	Markedly diminished interest and activity	Hypervigilance
	Reduced range of emotions Feelings of detachment or estrangement from others Sense of foreshortened future	Exaggerated startle response

states, which do not match full diagnostic criteria for PTSD, may be just as disturbing and disabling to those who suffer them (O'Brien, 1998).

PTSD, or other post-traumatic illnesses, may be classified as acute or chronic according to whether the duration of symptoms is less or more than 3 months; and delayed if symptoms emerge more than 6 months after the traumatic event. For example, a significant number of World War II veterans have recently developed PTSD, their traumatic combat experiences apparently reactivated by commemorative events 50 years after the war.

Other psychiatric reactions to traumatic stress

Other psychiatric disorders may follow traumatic experiences, and may occur in isolation or comorbidly with specific post-traumatic disorders. These include phobic anxiety, abnormal grief, depression, substance misuse, and other risk-taking behaviours.

Phobic anxiety. A form of situational anxiety associated with patterns of avoidance. The person becomes acutely anxious in situations reminiscent of the traumatic event and may suffer panic attacks in which severe anxiety

symptoms are associated with fear of collapse or death. They then avoid the feared situation, to varying degree. For example, after involvement in a road accident the survivor may avoid driving in the weather conditions in which the accident happened, may stop driving altogether or, at the extreme, may be unable to leave the security of their home at any time.

Abnormal grief. More common after traumatic bereavement; that is sudden, unexpected and often violent death (particularly by accident, suicide or homicide), especially when the death is witnessed, or the body is severely mutilated or not recovered (Parkes, 1996). The opportunity to view the dead body may reduce the chance of pathological grief, provided that this is voluntary and sensitively arranged (Hodgkinson *et al.*, 1993). Abnormal grief is characterized by its intensity, chronicity, or the presence of associated symptoms such as depression or a delusional conviction that the dead person is actually still alive.

Depression. Common after the experience of significant loss, so it is not surprising that its incidence among victims of trauma is high. Depression may occur in conjunction with specific post-traumatic disorders. This, and the fact that sadness, withdrawal and insomnia may seem understandable after a traumatic experience, may hinder its diagnosis and treatment. Persisting low mood, loss of energy and interest, and irrational self-blame, are important diagnostic clues. There may be significant suicide risk, particularly after traumatic bereavement.

Substance misuse. May precede and sometimes contribute to the traumatic event; but it may start after traumatization, when it represents a maladaptive means of controlling anxiety symptoms. However, drug or alcohol misuse is likely to compound post-traumatic symptoms and may contribute to the lasting personality changes which are described below. Pre-existing alcohol or drug dependency will become evident in trauma wards when patients develop withdrawal states.

Guilt and shame. Although these are not identified in standard psychiatric classifications, they are also prominent symptoms after trauma. 'Survival guilt' is an irrational conviction that one should not have survived where others died, and is particularly prevalent after mass disasters such as the holocaust. Shame is usually associated with one's perceived failings at the time of the traumatic event, or after, for example believing that one failed to do enough to save others from injury or death. There is growing evidence that shame is a powerful factor in perpetuating post-traumatic psychopathology.

Enduring personality change after catastrophic experience (ICD-10)

Adverse personality change may become evident, with or without features of PTSD, following exposure to catastrophe or prolonged, repeated (type II) traumatic ordeals such as torture. This condition, diagnosed after at least 2 years' duration, is often identified by the emergence of inflexible and maladaptive patterns of interpersonal behaviour which were not apparent before the traumatic experience.

Suggestive characteristics include:

- hostile or mistrustful attitude towards others and the world
- feelings of emptiness or hopelessness
- chronic feelings of threat
- sense of estrangement, even from those to

  whom hitherto one was closest
- social withdrawal
- substance misuse
- risk-taking behaviours.

Diagnosis of enduring personality change requires exclusion of pre-existing personality disorder, so can only be made reliably if significant personality change is confirmed by an informant. In severe cases this is difficult because the patient will have broken off all contact with family and friends.

Epidemiology

Psychiatric disorders occur in a significant proportion of people exposed to traumatic stress. Acute stress disorder was found in 33% of patients in the 4 weeks following injury in a road accident (Murray, 1997). Murray also found that 45% of those who suffered acute stress disorder fulfilled diagnostic criteria for PTSD at 24 weeks; though 15% who did not develop acute stress disorder also had PTSD at the same point.

A quarter of patients injured in road accidents were found to have psychiatric disorders in the following year, of three overlapping diagnostic types: mood disorders 10%, phobic travel anxiety 20% and PTSD 11% (Mayou *et al.*, 1993). The same research group has recently shown higher prevalence figures for PTSD in road accident victims of 23% at 3 months, and 17% at 1 year (Ehlers *et al.*, 1998).

Similar prevalence figures are found following comparable traumatic events, though higher figures have been demonstrated in the survivors of rape, combat and mass disaster.

Preventive and treatment interventions

Early preventive intervention

In view of the high incidence and morbidity of post-traumatic disorders there has been much interest in the potential preventive value of early psychological interventions, particularly psychological debriefing.

Psychological debriefing is an active early intervention which encourages survivors to review the traumatic episode with the aim of facilitating emotional and cognitive processing of their experience (Parkinson, 1997). Originally developed as a group method for helping emergency services or military personnel to come to terms with traumatic incidents (Mitchell and Everly, 1995), psychological debriefing has since been applied enthusiastically to individual survivors of traumatic events as diverse as rape, road accidents and prolonged hostage detention.

Group debriefings are usually welcomed by participants, but there is no scientific evidence to demonstrate that they reduce post-traumatic psychopathology. A recent survey of emergency services personnel who had participated in debriefings after involvement in traumatic incidents found that the perceived helpfulness of the intervention correlated negatively with the severity of the trauma, i.e. those exposed to the most stressful incidents reported the intervention to be least helpful (Orner, 1997). Research studies of individual psychological debriefing for victims of physical assault (Rose *et al.*, 1998) and patients injured by burns (Bisson *et al.*, 1997) or road accidents (Hobbs *et al.*, 1996) have not demonstrated any preventive benefit; and indeed there is some evidence to suggest that a single early intervention may be harmful to some patients, probably because it cuts through the early numbness which may serve a protective function.

As the limitations of generic models of debriefing are recognized, attention has turned again to programmes of crisis intervention which are tailored to the needs of the individual (Bordow and Porritt, 1979; Schnyder, 1997). This involves the provision of emotional and practical support, mobilization of the patient's social network, promotion of the patient's own adaptive patterns of coping, and review of the critical experience in order to develop a strategy for progressive adjustment. Unlike debriefing, crisis intervention usually involves several treatment sessions over the weeks following adverse or traumatic experience.

Intervention: treatment or support?

Recognising that individuals who have been traumatized need safety, security, sympathy and support (both emotional and practical) – the four Ss – current thinking emphasizes the value of supportive contact in the early aftermath of trauma, rather than active psychological interventions (Figure 15.1). For most people,

relatives and friends provide this supportive presence, but emergency service workers may provide crucial comfort and support during rescue and the immediate aftermath of traumatic events. After large-scale disasters there is also a role for voluntary workers, and organizations such as the Red Cross have an important supportive function.

In the hospital setting, nurses and other staff contribute substantially to the emotional support of patients, in part just by their reassuring presence. This facilitates the engagement of the patient, whose avoidance may otherwise lead to emotional distance and detachment. The willingness to listen to the patient, even when they express the same thoughts and feelings repeatedly, and the capacity to comfort without intrusiveness or emotional over-involvement, promotes the patient's sense of security and relatedness to others.

Staff can also help to mobilize the patient's social network, encouraging family and friends to provide a comforting but not intrusive presence, to listen sympathetically to the patient's account of their ordeal and to remain tolerant of their distress (Table 15.7). Many loving relatives unwittingly fuel distress by suggesting that the patient should just be glad to be alive; or, after a few days or weeks, that they should have put the experience behind them. Such comments are upsetting and alienating to someone who is still frightened, in pain and in the grip of vivid intrusive recollections of the trauma.

Table 15.7 Psychological role of trauma unit staff

Reassuring presence (emotional security)
Engagement (emotional relatedness)
Listening and comforting (emotional support)
Mobilization of social network
Information and advice about reactions to trauma
Screening for risk factors
Recognition of abnormal reactions
Referral for specialist psychiatric assessment
Involvement in psychiatric treatment programme

Accident department staff have another valuable role in advising patients, particularly those who are not admitted or who are discharged early, about the best ways of managing stress. Psychological first-aid includes information about normal psychophysiological reactions to

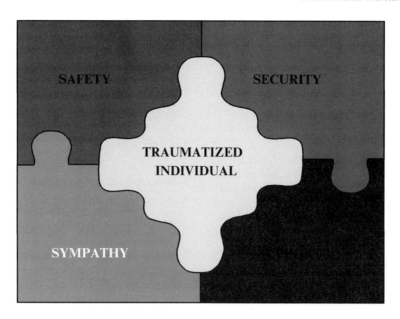

Figure 15.1 Principles of early management

trauma, and advice about the dangers of excessive use of caffeine or nicotine (which heighten physiological arousal, and thereby potentiate anxiety and avoidance behaviours) and alcohol (which generally does little to reduce distress, but obstructs psychological appraisal and processing of the traumatic experience); the value of both gentle exercise and sleep; and the potential benefits of talking about the experience. Written information, for example in the form of self-help pamphlets (e.g. Herbert, 1995), is a useful means of reinforcing verbal advice.

A further role for staff in a trauma unit is in the early recognition of adverse psychological reactions such as severe dissociation. Informal screening of patients for vulnerability factors, e.g. previous psychiatric disorder or social isolation, may facilitate the targeting of professional support on those who are most at risk. **Nursing and other staff can be trained to identify those clues and cues which are indicative of pathological reactions, and both increase their own psychological care of the patient and, where necessary, initiate referral to a liaison psychiatric service.** Early recognition of psychiatric problems is particularly important because chronic post-traumatic states may be more difficult to treat. Psychiatric problems may also hinder physical rehabilitation and recovery.

In most general hospitals the psychological work of trauma unit staff will be supported by social workers, the hospital chaplain or (where appropriate) bereavement counsellor, and liaison psychiatric service. Where psychiatric symptoms emerge after discharge from hospital, or are identified in patients who are not admitted, general medical practitioners and outpatient medical and nursing staff are responsible for instigating psychiatric assessment and treatment. Psychiatric follow-up may form an important part of the rehabilitation programme for injured patients. Arrangements for this vary from one place to another.

Treatment of post-traumatic disorders

Both physical and psychological methods are used in the treatment of post-traumatic psychiatric disorders (O'Brien, 1998).

Acute stress reaction and disorder

Nursing in a calm and supportive environment is essential for highly distressed patients. However, sedative medication may be required to reduce the high levels of psychophysiological arousal associated with acute stress reaction. Brief cognitive behavioural therapy (CBT) has been shown to be effective in the treatment of acute stress disorder, whereas non-directive supportive counselling is largely ineffective (Bryant *et al.*, 1998). This suggests that emotional support, however useful an adjunct to specific methods of treatment, is not itself therapeutic.

Depression

Medication may have an important role in the treatment of depression following trauma. There is some evidence that antidepressant medications also have a beneficial impact on the intrusive symptoms of PTSD (O'Brien, 1998). Cognitive behavioural therapy is an effective treatment for depression, though it has yet to be evaluated as a treatment for mood disorder following trauma.

Depression may compound grief, perhaps particularly after traumatic loss, and may diminish its responsiveness to grief counselling (Worden, 1991).

Anxiety disorders

Cognitive behavioural therapy is the treatment of choice for phobic anxiety and panic disorder after trauma, but drugs (specific tricyclics and selective serotonin re-uptake inhibitors) are also effective. Medication has a significant role in the treatment of hospitalized patients for whom psychological treatment programmes, especially those based on exposure and desensitization to the feared and avoided situation, are less feasible.

Post-traumatic stress disorder

Treatments for PTSD are the subject of much current research (O'Brien, 1998). The only methods for which there is already compelling research evidence of effectiveness are behavioural therapies based around exposure and desensitization of the traumatic memories and strategic reintroduction to avoided situations. Cognitive behavioural therapy, in which distorted beliefs (e.g. guilt, helplessness or hopelessness) are also actively restructured, appears to be promising. As noted above, antidepressant medications reduce intrusive re-experiencing symptoms, but are not effective in reducing avoidance behaviours (Sutherland and Davidson, 1994).

Traumas, and the psychiatric states to which

they give rise, are very varied. Clinical experience suggests that different treatment approaches tailored to the needs of the individual patient may be necessary for different clinical presentations.

Other issues

Compensation

There is an increasing trend, actively encouraged by some solicitors, for people who are injured physically and/or psychologically by accident or assault to claim compensation for their injuries and associated financial losses. It was long thought that involvement in personal injury litigation, which is usually prolonged, would delay recovery from injury. The basis of 'compensation neurosis' was that, consciously or unconsciously, psychological factors could perpetuate the disabling effects of injury.

While it would be understandable for people who are seeking compensation to emphasize or even exaggerate their injuries or disability, **there is no evidence that litigation delays or prevents recovery from the psychiatric impact of trauma** (Mendelson, 1995). There is little doubt, however, that the prolonged frustration, repeated reference back to the traumatic event, and adversarial nature of legal procedures can compound the distress which follows trauma. This, and other prominent reminders of the accident such as continuing physical problems or financial hardship, are often associated with chronicity of PTSD (Mayou *et al.*, 1997).

Major incidents or disaster

A disaster is a destructive event or circumstance, the scale of which in terms of deaths, injuries and disruption threatens or overwhelms the coping resources of the individuals, families and communities affected by it (Raphael, 1986; Hodgkinson and Stewart, 1991). Disaster also has a significant emotional effect upon the whole society in which it occurs. The psychosocial impact of a disaster is more than the psychological reactions of the many individual people who are traumatized directly by it.

A major incident can be defined operationally as any destructive event which, by virtue of the scale of injuries and deaths, challenges the capacity of the emergency services to respond to it. **Health services have emergency plans for managing the physical effects of major incidents; and, in just the same way, health and social services need to plan for the psychological effects** (Gibson, 1994; Hobbs, 1995).

Planning a psychosocial response for disaster involves more than planning for the management of those directly affected by it, the primary victims who, whether injured physically or not, may develop early or later psychiatric problems. An organized response is needed which will identify the many other people who are affected psychologically by the incident (see Table 15.2), including relatives of the primary victims, those who witness the event or its immediate aftermath, and the front-line workers who respond to the incident.

Studies have demonstrated that emergency service and front-line hospital and other staff are more likely to develop psychiatric problems after dealing with large-scale traumatic incidents (Raphael, 1986), but that experience and training for harrowing assignments can minimize psychiatric reactions (Alexander and Wells, 1991). Effective organizational systems are also important in reducing the misunderstanding, communication failures and role uncertainty which so often undermine the effectiveness and morale of staff dealing with mass emergencies, thereby increasing their vulnerability to psychological traumatization .

Traumatization of staff following disaster

Professional workers have been described as the 'hidden victims' of disasters. They face high levels of stress and may be traumatized during the rescue, resuscitation and treatment of the primary victim (Table 15.8).

Table 15.8 Causes of traumatic stress in staff

Suddenness of challenge – the lack of warning
Scale of injuries, death and destruction encountered
Identification with victims and anguished relatives
Intensity of demand on services
Disruption of usual routines
Inadequacy of training, organization and preparation
Lack of role and task definition for major incidents
Failures of communication – interpersonal and systems
Interdepartmental and inter-agency rivalry

Raphael (1986) reported that, of rescuers engaged in disaster work, 70–80% experienced transient symptoms of traumatic stress. Typically, 5% develop long-term psychiatric problems, including PTSD. However, a significant number later report that they were able to view the experience positively (Hodgkinson and Stewart, 1991). A positive perspective is more likely if the rescuer felt able to do something constructive to help others, even if only to recover for burial the bodies (or body parts) of those who died.

The factors which undermine the effectiveness of rescue and hospital staff are those which reinforce the negative feelings which are so common in the face of disaster, such as uncertainty about role and task, loss of confidence in their professional skills (de-skilling), helplessness, hopelessness and uselessness. This adverse reaction to the challenge of the situation may predispose staff to subsequent feelings of guilt or to the 'counter-disaster syndrome', the characteristics of which are listed in Table 15.9.

Table 15.9 Characteristics of the 'counter-disaster syndrome'

Over-identification with the victims of disaster
Over-involvement with the victim/patient
Overwork
Omnipotence
Indispensability
Eventual burn-out

Much can be done to reduce the traumatic impact of major incidents and disasters on the staff who respond to them, especially through ensuring that the organization and systems are in place to cope with the sudden, intense and dramatic demand. Clear, tested lines of responsibility and communication are essential, as is the planning and leadership that ensures that staff know what they are expected to do if faced by a major incident, for example where, with whom, and for how long. This last question is important, for staff also need rest breaks, refreshment and eventually to go off duty if they are going to be fit to return to work the next day. Disasters are never dealt with in one day.

Traumatization of staff by everyday critical incidents

The psychological impact on the front-line staff of a major incident is readily understood. Less obvious are the personal emotional reactions of trauma unit staff whose daily work involves the care of patients who have been severely injured, physically and psychologically. This is recognized increasingly in accident departments, but here the contact between nurse and patient is usually short, albeit intense. Nevertheless, the impact on staff of critical incidents such as a severely injured child, or a sudden death, can be highly distressing.

On trauma wards, however, relationships develop over longer periods between staff (particularly nurses and physiotherapists) and patients. They have daily contact with severely injured patients and their families, who may be struggling to accept and adapt to devastating injury, and who may be severely traumatized psychologically. Even the most resilient staff will be touched emotionally by this continuing contact with fear, pain and death. The empathic contact which is the hallmark of the nurse-patient relationship is the medium through which the patient's distress is felt by the nurse. If the patient is traumatized psychologically, the staff may be traumatized by their close empathic contact. **Trauma is contagious**.

The traumatic effect of this work may not be felt immediately. Often the impact is cumulative, the level of stress rising with successive incidents over a long period. Eventually one critical incident, itself no more stressful than many before, may prove too much to bear. The staff member goes off sick, sometimes never to return.

As for patients, staff will be more vulnerable to traumatic stress if they are socially isolated, or struggling with other stresses such as loss or illness. Perhaps unfortunately, the culture of many trauma units makes it difficult for staff to disclose their personal vulnerability, exposing them to increased risk.

Supporting staff in trauma units

The importance for staff support of effective organizational structures, communication and training has already been emphasized. Of less clear value are the various psychological interventions which have been promoted in recent years, ostensibly to support those affected by traumatic incidents, including professional workers, to prevent post-traumatic psychiatric disorders. Of obvious value is the opportunity before leaving the workplace after a traumatic incident to talk it through with other members of the team. This 'defusing' may help to promote communication, a wider perspective and understanding of the traumatic event and the team's response to it, thereby reinforcing team cohesion and encouraging mutual support. It may also present an opportunity for identifying those staff who may be particularly vulnerable to traumatization, such as those who are socially isolated or those are struggling with concurrent stresses such as bereavement or marital breakdown. They may need extra support.

As noted above, there is no evidence that debriefing interventions, even though often valued by staff groups, are effective in preventing post-traumatic psychiatric problems. More thought and research is required to determine the most effective ways of supporting the hospital staff who work with the injured victims of small- and large-scale traumatic incidents.

References

Alexander, D. A. and Wells, A. (1991) Reactions of police officers to body-handling after a major disaster: before and after comparison. *British Journal of Psychiatry*, **159**, 547–555.

American Psychiatric Association (1994) *Diagnostic and Statistical Manual of mental disorders*, DSM-IV. APA.

Bisson, J., Jenkins, P. L., Alexander, J. and Bannister, C. (1997) Randomised controlled trial of psychological debriefing for victims of acute burn trauma. *British Journal of Psychiatry*, **171**, 78–81.

Blanchard, E. B., Hickling, E. J., Mitnick, N. *et al.* (1995) The impact of severity of physical injury and perception of life threat in the development of post-traumatic stress disorder in motor vehicle accident victims. *Behavioural Research and Therapy*, **33**, 529–534.

Bordow, S. and Porritt, D. (1979) An experimental evaluation of crisis intervention. *Social Science and Medicine*, **13**, 251–256.

Breslau, N. and Davis, G. C. (1992) Post-traumatic stress disorder in an urban population of young adults: risk factors for chronicity. *American Journal of Psychiatry*, **149**, 671–675.

Bryant, R. A., Harvey, A. G., Dang, S.T. *et al.* (1998) Treatment of acute stress disorder: a comparison of cognitive behaviour therapy and supportive counselling. *Journal of Consultant and Clinical Psychology*, **66**(5), 862–866.

Cherpitel, C. J. (1993) Alcohol and injuries: a review of international emergency room studies. *Addiction*, **88,** 923–937.

Dunmore, E., Clark, D. M. and Ehlers, A. (1997) Cognitive factors in persistent versus recovered post-traumatic stress disorder after physical or sexual assault: a pilot study. *Behavioural and Cognitive Psychotherapy*, **25,** 147–159.

Ehlers, A., Mayou, R. and Bryant, B. (1998) Psychological predictors of chronic PTSD after motor vehicle accidents. *Journal of Abnormal Psychology*, **107**(3), 508–519.

Garland, C. (1991) External disasters and the internal world: an approach to psychotherapeutic understanding of survivors. In *Textbook of Psychotherapy in Psychiatric Practice* (J. Holmes, ed.). Churchill Livingstone.

Gibson, M. (1994) Managing people's social and psychological needs after a disaster: experiences from Belfast and the M1 plane crash. In *Management of Disasters and their Aftermath* (W. A. Wallace, J. M. Rowles and C. L. Colton, eds). BMJ Publishing Group.

Herbert, C. (1995) *Understanding Trauma.* Clinical Psychology Department, Warneford Hospital. Oxford.

Hobbs, M. (1995) A district framework for managing psychosocial aspects of disaster. *Advances in Psychiatric Treatment*, **1,** 176–183.

Hobbs, M., Mayou, R. A., Harrison, B. and Worlock, P. (1996) A randomised controlled trial of psychological debriefing for victims of road traffic accidents. *British Medical Journal*, **313,** 1438–1439.

Hodgkinson, P. E. and Stewart, M. (1991) *Coping with Catastrophe: A Handbook of Disaster Management.* Routledge.

Hodgkinson, P. E., Joseph, S., Yule, W. and Williams, R. (1993) Viewing human remains following disaster: helpful or harmful? *Medicine, Science, and the Law*, **33,** 197–202.

Janoff-Bulman, R. (1992) *Shattered Assumptions: Towards a New Psychology of Trauma.* Free Press.

Joseph, S., Williams, R. and Yule, W. (1997) *Understanding Post-traumatic Stress: A Psychosocial Perspective on PTSD and Treatment.* Wiley.

Koopman, C., Classen, C., Cardena, E. and Spiegel, D. (1995) When disaster strikes, acute stress disorder may follow. *Journal of Traumatic Stress*, **8,** 29–46.

Malt, U. F. and Olafsen, O. M. (1992) Psychological appraisal and emotional response to physical injury: a clinical, phenomenological study of 109 adults. *Psychiatric Medicine*, **10,** 117–134.

Mayou, R. A., Bryant, B. M. and Duthie, R. (1993) Psychiatric consequences of road traffic accidents. *British Medical Journal*, **307,** 647–651.

Mayou, R. A. and Bryant, B. (1994) Effects of road accidents on travel. *Injury*, **25,** 457–460.

Mayou, R. A., Tyndel, S. and Bryant, B. (1997) Long term outcome of motor vehicle accident injury. *Psychosomatic Medicine*, **59,** 578–584.

McDonald, A. S. and Davey, G. C. L. (1996) Psychiatric disorders and accidental injury. *Clinical Psychology Review*, **16,** 105–127.

Mendelson, G. (1995) 'Compensation neurosis' revisited: outcome studies of the effects of litigation. *Journal of Psychosomatic Research*, **39**(6), 695–706.

Mitchell, J. T. and Everly, G. S. (1995) Critical Incident Stress Debriefing (CISD) and the prevention of work-related traumatic stress among high risk occupational groups. In *Psychotraumatology* (Everly, G. S. and Lating, J. M. eds). Plenum.

Murray, J. (1997) *Trauma and Dissociation.* D.Phil. Thesis. Oxford University. (unpublished).

O'Brien, L. S. (1998) *Traumatic Events and Mental Health.* Cambridge University Press.

Orner, R. (1997) Emergency service may abandon Critical Incident Stress Debriefing. *Traumatic Stress Points*, (International Society of Traumatic Stress Studies), Winter, 5.

Parkes, C. M. (1996) *Bereavement: Studies of Grief in Adult Life.* Routledge.

Parkinson, F. (1997) *Critical Incident Debriefing: Understanding and Dealing with Trauma.* Souvenir Press.

Raphael, B. (1986) *When Disaster Strikes: A Handbook for the Caring Professions.* Unwin Hyman.

Rose, S., Brewin, C. R., Andrews, B. and Kirk, M. (1998) A randomised trial of psychological debriefing for victims of violent crime. *American Journal of Psychiatry*, **156**(3), 360–366.

Schnyder, U. (1997) Crisis intervention in psychiatric outpatients. *International Medical Journal*, **4,** 11–17.

Sutherland, S. M. and Davidson, J. R. (1994) Pharmacotherapy for post traumatic stress disorder. *Psychiatric Clinics of North America*, **17,** 409–423.

Terr, L. C. (1991) Childhood traumas: an outline and overview. *American Journal of Psychiatry*, **148,** 10–20.

Worden, J. W. (1991) *Grief Counselling and Grief Therapy: A Handbook for the Mental Health Practitioner.* Routledge.

World Health Organisation (1992) *International Classification of Diseases (ICD-10).* WHO.

Part III

The needs of the injured person

16

Diagnostic investigations in trauma

Philip Chapman-Sheath

Introduction

Trauma remains the leading cause of death in the first four decades of life and is responsible for major morbidity and disability in those who survive (Report of Chief Medical Officer of Health, 1984). It has been estimated that trauma is directly responsible for up to 165 000 deaths annually in the USA and up to 430 000 cases of disability of varying proportions (National Academy Press, 1985). In the UK there are around 18 000 trauma-related deaths per annum, one-third of these related to road traffic accidents which also lead to a further 60 000 trauma admissions to hospital (Westaby, 1989).

Identification of the trimodal distribution of trauma deaths has enabled a system of trauma resuscitation based on the principles outlined by the American College of Surgeons, 1997.

The first peak of deaths occurs early, within minutes, and is caused by major neurological and vascular injury. Patients in this category will die unless specialist attention is provided at the scene of the injury. The second peak of trauma deaths occurs minutes to hours after the event, caused by raised intracranial pressure and intracranial haemorrhage, respiratory compromise, major visceral damage, musculoskeletal trauma or hypovolaemic shock. By means of appropriate rapid resuscitation, investigation and management, a proportion of these lives will be saved. The third group of deaths occurs days to weeks after the initial event, most commonly due to sepsis and multiple organ dysfunction, which can be diagnosed and treated by use of a series of investigations leading to prompt and appropriate management.

It is the prompt resuscitation, assessment, investigation and diagnosis of these dysfunctional systems in the initial clinical setting that will help to optimize patients' chances of survival and help to reduce late deaths or subsequent morbidity.

Why are tests done?

At the same time as the initial resuscitation and management of a trauma patient, a careful assessment is required to elucidate the full extent of injury and the adequacy of any resuscitative procedures.

The full history, often from witnesses or paramedical staff, and clinical examination are coupled with investigations in this process of data gathering in order to diagnose pre-existing medical conditions, elucidate current organ dysfunction, prevent secondary complications caused by inadequate or inappropriate treatment and lastly to assist with the initiation of treatment and the patient's fitness for surgery.

A patient arriving in the trauma department is firstly triaged (categorized) by suitably qualified and trained personnel, to decide on the nature and extent of the likely injuries. It also enables other staff to assess and treat those with life-threatening injuries as a matter of urgency in an appropriate environment within the hospital.

This process of triage categorizes patients into injury severity and treatment priorities, and the multiply-injured or polytrauma patient will require immediate resuscitation, investigation and management.

Those patients with single system dysfunction or isolated injuries will be investigated and managed as their injuries dictate and may not require the full spectrum of investigations outlined in this chapter.

Use of tests

1. Diagnosis of injury.
2. Assessment of injury severity.
3. Identification of pre-existing medical conditions.
4. Adequacy of resuscitation.
5. Fitness for further treatment or surgery.

Types of tests

1. Radiological investigations.
2. Haematological and biochemical investigations.
3. Additional specialist investigations.

Radiological investigations

Radiological investigations are part of the first line of tests that trauma patients undergo and are critical in the prompt diagnosis of injury, the assessment of injury severity and in the identification of pre-existing pathology or previous surgery to the skeleton.

The radiological investigation of trauma patients is based on a number of recognized principles (Perry and Lewars, 1991), namely that:

- Plain radiographs are the most useful and moreover the most available in an acute trauma setting.
- Polytrauma patients require an initial 'trauma series' of three films (lateral cervical spine, chest and pelvis) before continuing with other investigations. This is based on the fact that major abnormality in these views reflects serious organ injury that may be life-threatening in terms of major neurological injury, re-

spiratory compromise or haemorrhagic shock.

- Exclusion of a fracture requires two different views of the affected bone (ideally at 90 degrees to each other).
- Soft tissue swelling may be the only indication of injury.
- Imaging must not interfere with the resuscitation or treatment of the patient.
- Senior radiological opinion is useful at an early stage in resuscitation and investigation.

At present, all trauma patients should ideally be assessed along current ATLS guidelines. These are based on the ABC resuscitation protocols which include the use of the three trauma series radiographs.

Trauma series radiographs

1. *Lateral cervical spine.*
2. *Chest* (supine anteroposterior – the most commonly obtained).
3. *Pelvis* (supine anteroposterior).

Any further radiological investigations would then be dictated by location and severity of injury as well as clinical availability (Table 16.1). These may include the following plain radiographs:

- skull
- facial bones
- cervical spine (anteroposterior and peg views)
- thoracic and lumbar spine
- chest (posteroanterior and lateral)
- abdomen
- extremities.

Initial trauma radiographs

Lateral cervical spine

All multiply-injured patients should be assumed to have an unstable cervical spine injury until proved otherwise by clinical or radiological investigation. Furthermore, any evidence of injury at or above the level of the clavicles should immediately raise the possibility of a cervical spine injury.

Table 16.1 Special investigations for trauma patients

Specialized radiographs	Specialized views directed at specific skeletal sites of injury
Ultrasonography	High-frequency sound waves used to generate a two-dimensional picture of visceral structures, used particularly in abdominal injury
Computerized tomography (CT)	A diagnostic technique involving the recording of 'slices' of the body with an X-ray scanner
Magnetic resonance imaging (MRI)	A diagnostic technique utilizing the phenomenon of nuclear magnetic resonance to obtain a biochemical profile of tissues, e.g. muscle.
Vascular imaging – angiography	Intravenous or intra-arterial injection of radio-opaque contrast material used to delineate vascular integrity and occlusion
doppler ultrasound	Specialized ultrasound used to determine direction and rate of flow of blood within the vascular system
Urological imaging – intravenous urography	Intravenous contrast injection filtered by kidney used to identify integrity of renal vasculature, adequate blood flow and functioning of renal system
– cystography/ urethrography	Contrast studies used to evaluate integrity of bladder and urethra
Gastrointestinal imaging – endoscopy	Direct visualization of intestinal lumen for sites of penetration or haemorrhage.
– contrast radiographs	Radiographs with intraluminal contrast to delineate the integrity and continuity of the gastrointestinal tract
Diagnostic peritoneal lavage	Instillation of saline into the abdominal cavity via a small catheter inserted surgically, to determine either haemorrhage or viscus perforation
Laparoscopy	Surgical keyhole operation to inspect the abdominal cavity for haemorrhage or visceral injury

The absence of radiological abnormality alone does not exclude the presence of a significant neurological injury. However, it does affirm that the spinal cord is not at risk from secondary damage caused by abnormal motion,

provided that full cervical spine immobilization is continued. Injury must be excluded by a combination of clinical assessment and radiological investigation (Table 16.2).

Soft tissues

The presence of soft tissue swelling can be extremely useful in diagnosing cervical spine injury in the 10% of cases where radiographs show no fracture; it is particularly visible on the initial lateral cervical film.

The prevertebral soft tissue shadow on this view has certain characteristics and standard measurements which, if disrupted, indicate possible injury. This soft tissue swelling may reflect underlying muscle oedema or haematoma formation. The presence of air or gas in the tissue planes visible on the radiographs may reflect an underlying open fracture or penetrating injury.

In addition, the anteroposterior radiograph yields valuable information regarding fractures and rotational injuries of the cervical spine which may be associated with respiratory injury, such as tension pneumothorax, reflected in tracheal deviation or the presence of a mediastinal haematoma.

Chest

The trauma patient with evidence of thoracic injury must be managed carefully and promptly, as up to a quarter of total trauma-related deaths occur secondarily to thoracic causes (Perry and Lewars, 1991). In addition, studies have shown that up to 16% of high-energy road traffic accident victims sustain some form of aortic injury (Westaby, 1989).

Rapidly lethal injuries which must take clinical priority in diagnosis and treatment include:

- airway occlusion or obstruction by foreign bodies
- tension pneumothorax
- massive haemothorax
- flail chest
- cardiac tamponade
- aortic injury or transection.

The electrocardiogram (ECG) is an invaluable investigation in the acute trauma setting, as it is capable of highlighting underlying and acute

Table 16.2 Cervical spine radiograph

View	Findings
Lateral	Commonly reveals 70–90% of important bone and soft tissue injuries
	Radiographs must show adequate view from skull base to C7/T1 junction (i.e. all seven cervical vertebrae)
	If radiograph is inadequate or of poor quality, then further radiographs required
	– swimmer's view (lower cervical/upper thoracic vertebrae)
	– anteroposterior
	– open-mouth (odontoid peg)
	– oblique (for facet joint fracture and dislocations)
Open-mouth (odontoid peg)	Visualizes the odontoid peg, lateral masses of atlas (C1) and vertebral body of axis (C2)
	Used to complete visualization of cervical spine
	Used if any other views are inconclusive or reflect abnormality
Anteroposterior	Demonstrates cervical vertebrae in entirety
	Used to complete visualization if suspicious of injury or if other views inconclusive or abnormal
	Used to diagnose burst fractures of vertebral bodies or rotational malalignment

Table 16.3 Radiological features of major thoracic injury

Radiological feature	Injury sustained
Mediastinal widening	Aortic arch vascular penetration or rupture
Mediastinal shift	Tension pneumothorax or haemothorax
Mediastinal or soft tissue air (surgical emphysema)	Penetrating neck or pulmonary injury
Multiple rib fractures	Reflecting major injury to head, lungs or spine
– first or second ribs	Associated with local neurovascular injury
– lower ribs	Associated with visceral injury
Pleural effusion	Pulmonary contusion, laceration or haemothorax
Irregular or indistinct cardiac and aortic outline	Cardiac contusion, laceration, tamponade or major vascular injury
Pulmonary opacities or segmental lung collapse	Adult respiratory distress syndrome (ARDS) or pulmonary contusion
Indistinct diaphragmatic outline or abdominal contents in thoracic cavity	Diaphragmatic rupture or direct laceration

cardiac pathology. This includes the presence of cardiac dysrhythmias, infarction or contusion which may occur as the cause or effect of the trauma sustained. If abnormality appears on the initial ECG, then further investigation such as 24-hour ECG traces or cardiac imaging using echocardiography or angiography can be undertaken as necessary.

Plain chest radiographs

The most useful view is the posteroanterior (PA) erect chest radiograph, which visualizes the lung fields, soft tissues, skeleton, cardiac and pulmonary vascular systems. It also may reveal the presence of free intraperitoneal air, indicating abdominal viscus perforation or an open penetrating injury of the abdomen. The gastric shadow may also reveal the presence of

gastric stasis with a dilated stomach, which requires aspiration via a nasogastric tube to prevent pulmonary aspiration of stomach contents or ultimately rupture of the stomach.

This PA radiograph is often difficult to achieve in the acute trauma setting due to the patient having either a reduced conscious level, therefore being unable to cooperate voluntarily during the procedure, the clinical condition preventing movement, or the patient being immobilized with cervical spine precautions. In these conditions, the most commonly available radiograph is the anteroposterior (AP) supine film. This has the disadvantage of magnifying the cardiac outline, thereby making an assessment of the mediastinal diameter and cardiothoracic ratio more difficult. The supine position also makes assessment of the lung bases and any fluid or blood in the pleural space, reflecting pulmonary contusion or hae-mopneumothorax, harder to identify.

Table 16.3 lists the radiological features of major thoracic imagery and Table 16.4 some special thoracic investigations.

Table 16.4 Special thoracic investigations

Lateral chest radiograph	Delineates cardiac and mediastinal outlines and localizes pulmonary contusion and masses
CT scan/MRI scan	Visualizes skeletal and vertebral fracture pattern and extent and delineates pulmonary, vascular, mediastinal and neurological structures
Angiography	Investigates pulmonary, systemic and cardiac vascular injury
Bronchoscopy	Direct visualization of pulmonary structures
Radioisotope scans	Quantification and diagnosis of pulmonary and vascular filling defects

Pelvis

Pelvic fractures can be divided into many different categories depending on the aetiology and velocity of the injury, the age and general condition of the patient, the relative stability of the pelvic ring after injury, or whether the fracture is defined as 'open' or 'closed'.

An open fracture occurs when a fractured bone or its adjacent haematoma is in direct communication with a surface lined with epithelium, which most commonly means the skin (but communication with the epithelial lining of the bladder or bowel is also defined as an open fracture).

A stable pelvic injury is one in which the pelvic ring and supporting ligaments can withstand further deforming forces if applied, and usually results from a single fracture at one site in the bony ring. These injuries may be treated conservatively with analgesia and a period of limited weight-bearing until fracture healing occurs. An unstable pelvic fracture is one in which there is potential for further displacement and therefore further damage to internal structures. In practice it occurs when the bony ring is disrupted in two or more places, or if there is a single fracture associated with major

ligamentous disruption.

The velocity and nature of the deforming forces that are applied to the pelvic ring will cause different fracture patterns. A relatively low-velocity injury, such as a fall from the standing position in an elderly osteoporotic patient (a fairly common occurrence), may result in a closed, stable pubic ramus fracture. On the other hand, a high-velocity injury, such as a fall from a height, crush injury or road traffic accident, will result in more extensive injuries and a different fracture pattern.

General bone density, related to the increasing age of a patient and to underlying medical conditions, also has a major influence on the incidence and nature of a pelvic fracture. For instance, a fall from standing in a young patient will often result in no fracture, but a similar fall in an elderly osteoporotic patient may result in a significant fracture.

A high-energy pelvic fracture in a patient of any age may be life-threatening. Several studies report mortality rates varying from 5% to 20% for closed isolated pelvic fractures (Pennal *et al.*, 1981; Poole *et al.*, 1991), rising to 50% or more for open pelvic fractures (Rothenberger *et al.*, 1978). The latter is due to the higher energy imparted to the pelvis which results in the greater displacement of fragments into other structures, leading to haemorrhage and a higher risk of deep infection from the skin or gastrointestinal tract.

Imaging of a suspected pelvic fracture therefore takes priority and the supine anteroposterior pelvic radiograph is taken in the trauma series during the initial resuscitation of the injured patient. This radiograph gives valuable information about the integrity of the pelvic ring and its stability, and also visualizes the hip joints and proximal femora which may also have been injured. The severity and pattern of fractures thus identified give an indication as to the likelihood of other associated injuries such as to the abdominal contents or neurovascular structures.

Both pelvic fractures and fractures of the acetabulum can easily be diagnosed on the plain radiograph, but more detailed information can be gathered later by the use of specialized radiographs (such as Judet views of the acetabulum and pelvic oblique and inlet/outlet radiographs) or by the use of more sophisticated imaging (CT scanning and MRI).

As previously mentioned, the presence of a

Table 16.5 Indications for plain skull radiographs

Penetrating injury	To detect intracranial air or foreign body
Focal neurological signs	To detect possible fracture
Loss of consciousness (significant)	To diagnose fracture which indicates a higher risk of subsequent intracranial haemorrhage
Cerebrospinal fluid leak (ears or nose)	For evidence of fracture
Inability to assess clinically (due to severe head injury, polytrauma, obtunded conscious level – drugs, medications, epilepsy, alcohol)	To exclude fracture and foreign body

pelvic fracture may result in major haemorrhage, often measured in litres. This bleeding may be obvious (overt), or hidden (covert) if it occurs into the retroperitoneal soft tissues of the pelvis. A displaced or unstable pelvic fracture may act as a source of continued haemorrhage or explain the signs of hypovolaemic shock in a trauma patient. Up to 85% of the haemorrhage is thought to originate from the fracture surfaces and minor pelvic veins and the rate of haemorrhage from these sites can be slowed by adequate reduction and stabilization of the fracture fragments. This stabilization can be achieved in the emergency setting by the application of a pelvic external fixator, prior to further resuscitation or life- and limb-saving surgery. The remaining 15% of the haemorrhage occurs from larger vascular structures (both venous and arterial) and from disrupted viscera. The stabilization of the pelvis in these cases may not be sufficient to reduce the rate of haemorrhage; therefore further intervention, including angiographic visualization and embolization of the bleeding vessels, may be required.

Any pelvic fracture or major joint dislocation (such as the hip) will also raise the possibility of internal organ derangement to the urological, lower gastrointestinal (especially rectum or anal canal), vascular or reproductive systems – all of which may require further specialist investigation at a later stage.

Further urological investigation is relatively commonplace due to the high incidence of renal and lower urological trauma associated with a pelvic fracture. These include the use of intravenous urography to visualize the kidney and ureter, together with cystography and urethrography to assess the integrity of the bladder and urethra respectively.

Additional acute emergency room investigations may also include ultrasonography of abdominal organs and intraperitoneal fluid, especially if the patient is not stable enough, either cardiovascularly or neurologically, to proceed with CT or MRI scanning.

If the clinical situation permits, CT and MRI scanning will be able to visualize further any musculoskeletal or visceral injuries.

Head injury

Trauma patients often have evidence of injury to the head and facial skeleton as a result of high-energy impact following road traffic accidents, falls and assault. The history of mechanism of such injury and detailed neurological status is vital in the resuscitation and management of these patients.

The initial assessment includes the clinical observation of obvious blunt or penetrating injury, followed by detailed and thorough clinical examination of the head and neck, maintaining cervical spine immobilization until injury to the cervical spine is excluded.

Neurological assessment begins during the primary survey, accurately detailing the conscious level and pupillary reflexes. It continues during the secondary survey which includes a detailed neurological examination, Glasgow Coma Score (GCS) (Teasdale and Jennett, 1974) and, if appropriate, more specialized reflexes such as the brainstem reflexes including respiratory pattern, oculocephalic (doll's eye) and oculovestibular (caloric).

Indicators of severe neurological injury include an alteration in the conscious level; a GCS below 6 (15 being the maximum) is defined as a severe head injury. In the case of an unconscious patient, if a correctable and easily reversible cause cannot be found (hypoxia, drugs, hypoglycaemia), they would invariably require further investigation by means of CT or MRI scanning.

An abnormal pupillary reflex (such as an asymmetry) can result from an expanding intracranial haematoma or raised intracranial pressure; the patient requires CT scanning, if the clinical circumstances permit, in order for treatment to be given.

Injury to the spinal cord will result in flaccid motor tone and absent motor reflexes below the level of the lesion. Adequate radiological imaging with anteroposterior and lateral radiographs of the entire spine (to exclude multiple level injury) and later CT or MRI scan will be required to delineate the level, type and severity of injury sustained (Tables 16.5 and 16.6).

Table 16.6 Indications for CT scan of head

Sustained reduction in GCS < 6 after resuscitation
Deteriorating conscious level (GCS reducing)
Focal neurological signs
Post-traumatic epilepsy
Depressed skull fracture
Penetrating injury
Persistent cerebrospinal fluid (CSF) leak
Investigation of facial skeleton fracture
Suspected hydrocephalus, infection or haematoma formation
Investigation of patient who cannot be evaluated clinically (sedated, ventilated) to exclude treatable cause

Maxillofacial

Fractures of the facial skeleton vary from simple isolated fractures to complex unstable fracture patterns. Complex fracture patterns frequently lead to compromised respiratory effort as a result of haemorrhage into adjacent soft tissues, progressing in some instances to airway occlusion. During the primary survey of the injured patient, it is crucial to assess that the airway is viable and patent and the ventilatory effort is adequate, before commencing with other assessments or investigations.

In the initial investigation of the maxillofacial region only four specialized radiographs are required for initial diagnostic purposes, these are:

1. 10° occipitomental (assesses inferior displacement of the facial skeleton).
2. 30° occipitomental (assesses posterior displacement).
3. Lateral facial (visualizes most facial fractures).
4. Soft tissue lateral (visualizes nasal bones, teeth and foreign bodies).

Often other specific views are required to visualize a fracture in more detail, but the best investigations are CT scanning, which helps to visualize the pattern and extent of the fracture and helps in the planning of surgical reconstruction, and MRI scanning, which helps to visualize soft tissue and ocular pathology.

Abdomen

Isolated abdominal injury only accounts for around 1% of hospital admissions, but the abdomen is commonly involved, to a greater or lesser degree, following trauma.

Abdominal injury is associated with high-energy trauma and therefore is seen commonly with head injury, thoracic injury and fractures to either the pelvis, spine or extremities.

The abdomen can be injured by several means including:

- direct blunt trauma
- indirect pressure from blasts and crushing
- shearing forces such as rapid deceleration
- penetration by sharp objects or fracture fragments from the skeleton.

Radiological assessment

The first-choice investigation in the trauma setting would be either CT or MRI scanning. These modalities may be used to diagnose the presence of free intraperitoneal blood or the nature and extent of ruptured viscera and, in conjunction with contrast studies, can delineate both vascular and gastrointestinal pathology.

If these modalities are unavailable, or the patient is unable, due to clinical condition, to travel to the site of the scanner, then an erect and supine plain abdominal radiograph should be taken. These can usefully reveal the presence of free intraperitoneal gas (either from a ruptured viscus or penetrating injury to the thorax or peritoneal cavity), soft tissue swelling (to direct further investigation to a particular region or organ) and diaphragmatic integrity.

In addition, ultrasonography is a very useful adjunct – it is portable and rapid, and therefore more easily available in the emergency room setting.

Other investigations

These investigations may include:

- urinanalysis – to detect microscopic haematuria
- arteriography/venography – to diagnose vascular occlusion, flow to organs and haemorrhage
- gastrointestinal contrast studies
- upper and lower gastrointestinal endoscopy
- diagnostic peritoneal lavage
- laparoscopy
- urological contrast studies (intravascular and intraluminal)
- urological endoscopy.

Special mention must be made of diagnostic peritoneal lavage (DPL), used to diagnose the presence of free intraperitoneal blood or perforated abdominal viscus. The technique involves the passage of a fine catheter into the peritoneal cavity by a skilled clinician, and the subsequent instillation and later retrieval of saline solution. The presence of free blood or bowel contents is usually obvious to the attending clinician, but further biochemical and microscopic evaluation can confirm the presence of either of these contents or of pancreatic amylase (indicating blunt retroperitoneal trauma) in diagnostic quantities. The accuracy rate for detecting free intraperitoneal blood has been calculated at over 90% (Olsen, 1972) and, when used for the diagnosis of continued pelvic haemorrhage following fracture, has a positive predictive value of 98% (Mendez *et al.*, 1994).

Extremities

It has been stated that 'there are no emergencies in orthopaedics, only priorities in management' (Bulstrode *et al.*, 1989). The relief of tension on soft tissues, the manipulation of a deformed limb with vascular compromise to restore normal circulation, the surgical decompression of a compartment syndrome and the cessation of major haemorrhage all take immediate priority. Attention can then be directed at the reduction of major joint dislocation, the splinting and stabilization of long-bone fractures and the dressing of open wounds. Only after these have been addressed can the patient be considered for fracture fixation surgery.

Musculoskeletal injury is extremely common in the multiply-injured patient and occurs in over 70% of cases, with up to 50% of the total sustaining extremity injury: nearly the same as the incidence of head injury; twice that of thoracic trauma; and four times that of abdominal trauma. The investigation of trauma patients with musculoskeletal injury commonly occurs at the same time as the investigation and management of other organ system injury. This forms the basis for the rest of the chapter.

The initial radiographs required will be determined by the site and severity of the injury sustained. Fracture of the upper and lower limbs depends on two types of variables:

1. The biomechanics of the force of the injury applied to the bone – the direction, speed of loading of the bone, velocity and magnitude of force and position of the skeleton relative to the force.
2. The individual patient characteristics – such as mobility of surrounding joints, bone density, sites of previous fracture and orthopaedic implants and bone pathology.

The general principles of radiological investigation, as outlined previously, apply particularly to fractures of the long bones and joint dislocations, and the mainstay of investigation remains the plain radiograph, with at least two views taken 90 degrees apart.

The importance of initial appropriate radiology is demonstrated by the evidence that the early stabilization of long-bone fractures, particularly femoral shaft and pelvic fractures, improves the outcome for trauma patients by reducing the incidence and severity of the known complications of major haemorrhage, fat embolus and the subsequent development of adult respiratory distress syndrome (ARDS) (Bone *et al.* 1989). Moreover, any fracture that is by definition 'open', in that it communicates with an epithelially lined surface, must be surgically debrided and stabilized as soon as possible after the event, ideally within 6 h, to reduce the incidence of infection and subsequent morbidity or mortality (Gustillo and

Anderson, 1976).

Other investigations useful in assessing extremity trauma include:

- angiography and doppler ultrasound – to diagnose and assess vascular injury preoperatively, perioperatively and postoperatively
- CT and MRI – to delineate extent and nature of soft tissue and skeletal injury
- electrophysiological studies – to diagnose the nature, site and severity of neurological injury.

Haematological and biochemical investigations

The use of haematological and biochemical investigations in the assessment of the trauma patient is well recognized. Specifically, these tests are used to gather information regarding the nature of injury and organ dysfunction as a baseline result before resuscitation fully commences to assess injury severity, organ system dysfunction and previous pathology, to monitor the adequacy of resuscitation procedures, to assess the patient's fitness for surgery and to monitor the patient both perioperatively and after definitive treatment.

Purpose of blood tests

- Diagnosis of injury.
- Assessing the severity of injury.
- Assessing the adequacy and appropriateness of resuscitative procedures.
- Diagnosis of pre-existing medical conditions and drug treatments.
- Assessing fitness for surgery.
- Monitoring the patient during procedures and recovery.

Types of initial blood tests

- Full blood count (FBC).
- Urea and electrolytes (U&E).
- Group and save (G&S) or blood cross-match.
- Glucose.
- Liver function tests (LFT).
- Amylase.
- Blood clotting.
- Arterial blood gases (ABG).

Additional investigations

- Blood autoantibodies – for transfusion reactions and detailed blood typing.
- Cardiac enzymes – a marker of myocardial muscle damage (e.g. infarction or blunt trauma)
- Infection screening – such as hepatitis and HIV serology.

Diagnosis and severity of injury

Blood investigations are performed during the initial resuscitation phase of management. Most of these initial tests are often not initially diagnostic of organ system dysfunction or of anaemia secondary to haemorrhage because there has not usually been sufficient delay in time between injury and testing to allow a change in the blood profile. However, these investigations are still useful as they can act as a baseline for any subsequent changes, reflecting evolving organ dysfunction, or in the assessment of the response of the body to resuscitation and treatment.

There are, however, some investigations which may show a relatively rapid change secondarily to trauma or stress (Table 16.7).

Response to resuscitation

The adequacy and appropriateness of any resuscitative procedure can be monitored by the use of serial blood investigations. After a time delay (which could be hours or days), the injured patient may show an alteration in the values of initial blood tests from the normal range. These changes vary with the severity and nature of the injury, as mentioned previously, and also with the time delay prior to the commencement of adequate and appropriate resuscitation. Throughout this period of resuscitation and then throughout the entire management of the trauma patient, it is vital to monitor for any of these secondary changes. These changes may reflect either an improvement in condition, and therefore the effectiveness of treatment, or indicate a deterioration in clinical condition which, if rapidly diagnosed and corrected early, may be fully reversible.

Table 16.7 Common changes in the initial blood results

Full blood count (FBC)	Anaemia – low haemoglobin Neutrophilia – response to stress hormones Dehydration – raised haematocrit and platelet count Infection – raised total white cell count
Urea and electrolytes (U&E)	Electrolyte alteration – secondary to abnormal renal functioning or as a result of inadequate resuscitation Dehydration – raised urea Renal failure – abnormal electrolytes and raised urea and creatinine level
Glucose	Diabetes – either high (response to stress hormones) or low (poor oral calorie intake)
Amylase	High level – response to pancreatic inflammation (alcohol, drugs) or direct trauma (blunt, penetrating)
Liver function tests (LFT)	Deranged as a result of damage, failure or inflammation of liver
Clotting	Prolonged clotting times – reflect either loss of clotting factors by haemorrhage or inability to produce them (liver disease or failure). May reflect development of disseminated intravascular coagulation (DIC) development
Arterial blood gases (ABG)	Reflect pulmonary function and efficiency and the adequacy of ventilatory resuscitation and support

The effect of pre-existing medical conditions post-trauma

The investigation of trauma patients will act as an adjunct to the medical history obtained from the patient, clinical notes or relatives, in order to diagnose and also to assess the current state of previous medical conditions. Conditions that are important to investigate include:

- pulmonary dysfunction
- anaemia
- infection
- malignancy
- renal dysfunction
- dehydration
- endocrine abnormalities
- diabetes
- liver disease
- blood dyscrasias
- alcohol level
- drug therapy
- pancreatic disease.

These conditions may all have a negative effect on the long-term morbidity and mortality of the traumatized individual if they are not diagnosed and treated appropriately.

Pulmonary dysfunction

The function and adequacy of ventilation is critical in the outcome of a traumatized patient.

Any underlying pulmonary disease, if unrecognized or unsuspected, may adversely affect the outcome of resuscitation. For instance, a patient with underlying chronic lung disease or asthma may require more aggressive ventilation or even intubation if they were to suffer multiple rib fracture or significant thoracic trauma. In these cases, the judicious use of both oxygen saturation monitoring or arterial blood gases can be extremely useful.

Anaemia

This may affect the tissue and organ response to trauma and surgery, as there must be an adequate supply of oxygenated blood, often in an already hypovolaemic patient, both to the vital organs (central nervous system, heart, kidneys) and damaged tissues in order to effect repair and normal homeostasis. A chronically anaemic patient will show signs of respiratory and cardiac compromise after relatively little blood loss and may require restoration of normal blood parameters prior to any surgical procedures.

Infection

A raised total white cell count can indicate current sepsis which, if severe, may preclude the internal fixation of open fractures or total joint arthroplasty, as there is a higher risk of deep-seated metalwork or prosthesis infection in those with active bacteraemia. However, the release of stress hormones secondary to trauma may often result in a transient neutrophilia, as mentioned previously, and this response is a normal occurrence not indicating infection. Occasionally as a result of trauma, an underlying or induced infection may become worse, leading to the development of ARDS or multiple organ failure – both with serious morbidity and mortality.

Renal disease

Dehydration secondary to reduced oral fluid intake post-injury or secondary to hypovolaemia will be revealed in abnormal serum electrolytes. These acute changes of fluid shift may result in reduced kidney perfusion by blood pressure changes which may exacerbate any chronic renal insufficiency and may be the precursor to acute renal failure, requiring active renal support including drug treatment and dialysis. The serum electrolyte balance is vital for adequate tissue homeostasis and acute changes in blood biochemistry can eventually lead to organ system dysfunction (e.g. cardiac dysrhythmias or arrest or neurological seizures and coma).

Endocrine disease

There is a wide range of inherited and acquired diseases which can alter the endocrine (hormone) system and which, therefore, will have profound effects on the internal cellular environment and cellular functioning. Many of these hormonal imbalances can lead to alterations in blood biochemistry, particularly the serum sodium and potassium concentrations important for normal cell functioning, or the systemic hormonal response to trauma by the overproduction, deficiency or inappropriate release of hormones.

The scope of this chapter does not allow for full elucidation of specific changes, but some of these imbalances can be rapidly fatal if left unrecognized and therefore uncorrected. Most hormonal imbalances should be addressed and corrected as soon as possible, and preferably prior to any definitive surgery. Examples include: the inappropriate release of antidiuretic hormone (ADH) as a direct response to trauma, which alters the serum sodium concentration; the lack of endogenous cortisol release in those

receiving oral steroid drug treatment, which affects the ability to cope with further tissue insult; and conditions of altered thyroid function which can have wide-ranging effects on many other organ systems.

Diabetes

Diabetic patients pose a special problem in trauma. A hypoglycaemic event may have lead to an altered conscious state which pre-empted the 'trauma'. Normal blood glucose control can also be altered as a result of the surge in stress hormones (mainly cortisol, glucagon and adrenaline) secondary to trauma. Patients with diabetes are also more susceptible to both infection and poor wound healing, due to abnormal glycaemic control, altered immune regulation and the microvascular arteriosclerosis to which they are prone.

Hepatic dysfunction and blood clotting

Patients with congenital or acquired liver disease, alcoholic liver disease or liver disease resultant from drug therapy may have deranged liver function tests and blood clotting due to alterations in blood biochemistry, hormonal control and clotting factor production. The liver is a highly complex organ with many functions and it is important to identify any derangement early. If possible, such derangements should be corrected as a matter of urgency to prevent further morbidity such as liver failure, hepatorenal syndrome or bleeding problems secondary to clotting factor deficiency.

Any blood-clotting problems should be recognized and treated promptly in order to arrest any haemorrhage resulting from open or closed trauma. A fractured bone will bleed into the surrounding tissues at a rate dependent on blood flow, site affected, severity of bone and soft tissue trauma, and ability of the clotting mechanism to arrest the loss. Continued haemorrhage will obviously lead to reduced cellular oxygen delivery and subsequent functioning and can, if severe, herald the syndrome of disseminated intravascular coagulation. This a potentially lethal derangement of blood-clotting mechanisms which leads to multiple intravascular thrombus formation and total depletion of intrinsic blood-clotting factors which can be fatal.

Fitness for surgery

As discussed previously, the trauma patient requires adequate and appropriate resuscitation prior to surgery in order to optimize biochemical and haematological parameters that may be long-standing (reflecting chronic illness) or acute changes (secondary to the traumatic event). The normalization of these parameters reflects adequate resuscitation and the establishment of normal tissue perfusion and homeostasis, thereby reducing the likelihood of further morbidity and mortality resulting from general anaesthesia and surgery above that of the initial traumatic event.

The most important parameters are the haemoglobin concentration, platelet count, serum urea and electrolytes, arterial blood gases and clotting profile. The individual clinical situations and patients themselves will dictate which parameters and how rapidly normalization should occur, but in polytrauma situations any life- or limb-saving procedures may have to occur before or during the correction of deranged parameters.

Conclusion

The acute trauma patient requires a rapid, comprehensive, appropriate and efficient series of investigations in the initial stage of resuscitation and management. This chapter outlines some of the major investigations based on radiological, haematological and biochemical parameters and later discusses some of the specialist investigations of specific organ systems and problems.

It would be impossible in this short chapter either to encompass all of the investigations that may be required in the trauma setting, or the specific combinations required for each clinical scenario, and a detailed summary of the use of specialist clinical investigations during the assessment and resuscitation of the trauma patient would add another dimension to this chapter. Therefore, the use of other specialist investigations and techniques that have not been mentioned, such as intracranial pressure monitors, aspiration pericardiocentesis, cardiac and pulmonary vascular pressure monitors, endoscopic assessment of the gastrointestinal, urological, pulmonary and reproductive systems, which are now commonplace, are beyond the scope of this chapter.

Suffice it to say that the history, clinical examination, laboratory and radiological investigations go hand-in-hand with other specialist clinical investigations, the nature of which depend upon the clinical situation and resources available to the clinician to resuscitate, diagnose and treat the injured patient.

References

American College of Surgeons Committee on Trauma (1997) *Advanced Trauma Life Support Student Course Manual*. ACSCT.

Bone, L. B., Johnson, K. D., Weigelt, J. and Scheinbeng, R. (1989) Early versus delayed stabilisation of fractures: a prospective randomised study. *Journal of Bone and Joint Surgery*, **71A**, 336–340.

Bulstrode, C. J. K., Ecker, J. and Laws, G. (1989) Musculoskeletal injuries. In *Trauma: Pathogenesis and Treatment* (D. Skinner, P. Driscoll and R. Earlham, eds). Oxford: Heinemann Medical Books.

Department of Health and Social Security (1984) *On the state of the public health: the annual report of the chief medical officer of the DHSS for the year 1983*. HMSO.

Gustillo, R. B. and Anderson, J. T. (1976) Prevention of infection in the treatment of one thousand and twenty-five open fractures of long bones. *Journal of Bone and Joint Surgery*, **58A**, 453–458.

National Academy Press (1985) *Injury in America* Washington DC: NAP.

Mendez, C., Gubler, D. and Maier, R. V. (1994) Diagnostic accuracy of peritoneal fractures in pelvic fractures. *Archives of Surgery*, **129**, 477–482.

Olsen, W. R. (1972) Quantitative peritoneal lavage in blunt abdominal trauma. *Archives of Surgery*, **104**, 536.

Pennal, G. F., Tile, M., Waddell, J. P. and Garside, H. (1981) Pelvic disruption: assessment and classification. *Clinical Orthopaedics*, **151**, 12–21.

Perry, N. M. and Lewars, M. D. (1991) Radiological assessment. In *ABC of Major Trauma* (D. Skinner, P. Driscoll and R. Earlham, eds). BMJ Publishing.

Poole, G. V., Ward, E., Muakkassa, F. *et al*. (1991) Pelvic fracture from blunt trauma: outcome is determined by associated injury. *Annals of Surgery*, **213**, 532–539.

Rothenberger, D., Velasco, R., Strate, R. *et al* (1978) Open pelvic fracture: a lethal injury. *Journal of Trauma*, **18**, 184–187.

Teasdale, G. and Jennett, B. (1974) Assessment of coma and impaired consciousness: a practical scale. *Lancet*, **2**, 81–84.

Westaby, S. (1989) Blunt injuries to the chest. In *Trauma: Pathogenesis and Treatment* (D. Skinner, P. Driscoll and R. Earlham, eds). Heinemann Medical Books.

17

The impact of trauma on the respiratory system

Helen Disley, Helen McDermott and Deborah Langstaff

Introduction

The aim of this chapter is to highlight and discuss the management of chest injuries, together with the complications that can ensue following such trauma. Case study scenarios are used to provide examples of some of the case mix variety and complexity that is encountered within the speciality. Oxygen therapy, the management of chest drains and tracheostomy care are afforded special consideration given that these therapeutic interventions are increasingly encountered within the acute ward environment, the last two no longer being solely within the domain of high-dependency unit care provision.

While the physiology of respiration is not given extensive coverage, aspects are included where relevant as an adjunct to the specific topic under discussion.

What is respiration?

Respiration has three phases:

1. Exchange of gases between the blood and external air.
2. Transport by the blood of dissolved gases from the lungs to other cells and tissues in the body.
3. Exchange of gases between the blood and body cells.

To burn nutrients as fuels and obtain energy from them, cells require dissolved oxygen for oxidation reactions, and they produce carbon dioxide by those reactions (Nason and Dehaan, 1973).

When, as a result of blunt or penetrating trauma, the mechanical or cellular elements of this process are disturbed or compromised, effective oxygenation must be restored and maintained. A variety of therapeutic interventions are available in order to achieve this aim, ranging from the administration of oxygen via a face mask, to intermittent positive pressure ventilation (IPPV) (Table 17.1).

The outcome following chest trauma varies with the individual and is influenced by a number of factors such as age, pre-existing respiratory or cardiac disease and the presence of additional bony or soft tissue injuries, as the following case study shows.

Case study

A 74-year-old man was admitted to hospital for 24-hour observation following a road traffic accident. He had been driving in good conditions at 30 mph, swerved to avoid a dog and crashed head-on into another car – combined impact velocity, 60 mph. His only injuries were bruising from the restraining effect of his seat belt, together with a minor degree of pulmonary contusion. Despite having suffered for many years from emphysema, prior to the accident he had remained active, tending his allotment and undertaking the role of housekeeper for his working son.

Initially he made good progress by the use of effective pain control and regular physiotherapy. However, by day three he was showing signs of respiratory distress, falling oxygen saturation levels, tachypnoea, pyrexia and intermittent confusion. He suffered a respiratory arrest, was transferred to ICU and required IPPV for a period of 2 weeks, following which he was extubated, remained stable for 24 hours and subsequently returned to the ward. Despite the continuation of all appropriate treatment measures his condition once again deteriorated, he suffered a second respiratory arrest and resuscitation attempts proved unsuccessful.

Signs and symptoms following injury

Respiratory rate. Note rate and depth of respiratory effort – increased shallow respirations could indicate signs of hypoxia due to chest injury (Royal College of Surgeons, 1997).

Heart rate. Variations in peripheral pulse could indicate tachycardia due to hypovolaemia, or bradycardia due to cardiac dysfunction.

Blood pressure. Hypotension could be due to hypovolaemia, septic or neurogenic shock.

Pyrexia. Indicating infection or due to immune response following trauma (Schrader, 1996).

Changes in skin colour, such as pallor, cyanosis, diaphoresis or flush should all be noted as they are signs of hypoxia and hypercapnia. Other significant signs are confusion, restlessness and anxiety, together with asymmetry of chest movement during respiration and unusual noises such as stridor. Obvious signs of chest trauma, such as bruising, grazes or marks over the chest wall should also be noted.

Action

An upright posture is the optimum position for lung expansion, and the administration of high concentrations of oxygen will make breathing easier. This should ease tachypnoea, dyspnoea and chest pain. A combination of analgesia and comfortable positioning will ease distress and, as a result, the body's demand for oxygen.

Chest x-ray to determine the nature and extent of injury will be required, and oxygen therapy must be commenced. In many instances arterial blood gas (ABG) analysis is indicated to determine po_2, pco_2 and blood pH, giving an accurate indication of the severity of hypoxia. In the case of many minor injuries, monitoring blood oxygen saturation via pulse oximetry may suffice. An oximeter monitors the patient's oxygen saturation continuously, rapidly detecting changes in oxygenation status (Odell Potter, 1989). A pulse oximeter measures the wavelengths of light transmitted through a pulsating arterial vascular bed, such as the fingertip. As the pulsating bed expands and relaxes, the light path length changes, producing a waveform. Because the waveforms are produced solely from arterial blood, the pulse oximeter calculates the exact, beat-by-beat arterial oxygen saturation without interference from surrounding venous blood, skin, connective tissue or bone. The finger receptacle is connected to a microcompressor that calculates and displays the saturation values. If the patient has a condition which significantly reduces peripheral vascular pulsations, such as hypotension or hypothermia, then a nasal probe should be used instead. Here the probe fits around the septal anterior ethmoid artery, where vascular pulsations are less easily disrupted (Odell Potter, 1989).

Prevention of complications

Normal respiratory effort is assisted by the normal muscular movements of everyday activity. A patient who is sitting or lying still is unable to expand their lungs fully, therefore optimum gaseous exchange and expectoration will not occur (Carola *et al.*, 1992). The cough reflex can be inhibited by pain; the patient suppresses the need to cough in order to avoid a painful jolt, but in so doing compromises the process of expectoration. Secretions collect, often in the lower lobes, creating an optimum site for infection.

Providing adequate analgesia allows the patient to move about comfortably and to comply with their physiotherapy programme. Complications can arise if insufficient regular analgesia is administered, especially in the wake

Table 17.1   Chest injuries and conditions

Injury/condition	Definition	Treatment
Fractured ribs	Rib fractures vary from an isolated fracture to multiple fractures, the severity of which may become life threatening.	• Oxygen therapy • Analgesia (oral, intramuscular – cautionary use of opiates) • Regional anaesthesia via the use of intercostal blocks • IPPV (in severe cases)
Flail segment	Fractures of two or more adjacent ribs in more than one place, or fractures of the ribs and sternum cause the detached segment of the chest wall to move inwards during respiration rather than outward – so-called paradoxical respiration.	This condition is severe, may become life-threatening and frequently requires IPPV
Fracture of the sternum	Isolated fractures of the sternum require symptomatic management only. However, the risk of damage to the myocardium or great vessels, or the development of cardiac tamponade, must be considered when a sternal fracture occurs in association with a fracture of the first rib.	• Analgesia • Oxygen therapy • Cardiac monitoring
Closed pneumothorax	A partial or complete lung collapse occurring when air enters the pleural space from within the lung, causing increased pleural pressure. The lung is prevented from expanding during normal respiration. The resulting ventilation–perfusion imbalance leads to hypoxia (Carola *et al.*, 1992).	If moderate to severe, an underwater sealed chest drain will be inserted which will allow air to escape from the pleural space, but not to re-enter (Gallon, 1998)
Haemopneumothorax	Significant blood loss into the pleural space	Insertion of underwater seal chest drain to allow the lung to re-expand and accumulated blood to drain away. Blood loss must be treated by intravenous fluid replacement or transfusion.
Tension pneumothorax	Caused by penetrating chest wounds, blunt chest trauma, occlusion or malfunction of UWS drainage tubing. Air enters the pleural space from within or without due to a sucking chest wound that creates a one-way valve. Air entering is trapped, accumulating pressure causes partial or total lung collapse with mediastinal shift and impaired venous return. Heart, trachea, oesophagus and great vessels are pushed to the unaffected side compressing the heart and contralateral lung. Without immediate action this condition is fatal	Immediate decompression is required, initially by the rapid insertion of a needle into the second intercostal space in the mid-clavicular line of the affected side. This manoeuvre converts the injury to a simple pneumothorax. Definitive treatment requires the insertion of a chest drain (ATLS, 1993)
Pulmonary contusion	This is characterised by damage to the lung parenchyma. The contusion causes haemorrhage and oedema in the affected area. Blood and colloid leak into the alveoli, severely compromising gaseous exchange. Impaired respiratory effort may lead to systemic hypoxia. Severe pulmonary contusion may predispose to ARDS	• Oxygen therapy • Physiotherapy • Respiratory support (in severe cases)
Adult respiratory distress syndrome	ARDS can be precipitated by trauma, shock and infection. Damage to the alveolar-capillary membrane results in increased permeability, allowing protein and water to leak into the interstitial space. Interstitial oedema decreases diffusion of gases and lung compliance leading to decreased lung volume. Respiratory alkalosis is followed by metabolic acidosis. ARDS is often fatal	Respiratory support via IPPV

ARDS, adult respiratory distress syndrome; IPPV, intermittent positive pressure ventilation; UWS, underwater seal

of fractured ribs or lung contusions. Careful consideration should be given to the choice of analgesia. Opiates can be given by continuous infusion with additional bolus injection as required (e.g. prior to physiotherapy). Epidural blocks can be used and are usually administered via a thoracic epidural catheter. Epidural opiates may also be used; however, vigilant monitoring of the patient's respiratory rate and depth should be carried out. Physiotherapy is essential for patients with chest injuries in order to clear secretions and thus reduce the incidence of infection. Physiotherapy aids lung expansion, thereby increasing oxygenation.

Complications and their management

Chest infection

Patients who have suffered a traumatic event, who are in pain and who have reduced mobility, are dehydrated and who are suffering from psychological shock are at a high risk of developing a chest infection (Odell Potter, 1989). A productive cough and pyrexia are also characteristic of the development of this particular complication. Antibiotic therapy is frequently indicated, together with physiotherapy.

Deep vein thrombosis

Reduced muscle pump activity of the lower limbs leads to a reduced volume of blood flow through the veins of the peripheries. Here, clotting of the blood may take place and deep vein thrombosis (DVT) occurs. Again, patients with reduced mobility and those who have experienced a traumatic event are specifically at risk. Thrombosis could also be due to local injury, such as a bruise or fracture (Odell Potter, 1989). Signs would include swelling, pain and redness of the affected area. DVT in itself may not be particularly serious, but the danger is that a fragment of clot may break off and lodge in the smaller vessels of the lungs or brain. Anticoagulation therapy is indicated.

Pulmonary embolism

If a fragment of clot breaks off and remains lodged in the smaller vessels of the lungs this is known as a pulmonary embolism (PE) or, in the case of multiple clots, emboli. Pleuritic chest pain, wheeziness, pyrexia, haemoptysis and inadequate blood oxygen saturation are all indicative signs. Anticoagulation therapy, reoxygenation and physiotherapy are all required. Anticoagulants include heparin, dalteparin, warfarin and aspirin, and are used as treatment and prophylaxis.

Aspirin is commonly used as DVT prophylaxis post-injury unless contraindicated. High-risk patients, or those for whom aspirin is contraindicated, receive dalteparin, subcutaneous heparin or intravenous heparin via continuous infusion. Exercises are encouraged to stimulate venous return and anti-embolic stockings are used, particularly following spinal or pelvic injury.

Anticoagulants are contraindicated in patients with underlying abnormalities of haemostasis, i.e. active peptic ulceration, severe liver disease, haemophilia and untreated hypertension. The main adverse effect with aspirin, heparin and warfarin is haemorrhage, although this may be more serious with warfarin as its half-life is much longer and clinical effects are apparent for a longer period.

Risk factors predisposing to the development of DVT or PE (Tritschler, 1994) are:

- surgery – particularly of the pelvis or hip
- obesity
- old age
- pregnancy
- oral contraceptive use
- previous DVT/PE
- malignancy
- immobility
- smoking.

Those directly related to trauma (Bayley and Turcke, 1992) include:

- shock, resulting in inadequate tissue perfusion
- fractures of pelvis or lower extremities
- multisystem trauma
- vascular, spinal cord or head trauma
- prolonged immobiliztion.

Fat emboli syndrome

One of the more serious complications associated with multiple trauma is fat emboli syndrome. A fracture initiates the pathophysiological process that leads to pneumonitis from lipase release. This may occur 24–72 h after injury. Prompt treatment is required in order to prevent acute respiratory distress and death.

Signs and symptoms include altered mental state, petechiae, pyrexia and muscle weakness.

Treatment includes intravenous fluid replacement to prevent shock and to dilute free fatty acids. Steroids may be used to counteract the inflammatory response to the free fatty acids. Drugs may be used to increase the patient's cardiac output. Reassurance is needed as the patient may be frightened and anxious due to hypoxaemia.

Oxygen therapy

Oxygen is required in aerobic metabolic pathways to produce biological energy from food fuels. Therefore tissues require oxygen for survival. Delivery depends on adequate ventilation, gas exchange and circulatory distribution. Tissue hypoxia can occur within 4 min following the failure of any of these systems, as the oxygen reserves in tissue and lung are relatively small. Thus, oxygen therapy is indicated whenever tissue oxygenation is impaired in order to allow essential metabolic reactions to occur and to prevent the development of complications associated with hypoxaemia.

The clinical application of oxygen can be a life-saving treatment (Bateman and Leach, 1998); however, it is a drug and must be used correctly. It is usually given as a temporary measure to relieve hypoxaemia, but does not replace the definitive treatment of the underlying condition.

The common clinical indications for oxygen therapy following trauma are:

- shock of any cause
- chest trauma, i.e. pneumothorax
- increased metabolic demands following burns, multiple injuries, severe infections
- postoperative states
- drugs, such as narcotics.

The administration of oxygen is achieved largely by face mask or nasal cannulae.

High-flow Venturi-type masks. These may individually offer separate low concentrations of oxygen, e.g. 24%, 28%, 35%, 40%. They are loose fitting, comfortable to wear and humidified tubing can be attached to them. Rebreathing of expired air is not an issue as the mask is flushed by high flow rates.

Low-flow masks. A concentration of up to 60% can be achieved with moderate oxygen flow rates.

Variable performance systems. Nasal cannulae are simple and convenient to use, and oxygen can be administered while the patient talks and eats. However, they can cause discomfort and drying of the nasal mucosa. The percentage of oxygen delivered via this route can decrease in patients who mouth-breathe.

Partial rebreathing masks. These incorporate non-rebreathing valves and reservoir bags which can provide concentrations greater than 60% at low oxygen flow rates. Prolonged use risks oxygen toxicity.

Face tent (bucket mask). This is a large, semi-rigid plastic half-mask which wraps around the chin and cheeks. The oxygen is delivered from the bottom of the mask and gases are exhaled through the open upper part. These masks are often of value with patients who are uncompliant due to confusion or restlessness.

Non-invasive assisted ventilation. This may be provided through tight-fitting nasal or full face masks during nasal IPPV and continuous positive airways pressure. These techniques can be used to support ventilation in sleep-associated hypoventilation, during weaning from mechanical ventilation and in respiratory failure.

Humidification of oxygen. The oropharynx or nasopharynx provides adequate humidification when oxygen is delivered at a flow rate of 1–4 litres/min. Humidification is usually necessary for patients receiving oxygen at flow rates in excess of this, in order to prevent drying of the nose and mouth. Oxygen can cause secretions to become sticky and difficult to expectorate. There are various ways of humidifying oxygen – all involve the use of sterile water. Humidifiers with inbuilt temperature regulators have obvious advantages, but are expensive.

Dangers of oxygen therapy

Fire

Oxygen promotes combustion. Facial burns and the deaths of patients who have smoked when using oxygen are well documented (Bateman and Leach, 1998).

Pulmonary oxygen toxicity

High concentrations of oxygen (over 60%) may damage the alveolar membrane when inhaled for more than 48 h. Progression to ARDS connected with high-protein alveolar oedema is associated with high mortality.

The management of chest drains

Chest drains are usually inserted in the fifth intercostal space in the anterior axillary line and are sutured into position (Skinner *et al.*, 1993). Here the chest wall is thin and any small scar is subsequently hidden. A chest drain is a large-diameter plastic tube with side holes at the end inserted into the patient. It is inserted through the chest wall and into the pleural cavity. The tubing is connected to an underwater sealed drain. The drainage bottle has a separate outlet pipe above the water level which is either left open to the atmosphere or attached to suction. If suction is used, the fluid in the chest drain bottle does not rise and fall with respiration. If the chest drain is left open to the atmosphere, air flow will be governed by the difference in intrapleural pressure and atmospheric pressure.

The chest drain remains *in situ* until the lung reinflates; often 24–72 h. Oxygen can be administered to speed resolution by increasing the absorption of pleural air.

It is important to note whether the fluid level in the tube fluctuates. If the level does not rise and fall with respiration, the tube may be obstructed or the lung may have re-expanded. Regular and thorough inspection of the system is essential; checking includes the following:

- machine is switched on
- pressure is correct
- tubing is patent
- chest drain bottle is below chest level
- clamps are nearby.

The reason the fluid bottle must be kept below chest level is to prevent fluid escaping into the pleural space (Campbell, 1993). Clamping of the chest drain tubing should only be carried out to change drainage bottles or in an emergency, i.e. disconnection. Tension pneumothorax may develop if the clamps are left on for long periods of time (Nicoll, 1983).

To decrease the risk of infection, the drainage bottles are only changed when full.

An occlusive dressing is used around the drain insertion points as it is secure and prevents leakage, and should be changed as required.

Removal of chest drains is the responsibility of the nurse if a purse-string suture is *in situ*. However, problems may arise when purse-string sutures fail, resulting in increased and unnecessary stress, anxiety and pain for the patient, and leaking drain sites. There is debate as to whether purse-string sutures should be used at all due to the significant amount of scarring caused.

Adequate analgesia is administered prior to removal. Patients are advised to take a few deep breaths and then to hold a deep breath in while the drain is removed. Again, an occlusive dressing is used to prevent air being drawn into the pleural cavity. Throughout the procedure a nurse is present to provide emotional support for the patient. A chest x-ray is then performed to ensure the lung is completely reinflated. The chest drain site is observed over the ensuing days for signs of infection (i.e. increased localized pain, inflammation, exudate and pyrexia). The sutures are removed 5 days later.

Tracheostomy care

A tracheostomy is an opening into the trachea usually formed under a general anaesthetic. It is indicated in trauma for

- excessive swelling to the head and neck
- the removal of excessive bronchial secretions
- minimizing the risk of aspiration in the absence of laryngeal reflex
- inadequate self-ventilation.

In patients breathing through a tracheostomy tube, the presence of moist inspired air is

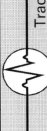

Trauma Service

Tracheostomy Management

EQUIPMENT

For replacement in emergency:
- Spare tube – 1 size smaller
- Tracheostomy dilators

Hygiene:
- Second tracheostomy tube
- Second inner tube

Dressings:
- Lyofoam tracheostomy dressing
- Velcro collar

Suction:
- Suction catheters: check appropriate size
- Wall suction: set at 100–120 mmHg
- Box gloves

Pressure:
- Tracheostomy cuff manometer: (inflate to 12–22 cmH$_2$O)

CUFFED TRACHEOSTOMY TUBES

- Over-inflation of cuff will cause pressure necrosis
- Check pressure with tracheostomy manometer each shift 12–22 cmH$_2$O
- Correct pressure cannot be achieved by using a syringe and the cuff reservoir alone
- Do not deflate cuff without suction above – if there is any risk of aspirating secretions or food

CLEANING TUBES

- Remove inner tube and clean under warm running water
- Do not soak
- Alternate outer tubes every 2 weeks – ensure member of staff **experienced in airway management** is present e.g. ICLL Registrar at first tube change
- Alternate inner tube 1–2 hourly (or as needed)
- Do not leave without inner tube during cleaning
- Replace all 4 tubes every 6 months
- Change suction bottle every 24 hours or as required

TRACHY TUBE	SUCTION CATHETER
Size 10	Size 14
Size 9	Size 14
Size 8	Size 12
Size 7	Size 10
Size 6	Size 10
Size 5	Size 8
Size 4	Size 6
Size 3	Size 5

SUCTION

Technique of suction:
- Insert catheter gently, use intermittent suction when withdrawing to reduce negative pressure
- Do not rotate as this increases trauma to mucosa
- Check O$_2$ saturation – particularly in patients with compromised respiratory function
- It may be necessary to increase oxygen administration throughout procedure
- Use gloves – procedure is clean, not sterile

Frequency of suction:
- Duration of suction should not exceed 15 seconds
- Wait 2–3 minutes before repeating to allow blood gases to recover

Pressure:
- Recommended pressure in adults: 100–120 mmHg
- Set wall suction between LOW and MEDIUM (check reading on gauge)
- Higher pressure causes atelectasis, mucosal damage, catheter collapse
- It is no more effective or efficient in removing secretions

Secretions:
- DO NOT INSTIL SALINE TO LOOSEN SECRETIONS
- This causes much distress, irritates mucosa, cannot be aspirated
- Consider humidified oxygen, systemic hydration, nebulized saline

Size of catheter:
- Dictated by size of tube
- Too large – increases trauma to mucosa, hypoxia, stress
- Too small – increases frequency of suction as ineffective

Figure 17.1 Tracheostomy management (From The Trauma Service, Oxford Radcliffe Hospital NHS Trust)

essential to prevent the accumulation of dry secretions and the subsequent risk of airway obstruction.

Case study

A 53-year-old man was recovering from a moderate head injury and was mobile. He had a tracheostomy tube without an inner tube *in situ*, which had been inserted 5 days previously in ICU. He was becoming increasingly agitated and restless and therefore not tolerating the constant humidification the tracheostomy required. He was found collapsed in the toilet, cyanosed and in respiratory distress. Drying of tracheal secretions had occurred through lack of humidification, and subsequently the tube had blocked. Emergency procedures were initiated. However, the tube needed to be removed. A different tracheostomy tube was inserted with an inner tube which could be removed and cleaned when necessary.

Specialized small, plastic masks for delivering humidified oxygen and air to the tracheostomy tube are available. The patient will inspire less oxygen than delivered, as dilution of room air occurs. A T-piece can also be used. This is a simple, large-bore, non-rebreathing circuit attached directly to an endotracheal or tracheostomy tube. Humidified oxygen is delivered through one limb of the T and expired gas leaves via the other.

Humidification is indicated because the natural mechanisms of gas filtration, warming and moistening are bypassed. Within the literature there is conflicting evidence regarding the insertion of saline to loosen secretions. Ashurst (1992) believes it initiates a cough reflex and loosens sticky secretions. However, Wainwright and Gould (1996) suggest that this routine is not supported by research and could cause more harm than good. Figure 17.1 gives an example of tracheostomy care guidelines.

Conclusion

This chapter has given an overview of the impact of trauma on the respiratory system and, where relevant, the circulatory system. Seemingly minor injuries may result in life-threatening complications requiring complex and physiologically supportive interventions. All healthcare professionals contribute to these programmes of care, the instigation of measures to promote recovery, and in the recognition and treatment of complications. The uniqueness of each individual patient in conjunction with their specific injury will be the key determinants in relation to outcome.

References

Ashurst, S. (1992) Suction therapy in the critically ill patient. *British Journal of Nursing*, **1**(10), 485–489.

American College of Surgeons Committee on Trauma (1997) *Advanced Trauma Life Support Student Course Manual*. ACSCT.

Bateman, N. T. and Leach, R. M. (1998) ABC of oxygen: acute oxygen therapy. *British Medical Journal*, **317**, 798–801.

Bayley, E. W. and Turcke, S. A. (1992) *A Comprehensive Curriculum for Trauma Nursing*. Jones and Bartlett.

Campbell, J. (1993) Making sense of underwater sealed drainage. *Nursing Times*, **89**(9), 34–36.

Carola, R. Harley, J. and Noback, C. (1992) *Human Anatomy and Physiology*. McGraw-Hill.

Gallon, A. (1998) Pneumothorax. *Nursing Standard*, **13**(10), 35–39.

Nicoll, J. (1983) Management of underwater chest drainage. *Nursing Times*, **79**(8), 58–59.

Nason, A. and Dehaan, R. (1973) *The Biological World*. Wiley.

Odell Potter, D., Lasker, J. and Arlene, C. (1989) *Emergencies*. Nurses' Reference Library.

Schrader, K. (1996) Stress and immunity after traumatic injury: the mind-body link. *AACN Clinical Issues*, **7**(3), 351–358.

Skinner, D., Driscoll, D. and Earlam, R. (1993). ABC of major trauma. *British Medical Journal*.

Tritschler, I. (1994) Anticoagulation therapy. *Nursing Standard*, **8**(49), 54–55.

Wainwright, S. and Gould, D. (1996) Endotracheal suctioning in adults with severe head injury: literature review. *Intensive and Critical Care Nursing*, **12**, 303–308.

18

Pain management

Bridget Gray and Sarah Richards

Introduction

Pain management in the acute setting is a complex and specialist subject in its own right. The aim of this chapter is to give the reader some insight into the specific techniques and pain relief modalities which are commonly used in the care of patients following trauma. The physiology of pain will be included only in so far as it complements the discussion of clinical examples.

The development of acute pain teams, patient-friendly technology, assessment tools and protocols have contributed significantly to the advancement of practice. Increasing recognition is being given to the fact that a collaborative approach to both education and practice must be the way forward in the future.

National guidelines have been published in many European countries and the USA which provide detailed guidance on the provision of care and the organization of acute pain services. In the UK, 4-5 years after the publication of professional guidelines by the Royal College of Surgeons (1990), fewer than half the hospitals surveyed had implemented a key recommendation – to introduce an acute pain service – the principal obstacle being financial constraints (Harmer *et al.*, 1995). Newly qualified doctors were still under-educated about the management of acute pain (Gould *et al.*, 1994), and pain relief remained inadequate (Oates *et al.*, 1994).

The nature of pain

Pain is a universal experience and is intimately associated with trauma. Traditionally, it has been viewed as a symptom for which a cause is diagnosed – the pain is then eliminated by cure or controlling the cause. However, during the last two decades health professionals have begun to look beyond this approach, endeavouring to reach an understanding of the complexities of pain pathways in order ultimately to improve the treatment of the patient in pain.

There are many definitions of pain. None perhaps encompasses all aspects of the pain experience, but the following definition cited by French (1989) demonstrates the emotional, cognitive and sensory processes involved: 'Pain is subjective, individual, and modified by degrees of attention, emotional state and the conditioning influences of past experience.'

The experience of pain is unique and complex. It can be influenced by many variables. These may include intrinsic patient factors such as age, previous experience, culture, anxiety, fear, socialization and communication skills. Extrinsic factors in the patient's environment are also involved and include fear of dependency, rigid analgesic prescriptions, underprescribing by health professionals of analgesic regimens, and disbelief of the patient's description of pain. Thus, an alternative practical definition of pain could be said to be 'pain is

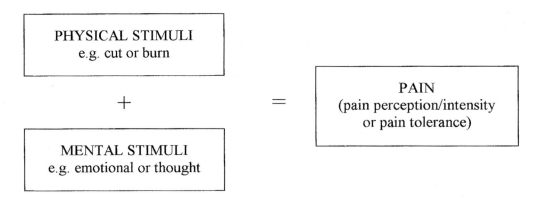

Figure 18.1   Physical trauma (Adapted from McCaffery and Beebe 1994)

what the patient says hurts'.

Hayward (1979; cited in Walding, 1991) identifies nine factors that contribute to an individual's perception of pain. Some factors are also intuitively understood by belonging to the same culture:

Biological factors

- Physical trauma.
- Age.
- Sex.

Social and cultural factors

- Education.
- Social background.
- Culture.

Psychological factors

- Personality.
- Suggestion.
- Anxiety.

Using this holistic framework it is helpful to explore the individual's response to pain in more detail.

Physical trauma

Most pain results from a combination of both physical and mental events; rarely is it purely psychogenic (mental) or physical in origin. Pain results from a total body response (Figure 18.1).

By way of further exploration it is helpful to consider the following. Endorphins produced in the pituitary and thalamic region of the brain are controlled by the cerebral cortex, which also plays a part in our emotions. It may also perhaps explain why emotion is such an influential factor in pain perception (Bowsher, 1993), in part accounting for the fact that individuals following traumatic amputation have been known to walk significant distances in order to get help.

Age

The influence of age on the pain experience is variable and this is echoed by Belville *et al.* (1971). However, the evidence is inconclusive. Donovan (1983) found that younger patients were more dissatisfied with their pain relief, and Woodrow (1972) found that pain tolerance decreased with age. McCaffery (1983) suggests that any relationship between age and pain may be due to how those individuals express rather than experience it.

Sex

Bendelow (1993) explored research into the role of gender in the development of beliefs about pain. A number of Bendelow's examples were perceptions about pain from men. To summarize, men felt they had to be stronger and tougher as that was how they believed society expected them to behave. This somewhat traditional view is also described by Jacques (1992). However, Bendelow (1993) also found that both sexes believed women coped better with pain.

Education

Education in Britain is largely influenced by social class (Cornwell, 1984). Bernstein (1961) identifies each social class as having a different code of language acquired during the course of their schooling. Davitz and Davitz (1975) found that nurses were better able to empathize with patients who were closest in situation to their own. The rigidity of class structure prevalent 20–30 years ago is perhaps no longer quite as influential as it was, so the applicability of such findings to today's practice might be open to question. However, it is only too easy for healthcare professionals to stereotype patients and thus respond to the 'type' rather than the individual.

Social background

Pain behaviour can be influenced by social, cultural and psychological factors (Helman, 1990). In general, attitudes towards pain are acquired early in life (East, 1992). Helman (1990) also highlights what is described as private pain and public pain. An individual experiencing private pain may never show any signs of this in public – perhaps due to the way in which he or she was brought up. Part of the decision about whether to translate private pain into public pain depends on the interpretation by the individual of the significance of that pain. It is also interesting to note how individuals in pain receive due attention and sympathy if their behaviour is consistent with society's view of how that pain should be exhibited, i.e. a subtle change of behaviour or an extravagant display of emotion. Within trauma the latter is commonly seen.

Culture

Culture is defined as 'a particular form, stage or type of intellectual development or civilisation' (Swannell, 1992). Individuals learn the appropriate response to pain in their sociocultural group through cultural values, social customs and family values (East, 1992). It is perhaps easier to understand the expression of pain in that context. If, however, the individual fails to conform, healthcare professionals must guard against making value judgements without taking into account the individual's unique response (Jacques, 1992).

Personality

If cognitive processes influence everything that we do and feel, and pain perception is no exception, personality must as a corollary be similarly influential. Bond (1979) suggests that an assessment of personality gives an indication of how individuals usually respond to stress in their lives. Of more concern to healthcare professionals is the fact that, as mentioned previously, we sometimes stereotype patients and then treat them according to those prejudices. The 'unpopular' patient may well get less sympathy, or even less analgesia, as a result (Gooch, 1989).

Suggestion

Any painful experience is invariably influenced by previous experiences (Hayward, 1979). Hayward (1975) identifies the importance of giving information to patients prior to the commencement of activities or procedures likely to cause pain. The expectation and anticipation of the severity of pain can be reduced through effective communication and an explanation of the methods available to minimize the pain. The patient is then afforded the opportunity to prepare themselves and achieve a degree of control.

Anxiety

The relationship of anxiety to acute pain is a major issue (Walding, 1991). There is also evidence to suggest that anxiety lowers pain tolerance (Melzack and Wall, 1988; Carroll and Bowsher, 1993; Fordham and Dunn, 1994). Twycross (1993) generalizes the treatment for reducing anxiety as 'understanding'. It is helpful to interpret this in terms of a professional and physiological understanding, but perhaps more importantly, personal and emotional understanding: 'Conveying that we care may be the most important thing we do' (McCaffery, 1983).

The role of the acute pain team

Pain control is highly relevant to both quality patient care and cost containment – effective pain management may improve recovery and therefore reduce length of stay (Fischer *et al.*, 1995).

Patients have the right to effective pain relief; failure to relieve pain is morally and ethically unacceptable. Liebeskind and Melzack (1987) state that, by any reasonable code, freedom from pain should be a basic human right limited only by our knowledge to achieve it.

However, many patients unnecessarily continue to suffer pain after surgery (Bostrum *et al.*, 1997); this is despite the introduction of new clinical modalities for treating acute pain, namely patient controlled analgesia (PCA) and epidural analgesia. Anaesthetists with expert knowledge of pain pathways and pain blocking techniques have taken a leading role in developing a collaborative approach to acute pain management – the so-called Acute Pain Services. Acute Pain Service teams are receiving extensive acceptance and support from many hospital trusts in the UK. The multidisciplinary team approach to pain relief involves anaesthetists, surgeons, nurses, pharmacists, physiotherapists and others, optimizing pain management (Audit Commission National Report, 1997).

The aims of the service are:

- to offer leadership and a pool of expert advice
- to improve the quality of patient specific analgesic regimens
- to expand the range of techniques used
- to increase the safety and efficacy of analgesia
- to provide the impetus for change.

Ready and Rawal (1996) believe that several principles should be applied:

- a belief in the importance of pain relief and the improvement in function that accompanies it
- recognition of the large degree of variability among surgical patients with regard to the amount of pain experienced
- a belief in the need to provide comprehensive education
- a belief that regular pain assessment and documentation are essential to improve post-operative analgesia
- a belief in the importance of a collaborative approach
- recognition of the importance of regular medical evaluation and availability of expertise
- recognition of the value of protocols for administering analgesia
- recognition that side effects associated with analgesic methods can interfere with optimal pain relief
- recognition of the need to monitor the quality and safety of the analgesia provided.

Education must remain a priority in order to increase knowledge, skills and awareness among healthcare professionals. The introduction of an Acute Pain Service can significantly improve the level of pain control for patients (Gould *et al.*, 1992).

Collaboration between anaesthetists, surgeons and nurses is the key to ensuring that patients are well informed and free from pain. Collaborative education is one route to the achievement of improved practice.

The Acute Pain Service addresses risk management issues, improving safety through the provision of education, protocols, guidelines and assessment tools, but the cooperation of all practitioners is essential.

A multimodal approach to acute pain management

A multimodal approach to acute pain management implies the use of pain-relieving techniques which act to reduce pain through a variety of actions. Figure 18.2 shows the different sites of action of some analgesics. By using several of these methods together, not only can overall analgesia be improved, but the total dose of each individual drug may also be reduced, thus limiting side effects.

Pain is a conscious interpretation of a noxious stimulus. It is conducted from receptors in the skin and other areas by fine myelinated and unmyelinated fibres. It is transmitted along the afferent component of peripheral nerves. There, neurons from the periphery synapse in the dorsal horn of the spinal cord with spinal interneurons, which in turn synapse with central neurons and pass up into the brain via the thalamus. From here, the pain stimulus is transmitted to the sensory cortex where it is perceived.

There is a large variation between the analgesic requirements of individual patients. A standardized analgesic regimen applied indiscriminately would prove to be ineffective for many patients. The importance of patient

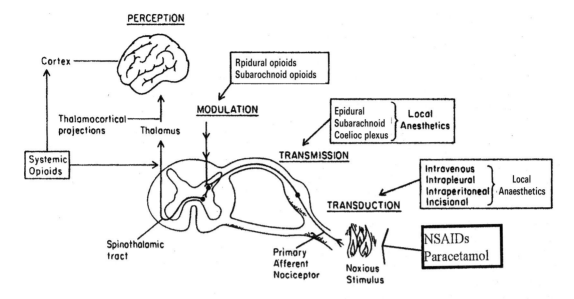

Figure 18.2 Pain pathways

selection for differing analgesic approaches cannot be over-emphasized, this fact having major implications for the cost-effectiveness of treatment rendered, together with post-injury and postoperative morbidity.

Due to their relatively low efficacy non-steroidal anti-inflammatory drugs (NSAIDs) are not suitable as sole analgesics immediately after major surgery. However, they may be of considerable value if used in conjunction with opioids and may lead to significantly reduced opioid requirements together with a concomitant reduction in the incidence of opioid-induced side effects. Therefore the use of NSAIDs in conjunction with PCA/epidural/IM/IV routes can contribute to more effective pain control.

The use of local anaesthetic agents administered for the purpose of operative surgery or during the course of general anaesthesia can also enhance pain control in the early postoperative period. A variety of local anaesthetic techniques may be utilized, for example local infiltration into the wound or a specific blockade.

In the last decade there have been significant improvements in the management of acute pain, but these have been brought about primarily by the introduction of new methods of delivery of analgesic drugs, such as PCA and epidural analgesia. Not all patients will have access to

these techniques, nor do all patients require them. It is just as important to improve the older and more traditional methods of analgesia as it is to introduce safely and effectively the more sophisticated and newer methods.

Given the variety of pain-relieving techniques currently available, it is helpful to consider their use in conjunction with the World Health Organization's analgesic ladder. The principles behind the use of the analgesic ladder are:

- professionals learn to use a few drugs well
- frequent evaluation is paramount
- move up or down the ladder – do not try alternatives from the same therapeutic group (Figure 18.3).

Some of the more familiar techniques will now be discussed using clinical guidelines and protocols as examples.

Intramuscular analgesia

It has been suggested that fear of addiction, dependence, tolerance and respiratory depression lead to under-treatment with opioids by all disciplines (Marks and Sachar, 1973; Cohen, 1980; Saxey, 1986; Seers, 1988). McCaffery and Beebe (1994) believe that this problem is compounded by under-prescribing by doctors, under-administration by nurses and under-

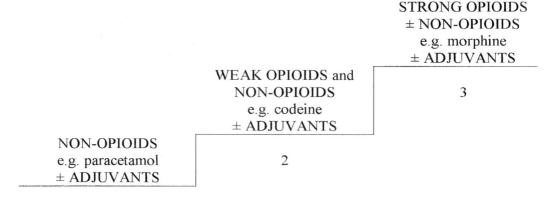

Figure 18.3   Therapeutic ladder (Adapted from Pearce, 1993)

reporting by patients.

One way to avoid such problems is through the use of an algorithm for intramuscular analgesia (Figure 18.4). The algorithm can be used in conjunction with a multifunctional pain assessment and observation chart (Figure 18.5). Table 18.1 details the observations required while the algorithm is in use.

Table 18.1   Algorithm observations

Observations required:

Pain score*	A pain score of 2–3 and above indicates moderate pain. Depending on patient need there may be a requirement for pain relief and the IM algorithm may be commenced
Sedation score	• A sedation score of 0–1 allows continuation of algorithm • A sedation score of 2 may indicate impending respiratory depression
Respiration rate	If respiration level is below 8, discontinue algorithm and contact doctor, give oxygen via face mask *NB. Naloxone 0.4 mg/3 ml of normal saline must be prescribed and administered at 0.1 ml over 30 s until respirations are 12*
Pulse rate and blood pressure	A systolic blood pressure of >100 mmHg is necessary prior to commencing the algorithm
Note the elapsed time since the patient's last intramuscular opioid injection	A period of 60 min must have elapsed before a further dose of opioid analgesia is administered, to exclude any potential harmful side effects

*If the pain score is below 4 for 4–6 hours, consider oral analgesia.

Patient controlled analgesia

The following are suggested drug regimens for use with PCA (Figure 18.6):

1. *Morphine*   1 mg bolus
   5 min lock-out
   If known sensitivity to morphine:
   Pethidine   10 mg bolus
   5 min lock-out
2. *Naloxone*   Should be prescribed for all patients receiving systemic opioids for the treatment of respiratory depression.
   40–80 μg IV boluses repeated every 5 min until respiratory rate is >8 per min and patient is more awake. Dilute 0.4 mg into a total of 10 ml with normal saline.

Safety guidelines

Respiratory depression is the single most life-threatening side effect of systemic opioids. Over-sedation is probably the best indicator of impending respiratory depression.

1. Do not give any systemic opioids during PCA administration.
2. The intravenous line for opioid infusions should be exclusive or have an anti-reflux valve *in situ*.
3. Give oxygen via face mask to all patients following major surgery for at least 12 h postoperatively.

Every patient receiving opioid systemic analgesia must have <u>an intravenous cannula in situ</u>

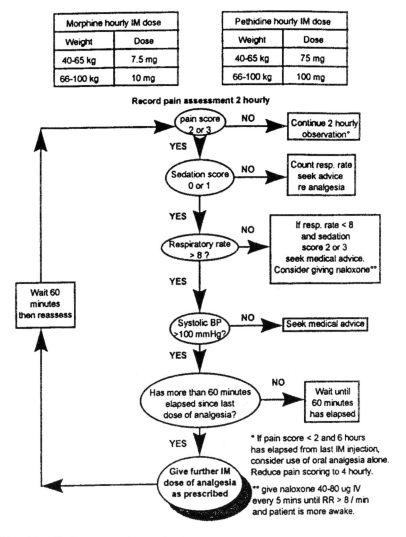

Morphine hourly IM dose	
Weight	Dose
40-65 kg	7.5 mg
66-100 kg	10 mg

Pethidine hourly IM dose	
Weight	Dose
40-65 kg	75 mg
66-100 kg	100 mg

Record pain assessment 2 hourly

pain score 2 or 3 — NO → Continue 2 hourly observation*

YES ↓

Sedation score 0 or 1 — NO → Count resp. rate seek advice re analgesia

YES ↓

Respiratory rate > 8 ? — NO → If resp. rate < 8 and sedation score 2 or 3 seek medical advice. Consider giving naloxone**

YES ↓

Wait 60 minutes then reassess

Systolic BP >100 mmHg? — NO → Seek medical advice

YES ↓

Has more than 60 minutes elapsed since last dose of analgesia? — NO → Wait until 60 minutes has elapsed

YES ↓

Give further IM dose of analgesia as prescribed

* If pain score < 2 and 6 hours has elapsed from last IM injection, consider use of oral analgesia alone. Reduce pain scoring to 4 hourly.

** give naloxone 40-80 ug IV every 5 mins until RR > 8 / min and patient is more awake.

Figure 18.4 Algorithm for intramuscular analgesia

4. Pulse oximetry may be a useful additional monitor, but note that in patients receiving oxygen, pulse oximetry is a poor indicator of respiratory depression.
5. Only the patient is permitted to press the PCA demand button.
6. Naloxone should be readily available on the ward.
7. Do not allow the patient to become over-sedated.

If the patient is difficult to rouse (sedation score 3) but has a respiratory rate ≥ 8 per min:

- remove PCA button from patient's reach
- give oxygen via face mask
- connect patient to a pulse oximeter
- perform quarter-hourly observations of respiratory rate, pulse and blood pressure
- do not recommence PCA until the patient is more awake and then consider a lower PCA dose.

If the patient is difficult to rouse (sedation score 3) and has a respiratory rate < 8 per min:

- stop PCA infusion

1. **Respiratory rate:** While the patient is at rest count the respiratory rate for one minute. Enter rate in box below.
2. **Sedation score:** Look at the patient and decide which of the following applies:

Awake   0
Dozing intermittently   1   Enter number in
Mostly sleeping   2   box below
Difficult to waken   3
3. Pain assessment score: "   Ask the patient:
No pain   0   "Which word best describes the pain
Mild pain   1   you have when you **move**?"
Moderate pain   2   Enter number in box below.
Severe pain   3
3. Nausea & Vomiting assessment score: Indicate which of the following applies.
None   0
Nausea   N   Enter rate in box below.
Vomiting   V

Record **pain, sedation** and **nausea** scores 2 hourly until pain score <2 for 6 hours then record 4 hourly.
For patients receiving PCA record number of patient **Tries**, number **Good, Total Dose given** and **Volume Remaining** in syringe.
If **IM analgesia** in use and pain score 2 or 3 refer to IM algorithm on reverse side of chart.

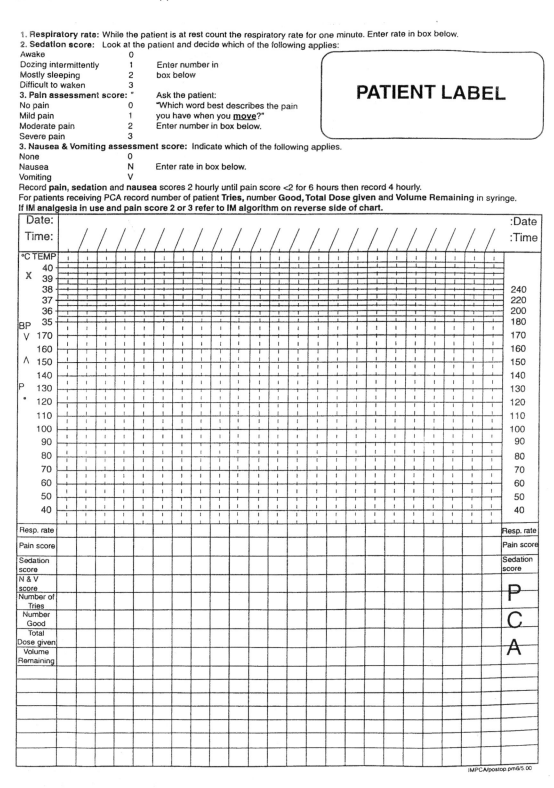

IMPCA/postop.pm6/5.00

Figure 18.5 Post-operative pain assessment and observation chart

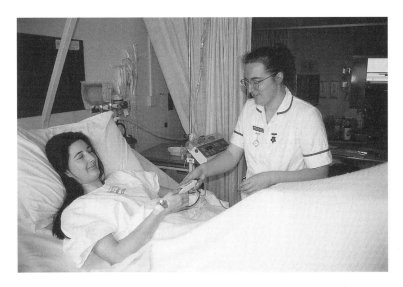

Figure 18.6 Patient-controlled analgesia

- give oxygen via face mask
- connect patient to a pulse oximeter
- call duty medical officer
- give naloxone as prescribed
- measure pulse and blood pressure and repeat observations quarter-hourly

If the patient's respiratory rate is < 8 per min but the patient is awake (sedation score of 0 or 1):

- continue PCA but observe closely for signs of over-sedation.
8. If nausea and vomiting is a problem give prescribed anti-emetics.
9. If itching is persistent consider use of antihistamines.

Remember that the regular use of non-opioid oral or rectal analgesics (NSAIDs and para-cetamol) with PCA will enhance pain management.

Epidural analgesia

Epidural anaesthesia and analgesia is established by the insertion of a narrow bore catheter into the epidural space.

Contraindications

- Patient on anticoagulation therapy.
- Shock or hypovolaemia.
- Use with caution in neurological disease.
- Systemic infection.

Drugs used in epidural analgesia

Generally, two classes of drug are used for epidural analgesia: local anaesthetic agents and opioids.

Local anaesthetics

Bupivacaine is the local anaesthetic most commonly used for epidural analgesia. It has a slow onset time of up to 30 min, but a long duration of action, approximately 2 or 3 h. It can be given as repeat boluses of 5–10 ml 0.25% every few hours or generally as a continuous infusion of 0.1–0.25% at 2–15 ml/h. Continuous infusions have the advantage of providing continual analgesia and reduced risks of toxicity.

Opioids

Almost every opioid has been given epidurally. The properties of opioids in the epidural space are dependent on their lipid solubility (Table 18.2). As the highly lipid soluble opioids spread only a short distance from the tip of the catheter in the epidural space compared with the less lipid soluble opioids, the correct placement of the catheter at the appropriate dermatomal level is essential to maximize analgesic effect. The low lipid soluble opioids can, over several hours, migrate up into the brain causing central effects such as respiratory depression. This can occur up to 12 h following administration.

By combining local anaesthetics and opioids less of each is used, which can reduce side effects while still maintaining high quality analgesia. However, in lower limb surgery the use of local anaesthetics alone has been shown to be as good as using combinations without the risks of respiratory depression.

Table 18.2 Physical properties of epidural opioids

	High lipid solubility	Low lipid solubility
Opioids	Fentanyl, diamorphine	Morphine
Onset time to effect	Short (5–10 min)	Long (30–40 min)
Distance spread from tip of catheter	Short	Long

Safety guidelines for epidural analgesia (Table 18.3)

1. All patients must receive intravenous fluids via an IV cannula for the duration of the epidural infusion.
2. If epidural opioids are administered the IV cannula must be left *in situ* for 12 h after discontinuing the epidural infusion.
3. Respiratory depression is the single most life-threatening side effect of systemic and epidural opioids. Over-sedation is probably the best indicator of impending respiratory depression.
4. Respiratory depression can occur up to 12 h following the administration of epidural opioids. The risk of respiratory depression is greater if systemic opioids are given as well as epidural opioids. **Therefore never give systemic opioids (IM/PCA) if epidural opioids have been administered unless under the direction of the Acute Pain Service.**
5. Give oxygen via face mask to all patients

following major surgery for at least 12 h postoperatively. Pulse oximetry may be a useful additional monitor. **In patients receiving oxygen, pulse oximetry is a poor indicator of respiratory depression.**

6. Naloxone and ephedrine should be readily available on the ward.

Conclusion

The conclusion to this chapter uses a case study to highlight the significant challenge that the achievement of effective pain control in a multiply-injured patient can present.

Case study

David, a 21-year-old student, had been involved in a road traffic accident. His injuries were complex, namely closed head injury, fractured right hemi-pelvis and fractured left acetabulum with damage to the sciatic nerve – he required specialist treatment.

The high degree of pain David experienced was not surprising – bone periosteum has a great number of nociceptors (pain receptors), and he had sustained multiple fractures.

Tissue damage causes a release of noxious substances, for example kinins and prostaglandins. These substances stimulate afferent sensory nerve fibres which cause an action potential (this is achieved through the interchange of potassium and sodium through the plasma membrane of the nerve cells), transmitting the impulse along the sensory fibres to the dorsal horn of the spinal cord. The structure of the nerve will determine the speed of this interchange. From here the impulse is interpreted and transmitted along the spinothalamic pathway to the thalamus.

David's requirements in relation to the effective management of his pain were complex. The nature of his injuries – fractures, nerve damage, the need for surgical intervention on a number of occasions, together with a degree of cognitive impairment as a result of his head injury – presented a significant challenge to those providing care. The following analgesic modalities were used in varying combinations during the course of David's treatment:

● oral analgesics, e.g. paracetamol and nefopam

Table 18.3 Safety guidelines chart

Complication and definition	*Action*
Retention of urine (a palpable bladder and no urine passed 6 h from end of surgery)	• If epidural opioids: try low-dose naloxone 30 μg • Urinary catheterization with antibiotic cover
High sensory/motor blockade (encourage patient to report changes in sensation and ability to move legs) Sensory level > T6 or degree of motor block progressively rising	• Stop epidural infusion and give oxygen via face mask • Measure BP, pulse and respiratory rate and repeat quarter-hourly for 1 h. Reassess sensory level/motor block quarter-hourly • If persistent high sensory/heavy motor block or vital signs unstable, seek medical advice • Once sensory level < T10/lower limb movement returned, restart epidural infusion at lower rate
Hypotension (systolic BP < 90 mmHg)	• Stop epidural infusion • Give oxygen via face mask and connect patient to a pulse oximeter • Give rapid infusion of 500 ml of either 0.9% saline, Hartmann's or Gelofusin over 15 min • Measure pulse and BP, and repeat observations quarter-hourly • Repeat rapid infusion if systolic still < 90 mmHg after 15 mins • Consider use of **ephedrine 15 mg IV if no improvement or systolic BP < 75 mmHg** • Seek medical assistance • Check for causes of hypotension, e.g. excessive blood/fluid loss, sepsis and cardiac failure • Restart epidural once systolic BP > 90 mmHg and vital signs stable
Respiratory depression/excessive sedation: (a) if patient sedation score is 2 (mostly sleeping)	• Give oxygen via face mask and connect patient to a pulse oximeter • Perform quarter-hourly observations of respiratory rate, pulse and BP • If no improvement after 1 h or vital signs deteriorate, then treat as (b) • Check for other causes of over-sedation, e.g. hypovolaemia.
(b) if patient sedation score is 3 (difficult to rouse)	• Stop epidural infusion • Give oxygen via face mask and connect patient to a pulse oximeter • Seek medical assistance • Give naloxone as prescribed if opioids have been administered • Measure pulse and BP and repeat observations quarter-hourly • Check for other causes of over-sedation e.g. hypovolaemia • Do not recommence epidural until the patient is more awake and then consider a lower infusion rate
Nausea and vomiting Itching	• Give prescribed anti-emetics • If persistent consider use of antihistamines • Pruritis due to epidural opioids can be treated with low-dose naloxone 30 μ IV
Infection at site of epidural catheter (marked erythema, induration, tenderness, purulent discharge)	• Stop epidural infusion • Remove dressing and take swab from entry site • Remove epidural catheter and send last 10 cm and tip for culture

- NSAIDs
- morphine via PCA
- bupivacaine via epidural
- amitriptyline, carbamazepine and diazepam
- Transcutaneous electric nerve stimulation (TENS).

Younger (1993) suggests that paracetamol produces analgesic effect by an unknown mechanism. Such drugs act by inhibiting cyclo-oxygenase, an enzyme necessary for the formation of prostaglandins. As prostaglandins sensitize the nociceptors and make them more likely to become activated by other chemicals released during trauma, the action of any inhibitory agent will be to reduce pain. NSAIDs can take a while to accumulate within the system, therefore their use in combination with morphine is often a good option. This was the treatment plan which was adopted each time David required surgery.

Morphine binds to opiate receptors on the membranes of nerve cells, slowing down the impulse and decreasing the pain. David felt that morphine helped his pain; however, he experienced peaks and troughs in terms of its effectiveness. For example, when he had a PCA he found that the morphine would be strong enough to relieve his pain so as to enable sleep, but he would wake in pain, press the PCA button, and have to wait for it to take effect. Similarly, with intramuscular morphine David would still experience peaks and troughs. The nursing staff expressed their concerns to the anaesthetist prior to David's fourth operation. It was decided that an epidural infusion should be used. In relation to analgesia following orthopaedic surgery, Lanz *et al.* (1982) found that the spinal route had various advantages, for example heightened alertness, and a reduction in the need for additional analgesia and sedation. David's continuous infusion of bupivacaine avoided the previous problematic peaks and troughs, providing a constant level of pain control. This proved to be extremely effective for him and, upon reflection, David appeared to be at his most comfortable.

Prior to the removal of the epidural catheter David was recommenced on his oral analgesic regimen, but at times this still seemed insufficient. Nefopam, an analgesic for moderate to severe pain, was commenced. This became David's preferred oral analgesic. As his ability to describe and discuss his pain improved, despite his head injury, it was apparent that there was still an element of pain which remained unrelieved, described by David as a constant, shooting, burning and aching pain in his left leg. This appeared to be neurogenic in origin, resulting from damage to his sciatic nerve. Amitriptyline and carbamazepine were prescribed. Amitriptyline given at night can improve sleep and reduce anxiety, it can also produce changes in adrenergic pathways by blocking the reuptake of noradrenaline. Carbamazepine acts by suppressing the abnormal nerve firings that occur as a result of nerve tissue injury.

David also experienced muscle spasms, perhaps as a result of anxiety-related muscle tension or from a pain-producing process such as a compressed nerve. A muscle relaxant and antispasmodic, diazepam, was effective in relieving these spasms.

However, it was still felt that David's nerve pain could be further relieved. Following a discussion with him, his family, physiotherapists and nursing staff, it was decided that transcutaneous electric nerve stimulation (TENS) would be tried. This method of pain relief was devised on the basis of the 'gate theory' (Melzack and Wall, 1988). They proposed that the transmission of nociceptive information could be modified during its passage through the dorsal horn of the spinal cord. They suggested that a specific circuit within the dorsal horn could act as a gate; if open it allowed the transmission of nociceptive information and ultimately, after central processing, pain was perceived. Conversely, closing the gate reduced or abolished central transmission, with an accompanying reduction in pain.

Descending impulses from the brainstem, cerebral cortex and thalamus may also have an effect on the gate. These modify the opening and closing of the gate through the descending dorsolateral spinal cord pathways. Inhibitory signals from the cortex, due to feelings of control or confidence, help to close the gate. Reducing anxiety, for example by providing the patient with information about when the pain will end or how to relieve it, will also close the gate.

David felt that in conjunction with his oral medication the TENS machine did relieve his nerve pain as much as he thought anything could. David's belief in the effectiveness of the TENS machine, even when the batteries had run down, intrigued the nursing staff, some of whom then questioned the severity of his pain. The mechanisms underlying the effectiveness of TENS are somewhat unclear (McCaffery and Beebe, 1994). TENS is a method of applying low-voltage electricity to the body via electrodes placed on the skin. It activates the gating mechanism and can increase the body's endorphin levels. The sensation experienced may be described as tingling, vibrating or pulsating. McQuay *et al.* (1997), in their studies of the effectiveness of TENS, fail to show any measurable difference between TENS and placebo stimulation.

However, whenever doubt is expressed regarding the severity of a patient's pain, the wisdom implicit within the following well-known definition must surely be our guide: 'Pain is what the person experiencing it says it is, existing whenever he or she says it does' (McCaffery, 1983).

References

Audit Commission National Report (1997) *Anaesthesia Under Examination.* Audit Commission.

Belville, J., Forrest, W. and Brown, B. (1971) Influence of age on pain relief from analgesics. *Journal of the American Medical Association,* **217**, 1835–1841.

Bendelow, G. (1993) Pain perceptions, emotions and gender. *Sociology of Health and Illness,* **15**(3), 273–294.

Bernstein, B. (1961) *Social Class and Linguistic Development: A Theory of Social Learning in Education, Economy and Society.* Free Press.

Bond, M. (1979) *Pain: Its Nature, Analysis and Treatment.* Churchill Livingstone.

Bostrum, B., Ramburg, T., Davis B. and Lidlund, L. (1997) Survey of post-operative pain management. *Journal of Nursing Management,* **5**, 341–349.

Bowsher, D. (1993) Pain management in nursing. In *Pain Management and Nursing Care* (D. Carroll and D. Bowsher, eds). Butterworth-Heinemann

Carroll, D. and Bowsher, D. (eds) (1993) *Pain Management and Nursing Care.* Butterworth-Heinemann.

Cohen, F. L. (1980) Post-surgical pain relief: patients' status and nurses' medication choices. *Pain,* **9**, 265–274.

Cornwell, J. (1984) *Hard-earned Lives: Accounts of Health and Illness from East London.* Tavistock Press.

Davitz, L. and Davitz, J. (1975) How nurses view patient suffering. *RN,* **38**(10), 69–74.

Donovan, B. (1983) Patient attitudes in post-operative pain relief. *Anaesthetic Intensive Care,* **11**, 135.

East, E. (1992) How much does it hurt? *Nursing Times,* **88**(40), 48–49.

Fischer, H. B. and Scott, P. V. (1995) Work is needed to show that good quality analgesia improves outcome for surgery. *British Medical Journal,* **311**, 1023–1024.

Fordham, M. and Dunn, V. (1994) *Alongside the Person in Pain.* London: Baillière Tindall.

French, S. (1989) Pain: some psychological and sociological aspects. *Physiotherapy,* **75**(5), 255–260.

Gooch, J. (1989) Who should manage pain – patient or nurse? *Professional Nurse,* March, 295–296.

Gould, T. H., Crosby, D. L., Harmer, M. *et al.* (1992) Policy for controlling pain after surgery: effect of sequential changes in management. *British Medical Journal,* **305**, 1187–1193.

Gould, T. H., Upton, P. M. and Collins, P. (1994) A survey of the intended management of acute post-operative pain by newly qualified doctors in the south west region of England in August 1992. *Anaesthesia,* **49**, 807–810.

Harmer, M., Davies, K. A. and Lunn, J. N. (1995) A survey of acute pain services in the United Kingdom. *British Medical Journal,* **311**, 360–361.

Hayward, J. (1975) *Information – A Prescription against Pain.* RCN.

Hayward, J. (1979) Pain: psychological and social aspects. *Nursing: The Add-on Journal of Clinical Nursing,* **1**(1), 21–27. cited in Walding, M. F. (1991) Pain, anxiety and powerlessness. *Journal of Advanced Nursing,* **16**, 388–397.

Helman, C. (1990) Pain and culture. In *Culture, Health and Illness.* Butterworth-Heinemann.

Jacques, A. (1992) Do you believe in pain? *Professional Nurse,* Feb., 249–251.

Lanz, E., Theiss, D., Reiss, W. and Sommer, V. (1982) Epidural for post-operative analgesia: a double blind study. *Anaesthesiology Analogue,* **62**, 236–240.

Liebeskind, J. C. and Melzack, R. (1987) The International Pain Foundation: meeting a need for education in pain management. *Pain,* **30**, 1–2.

Marks, R. M. and Sachar, E. J. (1973) Under-treatment of medical inpatients with narcotic analgesics. *Annals of Internal Medicine,* **78**, 173–181.

McCaffery, M. (1983) *Nursing the Patient in Pain.* Harper and Row.

McCaffery, M. and Beebe, A. (1994) *Pain: Clinical Manual of Nursing Practice.* Mosby.

McQuay, H. J., Moore, A. and Eccleston, C. (1997) Report to the Health Technology Assessment Programme on system review of outpatient services for chronic pain control. *Health Technology Assessment,* **1**(6), 1–135.

Melzack, R. and Wall, P. (1988) *The Challenge of Pain.* Penguin Books.

Oates, J. D. L., Snowdon, S. L. and Jayson, D. W. H. (1994) Failure of pain relief after surgery: attitudes of ward staff and patients to post-operative analgesia. *Anaesthesia,* **49**, 755–758.

Pearce, C. (1993) Care of the dying. In Carroll, D. and Bowsher, D., eds., *Pain Management and Nursing Care.* Butterworth–Heinemann.

Ready, L. B. and Rawal, N. (1996) Anaesthesiology-based acute pain service: a contemporary view. In *Textbook of Regional Anaesthesia and Analgesia* (D. I. Brown, ed.). W. B. Saunders.

Royal College of Surgeons of England and the College of Anaesthetists Commission on the Provision of Surgical Services (1990) *Report of the Working Party on Pain after*

Surgery. London: RCSE.

Saxey, S. (1986) The nurse's response to post-operative pain. *Nursing*, **3**(10), 377–381.

Seers, K. (1988) Factors affecting pain assessment. *Professional Nurse*, **3**(6), 201–206.

Swannell, J. (1992) *The Oxford Modern English Dictionary*. Clarendon Press.

Twycross, R. (1993) *Symptom Control in Terminal Cancer – Lecture Notes*. Sobell Publications.

Walding, M. F. (1991) Pain, anxiety and powerlessness. *Journal of Advanced Nursing* **16**, 388–397.

Woodrow, K. (1972) Pain tolerance: differences according to age, sex and race. *Psychosomatic Medicine*, **34**(6), 548–556. cited in Walding, M. F. (1991) Pain, anxiety and powerlessness. *Journal of Advanced Nursing*, **16**, 388–397.

Younger, J. (1993) Understanding paracetamol. *British Journal of Nursing*, **2**(20), 1027–1030.

19

Nutrition

Liz Purcell

Introduction

Nutrition is fundamental to optimal health and recovery post-injury or trauma. It is a vital aspect deserving of consideration by all health-care professionals.

Table 19.1 Malnutrition in hospitalized patients

	Incidence
Acute inflammatory bowel disease	30–50%
General surgery	50–65%
Cancer	44%
General medicine – surgery	31%

Numerous articles have been written which highlight the incidence of malnutrition in hospitals today (Table 19.1). Many of these have also demonstrated increased morbidity and a delayed recovery, especially in the elderly (King's Fund, 1992; Allan, 1993; Bettaway, 1995). Within this group, orthopaedic and trauma patients have been shown to be most severely undernourished or malnourished (Delmi, 1990; Allan, 1993). The King's Fund (1992) Report highlights that this group of patients receives the lowest quantity of dietary supplements. Those dependent on our average hospital diet have low food intakes and can develop 'hospital starvation' (Stableforth, 1986). Poor nutrition may prolong healing and reduce the quality of callus formation in bone injury

(Brown *et al.*, 1992). Furthermore, delayed tissue repair may result in increased pain and prolonged periods of stiffness and immobility, increasing rehabilitation and hospital stay. As a corollary, the risk of opportunistic infection and pressure sores also increases (Holmes, 1987). This is even more evident in patients who undergo surgery (Table 19.2). The worse the preoperative nutritional status, the more frequent the postoperative complications and deaths (Di Costanzo, 1995).

Table 19.2 Frequency of malnutrition in general surgery (Adapted from Hill *et al.*, 1977)

Minor surgery	12%
Pre major surgery	33%
Post major surgery < 1 week	13%
Post major surgery > 1 week	55%

Another group of patients at risk from malnutrition are those admitted following multiple injuries, frequently sustained as a result of road traffic accidents (RTAs). They experience a stress response which results in increased oxygen consumption, mobilization of muscle protein and a switch to lipid oxidation (Weekes, 1997). Consequently, their nutritional requirements are greatly elevated to meet the catabolic demands placed on their bodies. However, the hospital diet alone may be insufficient to meet these needs and this can lead to the complications mentioned earlier.

In comparison, supplementing the hospital diet or providing alternative diets (e.g. modified textures) where needed has been shown to reduce inpatient stay by a mean of 40% and secondary complications and mortality by some 43% (Delmi *et al.*, 1990; Brown *et al.*, 1992). The King's Fund (1992) Report suggested a potential saving of £266 million per annum with appropriate dietary intervention.

Generally, while the benefits of optimal nutrition in trauma patients may be well accepted, they are frequently poorly understood in practical terms. Subsequently, the delivery of nutrition as part of patient care is all too often undervalued or neglected. Reports previously mentioned, such as Hungry in Hospital (CMC, 1996) and the King's Fund (1992) Report aim to increase the awareness of this ongoing problem. They also cite evidence to suggest that the development of multidisciplinary teams improves patient selection for nutrition support, enhances clinical outcome and reduces complications and cost.

Success or failure is therefore largely dependent on the healthcare professional's understanding of the part that diet plays in the maintenance and promotion of health. Consequently, these reports make recommendations which include:

- more training in nutrition for doctors, ward staff and health visitors
- more clearly defined staff roles and responsibilities regarding mealtimes
- greater enforcement of existing guidelines regarding hospital catering.

In response to these recommendations many hospitals have now developed their own assessment or screening tool, their aim being to reduce the incidence of malnutrition in hospitals by an early recognition of those most at risk of becoming malnourished (Figure 19.1). These tools are designed for use on admission and throughout the hospital stay. Each nurse should screen his or her own patient. Based on the score received, a specific action plan should commence; for example, a low score may require a reassessment within 24–48 h, a higher score may constitute the initiation of supplemented drinks or additional snacks. A high score may indicate immediate referral to a dietitian.

On referral to the dietitian the patient's basal and total energy requirements are calculated. These are based on the patient's age, sex, estimated weight and clinical condition and encompass factors such as biochemistry, temperature and stress (Schofield, 1985; Elia, 1990). The dietitian will also calculate the patient's fluid and protein requirements and may consider additional factors such as electrolyte balance and vitamin and mineral status.

Total energy requirements

A patient's total energy expenditure can be divided into several different components:

- basal metabolic rate (BMR)
- post-prandial thermogenesis (PPT)
- physical activity (PA).

Basal metabolic rate

This is the metabolic activity needed to maintain life, which includes respiration, heartbeat and maintenance of body temperature (Weekes, 1997). Generally women have lower BMRs than their male counterparts due to a difference in body composition. Women have a lower percentage lean body mass and a higher proportion of fat, which is less metabolically active than muscle. BMR uses approximately 60–70% of the total energy expenditure (Weekes, 1997).

Post-prandial thermogenesis

This is the activity needed for the physical digestion, absorption and transportation of ingested nutrients. It generally contributes approximately 10% of the total energy expenditure (Weekes, 1997). This may be significantly less in some patients, for example those on long-term total parenteral nutrition (TPN) (McArdle, 1996).

Physical activity

This is probably the most variable of the contributors to total energy expenditure as it is dependent on an individual's activities throughout a typical day. Long-duration, low-intensity exercise such as standing and walking can actually contribute more to a day's energy

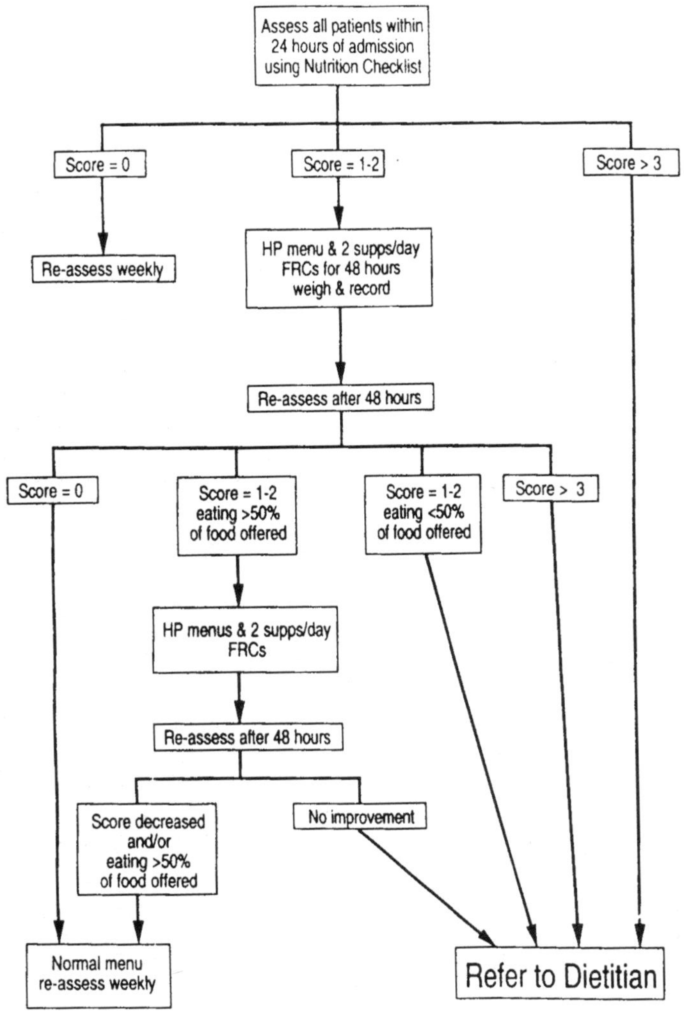

Nutrition checklist

Assess – first day on ward
– weekly thereafter

Appearance:

3 pressure sores or Waterlow > 20
1 obvious weight loss/cachexia
1 muscle wasting
1 sore mouth/tongue affecting oral intake
1 oedema (peripheral)
1 appearance (i.e. neglected)

Clinical Condition

3 ↓ level of consciousness
1 7 days pre or post op
1 history of XS alcohol intake
1 significant infection/trauma i.e. major surgery, pneumonia
1 therapeutic diet (i.e., diabetic)

Feeding difficulties

3 swallowing problems e.g. CVA
1 poor appetite/altered taste
1 poor ability to chew
1 difficulty feeding self
1 unwilling to eat

Weight

3 more than 10% unintentional weight loss in last 3 months

Figure 19.1 Screening tool, HP, high protein; supps, supplements; FRCs, food record chart

bus (Weekes, 1997). In an individual with normal muscular function, PA provides approximately 20–40% of the total energy expenditure. However, in disease and trauma there are additional complications, including pain – which is frequently underestimated (Wallace *et al.*, 1992) – pharmacological agents such as steroids and sedatives, psychological state, anxiety, tension and temperature. A temperature of 36–37°C is considered optimal; temperatures higher or lower than this can result in a rise in energy requirements due to the extra effort needed for sweating and shivering respectively (Weekes, 1997).

The calculations for energy requirements in a clinical setting, despite best efforts, are never 100% accurate due to the many changing variables, and therefore must be revised frequently.

Table 19.3 Differences in calories and protein when build-up drinks are introduced into the daily oral intake

Meal	Content	Energy (kcals)	Protein (g)
Breakfast	Cornflakes	70	1.5
	Milk and sugar	90	3.0
Mid-morning	Tea and milk	7	0.5
	Build-up milkshake	300	
Lunch	Soup	40	1.0
	Minced meat and mashed potatoes	260	15.0
	Peas	30	3.0
	Jelly	60	1.5
Mid-afternoon	Tea and milk	7	0.5
	Build-up milkshake	300	19.0
Dinner	Soup	40	1.0
	Build-up soup	150	8.0
	Egg sandwich	240	6.0
	Rice pudding	135	5.5
Supper	Tea and milk	7	0.5
	Total without build-ups	986	39.0
	Total with build-ups	1736	85.0

In the majority of cases, once assessment is completed the dietitian will recommend the most appropriate means of providing nutritional support. This may be something as simple as the provision of extra snacks or drinks to supplement the hospital diet and make up the potential calorie deficit, or the recommendation of tube or parenteral feeding if necessary. Whatever the chosen method of

nutritional intervention, the potential impact on a patient's well-being and the prevention of malnutrition and complications must be realized. Table 19.3 indicates the benefits that build-up drinks can have on a patient's calorie and protein intake, together with the somewhat lower calorie and protein alternative if nutrition support is not considered or initiated!

Hypercatabolism

Catabolism is part of the process of metabolism which describes the dynamic state of energy provision. The changes involved in the breakdown of tissues and their removal is catabolism. The opposite to this is the building of fresh tissue, which is called anabolism (Zainal, 1994).

Immediately post-injury the body goes into a hypercatabolic state where the rate of breakdown of body protein exceeds the rate of synthesis of new protein (Frayn, 1987). This is a prominent feature of the early post-injury stress response.

Catabolism occurs in a number of phases. First, the ebb phase. This occurs immediately post-injury and is characterized by rapid movement of stored fuels, predominantly glucose and fatty acids. This phase may begin even before the injury occurs, as in the 'fight-or-flight' response. This is when the sympathetic nervous system is activated and adrenaline is released from the adrenal glands. The ebb phase is unlike other states as there is no evidence of an increase in metabolic rate. The flow phase, which follows, is more prolonged and is associated with an increase in metabolic rate and catabolism (Frayn, 1987). The increase in energy demands correlates with the magnitude of the injury. Additionally, the rate of protein turnover appears to parallel the rise in metabolism and can lead to a negative nitrogen balance and an increased incidence of infective complications if adequate nutrition is not provided, or if malnutrition is already present (Rennie, 1985; Taylor *et al.*, 1998).

During the flow phase, the combination of catabolism of lean tissue, elevated metabolic rate and anorexia can lead to rapid weight loss and reduction of lean body mass. The patient's need for both an energy and a protein source is obvious (Frayn, 1987).

Therefore, over a week, this deficit has built up to 10 549 kcal. This is equivalent to a weight loss

Example: The nutritional cost of underfeeding – intravenous dextrose vs. nutritional support

A 58 kg female is given 2000 ml daily of 5% dextrose over a 7-day period post-surgery:

Basal metabolic rate	1315 kcal
Stress (BMR + 20%)	263 kcal
Activity (BMR + 25%)	329 kcal
Total daily requirement	1907 kcal
2000 ml 5% dextrose IV	400 kcal
Daily requirement less intake (1907 − 400) shows a deficit	1507 kcal

of 2 kg of muscle mass (most likely in catabolic patients) or 1.5 kg of fat.

Nutritional support is particularly important in the first week postoperatively or post-trauma, as the hypercatabolic state generally peaks around days 3–5.

How soon should nutritional support be considered? There are many conflicting views on this subject but, presuming the patient is haemodynamically stable, many authors have highlighted the benefits of early nutritional support. It is believed that starting nutritional support within 24 h of major surgery, injury or burns is ideal, while 48 h is considered to be acceptable (Minard and Kudsk, 1994). It has also been well documented that early initiation, especially via the enteral route, has a significant effect on septic complications in a wide variety of patients (Maynard *et al.*, 1992; Minard and Kudsk, 1994).

Similarly, Graham *et al.* (1989) randomized head injury patients to early jejunal feeding, i.e. less than 36 h, or delayed gastric/jejunal feeding, i.e. 3–5 days. He concluded that with early jejunal feeding there was a reduction not only in length of hospital stay, but also in the rate of infection.

Head injuries affect approximately 5000 people a year in the UK and are associated with an increased incidence of morbidity in survivors. Head injury induces a hypercatabolic state, as discussed earlier, resulting in increased nitrogen losses associated with increased infection. Although adequate early nutritional support reduces net nitrogen losses and is linked with improved clinical outcomes, a number of problems may limit the delivery of enteral nutrition. These include morphine and barbiturate use, severe infection, delays in gastric emptying due to increased intracranial pressure, or the development of an ileus due to shock or trauma (Taylor *et al.*, 1998). The latter is a common problem following major injury or surgery because ileus limits the ability of the gastrointestinal tract to tolerate feeding. However, it has now been recognized that this immobility is limited to the stomach and colon, leading to the development of techniques to take advantage of the small bowel's ability to absorb nutrients (Minard and Kudsk, 1994). This can be achieved with a jejunostomy tube positioned beyond the ligament of Treitz in the small intestine. It is believed that this region of the gut maintains normal motility and absorption even post-surgery. Another benefit of jejunostomy feeding is that, unlike gastric feeding which requires a 4-hour break in 24 h to allow the pH of the stomach to return to 2, administration of food can be continuous over 24 h. It has been suggested that patients fed by jejunostomy tube receive more of their estimated protein requirements a day. They also achieve a significantly greater percentage of their daily goal calorie intake (Montecalno *et al.*, 1992). A number of studies have also concluded that immediate jejunostomy feeding following major abdominal trauma is simple, safe and feasible. Early nutrition repletion reduces the incidence of septic morbidity and is therefore cost effective (Moore and Jones, 1986).

Potential advantages of enteral over parenteral nutrition

Infection

- Reduced overall.
- No feeding-catheter related sepsis.
- Preservation of systemic immune function.
- Preservation of gastrointestinal defence mechanism.

Metabolic

- Less risk of hyperglycaemia.
- Less risk of inadvertent fluid overload.
- Increased bile flow rate.

Gastrointestinal

- Lower risk of gastric 'stress' ulceration.
- Improved motility.
- Improved barrier and immunological function.
- Reduced permeability.

Miscellaneous

- Lower cost.
- No need for intravenous feeding line placement.
- Relatively simple feeding access.

Parenteral nutrition

Parenteral nutrition should be reserved for use in patients who are malnourished and in whom the gastrointestinal tract is not functional. 'If the gut works, use it', otherwise parenteral nutrition should commence as soon as possible and should continue for as long as necessary.

Conditions in which TPN is commonly used in adults include:

- postoperative states where enteral nutrition is contraindicated for more than 2–3 days
- short bowel syndrome
- gastrointestinal fistulae
- acute pancreatitis
- major sepsis
- severe burns
- inflammatory bowel disease.

Parenteral nutrition incorporates both vitramix and TPN.

Vitramix

This should always be administered via peripheral access and be used for no longer than 7 days. Vitramix alone is not nutritionally complete; therefore a daily addition of three phials – Additrace, Solvito and Vitlipid – is generally recommended to provide essential vitamins and minerals. Vitramix differs from TPN in that it is not tailor-made for individual patients.

A dietitian should be notified as soon as a patient is started on Vitramix. In the meantime, a regimen of 1 litre of Vitramix (plus previously mentioned additives) every 24 h should be commenced. This suggested regimen should run at a rate of 42 ml/h. Vitramix should not be fed via a central line at ward level, as it is not sterile.

Should intravenous feeding be necessary for a period longer than 7 days, access via a central vein using TPN should be considered and, if available, a TPN team or specialized dietitian should be notified. As with enteral feeding regimens, parenteral nutrition should provide:

- fluids – 30–35 ml/kg body weight
- energy – carbohydrates and lipids
- nitrogen – protein
- electrolytes
- vitamins – water and fat soluble
- minerals and trace elements.

Routes used for parenteral feeding

Central line

Central veins are used predominantly for longer term feeding (i.e. > 7 days) or if peripheral feeding is inappropriate. Central feeding allows the high osmolar and energy/nutrient density feed to be diluted rapidly, thereby reducing the risk of thrombophlebitis.

Venous access

This involves feeding through the internal or external jugular vein or the subclavian vein, the latter being one of the most common routes of insertion. A tunnelled catheter exit site is placed on the anterior chest wall, allowing more mobility and less discomfort for the patient. Contraindications to this route include a fractured clavicle, previous radical neck dissection or mastectomy (Taylor, 1992).

Key elements of nutritional support

Snacks/larger portions

Build-ups Milkshake drinks, high in calories and protein
Sip feeds Drinks which are milk or fruit juice based, high in calories, protein, vitamins and minerals

Enteral feeding *Orogastric*. Used temporarily if gastric emptying is adequate. Used to provide nutritional support where nasogastric feeding is contraindicated, e.g. basal skull fractures.

Nasogastric. Used if gastric emptying is adequate and tube feeding is likely to be short term.

Gastrostomy. Considered if feeding is to be long term, if the patient is unable to tolerate nasogastric feeding, or in the presence of an oesophageal abnormality. A gastrostomy is an artificial opening through the abdominal wall into the stomach, through which a feeding tube can be passed.

Jejunostomy. This type of feeding is appropriate when there is concern regarding aspiration or if there is abnormal gastric emptying or function. The most common indications are major upper gastrointestinal surgery.

Refeeding syndrome

Refeeding syndrome has been defined as severe fluid and electrolyte shifts, together with vitamin deficiencies in 'at risk' patients undergoing refeeding. At risk patients include the chronically ill and malnourished, patients suffering from alcoholism, patients on long-term diuretics, and those undergoing either enteral or parenteral refeeding (Solomon and Kirby, 1990).

Refeeding syndrome has been used to describe symptoms such as hypophosphataemia and other metabolic complications seen in malnourished patients undergoing refeeding. This change in metabolic state is governed by a stimulation of the glucose load in feeds, causing a shift from circulating glycogen to insulin. This insulin drives glucose, potassium, phosphate and magnesium into the cells, potentially leading to low serum levels.

Cardiac decompensation may also be seen. It has been suggested that hyperalimentation may be responsible for this decompensation by creating a repleted circulatory demand on a nutritionally depleted cardiac mass that has had, as yet, no time to 'catch up' (Heymsfield et al., 1978; Solomon and Kirby, 1990).

Finally, vitamin deficiency, in particular thiamine, can be a component of the refeeding syndrome. Thiamine (vitamin B1) is an essential coenzyme in carbohydrate metabolism. Its deficiency is most common in patients with chronic alcoholism. However, any patient with a poor nutritional state can become thiamine deficient and develop Wernicke's encephalopathy. This is the most severe form of thiamine deficiency and can also develop as a result of carbohydrate loading in patients with low thiamine stores. It has therefore been suggested that adequate thiamine should be provided prior to carbohydrate administration in susceptible patients. These may include patients suffering as a result of anorexia nervosa, prolonged fasting, refeeding after starvation, hyperemesis gravidarum and prolonged intravenous hydration.

The risks of providing high doses of thiamine are small, yet the benefits potentially life-saving (Solomon and Kirby, 1990). Table 19.4 lists some recommendations for avoiding refeeding syndrome.

Table 19.4 Recommendations for avoiding refeeding syndrome (Adapted from Solomon and Kirby, 1990)

1. Awareness
2. Recognition of patients at risk
3. Frequent serum electrolyte tests (especially potassium, magnesium and phosphate)
4. Correction of any electrolyte abnormalities before the initiation of nutritional support
5. Increasing calorie delivery slowly
6. Careful monitoring of electrolytes over the first week (potassium, magnesium, phosphate, glucose)

Conclusion

Nutritional support is a fundamental part of the therapy of most hospitalized patients. Early administration of nutrition, be it by the oral, enteral or parenteral route, has a significant effect on a patient's outcome. Early nutritional intervention can reduce the prevalence or risk of malnutrition, consequently reducing the likelihood of further septic or infectious complications.

An increased awareness and understanding among healthcare professionals of the part that diet plays in the maintenance and promotion of health will make a valuable difference to the outcomes for patients.

References

Allan, D. (1993) Adding food for thought, *Clinical Practice*, July, 632–637.

Bettaway, G. and Powell-Tuck, J. (1995) Malnutrition: Incidence, diagnosis, causes, effects and indications for nutritional support, *European Journal of Gastroenterology*, 7(6,), 494–500.

Brown, K. (1992) Effect of nutrition on recovery after fractured neck of femur, *Medical Audit News*, **2**, 1.

Burke, A. (1997) *Hungry in Hospital*, Health News Briefing, Association of Community Health Councils for England and Wales, Jan. 1997

Delni, M. (1990) Dietary supplementation in elderly patients fractured neck of the femur, *Lancet*, **335**(8696), 1013–6.

Di Costanzo, J. (1995) Influence of preoperative nutritional status on post operative morbidity, *Nutritional and Clinical Metabolism*, **9**, 168–175.

Elia, M. (1990) Nutritional support, *Medicine International*, 3392–3396.

Frayn, K. (1987) Fuel metabolism during sepsis and injury. *Intensive Therapy and Clinical Monitoring*, Nov./Dec., 174–180.

Graham, T., Zadrozny, D. and Harridgtont, T. (1989) The benefits of early jejunal hyperalimentation in the head injury patient, *Neurosurgery*, **25**, 729–735.

Heymsfield, S. Bethal, R. and Ansley, J. (1978) Cardiac abnormalities in cachectic patients before and during nutritional repletion. *American Heart Journal*, **95**, 584–594.

Hill, G. L. Blackett, R. L., Pickford, I. *et al.* (1977) Malnutrition in surgical patients: an unrecognized problem. *Lancet*, **1**, 689–692.

Kings Fund (1992) A positive approach to nutrition as treatment, Kings Fund Centre, London.

Maynard, N. and Bihari, D. (1991) Postoperative feeding, *British Medical Journal*, **303**, 1107–1108.

McArdle, W., Katch, F., and Katch, V. (1996) Exercise physiology, *Energy, Nutrition and Human Performance*, 4th Ed. Williams and Wilkins.

Minard, G. and Kudsk, K. (1994) Is early feeding beneficial? How early is early? *New Horizons*, **2**(2), 156–163.

Montecalno, M., Steger, K., Farber, H. *et al.* (1992) Nutritional outcome and pneumonia in critical care patients randomised to gastric versus jejunal tube feedings. *Critical Care Medicine*, **20**(10), 1377–1387.

Moore, E. and Jones, T. (1986) Benefits of immediate jejunostomy feeding after major abdominal trauma – a prospective, randomised study. *Journal of Trauma*, **26**(10), 874–879.

Rennie, M. (1985) Muscle protein turnover and the wasting due to injury and disease. *British Medical Bulletin*, **41**, 257–264.

Schofield, F. (1985) Predicting basal metabolic rate: New standard and review of previous work, *Human Nutrition: Clinical Nutrition*, **396**, 5–41.

Solomon, S. and Kirby, D. (1990) The refeeding syndrome: a review. *Journal of Parenteral and Enteral Nutrition*, **14**(1), 90–97.

Taylor, S. (1992) *Nutritional Support, A Team Approach*, Wolfe Publishing Ltd.

Taylor, S. and Fettes, S. (1998) Enhanced enteral nutrition in head injury: effect on the efficacy of nutritional delivery, nitrogen balance, gastric residuals and risk of pneumonia. *Journal of Human Nutrition and Dietetics*, **11**, 391–401.

Weekes, E. (1997) Energy requirements in adults. *Penlines*, **10**, 4–6.

Zainal, G. (1994) Nutrition of critically ill people. *Intensive and Critical Care Nursing*, **10**, 165–170.

20

Tissue viability, wound assessment and infection control

Julie Stewart-Smith and Kathryn Lewis

Normal skin integrity

Skin is the largest organ in the human body (Figure 20.1). It covers the entire body and has a surface area of 4.5–6.1 m^2 (15–20 ft^2). The skin varies in thickness from 0.5 mm to 4.0 mm or more in different parts of the body. It comprises two distinct regions, the epidermis and dermis. The epidermis is the surface coat and is made up from epithelial cells. The dermis, making up the main body of the skin, consists of connective tissue. The dermis is vascularized and nutrients reach the epidermis by diffusing through tissue fluid from the dermal blood vessels (Marieb, 1989). The hypodermis has a fatty composition and acts as a shock absorber and insulator, protecting the deeper body tissues from heat loss.

The epidermis has five different layers:

1. Stratum basale (basal layer).
2. Stratum spinosum (spiny layer).
3. Stratum granulosum (granular layer).
4. Stratum lucidum (clear layer).
5. Stratum corneum (horny layer).

The skin has many functions, preventing loss of body contents, thermoregulation and providing protection against mechanical injury due to the toughness and plasticity of the stratum corneum (Baker, 1989). Breaks in the skin, often caused by pressure, can lead to disruptions in this layer. Checking for skin integrity is a major component of patient assessment. Pressure sores can cause pain and discomfort, prolong

illness and lead to delayed discharge – all of which contribute to increased healthcare costs. It is the responsibility of all healthcare professionals to be aware of such issues, directing their efforts towards prevention and education.

The aetiology of pressure sores

Terms such as pressure sore, decubitus ulcer and bedsore are used interchangeably within the literature to describe areas of skin ulceration occurring as a result of unrelieved pressure. The term pressure sore, perhaps most accurately reflects the aetiology of the damage. They are caused by a combination of extrinsic and intrinsic factors.

Extrinsic factors

The three extrinsic factors in pressure damage are pressure, friction and shearing. Pressure is the most significant of the three and occurs particularly over bony prominences such as the sacrum, ischial tuberosities, trochanters, heels and elbows. If the pressure is significantly higher than capillary closing pressure, blood vessel occlusion will occur. Prolonged unrelieved pressure results in tissue necrosis. However, not all individuals who sit or lie on hard surfaces will develop a pressure sore. This is because ischaemia results in localized discomfort, often prompting the individual to change position. Such relief in pressure is then followed by reactive hyperaemia. As highlighted by

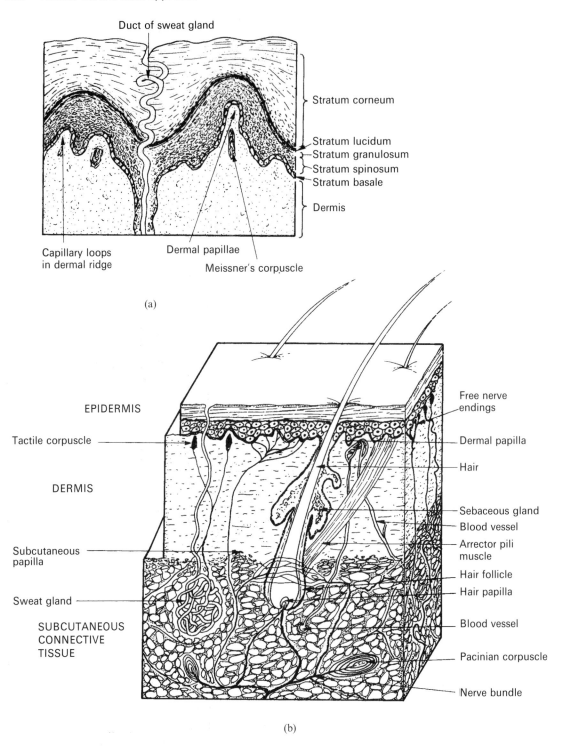

Figure 20.1 (a), Arrangement of the epidermal and dermal layers of the skin; (b) three-dimensional representation of the skin and subcutaneous connective tissue layer showing the arrangement of hair, glands and blood vessels (From Palastanga *et al.*, 1998, by courtesy of Dr R. W. Soames)

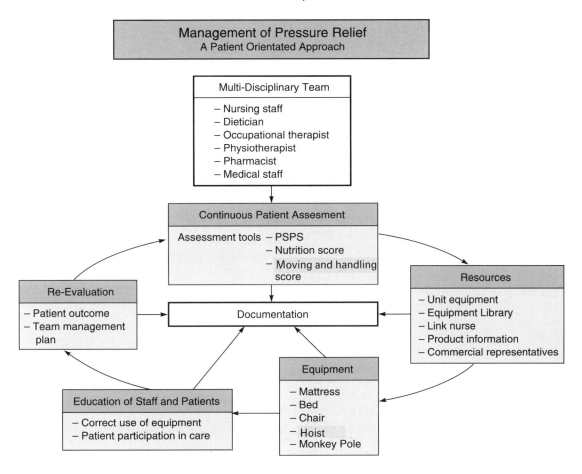

Figure 20.2 Management of pressure relief – a patient-orientated approach (from the Trauma Service Oxford Radcliffe Hospital NHS Trust)

Dealey (1997), there is no clear-cut evidence to define the pressure:time ratio at which pressure damage occurs.

Friction can also result in superficial damage, such as stripping of the epidermis. It is exacerbated by the presence of moisture (Kelly, 1994). Shearing can occur when a patient slides down the bed. The shear forces result in tearing of the capillary blood supply, which may then be followed by ischaemia and cell death (Gebhardt, 1995).

Intrinsic factors

There are a number of intrinsic factors that, combined, can predispose an individual to pressure sore development (Dealey, 1994a).

These include:

- age
- reduced mobility
- neurological deficit
- poor blood supply
- obesity/emaciation
- acute illness
- incontinence
- terminal illness.

Risk assessment

If pressure sores are to be prevented, a patient's at-risk status must be determined so that the effect of any predisposing factors can be ameliorated by early intervention (Alexander and Marsh, 1992). Pressure sore risk assessment scales attempt to determine an individual's risk status by quantifying a range of the most commonly recognized risk factors affecting the patient at a given time. Risk assessment scales were designed to assist, rather than replace, clinical judgement. The use of such assessment scales is believed to increase staff interest in pressure sore prevention, provide a focus for change (Hunt, 1993) and promote the effective use of resources (Birchall, 1987).

The earliest risk assessment scale was published by Norton initially in 1962 and again in 1975 (Norton *et al.*, 1962, 1975). Today, many such scales exist, such as the Waterlow Score (Waterlow, 1985), Braden Score (Bergstrom et al., 1987), Douglas Score (Pritchard, 1986), Lowthian Score or Pressure Sore Prediction Score (Lowthian, 1987). However, within the literature there is much discussion concerning their value. A major drawback with many scales is the lack of research to establish the reliability and validity of these tools (Barratt, 1987; Hamilton, 1992; Flanagan, 1993). Flanagan (1995) highlights the problem of implementing these scales in clinical areas for which they were not intended. Completion of the scoring system may be simply a paper exercise and lack of prevention may ensue. It would appear from the literature that certain risk assessment scales are more suited to particular clinical settings, so the choice of one specific risk assessment scale for general use within a particular healthcare facility is not appropriate and should be avoided.

Within the author's place of work a patient-orientated approach to the management of pressure relief has been developed (Figure 20.2). Within this cycle the use of a risk assessment scale is only part of the process.

One of the main problems in validating the usefulness of any risk assessment tool is that preventative measures would need to be modified during the research phase. From an ethical standpoint this would be unacceptable.

Despite their limitations, risk assessment scales are both practical and useful in promoting the systematic evaluation of a patient's risk factors. A single assessment on admission, however, is not adequate. Risk assessment should be ongoing, thereby reflecting changes in a patient's condition. Following the identification of the said risk, appropriate preventative measures should be implemented. As highlighted by Dealey (1997) 'failure to take due care constitutes negligence'.

Choice of risk assessment tools

The choice of risk assessment tool must reflect the clinical speciality and environment within which it is to be used. The Pressure Sore Prediction Score (PSPS) developed by Lowthian (1987) aims to address the specifics of risk assessment in the orthopaedic/trauma patient. Factors such as mobility, level of consciousness, general health and continence all feature in the scoring process. One criticism which has been levelled at this particular scale is the absence of nutritional status as a factor for consideration. This should not be considered an omission; the importance of nutrition is such that this aspect of care warrants its own assessment tool. The clarification and grading of pressure sores must also be addressed as part of the audit cycle. The Stirling Pressure Sore Severity Scale (Reid and Morison, 1994) is one example of a comprehensive and easy-to-use tool.

Cost of pressure sores

The cost of pressures sores is a huge issue for the National Health Service (NHS). Estimates of the annual financial burden placed on the NHS range from £60 million (Department of Health, 1992) to £300 million (Waterlow, 1988). The cost of prevention and treatment may not, however, be the only cost incurred by hospitals. There is an increasing tendency towards litigation by patients and relatives. In 1987 a patient was awarded £78 000 damages following the development of a hospital-acquired pressure sore. As highlighted by Dealey (1997), other litigants have since been successful, but many have accepted out of court settlements and damages are therefore unknown.

While the total cost of pressure sores is uncertain, indirect costs to patients and families are considerable. These can include pain, discomfort, psychological stress and lost patient/family income. Costs associated with pressure sore prevention include indirect costs, for example the implementation of new environmental health regulations pertaining to lifting and handling which may involve organizations in substantial implementation and adjustment costs.

Education

As highlighted by Dealey (1997), it should not

be assumed that all healthcare professionals have adequate knowledge regarding the causes, prevention and management of pressure sores. Such a statement is reinforced by the studies of Sutton and Wallace (1990) and Bennett (1992), who concluded that doctors and medical students have a limited understanding of the topic and tended to see pressure sores as a nursing problem. Gould (1992) found that a number of nursing colleges failed to give pressure sore prevention and management a high priority.

Today, however, there is much greater interest in pressure sores: short courses, diplomas and degrees in tissue viability are all available. Sadly, demand for such specialist courses in the UK has been, in the main, from the nursing profession only.

Information for patients and their carers

Patients are now seen to be more than just passive recipients of care. Patient education should be an essential part of care planning. Information provided to patients and carers in relation to pressure sore prevention can be summarized as follows:

- awareness of risk factors and their implications
- strategies for prevention
- support services available on discharge
- awareness of equipment and usage.

The Audit Commission Review (1991) suggested that the incidence of pressure sores could be used as a marker of quality standards within a hospital, and later *The Health of the Nation* document (Department of Health, 1992) recommended that one of the health targets should be an annual reduction in the incidence of pressure sores. The concept of pressure sores is now a national agenda item in the NHS and statistics can be used by purchasers and providers (Dealey, 1997).

The terms incidence and prevalence are often used interchangeably, but Dealey (1993) suggests that they have different meanings:

- *Prevalence* is the number of persons with a specific disease or condition as a proportion of a given population, measured at a specific point in time or over a specific period of time.

- *Incidence* is the number of persons developing a specific disease or condition as a proportion of the given population, measured over a period of time.

A prevalence survey provides a snapshot of the current situation. The Oxford Radcliffe Hospital conducts an annual pressure sore prevalence survey. The results are available to all hospital wards and departments and are presented to the Hospital Board. The results have shown that the increased use of pressure-relieving mattresses significantly reduces the incidence of pressure sores. Such a survey can provide baseline data about a patient population and can highlight areas where patients are at particularly high risk. It can also be used over time to measure the effects of prevention policies (Dealey, 1997).

Within the Oxford Radcliffe Hospital the equipment is coordinated and maintained by the 'Equipment Library'. This was created in 1992 (Fox and Delve, 1994). All equipment, such as infusion pumps, monitors and therapeutic mattresses, was pooled. The majority of hospital equipment is therefore stored in a central area where specialist staff are employed specifically to loan, maintain and monitor that equipment. The benefits of such a service are legion: well-maintained and up-to-date equipment; improved availability and utilization (no equipment hoarding); education and training, together with coordinated new product trials.

Wound assessment

Assessment is an integral part of the wound management process and should reflect a holistic and multidisciplinary team approach to patient care. The starting point in the assessment process is the general assessment of the patient. This includes assessment of the following:

- overall health and any ongoing disease process
- pain
- nutritional status
- sensory functioning
- medications
- physiological factors
- understanding of wound aetiology and the associated treatment.

All these issues are relevant to the process of wound healing. However, the following discussion will focus particularly on wound assessment.

Wound assessment offers practitioners a framework upon which to base clinical decisions aimed at maximizing healing potential. As highlighted by Flanagan (1997), accurate wound assessment is 'dependent on an understanding of the physiology of healing and the factors that delay this process, as well as the optimal conditions required at the wound surface to maximise healing'.

Wound healing is a highly complex process; therefore, appropriate wound assessment and subsequent management should be based upon an understanding of the normal process of repair and the factors which affect it.

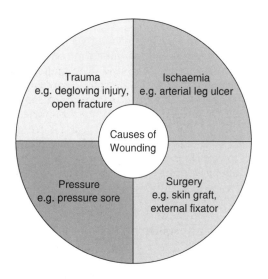

Figure 20.3 Causes of wounding

Normal wound healing

Any damage leading to a break in the continuity of the skin can be called a wound. There are several causes of wounding and these are shown in Figure 20.3. Wounds in the skin or deeper tissues have been described in a number of ways:

Superficial wounds. The epidermis has been damaged.
Partial thickness wounds. The epithelium and part of the dermis is destroyed, with partial damage to the sweat glands and hair follicles. When these wounds have a large surface area, hair follicles and sweat glands produce epithelial cells during epithelialization which form islets of cells on the wound surface, thus speeding the healing process.

Full thickness wounds. All of the epidermis is destroyed. Deeper tissues such as muscle, fascia or bone may also be involved. Healing may be slow if there has been extensive tissue loss.

The process of wound healing can be divided into four phases:

1. Inflammation.
2. Proliferation.
3. Epithelialization.
4. Maturation.

These phases do not occur in isolation; there is considerable overlap between them and they may last for varying lengths of time. Careful assessment can help to identify each of these stages, which is important as treatment objectives may vary at each stage.

Inappropriate wound management occurs as a result of practitioners failing to identify correctly the stage of healing a wound has reached, or failure to differentiate between the normal and abnormal characteristics associated with this process.

Phases in the process of healing

Inflammation

The inflammatory response is a non-specific local reaction to tissue damage and/or bacterial invasion.

The body's immediate response to injury is to re-establish haemostasis. Damaged cells and blood vessels activate coagulation factors and encourage clot formation. This gradually dries out to form a scab which temporarily closes the wound. At this stage wounds will usually produce large amounts of blood or serous fluid which act as natural cleansing agents. Tissue damage and the activation of clotting factors trigger the release of various substances that cause local blood vessels to become more permeable and to dilate. This inflammatory reaction can be observed clinically by the presence locally of erythema, heat, oedema, discomfort and functional disturbance. As highlighted by Flanagan (1997), inflammation is part of the normal protective response to injury and, although the clinical signs are similar, they should not be confused with infection.

Proliferation

During this phase the wound is filled with new connective tissue. Growth factors attract fibroblasts to the wound and stimulate them to divide and later to produce collagen fibres. The activity of fibroblasts depends on the local oxygen supply. If the tissues are poorly vascularized the wound will not heal.

Granulation is the term given to the formation of new capillaries in the wound bed which in turn support the development of new connective tissue. It is so called as the appearance of healthy granulation tissue in the base of a wound is granular and slightly uneven. The condition of granulation tissue is often a good indicator of wound healing. Granulation tissue that appears dark in colour is often a sign that a wound is poorly perfused.

Flanagan (1997) highlights the characteristics of healthy and unhealthy granulation tissue in Table 20.1

Table 20.1 The characteristics of health and unhealthy granulation tissue

Healthy	Unhealthy
Bright red	Dark red/bluish discoloration or very pale
Moist	Dehydrated
Shiny	Dull
Does not bleed easily	Bleeds easily

The process of wound contraction does not occur in wounds healing by first intention (i.e. where there is little tissue loss following surgical incision), but does play a significant part in the healing of large open wounds healing by secondary intention (i.e. in open wounds where there is significant tissue loss). Wound contraction occurs once a wound bed has filled with healthy granulation tissue. As a cavity wound shallows out with granulation tissue, the process of epithelialization combines with wound contraction to reduce the overall size of the wound. In open unsutured wounds the proliferation phase may exceed the 3–24 days that is considered normal for sutured wounds since more collagen is required to repair the tissue defect.

Epithelialization

During this stage of wound healing epithelial cells from the wound margin, sweat glands and hair follicles migrate over new granulating tissue until they form a continuous layer of cells and close the wound.

The process of epithelialization is very delicate and is dependent on the provision of a moist wound environment (Winter, 1962). Newly formed epithelial cells have a translucent appearance and are usually whitish pink (Englstein, 1985; Field and Kerstein, 1994).

Maturation

This is the final stage of wound healing and occurs once the wound has been closed by connective tissue and epithelialization. During this phase, type III collagen – a soft gelatinous collagen – is gradually replaced with stronger, more highly organized collagen. The process of remodelling continues with fibroblasts migrating from the wound site, and rationalization of the numerous blood vessels, resulting in shrinking and thinning of any scarring.

The normal process of wound healing ensures that the majority of wounds heal quickly and without complication. However, not all wounds heal without complication or delay. The multidisciplinary team is often challenged by patients with non-healing chronic wounds. Such wounds can have a profound effect on the quality of life of a patient and his or her family and friends.

Table 20.2 Factors adversely affecting the wound healing process

Age
Disease processes
Drug therapies
Infection
Poor surgical technique or wound care
Malnutrition
Smoking
Psychological status
Radiotherapy

Key factors adversely affecting normal wound healing are listed in Table 20.2. Factors such as those identified in the table may be treatable or preventable and, following identification of the problem, treatment should be given. Where this is not possible the likelihood of delayed healing should be planned for.

Clinical appearance of wounds

A method frequently utilized to assess wounds is direct observation of the characteristics of the wound surface and predominant colour (Cuzzell, 1988). This approach could be criticized for its oversimplicity; however, it is quick, relatively easy to do and has minimal resource implications.

The appearance of the wound gives an indication of the stage of healing that it has reached or of any complications that may be present. Wounds healing by secondary intention can be categorized as

- necrotic
- sloughy
- infected
- granulating
- epithelializing

Necrotic wounds

Necrotic wounds are covered with devitalized tissue that is usually black or brownish in colour. Necrotic tissue prolongs healing (Benbow, 1995; Flanagan, 1997; Morison *et al.*, 1997) and increases the risk of clinical infection.

The treatment objective for this type of wound is to remove the necrotic tissue. The quickest method of removal is surgical debridement. This is not however appropriate in all cases. An alternative method of treating these wounds is to rehydrate and soften the necrotic tissue, thereby promoting autolytic debridement. Autolysis describes the body's natural ability to break down and liquefy devitalized tissue, a process which is enhanced by moisture-retentive dressings. Alvarez (1988) argues that the maintenance of a moist wound surface helps to promote the rehydration of slough and necrotic tissue while allowing leucocytes and enzymes present in the exudate to break down avascular tissue.

Wound management products such as amorphous hydrogels or hydrocolloids may be used to soften and liquefy necrotic tissue. Enzymatic preparations may be utilized, but many are not universally available.

Sloughy wounds

Slough is formed when dead cells accumulate on the wound surface. In some chronic wounds, areas of fibrous tissue can cover the wound's base, often combining with slough, making it difficult to remove.

The treatment objective is to cleanse and debride. A variety of wound management products available for treating sloughy wounds include hydrogels, hydrocolloids, alginates (if exudate is present), polysaccharide dressings and enzymatic agents. Recently, the use of larval therapy has been utilized for the rapid removal of slough and necrotic tissue (Thomas *et al.*, 1996). Whichever technique is selected, desloughing should be carried out with caution as it may cause unnecessary trauma and prolong the inflammatory response.

Infected wounds

Wound infection may occur at any stage in the healing process and all types of wound can become infected. All wounds are colonized with bacteria which do not necessarily affect healing. Pathogenic organisms growing in large numbers are likely to produce wound infections.

Managing infected wounds is problematic, largely due to the lack of empirical evidence on the most effective management strategies. In the case of wound infections, systemic antibiotics are often the first choice of treatment. Antibiotic resistance is a growing problem, however, and Appleton and Leaper (1992) contend that antibiotics for wound infection should be prescribed only if there is spreading cellulitis or systemic toxicity.

Within the literature, research regarding the effectiveness of antiseptics on open wounds is conflicting. Interpretation of the findings is difficult due to small sample sizes, animal models and *in vitro* techniques. It would appear that the significance of these results for human tissue and the implications for clinical practice remain unclear. Morison *et al.* (1997) highlight that when considering the use of antiseptics it is important to balance the potential cytotoxicity of the bacteria against the potential cytotoxicity of some antiseptics. It is believed by Goldheim

(1993) and Gilchrist (1997) that although there should not be widespread and indiscriminate use of antiseptics, recent research supports consideration of their use in the management of infected wounds. New antiseptics which should be considered include cadexomer iodine, silver sulphadiazine and mupirocin.

Granulating wounds

Granulation tissue is highly vascular, giving it a characteristic deep pink-red colour. These types of wounds vary in size and in the amount of exudate they produce.

The management objective with granulating and epithelializing tissue is protection and the continued provision of warm, moist and clean conditions at the wound surface. Appropriate dressing products for granulating wounds include alginates, foams, hydrogels and hydro-colloids.

Epithelializing wounds

The process of epithelialization can be recognized by the presence of pink-whitish tissue migrating from the wound's margin or from the remnants of hair follicles in the dermis. Delicate epithelial cells can be partly translucent and may be confused with macerated skin. Dressing options including alginates, hydrocolloids, films and silicone-coated dressings.

Traumatic wounds

Traumatic wounds differ from surgical or chronic wounds in a number of ways. They can often be contaminated by various combinations of dirt, bacteria, foreign bodies, fungi or spores (Morison *et al.*, 1997). Management of such wounds requires thorough cleansing and debridement of the wound and surrounding skin by irrigation (Bale and Jones, 1997). After thorough wound cleansing, depending on the extent of contamination, surgical debridement under local or general anaesthesia is often required in order to facilitate the removal of any foreign bodies or devitalized tissue. All traumatic wounds, however superficial, require careful exploration in order to exclude the possibility of even the smallest foreign body, such as grit or splinters, remaining in the tissues providing a focus for infection.

Dressing selection

As highlighted by Thomas (1997), no single dressing is suitable for the management of all types of wounds, with few suitable for all stages of healing.

For successful wound management a flexible approach to the selection and use of products is required. It is, however, essential to combine an understanding of the process of healing with a knowledge of dressing materials. It is currently believed (Turner, 1982; Thomas, 1990) that for healing to take place at an optimum rate a dressing should ensure that the wound remains:

- free from clinical infection and excessive slough
- moist with exudate, but not macerated
- free from particles and toxic wound contaminants
- at an optimum pH value.

Other factors for consideration are whether the dressing is:

- acceptable to the patient
- appropriate to the current stage of healing
- cost-effective and available
- easy to apply.

The range of dressings available on the market today is extensive. Therefore within the author's place of work members of the multidisciplinary team believed that a collaborative approach to wound management was necessary. It was concluded that the provision of a framework enabling healthcare professionals to access information would subsequently improve practice. Wound management guidelines were produced (Figure 20.4). Guidelines, rather than protocols, were provided with the aim of enhancing, rather than replacing, clinical judgement. Dressing selection guides in the form of laminated pocket cards were also provided for staff to use at the bedside (Gray, 1996) and these are shown in Figure 20.5.

Cost of wound healing

On examining the true costs of healing, the cost to healthcare facilities has to be considered in terms of delayed healing or complications delaying recovery. Causative factors include surgical wound infection and pressure sores.

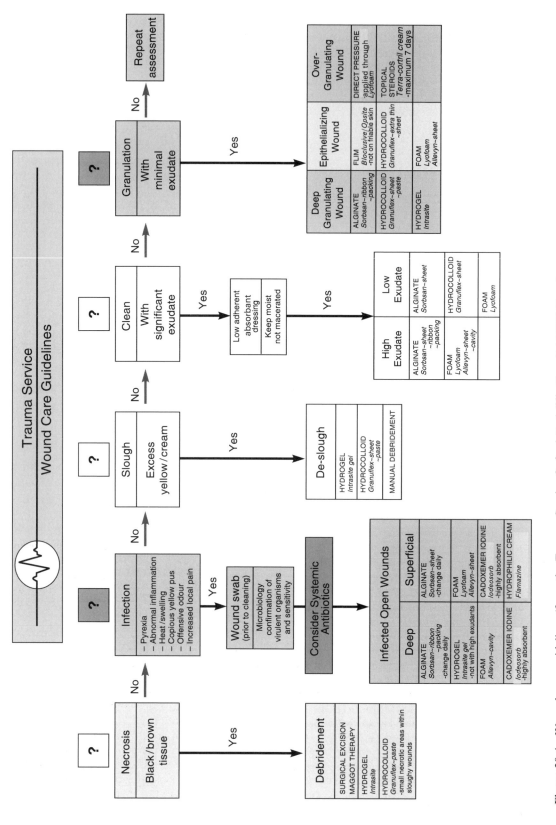

Figure 20.4 Wound care guidelines (from the Trauma Service Oxford Radcliffe Hospital NHS Trust)

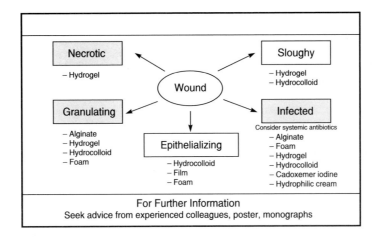

Figure 20.5 Dressing selection guide (from the Trauma Service Oxford Radcliffe Hospital NHS Trust)

Optimum Dressing	Nursing Implications
Maintain high humidity	Avoid dry dressings on open wounds
Remove excess exudate	Use absorbent dressings–avoid maceration
Provide thermal insulation	Expose wound for minimum of time
Ensure impermeability to bacteria	Apply strapping like a picture frame When strike through occurs–repad or redress with additional dressings
Keep free of particulates and toxic wound contaminants	Avoid cotton wool, lint, cut gauze Do not use key hole dressings
Prevent traumatic dressing removal	Avoid dressings drying out NB: JELONET Consider friable skin at wound edges

The development of postoperative wound infection and pressure sores can lead to cancelled admissions due to reduced bed availability, and can increase length of stay for patients who experience such complications.

Cost to the patient is another area for consideration. For a patient suffering from an acute or chronic wound, their pain and suffering cannot be quantified. However, the cost to an individual is not only in pain and altered body image, but may also result in loss of earnings which may cause considerable hardship and possibly affect future employment.

Role conflicts

Within the last 20 years, changes and developments in the understanding of wound healing and the management of wounds has been immense. An essential aspect of wound management is wound assessment and the planning of appropriate treatment. Today the debate as to which professional should make these decisions continues.

Harding (1992) believes that in matters of wound care there are no obvious experts. There are, however, many anecdotal reports of conflict between doctors and nurses over what constitutes an appropriate dressing. Dealey (1994b) states that many nurses will carry out medical prescriptions in wound management even if they do not believe them to be appropriate. The prescriptive authority doctors have over nurses does not, however, absolve nurses from the consequences of their actions. Should a nurse apply an inappropriately prescribed dressing it could give rise to the argument that it would break the nurses' Professional Code of Conduct set by the United Kingdom Central Council (UKCC, 1992), as the nurse would demonstrate failure to 'act in such a manner as to promote and safeguard the interests and wellbeing of patients'. Tingle (1992) states that medical staff may be unaware of the constraints of this code and the dilemma faced by the nurse if the medical prescription does not comply with her professional judgement.

It could be argued, however, that the debate between medical and nursing staff regarding wound management perhaps masks the more fundamental issue of interprofessional power. Despite such problems, in order to provide effective wound management and ensure the welfare of patients, a collaborative relationship between the professions based on mutual respect is required.

Infection

Infection is one of the risks resulting from trauma surgery. Cruse (1986) identified four categories, each associated with different risk of infection. It was found that clean operations (surgical incision into non-inflamed tissue) such as elective orthopaedic surgery (i.e. hip and knee replacements) resulted in wound infections of only 1.5%. This number is greatly increased following traumatic injury, especially in the case of open fractures where injuries are contaminated by road dirt, particles of clothing and chemicals (Cooper and Lawrence, 1996). Cruse classed these contaminated traumatic wounds as 'dirty' and these operations were found to have wound infections of up to 40%.

Despite advances in surgical techniques and antimicrobial therapy, sepsis remains a major cause of late death following trauma (Goris and Draaisma, 1982). The risk of infection is determined by three factors:

1. The organisms present.
2. The pathophysiological conditions at the site of contamination.
3. The state of host defence mechanisms – these can be depressed following trauma, as the polymorphonuclear function is abnormal and phagocytic capacity is reduced in the 24 h following trauma.

Antibiotic usage prior to surgery (on induction) provides adequate antibiotic cover when new tissue planes are opened. Second-generation cephalosporins, for example cefuroxime, reach high levels in bone following intravenous injection (Hughes *et al.*, 1981). Prompt diagnosis of acute bone infection is essential (Kinnard, 1985). Failure to identify causative microorganisms and begin appropriate antimicrobial therapy can result in further bone destruction and an increase in morbidity (Septimus and Musher, 1979).

The consequences of infection following traumatic injury are many and varied, for example increased length of hospital stay and increased cost of treatment. One of the main complications of infection is the delaying of wound healing. Wound infection has been found to cause 290 additional bed days for one group of surgical patients (Cutting and Harding, 1994). Toxins that are secreted into the wound environment by bacteria affect the synthesis of collagen, one of the constituents of granulation tissue (Kloth *et al.*, 1990). Bacteria also compete with cells in damaged tissue for oxygen and other nutrients.

Thomson (1995) defines infection as an 'invasion and multiplication of micro-organisms in the body tissue'. A patient's resistance to infection can reduce with age, surgical stress, length of hospitalization, steroid therapy, malignancy, the presence of a foreign body and a poor nutritional intake (Sawyer and Pruett, 1994).

When assessing wounds for evidence of infection, some signs can often be mistaken for the body's natural response to wound healing, these being inflammation, redness, heat, swelling and pain. The presence of pus with inflammation is a common indicator that infection is present. Other indicators which should also be considered are listed in Table 20.3.

Table 20.3   Infection indicators

New or increased pain in or around the wound
Increase or change in discharge from the wound
Granulation tissue which bleeds easily
Wound breakdown, dehiscence
Inflammation and raised skin temperature around the wound
Unusual exudate on the wound dressings
Patient feeling generally unwell

If a wound is thought to be infected it is necessary to take a swab from the infected area and send it to the laboratory for culture and antibiotic sensitivity. If infection is present, a course of antibiotics may be prescribed.

Infection can be due to poor handwashing technique by the multidisciplinary team. Handwashing using soap and water removes most of the transient bacterial flora acquired from regular patient contact. Another effective way of preventing the transfer of organisms to and from the hand is the use of universal precautions.

The use of Universal Infection Control Precautions (UICP)

Universal precautions were initially advised by the Centre for Disease Control (1987), in Atlanta, in response to the problems of identifying individuals infected with HIV. The purpose of UICP is to reduce the risk of nosocomial infection to patients, while protecting the healthcare worker from blood-borne viruses and pathogenic microorganisms in body fluids.

UICPs have now become a recognized standard in good infection control (Wilson and Breedon, 1990) whereby all blood and body fluids are treated as potentially infected. The policy does not prescribe the use of gloves and aprons for all procedures, but the healthcare worker is expected to assess the risk to which they may be exposed during the course of their working practice.

The options for long term intravenous antibiotic therapy

UICPs offer a way in which to minimize the risk of cross-infection. Unfortunately, it is impossible to eliminate totally the risk of infection, and outbreaks inevitably occur. Superficial wound infections are often treated with a short course of intravenous (IV) antibiotics, but deep wound infections often have to be treated more aggressively with long courses, often in excess of 6 weeks. A decision to instigate this type of treatment is made by medical staff in conjunction with microbiologists and specialists in infectious diseases.

A 6-week course of IV antibiotics has serious implications for the patient; it involves commitment to their treatment. A major problem

experienced by many patients is the issue of patent venous access. Peripheral access over this length of time is not appropriate. One option offered to patients who have to undergo long-term IV antibiotic therapy is the insertion of a central venous catheter or a percutaneous intravenous central catheter line (PICC).

These lines can be kept in place for long periods of time and, in the author's place of work, are inserted on the ward by a team of specialist nurses. They are inserted under light sedation (midazolam) and therapy can commence as soon as the position of the line has been verified by x-ray.

Nurses have produced information booklets for patients and their families which help them to understand the purpose and subsequent care of these intravenous lines.

In Oxfordshire, a scheme has been developed to enable some patients to receive their course of IV antibiotics at home. The Community IV Liaison Team work with the microbiologists and the Infectious Diseases Team educating and training community nurses, patients, or a willing and able family member to administer the antibiotics. Nurses and patients or family members are taught how to administer the drugs, together with caring for the line, learning how to observe for signs of infection and line occlusion. They are supported 24 hours a day by the IV Liaison Team.

If this community service cannot be offered to the patient, usually as a result of geographical location, the patient must remain in hospital for the duration of therapy unless suitably trained staff can offer the service as an outpatient at a community hospital.

Regular review as an outpatient is required in order to monitor the effectiveness of therapy. Key indicators suggestive of response to treatment would be reducing levels of creative reactive protein (CRP) and a fall in the erythrocyte sedimentation rate (ESR) measured via venous blood sampling. On completion of IV therapy the line is removed, but the patient may be required to continue with a course of oral antibiotics.

The implications of methicillin-resistant *Staphylococcus aureus* (MRSA)

The speciality of trauma has been identified by a working party report by the British Society of Antimicrobial Chemotherapy (1998) as a high-risk area for the prevalence of MRSA. Bowler (1997) illustrated the increase in the number of hospitals affected by MRSA from 25 in 1993 to more than 100 in 1996. The reasons for this are said to be due to increased pressure on hospitals to run at full bed occupancy. Maximizing bed occupancy leads to patients being on more than one ward throughout their hospital stay. Unidentified MRSA will have many contacts with staff and other patients.

MRSA is carried by 20–30% of the population (Griffiths, 1989), and when an individual is well it plays a non-invasive role as a commensal organism. When a patient is admitted to hospital following illness or injury, the bacteria may then present a significant risk. Risk factors for the acquisition of MRSA include duration of stay, the presence of wounds or ulcers and invasive devices, together with prior antibiotic therapy. The use of broad-spectrum antibiotics can increase the risk of acquiring MRSA as they can destroy some of the body's natural microbes, leaving areas on the skin for MRSA attachment. Any break in the integrity of the skin also provides the opportunity for MRSA to gain access to the body. The infection control team play an important role in the identification of patients with MRSA and the control of outbreaks. Patients who are known to carry MRSA are identified by flagged medical notes and it is generally accepted that in high-risk clinical areas they are nursed in isolation. This is another step in the prevention of cross-infection, as airborne particles contaminated with MRSA can be shed and dispersed into the environment.

In areas where patients are not routinely screened on admission, MRSA status is often not known. Controlling the potential spread of MRSA in these areas is frequently determined by good handwashing technique – the single most effective measure in infection control. The technique of handwashing should ensure thorough decontamination (Ayliffe *et al.*, 1978). The use of alcohol hand rub is also effective in removing MRSA. The working party report of the British Society of Antimicrobial Chemotherapy (1998) also advocates the following practices to help prevent the spread:

- the use of gloves and protective clothing
- daily damp dusting
- the rapid bagging of linen to help prevent dispersal of microorganisms into the

ward, and the treatment of linen according to hospital policy.

If several patients on a ward are identified as having MRSA, cohort nursing may be required. Here, new admissions are physically separated from those on the ward with MRSA and those known to have been exposed to it (Bowler, 1997). If this does not succeed in reducing the spread, then ward closure may be required.

The use of antibiotics with MRSA

MRSA demands the use of glycopeptides – vancomycin and teicoplanin. Vancomycin is a drug which requires the monitoring of serum blood levels, as toxicity can lead to impaired renal function. The dosage of antibiotics is modified in response to serum levels. If the spread of the organism is such that cohort nursing has been instigated, it is recommended that all patients undergoing surgery are given prophylactic vancomycin as opposed to the usual broad-spectrum antibiotics cefuroxime or cephradine. Measures such as these have serious cost implications relating not only to the cost of antibiotics, but also laboratory and nursing time. The need for effective infection control measures cannot be stressed too highly. It is therefore vital to minimize the occurrence of such infection.

The effects of isolation

Patients who are known to have MRSA or who are perceived to be in a high-risk category due to previous exposure should be nursed in a side room for the duration of their stay or until a negative MRSA status has been determined. Isolation, together with scrupulous UICPs, is known to reduce the spread of MRSA. The effects of isolation have been documented and can be seen to have both positive and negative effects on the physical and psychological well-being of the patient. Meers *et al.* (1997) suggested that isolation is expensive and disruptive to a patient's care. It may deprive the patient of special monitoring or treatment, as constant observation is not always possible and depends on the location of the side room within the ward environment. Knowles (1993) commented that although no deterioration in mental state had been found in patients who were in isolation using psychological scales, certain behaviours were observed such as agitation, aggression and depression. Patients commented that isolation encouraged feelings of loneliness and insecurity, as they perceived that they were not as visible to the nursing staff, thus getting less visits. Emotions such as anger were expressed as patients sometimes felt insignificant, comparing unfavourably with other patients due to the perceived stigma of their infection. Some individuals also missed contact with fellow patients. However, some patients enjoyed the experience of the side room as it enabled privacy and control of activities in the room, such as watching television and listening to the radio without headphones.

Meers *et al.* (1997) state that there is a lack of experimental evidence surrounding the need for isolation with patients who are known to have an infection, but that the physical barrier of a single room reminds staff to apply UICPs.

Conclusion

This chapter has attempted to explain some of the salient points pertaining to tissue viability in the trauma patient. Areas examined included an overview of the physiology of wound healing, wound assessment and management, risk assessment, infection control and infections associated with traumatic injuries.

A team approach is a fundamental requirement when addressing a patient's treatment and care needs in the complex area of tissue viability. Interprofessional collaboration is the basis upon which decisions should be made in the pursuit of excellence.

References

Alexander, C. and Marsh, L. (1992) Creating the optimum environment for pressure area care. *British Journal of Nursing*, **151**, 751–57.

Alvarez, O. (1988) Moist environment for healing: matching the dressing to the wound. *Ostomy/Wound Management*, 64-83.

Appleton, G. and Leaper, D. J. (1992) The infected wound. *Hospital Update*, **18**(3), 189–198.

Audit Commission Review (1991) *The Virtues of Patients: Making the Best of Ward Nursing Resources*. The Audit Commission for Local Authorities and the National Health Service in England and Wales.

Ayliffe, G. A. B., Babb, J. R., Taylor, L. *et al.* (1978) A test for hygienic hand disinfection. *Journal of Clinical Pathology*, **31**, 923.

Baker, H. (1989) *Clinical Dermatology*. Baillière Tindall.

Bale, S. and Jones, V. (1997). *Wound Care Nursing*. Baillière Tindall.

Barratt, E. (1987). Putting risk calculators in their place. *Nursing Times*, **83**(6), 65–70.

Benbow, M. (1995) Parameters of wound assessment. *British Journal of Nursing*, **4**(11), 647–651.

Bennett, G. (1992) Medical undergraduate teaching in chronic wound care (a survey). *Journal of Tissue Viability*, **2**(2), 50–51.

Bergstrom, N., Braden, B. and Languzza, H. (1987) The Braden Scale for predicting pressure risk. *Nursing Research*, **36**(4), 205–210.

Birchall, L. (1987) Making sense of pressure sore risk calculators. *Nursing Times*, **89**(18), 34–37.

Bowler, I. C. J. (1997) Is control of methicillin resistant staphylococcus aureus justified? *Quarterly Journal of Medicine*, **90**, 243–246.

British Society for Antimicrobial Chemotherapy (1998). Combined working party report: revised guidelines for the control of methicillin resistant staphylococcus aureus infection in hospitals. *Journal of Hospital Infection*, **39**, 253–290.

Centre for Disease Control (1987) Recommendations for prevention of HIV transmission in healthcare settings. *Morbidity and Mortality Weekly Report*, **36**, 28.

Cooper, R. and Lawrence, J. C. (1996) The prevalence of bacteria and implications for infection control. *Journal of Wound Care*, **5**(6), 291–295.

Cruse, P. (1986) Surgical infection: incisional wounds. In *Hospital Infections* (J. V. Bennett and P. S. Brachman, eds). Little Brown.

Cutting, K. F. and Harding K. G. (1994) Criteria for identifying wound infection *Journal of Wound Care*, **3**(2), 198–201.

Cuzzell, J. Z. (1988) The new RYB colour code. *American Journal of Nursing*, **88**, 1342–1346.

Dealey, C. (1993). Pressure sores: the result of bad nursing? *British Journal of Nursing*, **1**(15), 748.

Dealey, C. (1994a) *The Care of Wounds*. Oxford: Blackwell Scientific.

Dealey, C. (1994b) Monitoring the pressure sore problems in a teaching hospital. *Journal of Advanced Nursing*, **20**, 652–659.

Dealey, C. (1997) *Managing Pressure Sore Prevention*. Mark Allen.

Department of Health (1992) *The Health of the Nation*. London: HMSO.

Englstein, W. H. (1985) Experiences with biosynthetic dressings. *Journal of American Academy of Dermatology*, **12**, 434–440.

Field, F. K. and Kerstein, M. D. (1994) An overview of wound healing in a moist environment. *American Journal of Surgery*, **16**(7), 2–6.

Flanagan, M. (1993) Pressure sore risk assessment scales. *Journal of Wound Care*, **2**(3), 162–167.

Flanagan, M. (1995) Who is at risk of a pressure sore? *Professional Nurse*, **10**(5), 305–305.

Flanagan, M. (1997) A practical framework for wound assessment. *British Journal of Nursing*, **5**(22), 1391–1397.

Fox, P. and Delve, M. (1994) Equipped to care. *Nursing Times*, **90**(30), 46–47.

Gebhardt, K. (1995) What causes pressure sores? *Nursing Standard*, **9**(31), 48–51.

Gilchrist, B. (1997) Should iodine be considered in wound management? *Journal of Wound Care*, **6**(3), 148–150.

Goldheim, P. D. (1993) An appraisal of povodine iodine in wound healing. *Post-graduate Medical Journal*, **69**, 597–610.

Goris, R. J. A. and Draaisma, J. (1982) Causes of death after blunt trauma. *Journal of Trauma*, **22**, 141–146; cited in R. Coombes and R. H. Fitzgerald Jr. (eds) (1989). *Infection in the Orthopaedic Patient*. Butterworth.

Gould, D. (1992) Teaching students about pressure sores. *Nursing Standard*, **6**(26) 28–31.

Gray, B. L. (1996) Developing a model for clinical practice. *Journal of Wound Care*, **5**(9), 428–432.

Griffiths, G. (1989) Changing patterns of microbial disease. In *Applied Microbiology*. Scutari Press.

Hamilton, F. (1992) An analysis of the literature pertaining to pressure sore risk assessment scales. *Journal of Clinical Nursing*, **1**, 185–193.

Harding, K. (1992) Team effort. *Journal of Wound Care*, **1**(2), 5.

Hughes, S. P. F., Nixon, J. and Dash, C. H. (1981) Cephalexin in chronic osteomyelitis. *J. R. Coll. Surgery*, **26**, 335–339; cited in S. P. F. Hughes and R. H. Fitzgerald Jr. (eds) (1986). *Musculoskeletal Infections*. Yearbook.

Hunt, J. (1993) Application of a pressure area risk calculator in an intensive care unit. *Intensive and Critical Care Nursing*, **1**, 1–16.

Kelly, J. (1994) The aetiology of pressure sores. *Journal of Tissue Viability*, **4**(3), 77–78.

Kinnard, P. (1985) Diagnosis of acute bone infection. In *Current Concepts of Infection in Orthopaedic Surgery* (H. K. Uhthoff, ed.). Springer-Verlag.

Kloth, L., McCulloch, J. and Feeder, J. (1990) Wound healing: alternatives in management; cited in F. A. Davis (1997). The management of infected wounds. *Professional Nurse*, **12**(12), S8–S11.

Knowles, H. E. (1993) The experience of infectious patients in isolation, *Nursing Times*, **89**(30), 53–56.

Lowthian, P. (1987) The practical assessment of pressure sore risk. *Care Science Practitioner*, **5**(4) 3–7.

Marieb, E. N. (1989) *Human Anatomy and Physiology*. Benjamin Cummings.

Meers, P., McPherson, M. and Sedgewick, J. (1997) *Infection Control in Healthcare, 2nd edn*. Stanley Thornes Ltd, pp. 188–195.

Morison, M., Moffatt, L., Bridel-Nixon, J. and Bale, S. (1997) *Nursing Management of Chronic Wounds*. Mosby.

Norton, D., McLaren, R. and Exton-Smith, A. N. (1975) An investigation of geriatric nursing problems in hospital. *National Corporation for the Care of Old People*. Churchill.

Palastanga, N., Field, D. and Soames, R. (1998) *Anatomy and Human Movement* (3rd edn). Butterworth-Heinemann

Pritchard, V. (1986) Calculating the risk. *Nursing Times*, **82**(8), 59–61.

Reid, J. and Morison, M. (1994) Towards a consensus: a classification of pressure sores. *Journal of Wound Care*, **3**(3), 157–160.

Sawyer, R. G. and Pruett, T. L. (1994) Wound infections. *Surgical Clinics of North America*, **74**(3), 519–534.

Septimus, E. and Musher, D. (1979) Osteomyelitis: recent clinical and laboratory aspects. *Orthopaedic Clinics in North America*, **10**, 247; cited in Uhthoff, H. K. (ed) (1985) *Current Concepts of Infection in Orthopaedic Surgery*. Springer-Verlag.

Sutton, J. and Wallace, W. (1990) Pressure sore: the views and practices of senior hospital doctors. *Care Science Practice*, **8**(3), 115–118.

Thomas, S. (1990) *Wound Management and Dressings*. The Pharmaceutical Press.

Thomas, S. (1997) A guide to dressing selection. *Journal of Wound Care*, **6**(10), 479–482.

Thomas, S., Jones, M., Schulter, S. and Jones, S. (1996) Using larvae in modern wound management. *Journal of Wound Care*, **5**(1), 60–69.

Thomson, P. D. (1995). Wound microbiology. *Wounds*, **7**(2), 58–61.

Tingle, J. (1992) Some legal issues in wound management. *Nursing Standard*, **6**(34), Supplement on Tissue Viability.

Turner, T. D. (1982) Which dressing and why? *Nursing Times*, **78**(29), Supple., 1–3.

UKCC (1992) *Code of Professional Conduct, United Kingdom Central Council for Nursing, Midwifery and Health Visiting, 3rd edn*. UKCC.

Waterlow, J. (1985) A risk assessment card. *Nursing Times*, **81**(48), 49–55.

Waterlow, J. (1988) Prevention is cheaper than cure. *Nursing Times*, **84**(25), 69–70.

Wilson, J. and Breedon, P. (1990) Universal Precautions. *Nursing Times*, **86**(37), 67–70.

Winter, G. (1962) Formation of the scab and the rate of epithelialisation of superficial wounds in the skin of the domestic pig. *Nature*, **193**, 293–294.

21

Elimination

Catherine Evans

Introduction

Elimination via the gastrointestinal (GI) and urinary systems, along with respiration, is essential to remove the waste products of metabolism and digestion from the body, prevent disturbance of fluid and electrolyte balance and enable body systems to continue to function effectively (Marieb, 1998). It is a function that most people take for granted as a normal activity of daily living and do not think about a great deal. It is also a very personal and private matter for the majority of people and is therefore not often discussed.

The aim of this chapter is to describe how normal urinary and GI function are disrupted by injury. Discussion will include how the nurse uses assessment to identify current and potential problems relating to injury and how these are managed in the short and long term. As well as the physical impact of injury on elimination, the loss of independence and the reliance on others to maintain this function causes a great deal of anxiety and embarrassment for many patients. The nurse must recognize this and acknowledge the patient's worries while at the same time working with him or her to manage the problem, assisting a return to independence as quickly as possible.

Assessment

As part of the initial assessment on admission it is important to define the 'normal' or pre-injury elimination habits of individuals, including any recent changes such as pain on micturition, altered frequency or odour, and altered bowel habit. Are there any underlying urinary tract or GI disorders or infections, renal disorders or other disease such as diabetes that may affect urinary function? Is the patient constipated? Do they take aperients at home and are these effective? Are they taking any medication which may affect urine output (e.g. diuretics, anticholinergics) or bowel function (e.g. opiate analgesics)? Do they normally experience any urinary incontinence – if so, what type and how is this managed at home? Assess their diet and fluid intake, especially fluid balance – do they appear malnourished or dehydrated? A sample of urine is obtained on admission to provide a baseline screening tool. Any abnormal odour or appearance is noted and a dipstick test, such as Ames Multistix, performed. A normal fresh random urine sample will be clear with little odour. It will have a pH of 4.5–8.0 and contain no glucose, detectable protein or blood. If the sample tests positive for blood, protein, nitrites or leukocytes this is suggestive of a urinary tract infection (UTI), and a sample should be sent for microscopy, culture and sensitivity (Wells, 1997). However, there are many medical conditions that give rise to abnormal urinary constituents and these should not be ignored.

Assessment also includes the presenting condition to ascertain post-injury function. What injuries are present and what impact have they had or are they likely to have on elimination? Associated problems such as altered level of consciousness, limited mobility, changes in fluid and dietary intake, medication (analgesia, anaesthetics (Wynd *et al.*, 1996)) all affect elimination and must be considered.

Identification and management of problems relating to injury

Elimination can become a major problem for any individual post-injury; care must be taken to view the person as a whole and to take into account all the factors involved. Pain, anxiety and limited mobility can all contribute to alteration in elimination (Roper *et al.*, 1996), as well as more obvious complications such as trauma to the urinary tract itself or spinal cord injury affecting control of bladder emptying. If being rolled on and off a bedpan following a fractured neck of femur is a painful and traumatic experience, the individual may avoid drinking in an effort to decrease urine output or may even lie in a wet bed, as from their point of view it is preferable to being moved. It is therefore vital that pain is well managed and analgesia effective. Reassurance and support are also very important if the nurse is to gain the trust of the injured person, and an explanation of how individuals are to be moved and how they can help in the process may make them feel safer. Restricted mobility and positioning can also be a major hindrance; a man on flat bedrest may find it virtually impossible to pass urine lying on his back. Being logrolled to one side may help, but then he must attempt to pass urine in front of four nurses! Positioning, privacy and other issues surrounding this will be discussed later.

Pelvic fractures

Because of the anatomical position of the bladder and intestine, both are susceptible to injury if the pelvis is fractured and displaced. Lower UTI is one of the most common complications of pelvic fracture (Simpson-Meyer, 1989; Hefti, 1995). The most common injuries are rupture of the bladder, either puncture by bone fragments or due to sudden increase in bladder pressure, and stretching, partial or complete rupture of the urethra (Simpson-Meyer, 1989; McRae, 1989). Urethral injuries are more common in males than females (Simpson-Meyer, 1989). Signs of urinary tract injury include blood at the urinary meatus, haematuria, suprapubic pain, inability to pass urine and abrasions, lacerations or haematomas on flanks, genital or suprapubic areas (Genge, 1986; McRae, 1989). If these signs are present, a urethral catheter should not be passed until a urethrogram or cystography has been performed to determine injury (Simpson-Meyer, 1989; Dorozinsky, 1992). Bladder or urethral injury may need surgical repair and/or the insertion of a suprapubic catheter to allow healing (McRae, 1989; Hefti, 1995; Genge, 1989).

Tears to the rectum or small bowel may occur with open pelvic fractures. Abdominal rigidity or distension and absence of bowel sounds are signs of bowel involvement. The implications are very serious with risk of severe, life-threatening infection. Exploration and irrigation of the area and formation of a diverting colostomy (usually a loop colostomy) are essential (Genge, 1989; McRae, 1989; Brenneman *et al.*, 1997). Trauma patients rarely have pre-counselling and optimal siting of their stoma, as formation is invariably carried out during emergency surgery. However, the stoma is often a temporary measure to allow the bowel to heal and is likely to be reversed a few months later. As with all stoma patients, psychological support and teaching will be required in how to manage the stoma independently (Black, 1998); the extent of this will obviously depend on other injuries and physical limitations. Early liaison with a stoma care nurse who can provide support, information and advice will be beneficial to both the patient and family.

Spinal cord injury

Bladder emptying and defaecation are controlled by both autonomic and voluntary nerve impulses. When the bladder contains about 200–300 ml of urine, impulses are sent from stretch receptors in the bladder wall along afferent nerve fibres to the sacral region of the spinal cord. This causes a reflex response to the bladder from cord segments S2 and S3 along the cauda equina, resulting in contraction of the detrusor muscle and relaxation of the internal sphincter. In adults the afferent impulses also go to the cerebral cortex producing awareness of a full bladder and the need to urinate. Voluntary impulses return to the sacral centres allowing relaxation of the external sphincters and the voiding of urine (Marieb, 1998; McRae, 1989).

The defaecation reflex works in a similar way – movement of the faeces into the rectum causes distension and stimulation of stretch receptors. The sigmoid colon and rectum contract, and the internal anal sphincter relaxes. As with the urinary system, the external anal sphincter is under voluntary control (Marieb, 1998). As both these functions are under nervous control they will obviously be affected by spinal cord injury. Following acute spinal cord injury a period of spinal shock occurs resulting in the suppression of reflexes controlled by segments below the site of injury and flaccid paralysis occurs (Halm, 1990). This is due to disruption of impulses from higher centres of the brain and usually lasts 1–6 weeks, with gradual recovery of reflexes. During spinal shock the bladder loses all tonicity, and urinary retention with overflow occurs as it is unable to empty spontaneously (Nolan, 1994). In this situation catheterization is essential to prevent urinary stasis and over-distension. Urinary stasis due to retention or incomplete emptying of the bladder increases the risk of UTI and renal or bladder stones, especially when coupled with hypercalciuria and phosphaturia associated with prolonged immobilization (Young *et al.*, 1995). Perhaps more seriously, the urine may back up into the ureters and the renal pelvis causing renal infection and damage (Wynd *et al.*, 1996). Over-distension of the bladder can lead to breaking of the neuromuscular bridges between the fibres of the bladder, which are required for contraction. These may never recover and loss of contractility of the bladder may result (Dalton, 1993).

Long-term management depends on the level of cord injury; if the lesion does not affect the reflex arc of micturition (S2–S4) the bladder will contract in response to stimulation of stretch receptors, but the patient will have no voluntary control or sensation. In this case the bladder can be trained as part of rehabilitation. If the sacral arc is destroyed by lower motor neuron injury, the bladder does not contract, which leads to over-distension and overflow incontinence. Training of the bladder in this situation is not possible (Halm, 1990). It is possible to achieve long-term management of a non-contractile bladder by using intermittent catheterization. This should be introduced as early as possible, initially by nurses (Grundy *et al.*, 1986; Nolan, 1994), but eventually it should be performed by the patient – depending on level

of injury (Grundy *et al.*, 1986) – family or carer.

In the case of defaecation, as with urinary function, the level of injury determines outcome. Reflexic bowel occurs as a result of spinal cord injury (SCI) above the sacral arc (T12). The defaecation reflex remains, but the individual has no sensation to control defaecation and the external anal sphincter is spastic. During the period of spinal shock the rectum should be checked daily and any impaction removed using either suppositories or mild enemas (Halm, 1990). After spinal shock subsides and bowel function returns, a bowel programme should be commenced using stool softeners and bulk-forming agents (Nolan, 1994). Training of the bowel by the use of reflex stimulation techniques and increasing intra-abdominal pressure is possible (Halm, 1990). In lower motor neuron damage, where the sacral arc is disrupted, the defaecation reflex is destroyed and flaccid paralysis of the external sphincter occurs; the patient cannot pass formed stools but may experience incontinence of soft stool due to flaccid anal sphincter. There is a high risk of bowel impaction for patients with SCI (Halm, 1990) and regular manual evacuation may be required for those with poor anal tone (Nolan, 1994).

Head injury

Head-injured patients generally experience elimination problems due to a decreased level of consciousness or awareness. Awareness of the need to void or defaecate, awareness of socially acceptable behaviour, or the physical skills required to use a toilet, may be lost. Patients who are confused or disorientated may be unable to find the lavatory, especially at night (Roper *et al.*, 1996) and require assistance and reassurance. Fluid intake and output should be monitored as urine output may be altered by disturbances in antidiuretic hormone (ADH) secretion from the posterior pituitary lobe. This may cause diabetes insipidus or the syndrome of inappropriate secretion of ADH (SIADH), both of which put the patient at risk of fluid and electrolyte imbalance.

Restricted mobility and positioning

The most effective positions for bladder emptying are standing or sitting as, when supine, intra-abdominal pressure is reduced due to weakened abdominal muscles, restricted movement of the diaphragm and incomplete relaxation of the pelvic floor (Young *et al.*, 1995). This may result in an inability to pass urine or incomplete emptying. In females, gravity drains all urine from the urethra, but in males, voluntary contractions of the bulbocavernosus muscle expel the last drops (Carola *et al.*, 1992).

The ideal situation would be for an individual to get to the lavatory, either independently or with assistance, and maintain normal function as far as possible, using adaptive equipment such as a raised toilet seat or rails (Erdner and Kraftfine, 1992). This is often impossible due to the patient's injuries, so alternatives are therefore needed. If the individual is able to get out of bed they are encouraged to use a commode, thus promoting independence, mobility and better positioning. Using a commode should cause no more cardiovascular stress than using a bedpan (Roper *et al.*, 1996). However, it may take more effort and it may be more painful than using a bedpan, so this must be taken into account. For example, a patient with an unstable ankle fracture who is on bedrest may prefer to get out to the commode if the ankle can be kept safely elevated. However, in other situations, such as unstable pelvic or spinal injury, it is obvious that positioning would be very difficult and in spinal injury the level and stability of injury will determine whether the use of a bedpan is safe. For male patients, standing to pass urine is ideal if safety and mobility allows, but they may require physical support. The patient is encouraged to maintain normal function as far as possible, which requires the nurse to ensure that adequate analgesia, explanation, reassurance and assistance are given so that the patient feels safe and comfortable.

Constipation

By far the most common bowel associated problem experienced by trauma patients is constipation, defined as difficult and/or infrequent defaecation (Norton, 1996). Constipation may be due to disorders of the GI tract itself or may occur because of many other predisposing factors, the most common resulting from diet and fluid intake, medications, illness, reduced mobility, environmental and psychological factors. A low-fibre diet and inadequate hydration result in hard, dry stools that are difficult to pass. Changes in dietary patterns often occur as a result of hospitalization and surgery. Many medications are linked with constipation, but analgesics, particularly opiates, are the most common. Opiates cause hypersegmentation; the churning of food brings it repeatedly into contact with the intestinal mucosa so that nutrients and fluid are absorbed but no forward propulsion occurs, resulting in dry impacted faeces. Other significant, commonly used drugs causing constipation include antiparkinsonian drugs, calcium channel blockers, iron preparations and anticholinergics (Nazarko, 1996). Walking and moving stimulate peristalsis in the colon, therefore decreased mobility can cause constipation. An unwell or generally weak individual may be unable to generate enough abdominal effort to stimulate a defaecation reflex (Norton, 1996). As well as generalized decrease in mobility, diet and fluid intake associated with illness, certain conditions can cause constipation, for example neurological disease, depression and hypothyroidism (Nazarko, 1996). Lack of privacy, discomfort and embarrassment may cause the patient to ignore the urge to defaecate, leading to further absorption of fluid from the stool, making it harder to pass.

All these factors are relevant to trauma patients, and constipation is potentially a very real problem for many people admitted to hospital post-injury. Early management is essential and begins on admission with assessment of normal bowel function. Many factors are present in combination (e.g. altered diet, decreased fluid intake, reduced mobility, analgesia, lack of privacy, difficulty with positioning) and must be taken into account during the patient assessment. Patient involvement and education are important, so discussion regarding this potential problem should take place at an appropriate time. Intervention starts immediately; a protocol for bowel management has been developed (Gray and Nunn, 1996) within which four separate regimens can be followed – an individualized approach.

These groups are:

- patients on successful laxative therapy on admission
- patients over 70 years of age
- patients under 70 years of age
- patients not responding to the above.

These guidelines are used as an adjunct to

inform clinical judgement. An understanding of the causes of constipation, the use of non-drug therapy and the mechanism of action of laxative drugs is essential if nurses are to use the protocol effectively. The guidelines list drugs known to cause constipation, the laxatives in use, their mechanism of action and any side effects or contraindications.

Incontinence

Urinary incontinence is a relatively common problem for some patients following trauma. A large proportion of patients are aged over 70 and the majority will have their mobility limited; most will also have had surgery under a general or spinal anaesthetic. Many older people may experience a degree of incontinence (Royle and Walsh, 1992). In females this is often stress incontinence due to weakened pelvic floor muscles, while in males dribbling incontinence due to damage or degeneration of the urethral sphincter as the result of an enlarged prostate gland may occur. Pre-existing incontinence, especially urge incontinence, is exacerbated greatly by limited mobility and inability to reach the lavatory in time. Urinary incontinence among trauma patients is often short term or temporary and causative factors include decreased level of consciousness, disorientation, confusion (due to anaesthetic, analgesia, infection or hospitalization) and decreased mobility.

In the first instance management should involve regular offers of opportunities to use the lavatory, commode, bedpan or urinal and/ or the use of pads and pants or sheath catheters in males (Unsworth and Rowell, 1994). Regular inspection of skin integrity is essential and the use of barrier creams may be helpful. As well as the risk of maceration and abrasion to the skin during prolonged exposure to moisture (Kemp 1994), there are other problems associated with incontinence including distress and discomfort for the individual, risk of wound infection or breakdown and the possibility that the person may reduce fluid intake in an attempt to decrease urine output. Nevertheless, it is generally accepted that because of the inherent risks (Table 21.1), catheterization should be used in the management of urinary incontinence only as a last resort (Winson, 1997), and it is usually only indicated if there is a high risk of

impaired skin integrity, wound infection or maceration, or extreme discomfort. It should be viewed as a temporary measure and the catheter removed as soon as possible. Other indications for catheterization include the need for accurate fluid balance monitoring in haemodynamically unstable patients and, as already mentioned, urinary retention.

Table 21.1   Risks associated with catheterization

Infection
Trauma to urethra
Trauma to bladder
Blockage
Encrustation
Chemical allergy
Strictures
Bypassing of urine

The nurse should be aware of these risks and use research-based practice to minimize them (Table 21.2). The most common complication of catheterization is infection; UTI accounts for 30–40% of hospital-acquired infection and 10–20% of catheterized patients develop bacteriuria (Ward *et al.*, 1997).

Table 21.2   Recommendations for catheter care (After de Courcey-Ireland 1993; Getliffe 1994; MacKenzie and Webb 1995; Wilson and Coates 1996; Ward *et al.* 1997; Winson 1997; Lowthian 1998; Stewart 1998; Winn 1998; Penfold 1999)

Insertion

Antiseptic handwash before and after procedure
Clean meatal area with sterile water or saline
Aseptic technique for insertion
Sterile, water-soluble lubricant or anaesthetic gel for males and females
Appropriate choice of catheter

Care following insertion

Universal precautions and good handwashing technique
Meatal hygiene with soap and water
Maintain closed drainage system – use sample ports if necessary
Decontaminate drainage outlet with alcohol or chlorhexidine spray before and after emptying
Bladder washout (e.g. Suby-G) only if clinically indicated
Use of stands for drainage bag
Remove as soon as possible

Privacy and dignity

Elimination is an intensely private and personal matter for the majority of people, and the idea of using a commode or bedpan with only a curtain as separation from everyone else in the room is not a pleasant idea. Due to the high dependency and unpredictable nature of trauma admissions it is not always possible to ensure single-sex rooms, and this may cause further anxiety. For some people, even to talk about bowel function is embarrassing, so they are unlikely to express problems until the situation becomes unbearable. Wherever possible, patients should be wheeled out to a lavatory and given the privacy and time they need. Anxieties need to be recognized and addressed, and patients should be encouraged not to ignore the urge to defaecate or pass urine. Something as simple as turning on a radio or using a deodorant spray may make them less embarrassed about noises and smells, enabling the use of a commode or bedpan to become slightly more bearable. It is important that nursing staff acknowledge and understand the loss of dignity experienced by patients who need assistance to enable them to maintain normal bowel and bladder function.

The importance of good communication cannot be emphasized enough. It provides the basis for patient education regarding possible problems and management, empowering them to become involved in their own care and to retain some control in what can only be described as difficult and unexpected circumstances.

References

Black, P. (1998) Colostomy. *Professional Nurse*, **13**(12), 851–857.

Brenneman, F. D., Katyal, D., Boulanger, B. R. *et al.* (1997) Long term outcomes in open pelvic fractures. *Journal of Trauma*, **42**(5), 773–777.

Carola, R., Harley, J. and Noback, C. (1992) The urinary system. In *Human Anatomy and Physiology* (R. Carola, J. Harley and C. Noback, eds.) McGraw-Hill.

Dalton, J. R. (1993) Urologic management of the patient with a spinal cord injury. *Trauma Quarterly*, **9**(2) 72–81.

deCourcey-Ireland, K. (1993) An issue of sensitivity: use of anaesthetic gel in catheterising females. *Professional Nurse*, **8**(11), 738–742.

Dorozinsky, D. (1992) Abdominal and genitourinary injury. In *A Comprehensive Curriculum for Trauma Nursing* (E. Bayley and S. Turcke, eds). Jones and Bartlett.

Erdner, M. and Kraftfine, C. (1992) Rehabilitation. In *A Comprehensive Curriculum for Trauma Nursing* (E. Bayley and S. Turcke, eds). Jones and Bartlett.

Genge, M. L. (1989) Orthopaedic trauma: pelvic fractures. *Orthopaedic Nursing*, **5**(1), 11–19.

Getliffe, K. A. (1994) The use of bladder washouts to reduce urinary catheter encrustation. *British Journal of Urology*, **73**, 696–700.

Gray, B. and Nunn, R. (1996) *Protocol for Bowel Management* (unpublished) Trauma Service, Oxford Radcliffe Hospital NHS Trust.

Grundy, D., Russell, J. and Swain, A. (1986) ABC of spinal cord injury. *British Medical Journal*.

Halm, M. A. (1990) Elimination concerns with acute spinal cord injury: assessment and nursing interventions. *Critical Care Nursing Clinics of North America*, **2**(3), 385–398.

Hefti, D. (1995). Complications of trauma: the nurse's role in prevention. *Orthopaedic Nursing*, **14**(6), 9–16.

Kemp, M. (1994) Protecting the skin from moisture and associated irritants. *Journal of Gerontological Nursing*, **19**(2), 8–14.

Lowthian, P. (1998) The dangers of long term catheter drainage. *British Journal of Nursing*, **7**(7), 366–379.

MacKenzie, M. and Webb, N. (1995) Gynopia in nursing practice: the case of urethral catheterisation. *Journal of Clinical Nursing*, **4**, 221–226.

Marieb, E. (1998) *Human Anatomy and Physiology*. Benjamin Cummings.

McRae, R. (1989) *Practical Fracture Treatment*. Churchill Livingstone.

Nazarko, L. (1996) Preventing constipation in older people. *Professional Nurse*, **11**(12), 816–818.

Nolan, S. (1994) Current trends in the management of acute spinal cord injury. *Critical Care Nursing Quarterly*, **17**(1), 64–78.

Norton, C. (1996) The causes and nursing management of constipation. *British Journal of Nursing*, **5**(20), 1252–1258.

Penfold, P. (1999) UTI in patients with urethral catheters: an audit tool. *British Journal of Nursing*, **8**(6), 362–374.

Roper, N., Logan, W. and Tierney, A. (1996) Eliminating. In *The Elements of Nursing* (Roper, N., Logan, W. and Tierney, A. eds.). Churchill Livingstone.

Royle, J. and Walsh, M. (1992) *Watson's Medical-Surgical Nursing and Related Physiology*. Baillière Tindall.

Simpson-Meyer, P. S. (1989) Urologic complications associated with pelvic fractures. *Orthopaedic Nursing*, **8**(4), 41–44, 48.

Stewart, E. (1998) Urinary catheters: selection, maintenance and nursing care. *British Journal of Nursing*, **7**(1), 1152–1161.

Unsworth, J. and Rowell, R. (1994) Containing incontinence in males: an extra dimension. *British Journal of Nursing*, **3**(18), 936, 938–940.

Ward, V., Wilson, J. and Taylor, L. (1997) *Prevention of Hospital Infection: Clinical Guidelines – A supplement to Hospital Acquired Infection: Surveillance, Policies and Practice*, PHLS; cited in Stewart, E. (1998) Urinary catheters: selection, maintenance and nursing care. *British Journal of Nursing*, **7**(1), 1152–1161.

Wells, M. (1997) Urinalysis. *Professional Nurse*, **13**(2), 11–13.

Wilson, M. and Coates, D. (1996) Infection control and urinary drainage bags. *Professional Nurse*, **11**(4), 248–252.

Winn, C. (1998) Complications with urinary catheters. *Professional Nurse*, **13**(5), 7–10.

Winson, L. (1997) Catheterisation: a need for improved patient management. *British Journal of Nursing*, **6**(21), 1229–1252.

Wynd, C. A., Wallace, M. and Smith, K. M. (1996) Factors influencing postoperative urinary retention following orthopaedic surgical procedures. *Orthopaedic Nursing*, **15**(1), 43–50.

Young, M., O'Young, B. J. and McFarland, E. G. (1995) Rehabilitation of the orthopaedic trauma patient: general principles. *Physical Medicine and Rehabilitation: State of the Art Reviews*, **9**(1), 185–201.

22

Hygiene and mouth care

Helen Barnett and Jillian Heath

HYGIENE

'Leaving a patient unwashed was interfering injuriously with the natural process of health just as effectively as if she were to give the patient poison.' (Nightingale, 1859).

Introduction

The term hygiene is defined by the Wainwright (1992) as 'the science of health and the study of ways of preserving it, particularly by promoting cleanliness'. McLeod (1984) identifies hygiene as the 'principles and practice of health and cleanliness'. Therefore it can be argued that health and hygiene are inextricably linked and in the healthy individual are in equilibrium. If the balance of the equilibrium is altered by poor health status one can assume that the ability of the individual to meet their own hygiene needs will also be compromised.

In the wake of injury some patients will require emergency admission to hospital for treatment. Patients have no time to plan or prepare for hospitalization and this can be a bewildering and frightening experience if not handled sensitively and with care. Immediately post-injury, patients can be acutely ill requiring skilled medical, physiotherapy and nursing intervention. They will therefore require assistance with their activities of daily living as defined by Roper *et al.* (1981) in both the acute and rehabilitative phase.

This chapter aims to highlight the particular

challenges that injured people face with regard to maintaining their own skin and oral hygiene. Current trends and research relating to skin and oral hygiene will be discussed, together with other relevant practice issues. Topics covered include:

- The role of the nurse in assisting patients with their hygiene.
- Skin care.
- Individuality, dignity and respect.
- Oral hygiene.

The role of the nurse

The nurse may be required to assume total responsibility for a patient's hygiene requirements if they are unconscious or have multiple injuries. For those patients less seriously injured the nurse should work in partnership with the patient to encourage them to share this responsibility, thereby encouraging independence and rehabilitation. Hall and Wilson-Barnett, cited in McMahon and Buckledee (1992), suggest that the 'provision of hygiene and comfort is clearly part of nursing'. It can be argued that not only is it part of nursing, but that the provision of hygiene can be defined solely as the nurse's responsibility (in conjunction with the patient), whereas other aspects of patient care have multidisciplinary implications and accountability. The exception to this is the occupational therapist whose input relates in the main to assessment (rather than ongoing care), together with the provision of specialized equipment. The occupational therapist does have some input into assisting the patient with their hygiene needs by provision of equipment to assist the process, but does not assume total responsibility.

Wolf (1988) agrees that hygiene is the nurses' domain but goes further, stating that 'nurses own the hygienic care of their patients'. This somewhat exclusive approach also fails to accommodate the concept of patient participation. Saunders, cited in Cahill (1996), suggests that patient participation centres around the client becoming actively involved in 'performing clinical or daily living skills, or partaking in decision making skills'.

The concept of nurse 'ownership' in relation to their patients is a dangerous one. It can lead to paternalistic, ritualistic care which increases patient dependence, resulting in a loss of individuality, dignity and respect. The exception to this of course is when the patient is unconscious or so severely injured that they cannot actively participate in such care.

Bathing patients has long been viewed as a ritualistic daily task (Armstrong-Esther, 1981; Chapman, 1983; Gooch, 1987; Walsh and Ford, 1989; Spiller, 1992; Wolf, 1993; Jones, 1995), with nurses providing hygiene care as a ritual, rather than recognizing the therapeutic patient value, according to Barsevick and Llewellyn (1982). This is reflected throughout most hospital wards where more staff are assigned to an early shift than a late shift. It appears to be the norm for patients to have a wash or bath in the morning when there are more staff available to assist with hygiene needs. Later in the day when admissions and postoperative patients tend to be prioritized, hygiene may become a secondary consideration. This may not appear ideal when nurses are expected to provide individualized patient care, but, it is frequently the reality. Patients may find it frustrating that they cannot bathe independently and at a time which suits them. Jenkins and Price (1996) support the idea of 'patients and lay carers playing an active part in care negotiation'. This should be encouraged while the patient is in hospital as it lays down the foundations for any assistance which may be required at home following discharge. It may also highlight issues which the lay carer would otherwise not have encountered, enabling staff to address any problems during the course of discharge planning.

Spiller (1992) suggests that if 'patients are to be given greater choice as to when they bath, staffing levels may have to be redistributed'. Many patients prefer to wash or bath in the morning. For the injured patient, even activities as simple as washing and dressing can be strenuous and tiring – they may have the energy necessary to accomplish some of these tasks for themselves in the morning, but by the evening, following a day of therapy and treatment, many patients prefer just to rest.

Webster *et al.* (1988) conducted a small research study looking at the opinions of patients and nurses regarding bathing. The results showed that nurses and patients had divided opinions, with nurses placing greater importance on bathing than patients. Of the patients, 86% felt that nurses had far more important things to do than bath patients. Of the nurses, 91% felt bathing patients was important. **Wilson (1986) states that 'a bedbath facilitates listening and enables the nurse to pick up cues to a patient's anxieties and fears**. It provides the time and opportunity for the nurse to offer support and encouragement when difficult situations have to be confronted, solutions sought and decisions made'. Armstrong-Esther (1981) agrees with Wilson that the bedbath provides an ideal opportunity to 'improve communication through informal conversation'. The study by Webster *et al.* (1988) confirms that bathing a patient provides an ideal opportunity for nurses to engage in conversation. However, nurses placed a higher value on this than did patients. Patients 'merely agree that there is the existence of an opportunity' which is essentially placing a different emphasis on the importance of it.

The trauma patient has specific requirements in order to be able to meet their own hygiene needs, as they are often unable to wash and dress themselves independently. Showering and bathing are frequently impossible due to prolonged bedrest. Even relatively minor injuries can lead to major difficulties with washing and dressing. Nurses must be mindful of the privileged position they hold when providing intimate care to patients, and should be sensitive to patient concerns about washing personal areas of the body. Lawler (1991) raises the issue that it is embarrassing for patients to have intimate hygiene care performed by a stranger and that it is the nurse's uniform which makes it acceptable.

The nurse should ensure that she conforms to the patient's agenda and not her own when meeting hygiene needs. Seedhouse (1988), cited in McGee (1994), states that 'a broken arm is an impediment to autonomy in that it prevents the individual from carrying out certain choices'. As a nurse, one must assist the exercise of these choices, allowing them freedom to do this independently if possible. Higley (1986) maintains that if a 'healthy and safe balance of independence and dependence is maintained, then there is no loss of personal control or choice'. Vogelpohl (1996) warns of the dangers in not letting patients take risks and perform tasks independently resulting in 'caregivers contributing to loss of functional performance and dependency when they dress the person'. Sedgewick (1989) maintains that it saves time if staff make choices, whereas conversely Vogelpohl *et al.* (1996) argues that if the patient dresses himself, it 'requires less than one minute of additional caregiver time' but the benefits go beyond this. Obviously this depends on the patient's dexterity and speed and 'less than one minute' may well prove to be a conservative estimate in many instances. However, one should not underestimate the importance of allowing patients time to wash and dress themselves independently, albeit with supervision. It is more than likely that the task would be performed quicker by the nurse, but this would not contribute to promoting independence and fostering feelings of self-worth and achievement in the patient. The nurse should work in partnership with the patient, allowing them to perform the tasks which they can independently manage, the nurse assisting only with those components of care which require help.

The role of the occupational therapist

The role of the occupational therapist is to assess, plan, implement and then evaluate 'specific activities in order to help people reach their maximum level of function and independence in all aspects of daily life' (Wainwright, 1992). The occupational therapist assesses the patient's cognitive abilities as well as their physical capabilities. For example, a patient who is mildly confused may well require verbal prompting to do up the buttons on a cardigan, but can physically achieve this unaided. The occupational therapist can also provide aids and equipment to assist the patient in performing activities of daily living, such as a helping hand device to enable dropped items to be easily retrieved from the floor, a long-handled shoehorn, and a device to assist in putting on socks or stockings. Commodes can also be provided for those patients with limited mobility or no downstairs toilet. Perching stools are available for patients who cannot stand for long periods of time, so that they can sit at the sink while having a wash. The occupational therapist's assessment is a vital part of discharge planning in order to ensure a safe transition from hospital to home.

Skin care

The principal objective of skin care is to maintain the integrity of the skin and to ensure that there is no avoidable deterioration post-injury and during the recovery phase (Table 22.1). This section aims to look at normal skin and skin care. Abnormal physiological skin conditions which require specialist management are beyond the scope of this chapter.

It is well documented that 'excessive bathing has been reported to contribute to dry skin' (Armstrong-Esther, 1981; Porth and Kapke, 1983; Mairis, 1992; Frantz and Gardner, 1994; Hardy, 1996). Steinbaugh (1983) also claims that soaps which 'reduce the pH of the skin and remove natural skin oils also may be a contributing factor to dry skin'. Frantz and Gardner (1994) state that a 'soap with a documented low irritancy level' should be used to help prevent dry skin. According to Hardy (1996), the use of low irritancy level soaps may well be counterproductive as they have 'decreased cleansing ability' necessitating the use of an increased amount, thereby negating the low irritancy benefits.

Having a bedbath can prove hazardous to patients as they can end up being 'microbiologically dirtier after the bath than before' according to Greaves (1985). Nurses should be aware of these implications. If the water is not changed, 'dirty water is used to clean the skin, redistributing bacteria around the body' (Greaves, 1985). The problem is further compounded if one cloth is used to clean all areas of the body. The water then becomes 'a soup of soap and bacteria' (Greaves, 1985).

Table 22.1 Recommendations for skin care (After Porth and Kapke, 1983; Greaves, 1985; Gooch, 1987; Mairis, 1992; Sanderson and Weissler, 1992; Gould, 1994 and Skewes, 1996, 1997)

Daily baths can dry out the skin, so washing should be based on need rather than ritual

Patients should be encouraged to carry out their own hygiene needs in order to encourage independence

Limit the use of detergents, soaps and bubble bath as these can dry the skin

The choice of cleansing agents should depend on an assessment of the dryness of the skin

A cheap emollient can be used instead of soap for those patients who are elderly or have dry skin

Patients should bathe with warm to cool water, as hot water dilates superficial blood vessels and increases dryness and itching

Disposable flannels should be used where possible, but always when washing the perineum to reduce the risk of spreading bacteria from one area of the body to another Communal baths and hoists should be cleaned after each use and in accordance with local infection control policies.

Patients should be supplied with their own washbowls.

The bowl should be thoroughly washed with detergent and dried after use to reduce bacterial contamination and then stored inverted in the patient's locker

Early referral to an occupational therapist for a washing and dressing assessment is advised.

This is of importance if the patient has a wound which may subsequently become contaminated as a result of poor nursing practice. Many trauma patients have wounds (sustained at the time of the accident or due to subsequent surgical intervention) and these are particularly vulnerable to infection.

Gooch (1989) and Greaves (1985) advocate using disposable flannels, changing the water frequently and washing the perineum last. Ideally, two washbowls of different colours should be provided for each patient to reduce the risk of cross-infection. One bowl is used specifically for washing the genital and anal areas, the other used for the rest of the body, thus providing a more hygienic approach and reducing the risk of contamination. Gould (1994) highlights the bath as another source of cross-infection, and Murdoch (1990) reveals that bath hoists are also a potential source of bacterial contamination.

Hospitals should provide disposable flannels, soap, toothbrushes and paste, combs, razors, shaving foam, towels and nightwear. This is particularly important following injury, as patients have none of these personal items when they are admitted. Patients who are elderly or have relatives a long way away may also have difficulty in finding someone to bring in toiletries and nightclothes. Mairis (1994) concedes that if a patient is removed from recognizable surroundings (which may be sudden in the event of trauma, allowing little time to adjust to a new environment) and is without personal effects, then it is important to ensure dignity is maintained. Relatives and friends should be encouraged to bring in the patient's toiletries, nightwear and clothes as soon as possible. This allows the patient to have their personal belongings close to hand, enabling them to have greater control in caring and attending to their hygiene needs and allowing them dignity and respect.

'Washing patients to remove urine or faeces should be done with plain water or using a non-soda soap' advises Gooch (1987). Frequent washing of the incontinent patient with soap will dry the skin making it more prone to break down and increasing the risk of pressure sores in these vulnerable areas. Gooch (1987) claims that soap is not very effective in the removal of dried faeces and 'soap commonly used for toilet purposes is a soda soap which cannot function in a salinaceous medium such as that present in urinary incontinence'.

Handwashing facilities should be offered to the patient after using the bedpan or commode to prevent the spread of any microorganisms present on the hands. This is particularly important for bedbound patients who cannot walk independently to the lavatory to wash their hands. Rarely in practice are patients given the opportunity to wash their hands unless they specifically ask, yet one always washes one's own hands after a visit to the lavatory.

Sanderson and Weissler (1992) conducted a research study into coliform-type organisms recovered from the hands of nurses and patients in an orthopaedic hospital. The hands of both patients and nurses were found to carry coliforms from towels, clothing and other sources, including personal toilet. It is therefore important that patients should be given the opportunity to wash their hands frequently throughout the day, rather than once a day with the morning wash.

Bathing can be a pleasurable experience, providing warmth, quiet, relaxation and privacy as identified by Rader *et al.* (1996). However, often the experience in hospital is very different. The ward is noisy, the patient may be in pain, and ill-fitting curtains coupled with repeated interruptions offer little privacy. Careful consideration and forward planning can ensure washing is a more enjoyable experience, contributing positively to the patient's wellbeing.

Individuality, dignity and respect

Individuality, dignity and respect are pertinent to many aspects of nursing care. In hospital many patients conform to the 'sick role'. One manifestation of this is the wearing of night-clothes all day, despite the fact that the patient may be feeling well and sitting in a chair. Dean, cited in Sedgewick (1989), states 'it was felt that to be fully dressed is good for the morale, helps to maintain dignity, independence and status'. Patients should be encouraged to wear their own clothes during the day, as this fosters feelings of independence and wellbeing and contributes to increased self-esteem. Mairis (1994) concedes that 'self-esteem needs to be possessed and maintained in order that dignity should continue'.

For some patients it is not practical for them to be fully dressed, so it is important to encourage them to wear their own nightwear. If this is not possible, then patients should wear hospital nightwear as a last resort. If there are any colours to choose between, the patient should be asked their preference, even though as Sedgewick (1989) points out, it is often 'quicker and easier for the staff to make decisions on behalf of the individual'. Miller (1997) accedes that giving choice promotes independence and feelings of self-worth while maintaining some degree of individuality. Hospital nightwear with the words 'Hospital Property' clearly visible should be banned from use.

Levine, cited in McGee (1994), states that 'nursing care without respect dehumanises patients'. Browne (1993) believes that respect is a human right and is thus not conditional upon the approval of others. This is an important concept in the context of nursing –

mutual respect should exist between nurse and patient.

When considering hygiene needs, the issue of gender must be addressed. Nursing is a predominantly female profession, yet the ratio of male to female patients is more evenly balanced. The study of Webster *et al.* (1988) revealed that 55% of patients did not particularly object to being bathed by nurses and 73% did not feel embarrassed when being bathed. However, neither the gender of the nurse or patient were discussed. Both male and female nurses must be aware of the significance of gender and cultural issues in performing intimate hygiene care for patients. There are many women who would feel uncomfortable or refuse to be washed by a man for both personal and cultural reasons. Likewise, men may feel awkward when such needs are attended to by a female nurse. Every effort should be made to accommodate patients' preferences regarding the gender of the nurse carrying out their care, even if it requires reallocation of patients. The Royal College of Nursing (1994) is in agreement, stating that 'all patients in a mixed ward should be informed that they have the right to a nurse of the same sex'. In practice, most patients are ambivalent on this issue; however, for those patients or relatives who have expressed strong views or preferences, the necessary accommodation should be made.

Conclusion

Meeting hygiene needs is often perceived as a ritualistic and task-orientated element of care. This chapter has highlighted the need for nurses to adopt a more individualized approach when caring for their patients' hygiene requirements. Within the concept of individualized patient care is the notion of patient participation, leading to the formation of a nurse–patient partnership. This partnership consists of 'care negotiation' as identified by Jenkins and Price (1996) with both parties working towards the same end goal.

A team approach to discharge planning creates an environment of patient independence rather than dependence, resulting in increased self-esteem, dignity and respect. It enables patients to have greater confidence in their own ability to achieve, thus aiding the rehabilitation process.

MOUTH CARE

Introduction – why the need for mouth care?

'Mouth care, considered to be a part of routine nursing care, is not always performed routinely. This simple procedure, however, increases appetite, adds to the general comfort of the patient, and can prevent systemic illness' (Blarney, 1986). It is perhaps another example of nursing care that has become little more than banal, ritualistic practice (Page *et al.*, 1987). As discussed by Crosby (1989), it does appear that the healthcare professional's lack of knowledge can largely be attributed to the lack of research available concerning mouth-care procedures and products. Clearly, the more seriously ill or injured a patient is, the more reliant they will be upon the nurse for oral hygiene.

The principal objective of mouth care (Table 22.2) is to maintain the mouth in good condition; comfortable, moist and free from infection (Howarth, 1977). A dry mouth feels uncomfortable, reduces appetite and may contribute to the development of oral infection. **Oral problems can cause misery quite disproportionate to the size of the affected area, as discussed by Hilton (1980).** This can lead to poor nutrition through anorexia, dysphagia and loss of taste. However, the most simple mouth-care procedures can have 'returns for the patient significantly greater than the time and energy invested' (Richardson, 1987).

One additional objective is to empower individuals (if possible) to manage their own oral care; by providing health education at an appropriate level, suitable equipment and support at all stages.

Table 22.2 Aims of mouth care (After Howarth, 1977; MacMillan, 1981; Jenkins 1989)

Achieve and maintain a healthy, clean oral cavity
Prevent the build-up of plaque on oral surfaces
Keep the oral mucosa moist
Prevent infection
Prevent broken or chapped lips and areas surrounding the oral cavity
Promote patient dignity, comfort and well-being

Common disorders

The mouth harbours many varieties of bacteria which, suspended in saliva, do not pose a major problem for the various tissues in the mouth. However, once these organisms attach themselves to teeth, gums and the surfaces of the tongue via a mucopolysaccharide glue (which is insoluble in water), problems begin. These deposits cannot be rinsed away and dental plaque forms on the surfaces (Clarke, 1993). It is well known that plaque causes dental cavities and periodontal disease. Plaque is thought to release toxins which cause a local immunological response to occur with bacterial proteins, which in turn destroy the teeth and gums. If plaque can be thoroughly removed from all tooth surfaces daily, the mouth will remain healthy (Block, 1976; Gooch, 1985). Plaque takes about 24 hours to form and, if not removed, patients are at risk from the development of dental decay or gum disease while in hospital. Ultimately, if oral care is not carried out, changes will occur within the normal oral flora, thus allowing the growth of strains of bacteria such as streptococcus, which can spread systemically (Shepherd *et al.*, 1987).

Other common disorders of the mouth include dryness, furring, soreness, thrush and halitosis. If a dry mouth continues for long enough, it can be associated with dry, cracked and painful lips. Alert patients can obviously report these symptoms, but observation is needed for confused or unconscious patients. Furring of the tongue is sometimes associated with a dry mouth. Soreness is a sure sign of advanced problems such as ulcers or inflammation.

Thrush is often observed by the nurse prior to a patient complaining of any discomfort. It appears as small white spots or reddened oral tissue and can become very painful (Sutton, 1989). This is not uncommon in terminally ill patients and can also result from antibiotic therapy which may disrupt the flora of the mouth.

Factors which may contribute to poor oral hygiene following traumatic injury

The pressures associated with a busy acute ward environment all too often have an effect upon standards of care, despite efforts of the utmost diligence. As Meckstroth (1989) states, the mental and physical incapacities of patients, shortage of nursing personnel and the rapidly increasing elderly population all contribute to reduced quality and efficiency, especially when compounded by a lack of suitable equipment, funding and research based knowledge.

Principles of mouth care

As with any nursing procedure it is essential to start with an adequate assessment of the patient (Table 22.3). The goal of really effective mouth care is to ensure a shining, smooth, moist tongue and smooth, moist lips. Any pain, discomfort, furring or bleeding of any kind is abnormal. Therefore, any evidence of these abnormal signs requires particular attention. It is also vital to assess the particular needs of the individual according to their condition (Table 22.4). An unconscious patient will require the nurse to completely 'take over' the care of their mouth.

Table 22.3   Key points of oral hygiene

It is essential to carry out an assessment on admission to provide a baseline of information
The severe effects of plaque formation can cause cavities and periodontal disease
Toothpaste, toothbrushes and water are the cheapest and most effective tools for mouth care
Paediatric toothbrushes should be used as these will cause less damage to oral tissues
Oral care must be carried out twice a day and can be incorporated into the personal hygiene routine of the individual
Foam sticks and gloved fingers should no longer be used to clean a mouth, but can be used to moisten the oral tissues

Table 22.4   Groups at risk of poor oral hygiene (Adapted from Clarke, 1993)

Patients on certain drug treatments, such as antibiotic therapy, tranquillizers, antidepressants, diuretics, antihistamines, morphine, phenytoin, cytotoxic drug therapy and steroid preparations
Diabetics
The immunosuppressed
Patients with renal disorders
Anaemic patients
The elderly
The unconscious
Mechanically ventilated patients
Patients receiving oral suction
Patients receiving continuous oxygen therapy
Open-mouth breathers
Dehydrated or fluid-restricted patients

Mouth care should be planned daily and be based upon an individual patient assessment (Jenkins, 1989). On admission, it is imperative to establish a baseline of information from which any changes can be monitored. As Jenkins also stated, an early inspection of the mouth using a good light source should be carried out, noting dryness, colour and texture. The presence of any debris, plaque or bleeding should also be recorded.

Mouth care procedure for a patient requiring full assistance

Always ensure that gloves are worn to reduce the risk of infection to the nurse and the patient (Page *et al.*, 1987).

The teeth, gums and tongue should be brushed gently twice a day using a soft paediatric toothbrush and toothpaste containing fluoride. The action of brushing causes friction upon the mouth's surfaces, eventually removing bacterial plaque (Howarth, 1977; Liwu, 1989). Howarth and Liwu have studied the effects of foam sticks and gauze on plaque removal and have concluded that they are ineffective. In fact, the use of these tools may help to push plaque bacteria further into the teeth and gums. A small toothbrush will be less invasive and cause less damage to the tissues.

All excess water should be removed by gentle suctioning. It may be necessary to place the patient in the lateral position during this procedure to aid drainage and reduce the risk of aspiration (MacMillan, 1981).

It is essential to remoisturize the mouth by using foam sticks (this is the only time that the foam sticks should be used). This should be carried out on an unconscious patient every 2–3 h. Remoisturizing is essential to prevent discomfort and infection resulting from decreased salivary flow (Block, 1976). Clarke (1985) states that water is the best agent due to its pH level of 7 (neutral) as it causes minimal disturbance to the oral ecosystem.

Finally, soft paraffin should be applied to the lips to prevent them becoming dry, cracked and sore (Maurer, 1977).

Mouth care for the elderly

Older patients may well be able to maintain their own oral hygiene with just a little help from the nurse. They may require temporary assistance while recovering from surgery or illness, or they may require permanent help due to confusion or terminal illness.

If the patient is able to carry out their own care, assistance should be provided by placing the necessary articles in close proximity and by offering bowls of water and receptacles to spit into. For individuals requiring more assistance, the procedure for caring for an unconscious person should be followed. It is of course essential to provide a full explanation to reduce anxiety while the procedure is being carried out.

Denture care

Dentures should be cleaned daily using water, a soft toothbrush and either specialist denture cream or even hand soap (McCord and Stalker, 1988). If at any time dentures are not in use, they should be immersed in water or a denture cleansing solution. The water should be changed daily. Toothpaste is not suitable for cleaning dentures as it is too abrasive and will damage the surfaces (McCord and Stalker, 1988).

Conclusion

Oral hygiene is an essential part of care following traumatic injury. With an increasingly high patient turnover and reduced length of stay, less 'high profile' care may sometimes be overlooked. However, it can be shown just how essential oral care is, and how negligence can cause unnecessary harm.

References

Armstrong-Esther, C. A. (1981) Skin introduction. *Nursing*, 1st series, 1115.

Barsevick, A. and Llewellyn, J. (1982) A comparison of the anxiety reducing potential of two techniques of bathing. *Nursing Research*, **31**(1), 22–27.

Blarney, G. (1986) Mouth care – basic and essential. *Geriatric Nursing*, Sept./Oct., 242–243.

Block, P. (1976) Dental health in hospitalised patients. *American Journal of Nursing*, **76**, 162–164.

Browne, A. (1993) A conceptual clarification of respect. *Journal of Advanced Nursing*, **18**, 211–217.

Cahill, J. (1996) Patient participation: a concept analysis. *Journal of Advanced Nursing*, **24**, 561–571.

Chapman, G. E. (1983) Ritual and rational action in hospitals. *Journal of Advanced Nursing*, **8**, 13–20.

Clarke, G. (1993) Mouth care and the hospitalised patient. *British Journal of Nursing*, **2**(4), 225–227.

Crosby, C. (1989) Method in mouth care. *Nursing Times*, **85**, 35, 38–40.

Frantz, R. A. and Gardner, S. (1994) Clinical concerns: management of dry skin. *Journal of Gerontological Nursing*, **20**(9), 15–18, 45.

Gooch, J. (1987) Skin hygiene. *The Professional Nurse*, **2**(5), 153–154.

Gooch, J. (1989) Skin hygiene. *The Professional Nurse*, **5**(1), 13, 16, 18.

Gould, D. (1994) Helping the patient with personal hygiene. *Nursing Standard*, May, 8,34.

Greaves, A. (1985) We'll just freshen you up dear!' *Nursing Times*, March, 3, 4 and 7.

Hardy, M. A. (1996) What can you do about your patients dry skin? *Journal of Gerontological Nursing*, **22**(5), 10–18.

Higley, R. (1986) Independence vs dependence: whose decision? *ANNA Journal*, **3**(5).

Hilton, D. (1980) Oral hygiene and infection. *Nursing Times*, **76**(8), 340–342.

Howarth, H. (1977) Mouth care procedures for the very ill. *Nursing Times*, **73**(10), 354–355.

Jenkins, D. (1989) Oral care in ICU: an important nursing role. *Nursing Standard*, **8**(4), 24–28.

Jenkins, D. and Price, B. (1996) Dementia and personhood: a focus for care? *Journal of Advanced Nursing*, **24**, 84–90.

Jones, A. (1995) Reflective process in action: the uncovering of the ritual of washing in clinical nursing practice. *Journal of Clinical Nursing*, **4**(5), 283–288.

Lawler, J. (1991) *Behind the Screens*. Churchill Livingstone.

Liwu, A. (1989) Oral hygiene in intubated patients. *Australian Journal of Advanced Nursing*, **7**(2), 47.

MacMillan, K. (1981) New goals for oral hygiene. *The Canadian Nurse*, **77**, 40–43; cited in Clarke, G. (1993). Mouth care and the hospitalised patient. *British Journal of Nursing*, **2**(4), 225–227.

Mairis, E. (1992) Four senses for a full skin assessment observation and assessment of the skin. *Professional Nurse*, March, 376–380.

Mairis, E. (1994) Concept of clarification in professional practice – dignity. *Journal of advanced Nursing*, **19**, 947–953.

Maurer, J. (1977) Providing optimal oral health. *Nurse Clinical North America*, **12**(4), 671–685.

McCord, F. and Stalker, A. (1988) Brushing up on oral care. *Nursing Times*, **84**(13), 40–41; cited in Clarke, G. (1993). Mouth care and the hospitalised patient. *British Journal of Nursing*, **2**(4), 226.

McGee, P. (1994) The concept of respect in nursing. *British Journal of Nursing*, **3**(13), 681–684.

McMahon, R. and Buckledee, J. (1992) Skin problems beneath the breasts of in-patients: the knowledge, opinions and practice of nurses. *Journal of Advanced Nursing*, **17**, 1243–1250.

McLeod, W. T. (ed.) (1984) *The Collins Compact Dictionary*. Collins.

Meckstroth, R. (1989) Improving quality and efficiency in oral hygiene. *Journal of Gerontological Nursing*, **15**(6), 38–42.

Miller, F. M. (1997) Physically aggressive resident behaviour during hygienic care. *Journal of Gerontological Nursing*, **23**(5), 24–38.

Murdoch, S. (1990) Hazards in hoists. *Nursing Times*, **86**(49), 68–70.

Nightingale, F. (1859) *Notes on Nursing*. Harrison.

Page, C., Shephered, G. and Sammon, P. (1987). The mouth trap. *Nursing Times*, **83**(19), 24–29.

Porth C. and Kapke, K. (1983) Ageing and the skin. *Geriatric Nursing*, May/June, 158–162.

Rader, J., Lavelle, M., Hoeffer, B., and McKenzie, D. (1996). Maintaining cleanliness: an individual approach. *Journal of Gerontological Nursing*, **22**(3), 32–38.

Richardson, A. (1987). A process standard for oral care. *Nursing Times*, **83**(32), 38–40.

Roper N., Logan, W. and Tierney, A. (1981) *Learning to Use the Process of Nursing*. Churchill Livingstone.

Royal College of Nursing (1994) Mixed sex wards: the choice of patients. *Nursing Standard*, May, **8**(33).

Sanderson, P. J. and Weissler, S. (1992) Recovery of coliforms from the hands of nurses and patients: activities leading to contamination. *Journal of Hospital Infection*, **21**, 85–93.

Sedgewick, J. (1989) Dressed with dignity. *Nursing Times*, **85**(48), 30–31.

Skewes, S. M. (1996) Skin rituals that do more harm than good. *American Journal of Nursing*, **96**(10), 33–35.

Skewes, S. M. (1997) Bathing, it's a tough job! *Journal of Gerontological Nursing*, **23**(5), 45–49.

Spiller. J. (1992) For whose sake – patient or nurse? Ritual practices in patient washing. *Professional Nurse*, **7**(7), 431–432, 434.

Steinbaugh, J. R. (1983) Dry skin. *American Family Physician*, **27**, 171–174.

Sutton, R. B. O. (1989) Oral health problems in the elderly. *Geriatric Medicine*, **19**(3), 41–48.

Vogelpohl, T. S., Beck, C. K., Heacock, P., and Mercer, S. O. (1996) 'I can do it!' Dressing: promoting independence through individualised strategies. *Journal of Gerontological Nursing*, **22**(3), 39-42.

Wainwright, P. (ed.) (1992) *Oxford Reference Dictionary of Nursing*. Oxford University Press.

Walsh, M. and Ford, P. (1989) Rituals in nursing 1, 2 and 3. *Nursing Times*, **85**(41) 26–38, 42–43, 45–48.

Webster, R., Thompson, D., Bowman, G. and Sutton, T. (1988) Patients' and nurses' opinions about bathing. *Nursing Times*, September, **84**(37), 54–57.

Wilson, M. (1986) Personal cleanliness. *Nursing*, **3**(2) 80–82.

Wolf, Z. R. (1988) Nursing rituals. *Canadian Journal of Nursing Research*, **20**(3), 59–69.

Wolf, Z. R. (1993) The bath: a nursing ritual. *Journal of Holistic Nursing*, **11**(2) 135–148.

23

Casts, splints and traction

Tracy-Anne Enoch, Judith Harris and Mike Redrup

Introduction

The aim of this chapter is to give a brief overview of the many and varied options available for the immobilization of limbs following injury. Some of the techniques and casts are used as definitive treatments in their own right, others as an adjunct to surgical intervention in fracture management. The selection and application of a variety of traction systems will be addressed in a similar way.

Casting and splinting as an area of specialist expertise has developed significantly in recent years, due not only to advances in materials technology and the proliferation of companies offering ready-made adjustable splints, but also in response to advances in surgical fixation techniques.

The discussion relates specifically to the treatment and management of patients who have sustained injuries, rather than those undergoing elective orthopaedic procedures.

The history of casting

Plaster of Paris (POP) has been used since early Egyptian times, originally in wall decoration. It is made from gypsum, a naturally occurring mineral. The name, plaster of Paris, ostensibly originates from an accident to a house built on a deposit of gypsum near Paris. The house burnt down, and when rain fell on the baked mud of the floors it was noted that footprints in the mud set rock hard. This led to the rediscovery of the practice of heating gypsum to make a smooth covering for walls.

The use of POP applied to a continuous bandage in order to immobilize fractures was first credited to a Dutch army surgeon named Antonius Mathysen in the mid-1800s. These bandages were made by rubbing dry POP powder into coarsely woven cotton bandages, which were then soaked in water before being applied. They had to be freshly prepared before use. Prior to the commercial availability of such bandages in 1931, this was the only method of production.

The use of POP for the majority of fractures requiring immobilization continued through to the 1970s. At this point significant improvements were made in the manufacture of synthetic casting materials, providing lightweight alternatives to heavy, bulky plaster casts (Adkins, 1997).

Casts and splints

Reasons for using casts and splints:

- to support fractured bones, controlling movement of the fragments and resting damaged soft tissues
- to stabilize and rest limbs following ligamentous injury
- to support and immobilize joints and limbs postoperatively until healing is established, e.g. following nerve or tendon repairs

- to provide removable splints which enable mobilization or to prevent limb deformity
- to rest infected tissues, e.g. cellulitis
- to protect wounds and dressings from being disturbed if a patient is confused or agitated.

The choice of material

The material chosen for a particular cast will depend upon a number of different factors:

1. *The reason for the cast.* For example back slab, walking cast.
2. *The age and mobility of the patient.* When a patient is frail, a lightweight cast may be best and may enable the patient to mobilize more readily.
3. *The experience of the plaster technician or nurse.* The ultimate goal of cast immobilization is the prevention of joint motion or fracture angulation, together with the achievement of correct alignment. Synthetic casts 'set' quickly and should only be applied by experienced and competent individuals.
4. *The strength required in the cast.* Is weight-bearing required? Casts are frequently *in situ* for several weeks, so their durability must be given consideration. POP may be used in conjunction with a synthetic material in order to provide an additional, and often childproof, option.
5. *How long is the cast to remain in place?* POP remains the standard material for most casts. It is used in the initial management of new fractures. It is permeable to air and allows blood, pus and odour to pass through to the surface, thus facilitating observation. It accommodates a degree of tissue swelling and is easily removed. Once the swelling has reduced the POP is invariably changed to a lightweight synthetic cast.
6. *Likely exposure to water or soiling.* POP is not water resistant. Although lightweight synthetic casts are water resistant, they can cause skin maceration following immersion in water.
7. *Cost.* Synthetic casting materials which set quickly are lightweight, less bulky, strong and water resistant, but they cost more

than POP. However, their durability may well obviate the need for replacement, as may be the case following damage to POP casts, together with the inherent material and time costs associated with reapplication.

Plaster of Paris and synthetic casts

Plaster of Paris

POP consists of powdered calcium sulphate crystals incorporated into bandage. The bandage must be soaked in tepid water before application and this causes recrystallizing and interlocking of the powdered calcium sulphate crystals, resulting in a hardening of the bandage tape into the well-known plaster cast.

In the majority of cases POP is used for primary casting, while synthetic materials are used for definitive and specialist casts.

Fibreglass

Fibreglass was first applied as a casting material in 1970 (Southwick and Callaghan, 1985). This casting material consisted of a fibreglass tape impregnated with a light-activated resin; the tape hardened upon exposure to ultraviolet light. In 1978, the first water-activated cast was marketed by Cutter Biomedical.

The synthetic materials most utilized in casting today consist of:

- polyester/cotton knit
- thermoplastics
- fibreglass
- fibreglass-free polymers

Table 23.1 lists the advantages and disadvantages of various types of material used in casting.

Complications of casting

Tissue swelling

The limb should be elevated to reduce swelling. As most fractures are initially treated in a POP or backslab, the cast, together with all padding, should be split down to skin, enabling the swelling to be accommodated.

Table 23.1 The advantages and disadvantages of different types of casting material (Adapted from Adkins, 1997)

Cast type	Advantages	Disadvantages	Uses
POP	• Easily moulded • Strong • Inexpensive • Easy to remove • Smooth surface	• Not water resistant • Heavy, bulky • Long drying time • Long time to full weight bear	• Serial casting • Soft tissue oedema • Significant moulding • New fractures
Fibreglass	• Lightweight • Water resistant • Durable • Strong • Fast setting time and time to weight-bear	• Rough edges • Difficult to mould • Expensive • Latex/fibreglass exposure • Possible skin maceration with water	• Weight bearing casts • Long term casting • Simple fractures • Removable casts
Latex/fibreglass free	• As fibreglass • Latex/fibreglass free • Easy to mould	• As fibreglass	• As fibreglass • For patients with known or suspected latex allergy
Thermoplastics	• Water resistant • Fast setting time and time to weight-bear	• Difficult to mould • Heat activated for application • Cast softens with inadvertent heat exposure • Expensive	• When remoulding is needed without removal

Arterial occlusion

This can cause:

- pain – increased
- pallor
- paraesthesia – loss of sensation to the limb
- pulselessness – distal to fracture/site of injury
- pressure on an artery at the fracture site.

Nerve impairment

The cast may be too tight, causing pressure on nerves running in close proximity to bony prominences. Inadequate padding may lead to numbness and tingling as a result of pressure.

Pressure sores

A cast may be either too tight or too loose, leading to friction over bony prominences which can result in the breakdown of the skin's integrity. Putting foreign bodies inside the cast, such as knitting needles to ease itching, can also cause skin damage.

Loss of function

The immobilization of one part of the body may lead to problems in an adjacent joint due to the patient being reluctant to exercise, e.g. frozen shoulder following wrist injury.

Joint stiffness

This can result from long periods of immobilization while waiting for fracture union.

Depression

Long periods of immobilization or restricted mobility (often encountered during the course of staged reconstructive surgery post-injury), together with effects on lifestyle and activities, can lead to depression.

Observations following the application of a cast

When a cast is applied it is important that the affected limb is checked regularly in order to prevent many of the previously mentioned complications (Figure 23.1). Initially, check CSM hourly (C, colour; S, sensation, and M, movement.)

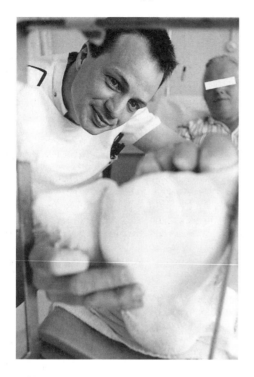

Figure 23.1   Neurovascular observations

Colour

- Check pulses.
- Check nail beds for capillary return.
- Check colour – fingers or toes should be pink and warm to touch.

Impaired colour could be due to arterial occlusion or a reduction in the blood supply to the limb caused by swelling. To reduce swelling the limb should be elevated and the plaster split.

Sensation

If there is an increase in pain this could be due to swelling within the cast. There could also be bleeding into the muscle fascia around the fracture site; this causes swelling and characteristically intense pain.

Paraesthesia or paralysis may occur. It is important to know if the patient can feel their fingers or toes being touched, as nerve damage or impaired circulation could be the cause.

Movement

Check whether the movement is normal. If it is not, this could indicate nerve damage.

Any alteration in colour, sensation or movement must be investigated immediately and reported to medical staff. The cast and padding should be split to reduce pressure and, if necessary, under appropriate supervision, removal may be required. A window cut into the cast may sometimes be considered, as it will allow the skin to be checked if there is any question of breakdown or pressure damage.

Proprietary brand splints

In recent years many proprietary brand adjustable splints have been marketed for the treatment, immobilization and support of limbs. Considerations for the care of patients treated in these splints are similar to those for patients in casts. The advantages of such splints are the ease of application and removal, together with the fact that removability facilitates skin inspection and hygiene (Figure 23.2).

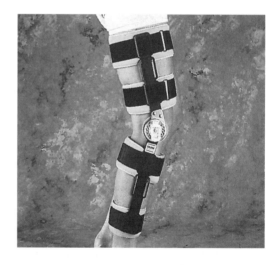

Figure 23.2 Ready made splint

Disadvantages include the potential for non-compliance on the part of the patient (due to ease of removal) and the fact that the build of some patients may not readily conform to the sizing and availability of such products.

Instructions and advice on discharge

On discharge it is important to give advice and

information to patients about caring for their cast or splint:

- Remember to exercise as instructed by the physiotherapist to help prevent joint stiffness and aid circulation.
- Elevate the limb when not mobilizing to reduce swelling.
- Do not get the cast wet.
- No foreign bodies, such as knitting needles, should be put inside the cast.
- Do not attempt to cut or remove the cast yourself.
- Any increase in swelling, pins and needles, loss of sensation or movement should be reported to your GP, or return to the Accident and Emergency Department.

A reflective account of the problems of compliance following injury

What can be done to encourage injured people to comply with recommended treatment or care? Being confined to bed, wearing a cast or splint, or using a walking aid involves a change in behaviour which is often not welcomed. How can healthcare professionals have a positive but understanding influence? How can we encourage people to accept healthy behaviour? This short reflective account aims to discuss the theory relating to non-compliance using a practice situation to highlight the difficulties.

Non-compliance within the speciality of trauma is frequently observed, although there is no literature relating to this specific area. The subject of non-compliance in relation to taking medication is well researched, so this literature is drawn upon and related to the care of the injured person in the acute setting.

Non-compliance is defined as 'not acting in accordance with a request or command' (Swannell, 1992). Weller and Wells (1990) go a step further by describing non-compliance as the decision made by a patient not to comply with a health regimen despite fully understanding the rationale for such therapy; a patient may fully understand the rationale of therapy, but chooses to ignore it. Becker and Maiman (1980) argue that non-compliance is a substantial obstacle to the achievement of therapeutic goals.

Example

Kate, a 20-year-old girl, sustained an ankle fracture in a road traffic accident. She was admitted to hospital for elevation of her ankle in order to reduce the swelling prior to internal fixation. Initially, oral analgesia and cryocuff therapy provided effective pain relief. The physiotherapist taught Kate how to transfer from bed to chair without putting weight through her foot.

It subsequently became apparent that Kate was spending a lot of her time either going to or returning from the smoking room. As a result, the elevation therapy was rendered ineffective, swelling did not reduce and her analgesic requirement increased to intramuscular morphine. A computerized tomography (CT) scan was performed which identified complex fractures. Kate was reminded to keep her leg elevated, but she continued to take frequent breaks from this. Could this be viewed as non-compliance?

Despite being fully informed, the visits to the smoking room continued at regular intervals. The consultant discussed the CT results with both Kate and her parents, outlining the possible complications in years to come. Following this, Kate tried to keep her ankle elevated for longer periods. Is this compliance? Kate now appeared to have a greater awareness and understanding of her position but she still persisted in taking breaks from elevation.

Given her sudden admission to hospital and the associated stress, Kate may have failed to appreciate the importance of elevation, or tried to cope by denying her injuries, exemplifying unintentional non-compliance, described by Hussey and Gilliland (1989) as inadequate understanding of a disease or condition. However, the importance of elevation had been stressed not only on admission, but regularly throughout her stay.

Could she have continued to be ignorant of the importance of elevation or was she making a conscious choice not to comply, thus suggesting intentional non-compliance? Hussey and Gilliland (1989) state that intentional non-compliance is when a patient makes a conscious choice to find another method of treatment, or chooses not to comply.

It is difficult to distinguish between unintentional and intentional non-compliance within the context of acute care. In the wake of injury, to a degree, a person suddenly has to relinquish control of their life. Perhaps visiting the smoking room was just a gesture of independence?

Perhaps Kate's nicotine craving superseded the need to keep her foot elevated? Perhaps she enjoyed the company of others in the smoking room? Or was she finding it difficult to accept that she had seriously injured her ankle?

If Kate had been more compliant with her regimen, the swelling would have reduced more quickly, her operation could have been performed sooner and she would have benefited by earlier discharge from hospital. The hospital would also have benefited, by an increase in bed availability.

Buchmann (1997) promotes the application of a structure that improves compliance and adherence to treatment, and which also aids in developing an understanding of relevant social and psychological influences (Cameron, 1996).

- *Knowledge and understanding*. For individuals motivated to comply, but who are ignorant of treatment programmes, the provision of information should be beneficial. For those who are already knowledgeable, but insufficiently motivated, additional information is unlikely to enhance compliance. The information given to Kate was basic, but perhaps initially the importance of compliance was not emphasized enough and therefore not taken seriously by her. Motivation could have been enhanced by emphasizing positive outcomes.
- *Quality of interaction*. Healthcare professionals can have a positive or negative effect on patient compliance. Communication in a busy ward can lead to rather rushed exchanges. Perhaps the staff lacked empathy, were unable to compromise or had other priorities?
- *Social isolation and social support*. Kate was in a side room and was alone for long periods. Her parents visited and were made aware of the importance of elevation, though they also wheeled her out to the smoking room on occasion.
- *Health beliefs and attitudes*. These have a significant influence on compliance. Emphasis should be placed on how effective a particular treatment can be, if adhered to. A simple outline of the treatment plan can reduce anxiety and increase motivation. Kate was encouraged to become involved in her care, specifically in relation to her analgesic requirements.

Rodin and Janis (1979) identify the specific responsibilities of the nurse (including the establishment of referent power) as being benevolent and caring, present where one can

be a frame of reference, and able to serve in the role of significant other. The nurse should be educated, knowledgeable, skilful and with enough experience to encourage efficacy – the desired effect. There are nine essential building blocks to referent power (Rodin and Jarvis, 1979):

1. Use acceptance statements to convey that the person is held in high regard.
2. Show unselfish willingness to provide help out of a sense of caring.
3. Encourage self-disclosure, increasing insight so that cognitive restructuring and learning can occur.
4. Give positive feedback if behaviour is complying with advice, and just accept if it is not.
5. Encourage a sense of personal responsibility.
6. Encourage other members of the interprofessional team to endorse the request.
7. Elicit commitment e.g. a number of hours of elevation before taking a break.
8. Maintain positive regard – avoid judging and encourage communication.
9. Plan early discharge as a motivating factor

The staff needed to avoid making judgements and help Kate become aware of her behaviours so that she could gain insight, learn and perhaps develop a more positive attitude. Helping Kate to admit to how much she smoked may have helped her to cut down so that she could maintain effective elevation for longer periods. A sense of personal responsibility must be promoted by all healthcare professionals, together with the provision of consistent information. Positive feedback can help to reinforce compliance, though making judgements must be avoided.

Nyatanga (1997) believes the paternalistic management of non-compliance is not successful and that more energy should be invested in understanding the reasons behind behavioural patterns related to non-compliance. He suggests that a patient may act according to their understanding. For example, Kate considers elevation and attaches a value to it. If the value outweighs the value she attaches to smoking, then she is more likely to comply. This underlines the importance of the patient understanding the benefits of compliance.

It can therefore be seen that compliance or non-compliance must be an individual's decision. It is the responsibility of all healthcare professionals to ensure that the patient is made fully aware of their situation in order that they may be active participants in treatment programmes, despite the traumatic circumstances of their admission to hospital.

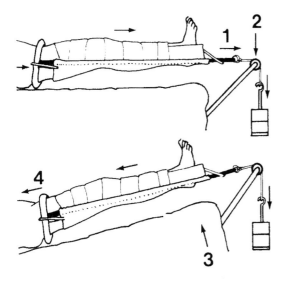

Figure 23.3 Traction and counter traction

against, or a force pulling in the opposite direction. This is known as counter-traction and is shown in Figure 23.3 (McCrae, 1989).

If a pulling force is applied in only one direction, the patient will be slowly pulled down the bed until the traction appliance hits the end of the bed. If the foot of the bed is elevated, the gravitational pull of the patient's body weight creates a force pulling in the opposite direction and effective counter-traction is achieved.

Traction is used for a variety of reasons:

- realignment of fractures or joint surfaces
- immobilization of fractures or joints
- to reduce or overcome muscle spasm.

Skin traction and skeletal traction

The application of a traction force is achieved in one of two ways – skin traction or skeletal traction.

Managing patients in traction

The continual developments in both internal and external fixation following traumatic injury have resulted in a dramatic reduction in the use of traction systems (Nichol, 1995). However, traction still has its place and it is important that the skills required to ensure safe maintenance and patient care remain current. A situation may arise where a patient is not fit to undergo lengthy surgery, or the nature of the injury is such that conservative treatment is felt to be preferable.

This section contains a brief overview of why and how traction systems are used and outlines the care of a patient in traction.

There is no mystery to traction. Simply put, traction is the application of a pulling force. To pull effectively there must be something to pull

Skin traction

The pull is exerted on a material (either adhesive or non-adhesive) applied to the patient's skin. It is important to consider the patient's skin integrity before choosing a traction set. If adhesive materials are used for elderly patients or those with friable skin, damage can be caused when the time comes to remove the traction. The pull is transmitted from the material through the skin to the underlying tissue and bone. This is shown in Figure 23.4.

This is likely to be the most well known of all traction systems as it is common practice in many areas to apply skin traction to patients who have sustained femoral neck fractures. The belief is that this will reduce the level of pain which the patient experiences. Some surgeons

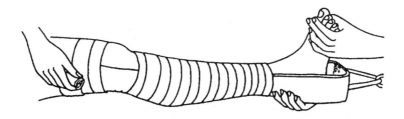

Figure 23.4   The application of skin traction (Taylor, 1987, by permission of Churchill Livingstone)

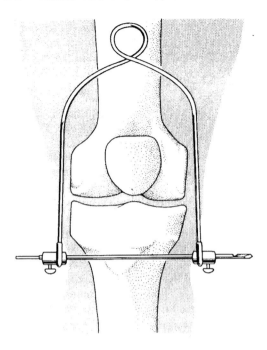

Figure 23.5 Tibial Denham pin (Miller and Miller, 1985)

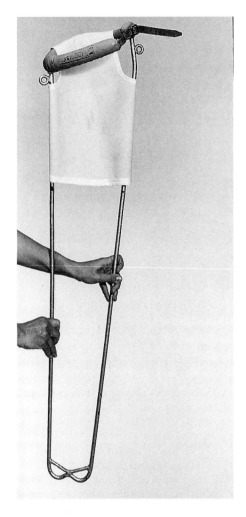

Figure 23.6 Preparation of a Thomas splint

also believe that the position of the fracture can be maintained or improved. There is increasing evidence, however, to support the view that there is no discernible benefit from traction for this client group (Finsen *et al.*, 1992; Anderson *et al.*, 1993; Needoff *et al.*, 1993).

The process of applying traction to a limb with an unfixed fracture can be painful, despite analgesia and careful handling. It is necessary to remove non-adhesive traction sets regularly to check skin integrity. Where non-adhesive sets are used it is possible to damage the patient's skin, as a shearing force is created if too much weight is used inadvertently. This is a particularly significant problem for the frail elderly who often have poor skin quality. Allergic reactions to strapping can also occur (Anderson *et al.*, 1993).

Such concerns, weighed against the negligible benefit, suggest that the use of this system must be carefully considered. The patient can probably be managed more effectively by the administration of regular, effective analgesics, comfortable positioning of the affected limb on a pillow or in a trough, and surgical fixation, ideally within 24 h.

Skeletal traction

The pull is exerted via a metal pin directed through an area of bone. This means that traction can be applied to almost any part of the body. For example, Denham pins are inserted through the proximal tibia to facilitate the application of traction for femoral shaft and femoral neck injuries. (Figure 23.5).

Skeletal traction systems often look complicated, but are actually quite straightforward. When correctly assembled and regularly checked, the systems are robust and comfortable enough to enable the patient, with assistance, to carry out most activities of living.

The form of traction applied varies according to its intended use – fixed or balanced.

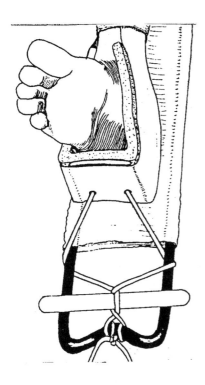

Figure 23.7 Fixed traction using a Thomas splint

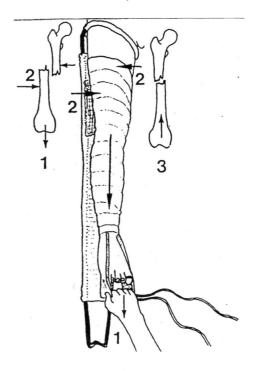

Figure 23.8 Establishing alignment – see text for explanation (McRae, 1989, by permission of Churchill Livingstone)

Fixed traction

This is where a force is exerted on that part of a limb which lies between two fixed points. The most common example of a use for fixed traction is the immobilization of a femoral shaft fracture using a Thomas splint (Figure 23.6). As shown in Figure 23.7, the two fixed points are the splint ring which presses on the patient's ischial tuberosity, and the cords tied to the distal end of the splint. As shown in Figure 23.8, realignment of the fracture is achieved by pulling against muscle activity (1) and bandaging the limb to the splint (2). An appropriate position (3) is maintained when the traction set is tied off to the splint end.

Balanced traction

Balanced traction is where a force is exerted on that part of a limb which lies between two mobile points. Traction is achieved by the attachment of weights via a pulley system, and counter-traction is introduced by elevating the foot of the bed to use the gravitational pull of the patient's body weight. Balanced systems are invariably used where lengthy periods in traction are required.

Fixed and balanced systems can be applied using either skin or skeletal methods. However, when its use is likely to be short term and the amount of weight required is small, skin traction is often used.

Some examples of traction systems include:

- *Balanced skeletal traction using a Thomas splint.* Commonly used for midshaft femoral fractures as shown in Figure 23.9. (a securing bandage would normally be *in situ* around the patient's thigh to incorporate the splint, but this has been omitted for clarity).
- *Perkins traction.* Used with a split bed, this system allows the knee joint to be actively exercised following a femoral shaft fracture while the traction is still *in situ*. Also used when the application of a straight pull is required, i.e. acetabular fractures. This is shown in Figure 23.10, where the weights have been set at different levels to control rotation.

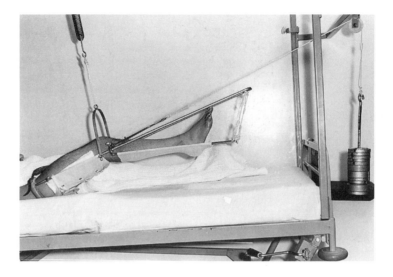

Figure 23.9   Balanced skeletal traction using a Thomas splint

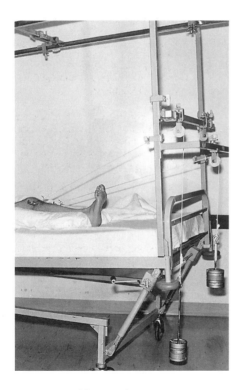

Figure 23.10   Perkins traction

- *Hamilton-Russell traction using a skin application*. Occasionally used for the non-operative management of patients following femoral neck fracture (Figure 23.11).

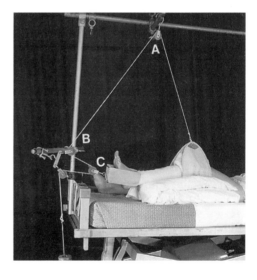

Figure 23.11   Hamilton-Russell traction

- *Halo traction*. Used for unstable cervical spine fractures (Figure 23.12).

Complications associated with the use of traction are related in the main to poor application. The risk of over-distraction or complete separation of the fracture segments leading to delayed union may be caused by the application of too much weight (Tables 23.2–23.4).

Checking the position of the fracture by x-ray is necessary each time adjustments are made.

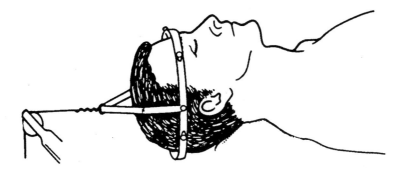

Figure 23.12 Halo traction

Table 23.2 General considerations for the care of a patient in traction (Adapted from Smith, 1984; Mallett and Bailey, 1996)

Potential problem	Possible cause	Action
Joint stiffness or muscle wasting	• Long periods of inactivity	• Liaise with physiotherapist to establish exercise programme
Delayed union or non-union	• Over distraction of fracture due to excessive weight	• Reduce weight following consultation with medical staff • Confirm correct position by x-ray investigation
Contact dermatitis	• Allergic reaction to traction set or bandaging	• Change to hypoallergenic bandaging • Change from adhesive to non-adhesive traction sets • Remove all bandages daily to check skin integrity
Pressure sores	• Long periods of immobility	• Encourage the patient to lift with aid of a monkey pole to relieve pressure • Increase the degree of elevation of the foot of the bed if patient is sliding down • Encourage adequate nutrition and hydration • Move patient 4-hourly to check skin condition • Use of appropriate aids such as pressure-relieving mattresses • Avoid and alleviate pressure from splints or any part of the traction apparatus

Table 23.3 Non-adhesive skin traction (Adapted from Smith, 1984; Mallett and Bailey, 1996)

Potential problem	Possible cause	Action
Disruption of skin integrity under traction set	• Shearing force due to excess weight or poor application • Inadequate padding over bony areas or bandaging too tight	• Ensure weight no greater than manufacturer's recommendation, i.e. 6 lb or below • Reapply bandaging • Ensure areas around malleoli are well padded
Altered sensation to the periphery of affected limb		• Check colour, sensation and movement hourly (initially) to ensure bandaging not too tight • Advise medical staff and reapply traction

Table 23.4 Skeletal traction (Adapted from Smith, 1984; Mallett and Bailey, 1996)

Potential problem	Possible cause	Action
Altered sensation to the periphery of affected limb	• Splint or bandage support too tight causing pressure on nerve	• Change splint after discussion with medical staff • Reapply bandaging
Development of drop foot	• Nerve palsy due to pressure on common peroneal nerve	• Check limb position – should not be externally rotated • Check position of padding and adjust as necessary • Release bandaging if too tight • Assess patient's ability to dorsiflex ankle and report if diminished • Check colour, sensation and movement
Development of sore under splint	• Splint too tight or inadequately padded	• Replace with splint of correct size • Apply dressing to any areas of skin breakdown • Repad • Check skin integrity 4-hourly in all areas where splint is in contact with skin
Discomfort from pin sites	• Pin site infection • Pin may be loose • Skin needs releasing	• Check pin sites daily and clean thoroughly, ensuring no scabbing develops. Skin should be mobile around pin and pain free. Report any signs of infection, exudate, inflammation or pyrexia • If pin slipping, report immediately. In cases where patient has poor bone quality a below knee cast incorporating the pin or the insertion of two pins joined with an external fixator block may prevent slipping • If skin adheres to pin it should be released. This involves incising the skin under local anaesthetic and is performed by medical staff

Vascular and neurological damage can be caused by constriction where bandaging is too tight or splints are ill-fitting. Foot drop can occur if there is undue pressure on the common peroneal nerve which supplies the muscles that dorsiflex the foot. This can be caused by inappropriate padding around the knee joint or pressure on this area by tight splinting.

These problems can be avoided by looking at and listening to the patient. A correctly applied traction system should cause no discomfort. Any complaints of pain or paraesthesia by the patient, or observation of pallor or pulselessness in the limb or extremities distal to the fracture, must be immediately investigated.

Constant checks of skin integrity must also be made, as blistering or pressure necrosis can occur from adhesive tape, the shearing effect of excess weight, over-tight bandaging or incorrect splint size.

Where the long-term use of traction is required, reduction of muscle activity can lead to muscle atrophy and/or joint stiffness. Early physiotherapy input is vital in order to maximize muscle bulk and joint mobility through exercise.

Conclusion

Care of the patient in traction is quite straightforward. Most of the aspects of care that need to be considered are those encountered by any patient on bedrest, such as constipation, deep vein thrombosis, chest infection, difficulty in maintaining hygiene, and boredom, although there are some special considerations, as detailed above. When caring for someone in traction it is important at all times to observe and listen to the patient. If they are uncomfortable, then poor application is invariably the cause.

References

Adkins (1997) Cast changes: synthetic versus plaster. *Paediatric Nurse*, **23**(4), 422-427.

Anderson, G. H., Harper, W. M., Connoly, C.D. *et al.* (1993) Pre-operative skin traction for fracture of the proximal femur. *Journal of Bone and Joint Surgery*, **75B**(5), 794-796.

Becker, M. H. and Maiman, L. A. (1980) Strategies for enhancing patient compliance. *Journal of Community Health*, **2,** 113-135.

Buchmann, W. F. (1997) Adherence: a matter of self efficiency and power. *Journal of Advanced Nursing*, **26**(1), 132-137.

Cameron, C. (1996) Patient compliance: recognition of factors involved and suggestions for promoting compliance. *Journal of Advanced Nursing*, **2**, 244-250.

Finsen, V., Borsetm, M., Buvik, G. E. and Hauke, I. (1992) Pre-operative traction in patients with hip fractures. *Injury*, **23**(4), 242-244.

Hussey, L. C. and Gilliland, K. (1989) Compliance, low literacy and locale of control. *Nursing Clinics of North America*, **24**(3), 605-611.

Mallett, J. and Bailey, C. (1996) *Manual of Nursing Procedures*. Blackwell.

McRae, R. (1989) *Practical Fracture Treatment*. Churchill Livingstone.

Miller, M. and Miller, J. H. (1985) *Orthopaedics and Accidents Illustrated*. Hodder and Stoughton.

Needoff, M., Radford, P. and Langstaff, R. (1993) Pre-operative traction for hip fractures in the elderly – a clinical trial. *Injury*, **24**(5), 317-318.

Nichol, D. (1995) Understanding the principles of traction. *Nursing Standard*, **9**(46), 25-27.

Nyatanga, B. (1997) Psychosocial theories of patient non-compliance. *Professional Nurse*, **12**(5), 331-334.

Rodin, J. and Janis, I. (1979) The social power of healthcare practitioners as agents of change. *Journal of Social Issues*, **35,** 60-81.

Smith, C. (1984) Nursing the patient in traction. *Nursing Times*, April, 36-39.

Southwick, J. R. and Callaghan, D. J. (1985) A study of blood drainage patterns on synthetic cast materials. *Orthopaedic Nursing*, **4**(2), 72–75.

Swannell, J. (1992) *The Oxford Modern English Dictionary*. Clarendon Press.

Taylor, I. (1987) *Ward Manual of Orthopaedic Traction*. Churchill Livingstone.

Weller, B. F. and Wells, R. J. (1990) *Baillière's Nursing Dictionary*. Baillière Tindall.

24

Moving and handling

Tracy-Anne Enoch

Introduction

The high incidence of back injuries among healthcare staff has long been recognized (Venning, 1988; Moffet *et al.*, 1993; Love, 1996; Smedley *et al.*, 1997). Many of these studies cite patient moving and handling as being the causative factors. Lack of risk assessment, inadequate provision of appropriate aids or equipment, and poor staff compliance towards lifting policies are highlighted as the main contributory factors.

Every year 80 000 staff sustain back injuries, of which an estimated 3600 hurt themselves so seriously that they are invalided out of the profession (Snell, 1995). The EC directive 90/269 (European Commission, 1990) on the minimum health and safety requirements for the manual handling of loads became law in January 1993. In Britain this legislation was implemented in the form of Health and Safety Regulations on the Minimum Requirements for the Handling of Loads (1992). The introduction of this legislation places new responsibilities on both employee and employer, aimed at reducing the risk of back and associated injuries brought about by patient handling activities. Of the 45 000 Health Service accidents reported to the Health and Safety Executive in 1988–90, 70% involved patient-handling situations.

The European Community regulations were designed to stop people being injured while moving loads at work. Corlett *et al.* (1992) described the aim of the legislation as an attempt to 'harmonise health and safety stan-dards throughout the European Community, such that competitive advantage cannot be gained by lowering standards'. The almost total abolition of manual lifting advocated by this legislation should have resulted in a dramatic reduction in back injuries and manual handling accidents.

Unfortunately, many healthcare staff are all too painfully aware that this is not in fact the case. The investigation of Smith and Seccombe (1996) showed that in 1992 a quarter of all nurses interviewed by the Royal College of Nursing reported some degree of back injury, with this figure increasing to a third by 1996. It would appear therefore that, irrespective of the introduction of legally supported guidelines to reduce the need for manual handling and the resultant injury to staff, this problem continues to grow.

In recent years, numbers of hospitals have developed specialist trauma units, thereby significantly improving the outcome for seriously injured patients (Backer *et al.*, 1985). 'Trauma can happen to anyone, from a fit twenty year old to a confused eighty year old, from minor injury to major. Each injury is unique and no fracture is the same' (Christie, 1994). As a result, every care situation is equally unique. The very nature of this speciality is associated with an increased demand for moving and handling patients; as a direct corollary, the potential for injury is also increased. The dependency of patients, even those who have sustained a seemingly minor injury, can be significant. The needs of the multiply-injured patient, the frail elderly and the immobile are challenging in their complexity.

This clinical speciality encompasses those areas of practice where the highest incidence of lifting and handling injuries are reported. This is supported by the paper by the Royal College of Nursing (RCN, 1996a), in which they profile selected practice areas and show distinct patterns regarding the incidence of various types of injury. Approximately 80% of injuries to staff in orthopaedic environments were handling related, with 70% in elderly care and 60% in surgery.

The speciality of trauma is a particularly high-risk area, highlighted in part by the previous statistics, but also due to the increasing numbers of elderly patients presenting for treatment (Newman, 1992).

The new legislation brought about by EC 90/ 269 requires employers to demonstrate a proactive rather than a reactive response to accident prevention in the area of manual handling, with the employee required to take responsibility for their own actions.

Responsibilities of the employer

The employer must

- Develop and implement a code of practice to cover all aspects of patient handling and loads in the workplace.
- Ensure that manual handling tasks are avoided wherever reasonably practicable. Where unavoidable, a proper assessment of the risks must be undertaken. This assessment must include the environment, how the task is done, the staff available, training and the load itself. Action should be taken to reduce the risk of injury. The assessment must be documented.
- Supply equipment to move the load safely.
- Make training for staff mandatory, both as part of their induction programme and yearly thereafter. All new staff must be trained before handling any loads.
- Record and monitor training. It is also the responsibility of the manager to ensure that training is being properly applied.
- Ensure that all employees are medically fit for work. This includes pre-employment medicals and assessment of fitness to

return to work following illness.
- Provide a uniform allowing full movement.

Responsibilities of the employee

The employee must

- Take reasonable care of his or her own safety and that of colleagues.
- Cooperate with the employer to develop a code of practice on the handling of loads. This includes the responsibility to report lack of staff, lack of or defective equipment, injury, illness or disability affecting the ability to lift.

One of the major difficulties in attempting to implement the HSE regulations based upon EC 90/269 in the speciality of trauma is the diversity of handling tasks encountered in this care setting. Many adult patients invariably exceed the safe load threshold and are unable to assist due to the nature of their injuries.

The complexity of providing training programmes, creating assessment tools and providing lifting aids which will meet all these needs is significant.

This chapter will discuss how to address issues of risk assessment, problems with staff compliance and training, and use of equipment, in order to offer suggestions as to how these needs can be met.

Risk assessment

All components of the EC 90/269 directive related to manual handling require some degree of risk assessment in order to establish the appropriateness of the procedure which is to be carried out, or the need to provide alternative options such as mechanical aids.

Employer's obligations

General provision

'The employer shall take the appropriate organisational measures, use the appropriate means or provide workers with such means in order to reduce the risk involved in manual handling.'

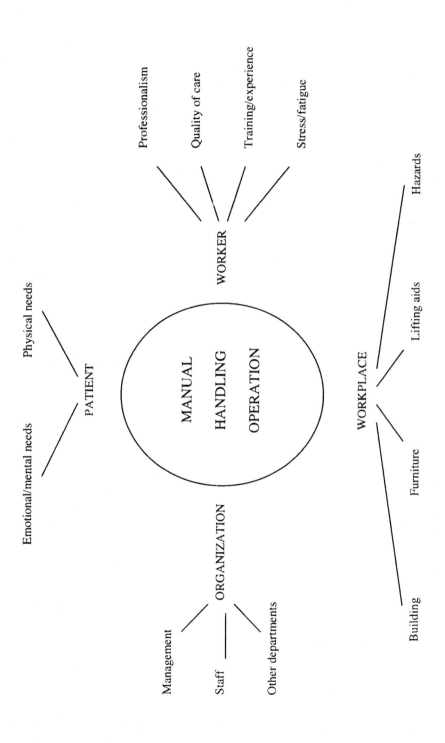

Figure 24.1   Proposition for a model of nurses' perceptions of factors that influence patient handling (Adapted from Hignett and Richardson, 1995)

Organisation of workstation

'Take care to avoid or reduce risk, particularly of back injury.'

Information for and training of workers

'Employers must ensure that workers receive information on the risk they might be open to.'

The Manual Handling Operations Regulation (HSE, 1992) requires risk assessment to be carried out 'if the employers cannot avoid the need for a manual handling action that involves risk of injury'. In response to these regulations both the HSE and the RCN produced documents providing guidelines to introduce risk assessment. The HSE (1994) document and the RCN (1996) guide offer basic outlines to facilitate the introduction of risk assessment.

There are an abundance of risk assessment tools available and it is necessary to review the components of any tool considered in order to establish which aspects are suitable for any given clinical environment. Pilling (1993) offers a risk calculator which aims to identify, measure and reduce risk, initially aimed at community care but offered as appropriate to hospital care settings. If adopted in the adult trauma care setting, every patient would be considered a high risk, as a patient need only be 6 stone (38 kg) and requiring orthopaedic surgery to pass Pilling's (1993) high-risk threshold. She suggests that in all high-risk situations preventative action and introduction of equipment should 'solve' the handling problem. In the community situation cited in her paper, handling risk was reduced by the provision of a hoist and through ceiling lift. The cost implication associated with the provision of such equipment to every patient in a clinical setting, it could be argued, makes such a tool unrealistic in its expectation. While the concept of the tool appears promising, it would need to be reviewed in order to reflect more accurately patient requirement in the trauma setting.

Barker *et al.* (1992) include two modules based on assessment and planning. These modules contain guidelines for staff to review lifting activities, identify problems and plan lifting action accordingly. What is not considered is the action that should be taken when a high-risk situation is identified, but where no

aids are available as an alternative to manual handling.

Perhaps the most useful component of the module related to the practice area under consideration is the review of Haynes (1986), cited in Barker *et al.* (1992), 'Patient Movement Hazard Code'. This code assesses patient environment and method of movement needed in much the same way as Pilling (1993), but allows for 'staff experience and instinct to categorise patients who are likely to behave in an unpredictable manner'. Its aim is to provide staff with a warning about both patient state/ability and potential environmental hazards, to be coded in the patient's notes without the need for lengthy documentation. It is interesting that the assessment tool which more closely fits the needs of a clinical environment such as trauma, with the unpredictability of its clientele, was developed sometime before, rather than in response to, EC directives and HSE or RCN guidelines.

Hignett and Richardson (1995) offer a paper which displays research findings to support their investigation into one particular aspect of risk assessment. They found that difficulties arose in translating HSE regulations to healthcare settings because the guidelines were developed for inanimate loads. The unpredictable nature of animate loads led them to question the relevance of HSE guidelines in this context. They chose a grounded theory approach using qualitative analysis to determine factors perceived by staff to be important when considering patient handling (Figure 24.1).

The advantage of this model is that it highlights where risks lie. It also has the potential to be used as a springboard to aid in the development of a tool specific to the trauma environment, which seems to require a combination of components selected from a variety of the tools under discussion. However, what is clear is that whenever risk assessment is carried out it is vital that, wherever possible, hazardous lifting situations are avoided. Full assessment must take place when this is not possible so that risk may be reduced as far as practicable.

Hignett (1994) outlines the Manual Handling Operations Regulations specific to risk assessment and this, linked with the tools reviewed, would perhaps provide the ideal basis for the design of a risk assessment tool that would be appropriate for use in the speciality of trauma.

Risk identification

- Is there risk of injury?
- Is it reasonably practicable to avoid moving the loads?

Risk assessment

- Is it reasonably practicable to automate or mechanize the operations?
- Carry out a manual handling assessment.

Risk management

- Determine measure to reduce risk of injury to the lowest level reasonably practicable.
- Implement these measures.

Safe practice

The objective must be to reduce manual handling, thereby reducing the risk of injury. However, sifting through the mountain of information available often leads to confusion regarding which handling techniques are 'safe'. Scott (1995) reviewed handling skills from a safety perspective and produced a selection of points for staff to consider when moving patients. These factors, highlighted in terms of their problem-solving approach, can be considered relevant to most clinical specialities and are of particular relevance to trauma care as they address both the patient as an individual together with their environment.

Points for staff to consider before moving a patient

Before moving a patient you should assess the situation as a whole, decide on the method, check the environment, organize yourself and/or team and above all explain the procedure to the patient.

Consider what you want to do and why, taking into account the following questions:

- Does the patient need to be moved at all?
- Can the patient move independently?
- Must the patient be lifted?

Consider the following factors before moving the patient:

- patient's age
- functional ability of the patient
- stage of rehabilitation
- patient confidence and cooperation
- mental state of the patient
- medical condition and clinical state of the patient
- size and weight of the patient
- working environment
- urgency
- number of staff needed and available
- whether there is any lifting/moving equipment available
- whether there are any mechanical aids available and functioning.

Remember:

- take into account task, load, working environment and the individual's capabilities
- learn the principles underlying the basic techniques and adapt these to each situation.

'There is no magic technique that works in every situation' (Scott, 1995).

Training programmes appropriate to each clinical environment are also vital if a change in attitude toward handling is to be achieved. Blamire (1995) highlights training as an important issue in ensuring that safe handling procedures are followed. Prescriptive, step-by-step routines designed to standardize practice and ensure uniformity and compliance are both impractical and inflexible when used to move anything other than inanimate objects. Once again there is a need to consider the uniqueness of each handling situation, together with the individual skills of those carrying out the manoeuvre.

Principles of training

The following are the principles of training for safe practice in moving and handling (Blamire, 1995):

- Training must be tailored to the needs of the different groups of trainees/clients.
- Aims and objectives must be clearly identified.

- The expected outcome of each training session must be clearly defined to prevent misleading assumptions.
- Some trainees will themselves be expected to become trainers and will require teaching skills.
- Manual handling skills should not be taught as a series of procedures designed to deal with single situations, but should be taught as principles to be adapted and modified.
- Assessments of situations and people's disabilities are the foundation of good decision-making, preparation and practice.
- Moving and handling disabled individuals must be managed in the context of promoting independence.
- There is a spectrum of assistance for the disabled, ranging from those who require minimal assistance to those who require lifting. The aim must be the right amount of the right kind of help. Lifting must always be a last resort and, when appropriate, a mechanical aid selected and used correctly.
- Manual handling skills are required in all activities, not just in the workplace.
- Training must be evaluated and audited to allow appropriate changes to be made.
- A full and accurate record must be kept of all training provided.

Once appropriate training has taken place it is important to ensure that staff adhere to the principles they have learnt.

Hack (1996) suggests that a three-fold strategy needs to be devised involving:

1. The constant reinforcement of principles of manual handling through remodelling, teaching and practical demonstration.
2. The updating of staff through rolling programmes.
3. The supplementation of practical teaching with written information.

To change existing habits she also suggests the introduction of:

- individual counselling, ward meetings and written information
- strategies to promote the positive benefits of change, such as reduction in incidence of injury
- observation and supervision at ward level.

Competence and safety in moving and handling procedures will only be achieved if reinforcement of training takes place. Thorough implementation of HSE (1992) regulations which provide a more explicit framework for risk assessment, while not eliminating the need to lift, would help to reduce the factors that hinder safe practice. It would appear that aiming towards a 'minimal risk' rather than a 'no lifting' policy would be more appropriate in the speciality of trauma. It is important to be aware of the availability of equipment that may be used to reduce the need to lift.

The shift in policy advocated by the new regulations requires greater emphasis on the provision and use of moving and handling aids. The EC 90/269 directive clearly states that 'dangers and hazards must be identified and equipment provided for safer working practice for staff and carers'. The key obviously lies in the provision of appropriate items of equipment for the task in hand. With the myriad of choice now available, it is often thought surprising that injuries continue to escalate (Owen and Garg, 1994). Could it be perhaps that the extent of this choice in some way creates its own problems, confusion abounding as to which might be the appropriate aid to use?

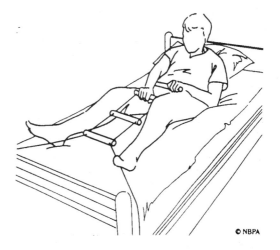

Figure 24.2 Ladder (From NBPA)

Numerous articles give an overview of the many products available (Tarling, 1992; Seymour, 1995; Trevelyn, 1996; Cowan, 1997), with each successive document providing a longer

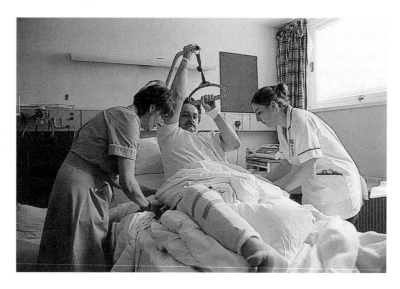

Figure 24.3 Monkey pole

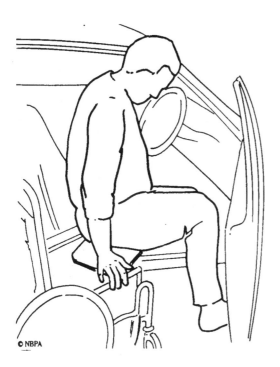

Figure 24.4 Transfer board (From NBPA)

patients must be carefully examined when considering the purchase of lifting aids in order to ensure adequate support for safe and painless transfer (Figures 24.2–24.8a,b).

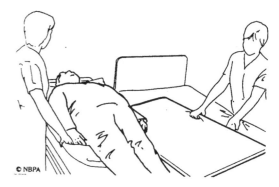

Figure 24.5 Board slide (From NBPA)

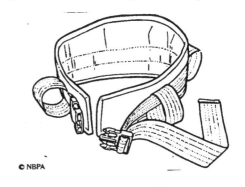

Figure 24.6 Handling belt (From NBPA)

list. For example, Cowan (1997) outlines the attributes of 16 hoists, 6 transfer boards, 5 sliding sheets and 14 other gadgets, from swivel cushions to transfer disks. It would seem the choice is limitless and the needs of trauma

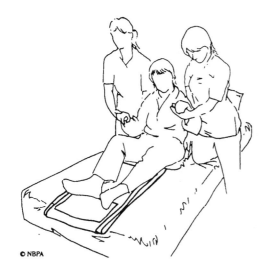
© NBPA

Figure 24.7   Sliding sheet (From NBPA)

A number of issues need to be considered when reviewing aids, such as ease of raising, lowering, stability, safety, comfort and dignity. More importantly, adequate training related to usage is vital.

Connolly *et al.* (1990) found that 22% of staff had no training in the use of aids, 61% had informal training only and 45% of nurses stated that they had neither a sufficient number, nor variety of aids to meet client needs.

The report found that 56% of staff did not use aids, as they felt that the aids available did not match client needs. This can be an issue in trauma, where patients with unstable injuries cannot be positioned or adequately supported in slings in order to enable safe transfer by such means. Many could also experience pain, as hoist slings can apply pressure at the exact point of injury.

Conclusion

As yet there is little evidence to suggest that the introduction of the EC 90/269 directive has had a great deal of effect on reducing the incidence of back injury, or indeed on influencing the amount of handling carried out.

Although advice abounds, there is little researched information available that gives clear, tried and tested guidance as to how to approach moving and handling. Indeed it could

perhaps be argued that it is this very abundance of advice that makes tackling the whole issue so complex.

Working towards the adoption of a no-lifting policy is perhaps over ambitious at this time, particularly in a speciality such as trauma. Tracy (1996) believes that patient handling still has a role, but that more emphasis should be placed on teaching the correct use of aids, as opposed to lifting techniques, in order to reduce risk. Willis (1996) would argue that it is not always reasonably practical to avoid manual handling altogether, and when this is the case the aim should be to take all appropriate steps to minimize risk.

Awareness of the uniqueness of each patient in the trauma setting must always be foremost in the minds of those carrying out handling tasks. Hignett (1994) refers to nursing as being 'typically a dynamic, heterogeneous job performed in multi-functional work stations'. She believes that this, combined with the handling of human beings and the inherent multitude of variables, prevents generic tasks from being identified. Specially applied to lifting, the task will be different on every occasion, affected by changes in the patient's condition, location within the ward, or the involvement of different staff members. These are the very issues encountered in a speciality such as trauma, where a risk assessment tool should be designed specifically to meet the needs of the clinical area in which it is to be used.

Staff intuition, together with experience, can influence practice. In valuing the experience and incorporating it within a tool, it may be possible more readily to encourage its use and overcome the problem of non-compliance. The tool itself should aim to identify and accommodate the unique needs of trauma patients in addition to the demands made on staff. Risk assessment should also give consideration to the variety of aids and equipment required, and how such provision might be funded.

The whole process of risk assessment must be supported by a training programme. The *Guide to Handling Patients: Introducing a Safer Handling Policy* (RCN, 1998) provides guidance in this area.

Within the field of trauma care, aiming to create a minimal risk code of practice may be the most appropriate direction to take in order to meet the needs of the unique patient population while acknowledging the require-

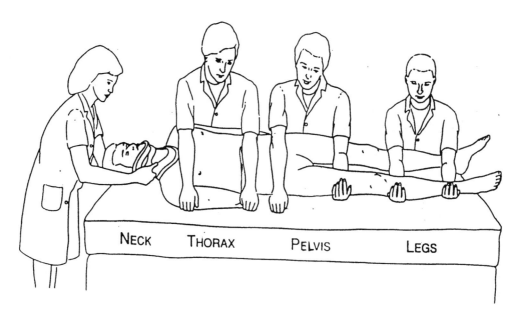

Figure 24.8a Preparing to log roll

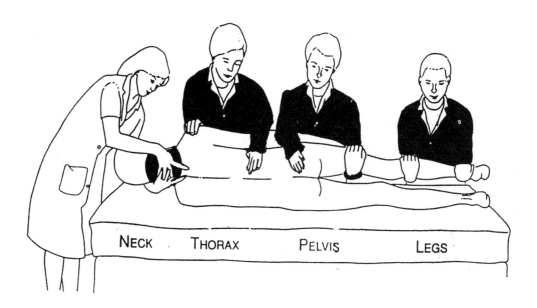

Figure 24.8b Log rolling

ments of the regulations laid down by both the EC and the HSE. The introduction of a code of practice, as opposed to a policy statement, is advocated as it would 'reflect the culture and work practices of a work environment, evolving in a local context to reflect the contextual biases of the setting it will serve' (Homans, 1951).

References

Backer, C., Degultis, L. and DeSantis, J. (1985) Impact of

trauma service on trauma care in University Hospital. *American Journal of Surgery*, **149**, 453.

Barker, K. L., Bell, R. E., Green, W. H. and Klaber-Moffet, J. (1992) *Trainer's Manual for the Prevention of Back Injury*. Nuffield Orthopaedic Centre.

Blamire, G. (1995) An educational framework for training in manual handling. *Physiotherapy*, March, **81**(3), 149–153.

Christie, J. (1994) *Trauma Nurses' Perception of Trauma Nursing*. MSc in Nursing. Unpublished.

Connolly, M. J., Wilkinson, E., Flanagan, S. and Mulley, G. P. (1990) Nurses' attitudes to and the use of patient hoists in hospitals. *Clinical Rehabilitation*, **4**, 13–17.

Corlett, E. N., Lloyd. P. V., Tarling, C. *et al.* (1992) *Guide to Handling Patients*. National Back Pain Association.

Cowan, T. (1997) Patient moving and handling equipment. *Professional Nurse*, June, **12**(9), 660–668.

European Commission (1990) Council directive on the minimum health and safety requirements for the minimal handling of loads where there is a risk, particularly of back injury, to workers. 90/269/EEC. *Official Journal of the European Communities*, **4**, 156–159.

Hignett, S. (1994) Shifting the emphasis in patient handling. *Occupational Health*, April, 127–130.

Hignett, S. and Richardson, B. (1995) Manual handling human loads in a hospital: an exploratory study to identify nurses' perceptions. *Applied Ergonomics*, **26**(3), 221–226.

Homans, G. C. (1951) *The Human Group*. Routledge Kegan Paul.

HSE (1992) *Manual Handling: Guidance on Regulations L.23. Manual Handling Operations Regulations*. Health and Safety Executive.

HSE (1994) *Five Steps to Risk Assessment*. Health and Safety Executive.

Jones, N. (1993) Lifting patients. *Community Outlook*, Jan., 12–14.

Love, C. (1996) Injury caused by lifting: a study of the nurse's viewpoint. *Nursing Standard*, **10**(46), 34–39.

Moffet, J. A. K., Hughes, G. I. and Griffiths, P. (1993) A longitudinal study of low back pain in student nurses. *International Journal of Nursing Studies*, **30**(3), 197–212.

Newman, R. J. (1992) *Orthogeriatrics: Comprehensive Care for the Elderly*. Butterworth–Heinemann.

Owen, B. D. and Garg, A. (1994) Reducing back stress through an ergonomic approach: weighing a patient. *International Journal of Nursing Studies*, **31**(6), 511–519.

Pilling, S. (1993) Calculating the risk. *Nursing Standard*, October, **8**(6), 18–20.

RCN (1996a) *Hazards of Nursing: Personal Injuries at Work*. RCN.

RCN (1996b) *Manual Handling Assessments in Hospitals and the Community*. RCN.

RCN (1998) *Guide to the Handling of Patients: Introducing a Safer Handling Policy*. RCN.

Scott, A. (1995) Improving patient moving and handling skills. *Professional Nurse*, **11**(2), 105–110.

Seymour, J. (1995) Handling aids: lifting and moving patients. *Nursing Times*. July, **91**(27), 48–50.

Smedley, J., Eggar, P., Cooper, C. and Coggon, D. (1997) Prospective cohort study of predictors of incidents of low back pain in nurses. *British Medical Journal*, **314**, 1225–1228.

Smith, G. and Seccombe, I. (1996) *Manual Handling: Issues for Nurses*. RCN/Institute of Employment Studies.

Snell, J. (1995) Raising awareness. *Nursing Times*, **91**(31), 20–21.

Tarling, C. (1992) The right equipment. *Nursing Times*, **88**(50), 38–40.

Tracy, M. (1996) Campaign for safer patient handling. *Occupational Health*, **94**, 127–130.

Trevelyn, J. (1996) Handling aids for nurses and carers. *Nursing Times*, **92**(8), 58–60.

Venning, P. J. (1988) Back injury prevention among nursing personnel. *American Association of Occupational Health Nurses Journal*, **36**(8), 327–322.

Willis, J. (1996) Moving and handling: guidelines for back care. *Nursing Times*, **92**(49), 48–50.

25

The consequences of altered body image following trauma

Kerry Davidson

Introduction

Altered body image (ABI) is usually associated with loss of physical function and cosmetic appearance. Wright (1986) defines ABI as 'a change in appearance or function of any part of our body which threatens our body image'. This change does not have to be scarring or disfigurement. Such a definition has wide implications for individuals post-trauma. Accidental injury, together with an unplanned admission to hospital, will lead to a change in a person's life and therefore an alteration in their perception of self. The trauma patient, according to Price (1986), has difficulty adapting to ABI due to the rapid change in image and the lack of psychological preparation for that change. These changes include a decrease in self-esteem, a role change, and the physical and psychological sequelae of injury in addition to an unexpected dependence on health professionals.

Cronan (1993) suggests that nurses are well placed to help patients deal with their ABI. However, in many instances the problem of ABI may not be managed as well as it could due to the fact that nurses may not have the knowledge to 'think past the scar'. Macginley (1993) states that without this essential knowledge and skill, nurses are unable to help patients obtain and maintain a positive body image. Conway (1994) suggests that the ideal type of nurse expert is one who uses both theory and practice in order to inform care. Experienced nurses have a wealth of practical knowledge, but for many the necessary and complementary theoretical knowledge, particularly in relation to an issue such as ABI, may well be lacking. The same could also be said of other disciplines.

Normal body image

Can ABI be recognized if the concept of normal body image (NBI) is not understood? Price (1990) argues that an understanding of NBI is critical if changes and problems associated with ABI are to be appreciated. NBI is something we all possess, but may never really recognize. Salter (1988) suggests that NBI is complex and continually changing, but rarely consciously confronted.

Price's model of body image (Figure 25.1) illustrates the three main components that make up NBI – ideal, reality and presentation. He suggests that these three components are in a state of dynamic balance. When one changes, the others change in order to maintain an equilibrium. There are many factors which influence these components including the ageing process (Janelli, 1986), culture and the environment (Macginley, 1993), society, peer pressure, media and fashion (Cronan, 1993).

Nurses and other healthcare professionals must develop an understanding of NBI before they can hope to address the greater complexities of ABI.

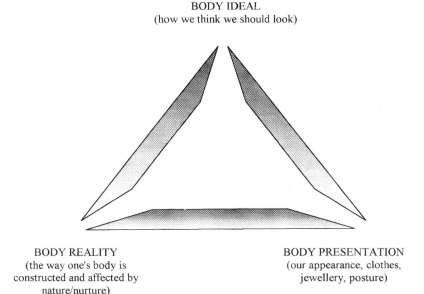

BODY IDEAL
(how we think we should look)

BODY REALITY
(the way one's body is
constructed and affected by
nature/nurture)

BODY PRESENTATION
(our appearance, clothes,
jewellery, posture)

Figure 25.1 The three main components of body image (From Price 1990)

Altered body image

According to Price (1986), following trauma, patients have difficulty adapting to ABI due to the fact that the change in image is so rapid and that inevitably there can be no psychological preparation for such a change. Sequelae that may contribute to ABI post-injury are highlighted in Figure 25.2. The many factors which impact on body image in addition to a patient's personal response are summarized in Figure 25.3.

When looked at together, both of these diagrammatic representations form a complete picture specifically from the patient's perspective. Griffin (1982) emphasizes that loss of control alters the concept of self. Webb (1985) suggests that just being in hospital and needing assistance with activities of daily living can affect body image.

The passage of reflection which follows explores the impact of ABI for one patient and her primary nurse. The patient's struggle towards acceptance and the nurse's struggle to care help link theory to reality, providing a good example of the effect that knowledge can have on practice.

Reflections of a nurse

I get up in the morning, look in the mirror and, I have to say, I am not usually happy with what I see. Too fat, too spotty, grey hair – the list seems endless, showing that on occasion I have a problem with my body image. Schilder (1989) defines body image as the picture of our body which we form in our mind, the way our body appears to ourselves. Simply put then, body image is the way we see ourselves. Perhaps I am unhappy with my body image because obviously it changes throughout life. Cronan (1993) suggests that body image problems arise naturally within the ageing process because of the conflict between feelings and looks. Much of the time I still feel inside as I did when I was twenty-two, the same moral values, beliefs and sense of fun. I feel young, but every day I look in the mirror and see my thirty years. What a conflict. Societal pressures also affect body image; as far as the media are concerned good-looking equals thin. Where is the room for the fat, birth-marked and teeth-braced people of the world? Salter (1988) suggests that society exerts great pressure on us to comply with a certain image, while Cronan (1993) specifies fashion, mass media, socialization, culture and peer pressure as factors affecting

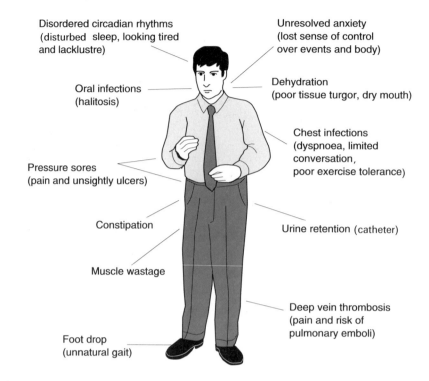

Figure 25.2   Sequelae that undermine body image (Adapted from Price, 1990)

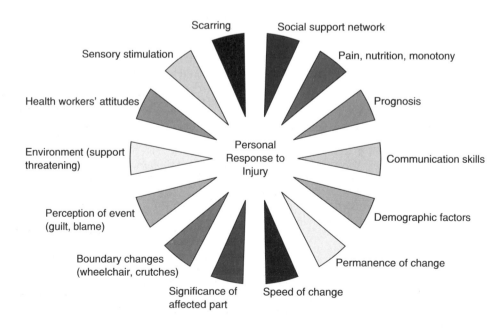

Figure 25.3   Factors impacting on body image (Adapted from Salter, 1988; Macginley, 1993; Price, 1990)

body image formation.

If I have problems accepting my own body image which is 'normal', how then can I hope to address the problems people with altered body image experience post-trauma? Wright (1986) suggests that any change in appearance or function of any part of our body threatens our body image. This change does not have to be obvious scarring or disfigurement. Following trauma, patients will have experienced some change in function which will affect how they feel about themselves. I want to develop insight into what I can do to help them come to terms with this change.

Example

Kim, a forty-six year old lady who had sustained multiple injuries, was admitted to the ward from ICU. Her fractures had been stabilized and split skin grafts had been applied to her right leg. She was to be on bedrest for a period of about 3 weeks prior to mobilization in a wheelchair. At the end of a 5-week stay she was still only allowed to partially weight-bear through her left leg. Initially, as Kim was so ill, she was extremely dependent. As nurses, we carried out all aspects of personal care, on many occasions giving her little choice. For example, 'I'm just going to help you with a wash'. Griffin (1982) states that forced dependency is a very significant stressor for critically ill patients. Kim must have felt no control over her situation. Griffin (1982) goes on to suggest that levels of control in daily life are incorporated into one's identity. My behaviour was fostering in Kim an attitude of dependence. Small changes such as 'Are you ready for a wash?', 'Which night-dress would you like to wear?' would have helped Kim to feel she had some control. I was not aware of the extent to which loss of control could affect body image.

This suggests that every person admitted to hospital following trauma will suffer from altered body image (ABI), not necessarily as a result of injury, but from loss of control and change in role. Webb (1985) is in agreement, stating that simply being in hospital and needing assistance with the activities of daily living can influence body image. Emerson (1983) recognizes that a crisis occurs when the previous equilibrium is upset. Unplanned admission to hospital following accidental injury would upset this equilibrium. Kim had been badly injured, endured role change, dependence and anxiety about her partner,

John, who was also injured in the accident. With that much to contend with, I would feel terrible too!

As Kim's condition improved, she became very aware of the physical aspects of ABI. Dewing (1989) suggests that body image has two components – the physical and psychological. This was very evident in Kim's case as she had to overcome many psychological barriers in order to accept her physical disabilities. Awareness of the skin grafts came the first time the dressings were changed. When I began to take the dressings down I explained that the grafts would look very red and raw and that if she did not want to look at them that would be fine. I had spent a few days building up a rapport with Kim to gain her trust. I felt that if she trusted me she would be able to cope more easily. I explained that her sites would not appear good from her point of view, but would probably look healthy and good from mine. Gaster (1995) suggests that the key characteristic in the relationships professionals have with clients is trust, and that the key values are integrity and fair conduct. I had not wanted to give Kim an unrealistic view of what to expect. She was devastated – 'pavement pizza' and 'raw meat' were her words. I spent a long time with her while she cried, looking back and grieving for what she had lost. I tried to reassure her that things would improve and that her leg would not look like that forever. Piff (1986) suggests that the reaction patients have to their disfigurement strongly influences how they cope in the future. Therefore inexperienced staff need to be aware of this and temper their own reactions accordingly.

A few days later an ex-patient was readmitted. Six months previously he had undergone significant skin grafting to his leg. I asked him if he would mind showing his grafts to Kim and he agreed. Kim did seem happier knowing that cosmetically the sight of her leg would improve. Drench (1994) states that interaction with people who have similar body image deficits, but lead active lives, seems to help an individual make the transition to a new and acceptable body image. I now thought that I was beginning to make headway with Kim, but she remained emotionally labile – one moment happy and the next sobbing uncontrollably. I spent a lot of time with her, listening and talking. Finally, I felt that I had built up a good trusting relationship. Trust, according to Macginley (1993) is very important if a nurse is to help a patient adapt to ABI.

One aspect of Kim's admission which proved

problematic concerned contact with her family and their involvement in her care. Kim and John's home was some 45 miles away from the hospital and, coupled with the fact that John himself had been hospitalized for 10 days, his injuries also prevented him from driving. As a result, he could only visit twice a week. Norbeck (1981) stresses the importance of the patient's own effective support network. I felt that the infrequency of John's visits meant that Kim was missing a vital element of her care, which could help her come to terms with her ABI. Kim attributed John's absence to the way she looked. This reaction is not uncommon. Goffman (1963) suggests that an individual with a physical deformity or disability becomes stigmatized, that person being 'reduced' in the mind of society. Kim felt that John was letting her down and, because of perceived value systems within society, she subsequently did not seem important to John or to herself. Smitherham (1981) states that the ideal body image in our society represents youth, beauty, vigour, intactness and health; anyone deviating from this ideal is likely to suffer from decreased self-esteem, insecurity and anxiety. Kim was continually upset and I think that Smitherham's ideas explain why she felt no one would love her any more, and that as a result she could not love herself. Media and peer pressure have a hinge effect on individuals and their self-image. Price (1990) suggests that self-image relies on approval from others. All the talking in the world did not improve Kim's emotional state. So, no more talking.

We began in earnest to educate Kim in how to become more independent, to increase her self-esteem and motivation. This was quite difficult at first, because of her forced dependency. We had pushed Kim into a dependent role. Therefore we began to set daily achievable goals such as rubbing cream into her donor site. This was beneficial, as Smith (1989) states that the use of touch can be developed to therapeutic effect. By touching Kim and encouraging her to touch her donor site and scars, we were increasing self-esteem. We encouraged her to get dressed and taught her to transfer from bed to wheelchair. We were re-establishing her independence in preparation for self-care and discharge. We praised her in order to acknowledge that progress was being made and we evaluated outcomes to increase self-esteem further. Meisenhelder (1985) states that it is not the actual self-care task, but rather the verbal feedback that provides an individual with positive self-appraisal and increased self-

esteem. We had kept Kim informed and aware of any telephone calls from her family in order to combat her feelings of family neglect and kept her up to date with her treatment plan. Wilson-Barnett (1980) suggests that giving information reduces anxiety and aids adjustment to stressful events before they occur.

I thought we were doing a good job in promoting Kim's acceptance of her ABI, but she continued to be very emotional and cried endlessly. We tried to get her to see a counsellor, with a view to helping her come to terms with her injuries, but she would not. I was beginning to become very judgemental, thinking 'why doesn't she just pull herself together? I haven't got time for this.' Macginley (1993) suggests that the nurse should be able to empathize with the patient's feelings in a positive and accepting manner, without being judgemental. I was no longer able to do this. I found it hard to care for Kim. Trying to deal with overwhelming feelings of despair and anger became difficult and occupied more and more time, until sometimes I just left her to cry because it was just too much for me to take. Mellor (1996) suggests that getting close to patients can be stressful and can lead to burnout. By this stage I did not even feel guilty about my actions – the whole nursing team had spent a great deal of time with Kim, yet it was still not enough.

At the point of discharge home Kim was still very emotional and prone to frequent bouts of crying. Overall she had done well and achieved a great deal; our involving her regularly in planning and evaluating her care had helped. Price (1986) advocates the involvement of patients in their care, concluding that they will be more likely to come to terms with their body image as a result. Kim went home and, despite the whole team having tried hard on her behalf, we had failed. No, not failed, but not quite made the grade.

Discussion

After reflecting on this episode, my reading has led me to realize that there were gaps in my knowledge of normal body image and the stages that a person with ABI goes through. In future, my care will be enhanced by the knowledge that I have subsequently acquired. Price (1990) states that a nurse must become more aware of the normal, as a patient who suffers abrupt body image change will not have had time for such reflection.

Price suggests that when one component

changes, all the components have to adapt. This was difficult for Kim as so much had changed. Her body reality was altered; her ideal had changed; she was now dependent and had lost her normal role. Her choice of clothing would now change as she felt she should cover up her legs. Macginley (1993) suggests body reality is constantly changing from birth to old age. Kim was also going through the menopause – another change she was having to endure. She wanted her HRT patches but, due to the risk of deep vein thrombosis and embolism, they were not prescribed. No wonder she had such a hard time. All these different components were trying to adapt to change, some associated with normal body image and some with ABI. Kim was quite a plump lady and her skin grafts appeared very sunken. Perhaps she already had negative feelings about her body without the additional burden of alteration. Salter (1988) suggests that people with a high self-esteem will have a more realistic picture of their body than people with low self-esteem. She goes on to say that those with high self-esteem will adapt more readily to change in body image. Meisenhelder (1985) defines self-esteem as a positive regard for oneself and describes it as a key component in restoring and maintaining mental and physical health. If these concepts had been considered during Kim's admission, we may have been able to facilitate more acceptance and motivation.

Smith (1985) discusses the concept of patient power; nurses being able to allow a patient to have control over their own destiny. Did we allow this? We did eventually, following a stage of complete dependence, but could we have utilized my new knowledge more effectively in practice? The answer has to be 'yes'. By developing insight into normal body image in relation to ourselves, as well as Kim, a more holistic care plan could have been drawn up. I am not saying that we did not have a realistic care plan, but we did prioritize her problems specifically as anxiety, motivation, mobilization and wound care. However, in the light of this new knowledge relating to control, self-esteem and how a person adapts to ABI, the care plan could have been improved.

The last aspect of this episode involves the application of Dewing's four-stage model (Table 25.1) to Kim's experience of traumatic injury. Kim had retreated into denial and emotional withdrawal. She displayed only two emotions – anger and sadness. I think Kim was still in 'retreat' when she was discharged. Perhaps it would have been easier for those

nurses caring for her if we had realized that she was still at this stage, rather than having doubts about the quality of care she had received. Brennan (1994) suggests that a thorough assessment, systematic planning and evaluation of interventions are needed in order to enable patients to accept ABI. We had achieved most of this, but not the acceptance. This has significant implications for practice. I would suggest that many patients leave hospital following trauma only having reached the stages of retreat or acknowledgement. We, as a profession, should realize that anger and denial are going to be directed at us and that these patients subsequently need support from general practitioners and healthcare workers in the community

Some time later Kim was readmitted to hospital for a bone graft and her emotional state had improved. She was now acknowledging her problems, reliving her accident and actively searching out information and knowledge to enable her to cope. I am hopeful that the next time I see her, Kim will be at the reconstruction stage and that she will be making plans for the future.

The most important thing I have learnt is from Stanley (1977): **'Until nurses understand their own body image and can anticipate their reaction to the alteration in the patient's changed state, they may retard rather than hasten the patient's acceptance of change.'** I am now more aware of how I feel about my body image as a result of my reflections and feel that my future care of such patients will be improved.

Table 25.1 The four stages encountered by patients challenged by altered body image (Adapted from Dewing, 1989)

Impact	Initial shock, anger, depression and pessimism
Retreat	Mourning for affected part and desire to return to previous self, denial and emotional withdrawal
Acknowledgement	Confrontation of the problem, reliving events, searching for a cause and seeking information to aid coping mechanisms
Reconstruction	Recognition of implications, accepting the use of aids and planning for the future

Reflections of a patient

The following passage is the account of a patient's experience of altered body image. Jane sustained an unstable fracture of her cervical spine in a car accident. She was treated in halo traction initially, but this was soon converted to a halo brace which she then wore for 3 months until the fracture united.

In a study of patients who had experienced wearing such a brace, 79% of the sample reported that the halo brace affected their feelings about their appearance, and 17% reported that they felt like a freak, an alien or a Martian (Olsen *et al.*, 1991).

When the halo traction was put on I didn't know anything about it and when I realized what was attached to me I didn't really have any reaction other than 'What the hell is this?' When I first saw myself in the mirror it was like 'Oh my God, what is this contraption? I look like a bionic woman made of metal'. I then called it my bondage equipment (my odd sense of humour).

I did feel very ugly and out of place and very self-conscious because people were staring at me. Even though most of them were, there were three different types of people: those who continually stared; those who looked out of the corners of their eyes when they thought you couldn't see them; and those who looked and asked you what it was and were very friendly – just curious really.

In the hospital what people thought of me wasn't really an issue. I was in a hospital and you expect to see strange things there. I felt safe and when people stared I just stared back and either smiled or stuck my tongue out at them! Some days if I was tired or fed up it would upset me, but it never really got to me. On the ward people would stop at my bed and have a chat about what had happened to me, which was much nicer and made me feel less of a freak.

When I left the hospital it was totally different. I felt very self-conscious and abnormal and wouldn't go out if I didn't have to. Everyone looked at me then. Some people would laugh, which made me cry and then I would get angry and rebel a bit.

Even in the car at traffic lights some people would point and stare, which really infuriated me. I think it made me become more of a recluse and I would only go out for appointments.

At the doctor's surgery I even went in through the back entrance so that nobody would see me. I wasn't embarrassed about what I had on me, just very vulnerable to what the outside world thought of me.

I couldn't make myself look nice. I couldn't wear nice clothes, just very baggy T-shirts which didn't help matters much. I felt very frumpy and because of the halo couldn't have my hair nicely styled.

Where my family were concerned, children were scared of me and wouldn't hug or touch me which made me upset. They got used to it after a while, as children do, but even now, 10 months on, they won't have a cuddle with Auntie Jane because they are scared to touch me.

Even now (without the halo brace) I feel paranoid that everyone is staring at me, which isn't true because there's nothing for them to stare at – it's just in my mind.

Frustration was the main thing I felt when I had the halo brace on. With it on I couldn't do the things I normally would. I couldn't retaliate to the people who stared as I would have done normally.

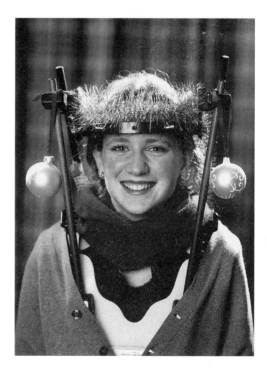

Figure 25.4 Patient with halo brace demonstrating a positive attitude to her predicament

This is the experience of one young woman. However, not all patients are alike. Figure 25.4

shows a different individual whose positive attitude to her 3-month sojourn was exemplified by the fact that the festive image shown in the photograph was a printed Christmas card!

References

Brennan, J. (1994) A vital component of care. The nurse's role in recognising altered body image. *Professional Nurse*, Feb., 298–303.

Conway, J. E. (1994) *Expert Nursing Knowledge as an Evolutionary Process*. PhD Thesis, Warwick University (unpublished).

Cronan, L. (1993) Management of the patient with altered body image. *British Journal of Nursing*, **2**(5), 257–261.

Dewing, J. (1989) Altered body image. *Surgical Nurse*, **2**(4), 17–20.

Drench, M. (1994) Changes in body image secondary to disease. *Rehabilitation Nursing*, **19**(1), 31–36.

Emerson, J. (1983) Living through grief. *Nursing Mirror*, **157,** 2–10.

Gaster, L. (1995) Quality in public services. *Manager's Choice*. Open University Press.

Goffman (1963); cited in Dewis, M. E. (1989) Spinal cord injured adolescents and young adults: the meaning of body changes. *Journal of Advanced Nursing*, **14,** 389–396.

Griffin, J. (1982) Forced dependency in the critically ill. *Dimensions of Critical Nursing*, **1**(6), 350–352.

Janelli, L. M. (1986) The realities of body image. *Gerontology Nursing*, **12**(10), 23–27.

Macginley, K. J. (1993) Nursing care of the patient with altered body image. *British Journal of Nursing*, **2**(22), 1098–1102.

Meisenhelder, J. (1985) Self-esteem: a closer look at clinical interventions. *International Journal of Nursing Studies*, **22**(2), 127–135.

Mellor, D. (1996) Altered body image. *Professional Nurse*, **11**(5), 296–298.

Norbeck, J. S. (1981) Social support: a model for clinical research and application. *Advanced Nursing Science*, July, 43–59.

Olsen, B., Ustanko, L. and Warner, S. (1991) The patient in a halo brace – striving for normalcy in body image and self-concept. *Orthopaedic Nursing*, **10**(1), 44–50.

Piff, C. (1986) Facing up to disfigurement. *Nursing Times*, **82,** 16–17.

Price, B. (1986) Keeping up appearances. *Nursing Times*, **82**(37), 58–61.

Price, B. (1990) *Body Image: Nursing Concepts and Care*. Prentice Hall.

Salter, M. (1988). *Altered Body Image: the Nurse's Role*. Wiley.

Schilder, E. (1989) Bodily perceptions and their influence on health. *Nursing Standard*, **4**(13), 30–32.

Smith, F. B. (1985) Patient power. *American Journal of Nursing*, Nov., 1260–1262.

Smith, S. A. (1989) Extended body image in the ventilated patient. *Intensive Care Nursing*, **5**(1), 31–38.

Smitherham (1981); Cited in Cronan, L. (1993). Management of the patient with altered body image. *British Journal of Nursing*, **2**(5), 257–261.

Stanley, I. (1977) Does your body image hurt patient care? *Registered Nurse*, **40**(12), 50–53.

Webb, C. (1985). *Sexuality, Nursing and Health*. Wiley.

Wilson-Barnett, J. (1980) Prevention and alleviation of stress in patients. *Nursing*, **1**(10), 432–436.

Wright, B. (1986). *Caring in Crisis*. Churchill Livingstone.

26

Communication – the foundation of successful care

Julie Wright

Introduction

Effective communication between patients, relatives and all members of the multidisciplinary team (MDT) is vital if the best possible outcomes from admission are to be achieved. Any breakdown in this system, or reduction in the quality of communication, will ultimately lead to less than satisfactory patient care (MacKay, 1993).

Successful communication is dependent on many factors – environmental, physical, cultural and professional – and 'involves all the senses' (Ford and Walsh, 1994) (Table 26.1). It is not only about practising learned interpersonal skills (Hartrick, 1997), but it allows the healthcare professional the opportunity to develop the necessary 'partnerships in care' (Wade, 1995).

What is communication?

Successful communication is the positive interaction of individuals by mutually understood means, in spite of those factors serving to prevent understanding (Bassett, 1993).

The communication process requires a sender, a message and someone to receive that message. This message is vulnerable to distortion during transmission, for example by background noise or the receiver's inability to concentrate and thus understand the communication (Shannon and Weaver, 1985). When the initial message has been received the communication process starts again, resulting in dialogue (Bowers and Moore, 1997).

According to Mikhail Bakhtin, a Russian philosopher, this 'dialogue' is greater than the simple exchange of spoken words. He believed that it includes non-verbal communication and portrays the individual in their entirety, at that moment. This allows any participant in the dialogue to relate to that person holistically (Bowers and Moore, 1997).

The messages or feedback can be in many forms: verbal, non-verbal or written. Verbal communication may be accepted as the spoken word (Jarrett and Payne, 1995). Non-verbal communication is the manner in which individuals truthfully convey their emotions using posture, facial expressions, gestures and position, i.e. 'all forms of human communication not controlled by speech' (Kacperek, 1997). It also includes para-linguistic cues such as laughter, sighs, groans and intonation (Brown, 1997). As such, body language can be used to facilitate or discourage communication (Brown, 1997). Also, the importance of silence should not be underestimated. When used in conjunction with verbal communication, it can be a powerful tool, sometimes transmitting more meaning than words (Lomax, 1997).

All members of the MDT must accept that the quality of their communication has a direct relationship to their success in treating a patient (Bassett, 1993). Not only must they have knowledge of those means of communication at their disposal (Table 26.2), but also an understanding of their profound effects (Table

Table 26.1 Factors influencing communication

Environmental	Physical	Cultural	Professional
Equipment noise	Inability to speak	Language	Self-awareness
General conversation	Patient position	Gender	Use of aids
Decor	Disorientation	Religion	Assessment of situation
Sleep deprivation	Unconsciousness	Social status	
		Education	

26.3). Each individual requires a significant degree of self-awareness in order to be effective in the provision of holistic care (Smith, 1995; Bowers and Moore, 1997).

Table 26.2 Means of communication

Verbal
Non-verbal
Para-linguistic cues
Touch
Reading
Writing

Table 26.3 Effects of communication

Give/gain information
Relinquish/assume control
Give/receive comfort and reassurance
Give/gain pleasure

The effects of trauma on communication

When an individual experiences or even witnesses an actual or perceived threat to life or limb, that person is shocked, frightened, totally unprepared and usually helpless (Herbert, 1995). An individual will react to a traumatic event in their own unique way, and thus each member of the MDT has a duty to assure them that these reactions are normal, orientate them to reality and encourage them to assume control (Groves, 1986; Herbert, 1995).

Having reviewed a significant number of studies, Teasedale (1993) has found that verbal and written information about a situation does little to relieve anxiety, promote comfort or assume control. He suggests that patients have the greatest opportunity to reduce their anxieties when presented with the means to control

their situation, such as relaxation techniques to control pain or the opportunity to 'reframe' their fears in a less threatening way (Teasedale, 1993).

> *Example*
>
> A young man, having sustained a fracture to his tibia, developed compartment syndrome. In discussion he was informed that there was a 20% chance of amputation. Given the opportunity to consider the information about his situation, he was later able to express his fears in a more positive manner. He told his family that there was an 80% chance his leg would survive.

However, it is important to remember that not all patients wish to collaborate with members of the MDT in making decisions about the direction of their care (Waterworth and Luker, 1990). If healthcare professionals are to treat these patients as autonomous individuals, they must be prepared to provide care in a more maternalistic fashion (May, 1995).

It may be difficult for a member of the MDT to communicate positively with a person following major trauma.

> *Example*
>
> A confident, competent and knowledgeable staff nurse arrived on duty and found she was to care for a young man who had sustained a fracture to his cervical spine following a road traffic accident. Despite immediate reduction and stabilization of the fracture, the man lost all power and sensation to his lower limbs, with significantly reduced power and sensation to his upper limbs. The nurse found it difficult to approach the patient initially, because she 'couldn't bear to look him in the eye' for fear of communicating 'how sorry she felt for him' in this apparently hopeless situation.

The nurse in the above example was obviously self-aware, conscious of those aspects of her behaviour which might have been detrimental to her forming a therapeutic relationship with the patient (Smith, 1995). She had also acknowledged the fact that non-verbal behaviour, especially eye contact, is a very powerful communication tool (Davies, 1994). This scenario also illustrates her unwillingness to deceive the patient and thus create a barrier to effective communication in the future (Teasedale and Kent, 1995).

Communicating with the trauma patient

Some means of communication with the trauma patient are as follows (Groves, 1986; Herbert, 1995; Brown, 1997):

- *Gain eye contact.* This will add humanity and sincerity to the situation.
- *Introduce yourself.* First names mean the patient can immediately call on you for support or clarification.
- *Provide a precise and brief account of the situation.* Repeat as often as is necessary, even if the patient is unconscious.
- *Explain procedures.* These explanations should be general initially, then in more detail prior to any procedure, even if the patient is unconscious.
- *Touch.* Only if permission is given or deemed appropriate to the situation.

Communication and the professional–patient relationship

It is unrealistic to expect every member of the MDT to form a therapeutic relationship with every patient (May, 1995); a therapeutic relationship being that which results from the professional using all the skills, experience and knowledge at their disposal, together with their concern for a fellow human in order to facilitate their progress towards health (Hockey, 1991; Savage, 1995).

Some patients are admitted for day surgery or short periods of observation following trauma. Such patients may feel it unnecessary to form any sort of personal relationship with those professionals providing them with physical care

(Baillie, 1996) and consider communication on a superficial level to be sufficient. Some patients may actively avoid sharing intimate details with a healthcare professional they have never met before, considering such conversations as intrusions into their privacy (May, 1995). In these circumstances, Muxlow (1995) believes it is still possible for the nurse to provide care at a more detached and professional level.

Baillie (1996) states that 'the level of involvement often depends on how much time the nurse spends with the patient'. This may imply that primary nursing, where the patient is provided with a greater opportunity to communicate with a smaller number of nurses, would be more likely to result in the formation of therapeutic relationships, thus leading to higher quality care. However, Ford and Walsh (1994) challenge this assumption by insisting that the quality of care is due to the knowledge, experience and ability of the nurse to practise reflectively, rather than the system of care delivery.

Example

A staff nurse caring for an elderly lady who had sustained a femoral neck fracture met her only 2 hours prior to surgery, and had spoken to the woman's daughter only once by telephone. The patient was frank regarding her wishes not to be resuscitated in the event of a cardiac or respiratory arrest. Perioperatively she suffered a cardiac arrest and, according to her wishes, was not resuscitated. The staff nurse arranged for her daughter to visit her in theatre. The woman's daughter later wrote, 'in a few short hours you helped Mum and myself in a way I will never forget'.

This example suggests that it is not always the amount of time spent with a patient that results in a caring relationship. It is the relating of two or more human beings, able to trust and accept one another's individuality, which results in the formation of this therapeutic bond and leads to satisfaction with care (Wade, 1995; Hartrick, 1997; Bowers and Moore, 1997).

Seemingly then, it is possible for a strong therapeutic relationship to exist between professional and patient. This intimate level of communication between individuals is not solely dependent on the amount of time spent together, but on whether these human beings connect. According to MacKay (1993) and Bassett (1993), this high quality of communication should result in excellent patient care. However, the emotional demands made on the professional in this close relationship may eventually cause them anxiety and ultimately have a detrimental effect on their ability to provide care of such an intimate nature (Muxlow, 1995; Baillie, 1996).

Deception, empowerment and effective communication

In order for a therapeutic relationship to exist between professional and patient, there must be a connection between the two individuals, some emotional investment and therefore an element of trust (Baillie, 1996; Hartrick, 1997).

In a limited study, Teasedale and Kent (1995) found that nurses rarely, then albeit reluctantly, used deception (i.e. lying and non-disclosure of information) in practice. Instances in which deception was identified involved non-disclosure of information related to diagnosis or prognosis, distorting the course of events and distracting patients with information not directly related to their anxiety (Teasedale and Kent, 1995). The most common reason for these forms of deception was that a family or consultant did not want a patient to know about their diagnosis or prognosis lest they 'give up', or become 'upset' or 'difficult to manage' (Teasedale and Kent, 1995; Woods, 1998). Aside from the moral and ethical implications, the use of deception presents a huge barrier to communication between healthcare professional, patient and family – especially when that deception is discovered. The element of trust in a relationship is inevitably lost (Teasedale and Kent, 1995; Woods, 1998).

Example

A middle-aged lady was admitted for cervical spine stabilization. She had been suffering pain, together with altered power and sensation in all limbs associated with vertebral collapse, pathological in origin. Her caring and attentive daughters met with the consultant for an update on their mother's diagnosis, prognosis and further treatment options. A malignant tumour was removed from the patient's spine and when she had recovered from surgery she was to be transferred for radiotherapy and other symptomatic treatment. Both daughters asked that the diagnosis and treatment plan be kept from their mother. The consultant (and subsequently the rest of the MDT) agreed that the information would not be disclosed.

In accordance with the findings of Woods (1998), this family were trying to protect their mother from information which they felt may harm and upset her. However, they were never told that their good intentions denied their mother autonomy and the opportunity to work with the healthcare professionals and her family, directing and influencing care as she felt was appropriate to her needs (Woods, 1998). She had been disempowered and the power to influence the direction of her future care remained with the MDT (Wright, 1995).

Members of the team, by colluding with the family, were left in the unenviable position of questioning their duty to care and their roles as patient's advocate (Teasedale and Kent, 1995; Woods, 1998). The nurses in particular would have been aware that this deception prevented them from communicating with this patient on a more intimate level, because it was impossible to relate in an honest, respectful and empathetic manner (Teasedale and Kent, 1995; Hartrick, 1997). The opportunity to form a therapeutic relationship was missed. The patient herself may well have been aware that her diagnosis and prognosis were grim, but decided to join her family and carers in the pretence in order not to distress them (Jarrett and Payne, 1995). In finding that her carers and family had knowingly deceived her, this lady may also have developed negative feelings about the quality of her care (Teasedale and Kent, 1995).

It appears that deception has no positive effects on the communication process between the healthcare professional and patient, and thus on their perceived quality of care (Teasedale and Kent, 1995). The patient described in the previous example may have perceived the MDT as having more power, knowledge and thus control over her life than she, resulting in a huge communication barrier. The elements of reciprocity and mutuality i.e. partnership, were absent (Wade, 1995). Individual professionals should reflect on their practice and, with the team, develop a culture which is honest, open and naturally discourages such deception (Woods, 1998).

The use of humour in communication

Humour is difficult to identify and define because its use and comprehension varies with individuals (Simon, 1988; Sumners, 1990). The majority of research into humour and its effects has been conducted by social scientists (Savage, 1995), who believe its effects range from managing stress and encouraging creative thinking, to altering the disease process (Mallet, 1993, 1996; Simon, 1998).

It is therefore surprising to find that relatively little research has been conducted into the use of humour by healthcare professionals in the course of their practice. Those studies in existence demonstrate that humour is used in nurse–patient communication (Mallett and A'Hern, 1996) and is generally accepted as an integral part of communication within that relationship (Simon, 1988; Sumners, 1990). Fosbinder (1994) believes that trading personal information and engaging in humorous dialogue is vital in the building of a therapeutic relationship. Savage (1995) agrees and suggests that the use of humour in communication creates an atmosphere whereby both professional and patient reveal more of their personalities. She believes that this helps both parties to negotiate ambiguous topics or areas of conversation regarding the intimacies of patient care. There is also some suggestion that the ability of a patient to use humour in communication indicates their recovery (Savage, 1995) and, in the older adult, satisfaction with life (Simon, 1988). However, the evidence is vague and varies significantly according to the persons involved in the relationship.

The potential for the therapeutic use of humour in communication appears to be great. However, Sumners (1990) states that injudicious use can be detrimental, conveying anger and resulting in the destruction of self-esteem. Hulatt (1993) warns that healthcare professionals should think about what they are aiming to convey before using humour to vent anger or frustration. However, Naish (1995) warns against the planned and possibly forced use of humour by health professionals as, without spontaneity, the many benefits may be lost.

Barriers to verbal communication

Having concentrated on and emphasized the importance of non-verbal communication in the formation of relationships, it is useful to consider the role of the spoken word in effective communication.

Despite the general acceptance that dialogue is a two-way process (Jarrett and Payne, 1995; Bowers and Moore, 1997), it seems unusual that many researchers have concentrated on the nurse's contribution and largely ignored that made by the patient (Jarrett and Payne, 1995). It was assumed that most nurses (and probably most other healthcare professionals) lacked effective communication skills, until Wilkinson (1991) suggested that nurses in particular were skilful manipulators of conversation. Dialogue was 'blocked' or 'facilitated' using non-verbal and verbal cues, steering the conversation to elicit more information from the patient or avoid potentially difficult areas as perceived by the nurse. This implies that the patient is a passive participant in any conversation. However, Jarrett and Payne (1995) argue that patients may also steer dialogue in order to receive or avoid disclosure of information to any healthcare professional.

Payne and James (1995) suggest that the use of 'professional jargon', together with the perceived social status and education of the participants, may constitute a barrier to effective communication. In a small study, they found that 33% of medical terms elicited contradictory responses from healthcare professionals and members of the general public. Therefore staff must determine whether the patient's understanding of any medical terminology used is actually that which the healthcare professional intended to convey (Payne and James, 1995).

Livingstone (1991) advocates that the healthcare professional should think before speaking, carefully explaining the use of any medical jargon or abbreviations. However, Bowles (1995) in a short, anecdotal article warns that the professional should never underestimate patients (or relatives), but be acutely aware of the limits of their own knowledge in order that their explanations are accurate.

A more obvious barrier to verbal communication is the fact that one may not be able to communicate with the patient in the same language. Despite our ability to communicate our attitudes and feelings non-verbally (Brown, 1997; Lomax, 1997), it is difficult, sometimes impossible, to impart or gain important information regarding an individual's treatment or diagnosis in the presence of a language barrier (Roberts, 1994). Roberts found that a language barrier also resulted in cultural misunderstandings, and ultimately the failure of nurses to form therapeutic relationships with patients. Even if a patient had some comprehension or ability to use the same language as the nurse, it was apparent to Roberts (1994) that an anxiety-inducing admission to hospital resulted in a reliance on their first language. There can be no greater anxiety-inducing admission than that following trauma.

Example

A 74-year-old lady, originally from a southern province of China, had been resident in the UK for almost 40 years. She and her family ran a successful restaurant and she was obviously a respected and supportive member of her small community. However, she spoke no English. Having slipped and fractured her ankle she required surgery and was admitted to hospital. On admission she was accompanied by her son who spoke fluent English as well as his native dialect. Her primary nurse quickly seized the opportunity to learn a few words and phrases of Chinese, asking her son to pronounce these as he wrote them on a clipboard. The son visited and stayed as often as possible and, in his absence, the nursing staff used the words and phrases jotted on the clipboard. Their vocabulary increased over time.

In this manner, both patient and nurses were able to communicate verbally, even if only in relation to a few key aspects of care. Nodding vigorously, clapping her hands and smiling, she obviously appreciated the nurses' attempts to communicate with her in her native language.

Roberts (1994) found that the majority of patients valued these instances of 'limited phrase switching', interpreting them as a means of demonstrating respect for a different culture. Patients also perceived those staff who attempted to communicate in their language as more 'intimate and homely' (Roberts, 1994).

Some of the physical and cognitive barriers to verbal communication encountered by patients following traumatic injury can be as a result of facial fractures, head injury, concomitant dementia/stroke, or the formation of a tracheostomy. Discussion of the specific communication issues associated with any of these barriers is beyond the scope of this chapter, the reader is advised to seek further information from the relevant specialist texts.

Conclusion

Communication is a complex process involving much more than the mere exchange of words. In acute care settings, and particularly in the speciality of trauma, the balance of power between the participants, patients and professionals could be perceived as being far from equal; the patient – unprepared, afraid, lacking information; the professional – knowledgeable, prepared and in a familiar environment. It is the responsibility of all professionals to redress this balance in order for both patients and families to become equal partners in the recovery process. Effective communication is the foundation of successful care, playing a key role in the achievement of optimal patient outcomes.

References

Baillie, L. (1996) How nurses view emotional involvement with patients. *Nursing Times*, **92**(9), 35–36.

Bassett, C. (1993) Communication with the critically ill. *Care of the Critically Ill*, **9**(5), 216–217, 219.

Bowers, R. and Moore, K. (1997) Bakhtin, nursing narratives and dialogical consciousness. *Advances in Nursing Science*, March, **19**(3), 70–77.

Bowles, L. (1995) Learning from patients. *Professional Nurse*, **10**(9), 600.

Brown, T. (1997) Body talk. *Nursing Standard*, **11**(30), 21–23.

Davies, P. (1994) Non-verbal communication with patients. *British Journal of Nursing*, **3**(5), 220–223.

Ford, P. and Walsh, M. (1994) *New Rituals for Old: Nursing through the Looking Glass*, Butterworth-Heinemann.

Fosbinder, D. (1994) Patient perceptions of nursing care: an emerging theory of interpersonal competence. *Journal of Advanced Nursing*, **20**, 1085–1093.

Groves, M. J. (1986) In *Trauma Nursing* (V. D. Cardona, ed.). Wright.

Hartrick, G. (1997) Relational capacity: the foundation for interpersonal nursing practice. *Journal of Advanced Nursing*, **26**, 523–528.

Herbert, C. (1995) *Understanding Your Reactions to Trauma: A Booklet for Survivors of Trauma and their Families.* Warneford Hospital, Oxford.

Hockey, L. (1991) In *Nursing as Therapy* (R. McMahon and A. Pearson, eds). Chapman and Hall.

Hulatt, I. (1993) Just a laugh? *Nursing Times*, **89**(36), 41.

Jarrett, N. and Payne, S. (1995) A selective review of the literature on nurse–patient communication: has the patient's contribution been neglected? *Journal of Advanced Nursing*, **22**, 72–78.

Kacperek, L. (1997) Non-verbal communication: the importance of listening. *British Journal of Nursing*, **6**(5), 275–279.

Livingstone, S. (1991) Watch your language. *Nursing Standard*, **5**(20), 44.

Lomax, B. (1997) Learning to understand a patient's silence. *Nursing Times*, **93**(17), 48–49.

MacKay, L. (1993) *Conflicts in Care: Medicine and Nursing.* Chapman and Hall.

Mallett, T. (1993) Use of humour and laughter in patient care. *British Journal of Nursing*, **2**(3), 172–175.

Mallett, T. and A'Hern, R. (1996) Comparative distribution and use of humour within nurse–patient communication. *International Journal of Nursing Studies*, **33**(5), 530–550.

May, C. (1995) Patient autonomy and the politics of professional relationships. *Journal of Advanced Nursing*, **21**, 83–87.

Muxlow, J. (1995) The relationship between nurse and patient. *Professional Nurse*, **11**(1), 63–65.

Naish, T. (1995) Taking fun seriously. *Nursing Standard*, **9**(29), 18–20.

Payne, S. and James, B. (1995) Can they understand you? *Nursing Management*, **2**(7), 12–13.

Roberts, G. W. (1994) Nurse-patient communication within a bilingual healthcare setting. *British Journal of Nursing*, **3**(2), 60–67.

Savage, T. (1995) *Nursing Intimacy: An Ethnographic Approach to Nurse–Patient Interaction.* Scutari Press.

Shannon and Weaver (1985) In *Planning and Producing Instructions Media* (J. E. Kemp and D. K. Dayton, eds). Harper and Row.

Simon, T. M. (1988) Humour and the older adult: implications for nursing. *Journal of Advanced Nursing*, **13**, 441–446.

Smith, C. (1995) Learning about yourself helps patient care: using self-awareness to improve practice. *Professional Nurse*, **10**(6), 390–392.

Sumners, A. D. (1990) Professional nurses' attitudes towards humour. *Journal of Advanced Nursing*, **15**, 196–200.

Teasedale, K. (1993) Information and anxiety: a critical reappraisal. *Journal of Advanced Nursing*, **18**, 1125–1132.

Teasedale, K. and Kent, G. (1995) The use of deception in nursing. *Journal of Medical Ethics*, **21**, 77–81.

Wade, S. (1995) Partnership in care: a critical review. *Nursing Standard*, **948**, 29–32.

Waterworth, S. and Luker, K. (1990) Reluctant collaborators: do patients want to be involved in decisions concerning care? *Journal of Advanced Nursing*, **15**, 971–976.

Wilkinson, S. (1991) Factors which influence how nurses communicate with cancer patients. *Journal of Advanced Nursing*, **16**, 677–688.

Woods, S. (1998) Ethics and communication: developing reflective practice. *Nursing Standard*, **12**(18), 44–47.

Wright, T. (1995) Can patients become empowered? *Professional Nurse*, **10**(9), 599.

Part IV

Role clarification and teamwork

27

The role of the primary nurse in managing care

Anna Leeman and Helen McDermott

Introduction

Traumatic injury by its very nature is sudden, unpredictable, unplanned, disruptive, unwelcome, inconvenient, shocking and painful (Morse and O'Brien, 1995). Trauma has been defined as 'a wound; an injury; an emotional shock; the state or condition caused by a physical or emotional shock' (Macdonald, 1972).

The experience of injury has both physical and psychological dimensions. An understanding of the impact of injury on these dimensions is essential if true adaptation and reintegration into society is to be achieved (Frese, 1985).

Accidents are the major cause of death in people under the age of 30 years in the UK (Department of Health, 1992). It is estimated that for every death on the roads, there are more than two victims with permanent disability (Baskett, 1990).

The cost of trauma encompasses the enormous cost of treatment, rehabilitation and welfare support, loss of expertise in the workplace, reduction in tax revenue and the physical and psychological debility of the victims and their families (Rice and Mackenzie, 1989). The World Health Organisation (1982) considers the cost of all accidents to be approximately equal to 1% of the gross national product of any country, whether developed or developing.

Recognition of the scale of the problem has prompted increased research and development into the management of trauma, which is leading to improvements in emergency and acute care management. Such advances are positively affecting survival rates from accidental injury (Strohmyer *et al.*, 1993).

The development of a trauma system where trauma patients are concentrated at specific hospitals has been shown to improve the outcome of the seriously injured (Driscoll, 1992). To many working within the healthcare setting, trauma is synonymous with orthopaedics and is not recognized within the UK as a discrete speciality (Baskett, 1990). Despite this, developments within other countries are challenging current practices. Trauma audit is highlighting the need for specialist knowledge and experience in the treatment of injury (British Orthopaedic Association, 1992).

The focus of this chapter will be to describe the role and contribution of the primary nurse in enabling individuals to adapt to the physical and psychosocial effects of injury.

In striving to provide a quality service, nurses need to recognize the uniqueness of their contribution within the speciality of trauma and develop expertise supported by research-based practice. Only through an understanding of the significance of the traumatic event and the injury, both for the individual and their family, can healthcare professionals assist the victims of trauma to cope with their experiences and adapt accordingly.

Nurses who choose to work within the speciality of trauma need to develop the ability to be flexible, adaptable and responsive to the needs of patients in their care.

The nature of primary nursing

In essence, primary nursing redefines traditional notions of responsibility within nursing, removing accountability for decision-making from the ward sister to the primary nurse. The patient no longer becomes the passive recipient of treatment, but is involved in decision-making and the planning of their care through their relationship with the primary nurse (Ersser and Tutton, 1991).

Hegyvary (1982) believes that primary nursing 'is both a philosophy and an organisational design. It is not simply a way of assigning nurses to patients, but rather a view of nursing as a professional, patient centred practice'. This belief is also supported by Marran (1974).

Medical advances in the treatment of trauma, increased patient turnover and shorter length of stay have all affected the delivery of nursing care. The acute nature and pace of the workload no longer allows for a hierarchy within nursing where a senior nurse holds all the information and subsequently makes decisions about care delivery. Society's expectations regarding healthcare have also changed; individuals wish to have information and to be involved in decisions about their health (Wright, 1987). Nurse education has adapted to accommodate the changing needs of the health service, and issues of accountability and autonomy are debated within the literature. Nurses are encouraged to question their practice and the practices of others, no longer following blindly the dictates of others (Ford and Walsh, 1994).

Reflections of a primary nurse: Confidently accept challenge and criticism of your own practice

Young male patient with multiple injuries including a moderate head injury. At times aggressive, most of the time restless and agitated. Immobile, though mobile within the confines of his bed. Thrashing around so much that it causes increased pain from various injuries. Spent four days in ICU prior to transfer to ward. Had been receiving a continuous morphine infusion prior to transfer. Drowsy on first day on ward, therefore only oral analgesia administered as patient did not display verbal/non-verbal signs of pain. However, restlessness increased and ability to verbalize pain also increased. Intramuscular opiate analgesia was subsequently administered in order to reach patient's pain corridor (McCaffery and Beebe, 1997).

The cumulative effect of 24 hours without sleep, recovery from head injury and the drowsiness caused by opiates resulted in the patient being awake for only short intervals during the day.

The criticism of my practice came from a senior physiotherapist who felt the patient was unacceptably drowsy following the administration of opiate analgesia, therefore preventing patient cooperation in chest physiotherapy and limb exercises.

From previous discussions with other multidisciplinary professionals regarding the potential effect of opiates I felt I had the experience to deal with this situation. My confidence came from extended knowledge gained from additional courses in pain management.

In the ensuing discussions with the physiotherapist, I acknowledged the importance of her intentions but was able to verbalize adequately and professionally my rationale for care, which was research based. The physiotherapist accepted this rationale.

Changing from the traditional system of task or patient allocation to that of primary nursing requires an enabling management style. Manley (1990) describes how clinical managers have to allow nurses to be accountable and act on decisions about care. They need to support and nurture, not control and command, thus aiding the decentralization of decision-making to the bedside.

Changing from traditional systems of care delivery to primary nursing requires planning and education. Nurses need to understand the issues surrounding accountability and feel prepared to take on the responsibilities inherent in the primary nurse role. Maas (1973) defines accountability as 'responsibility and answerability to authority for one's actions. The accountable individual is prepared to explain and to take responsibility for the results of his actions'. (Table 27.1).

The success of primary nursing rests on the commitment, education and expertise of the nurses involved. Bowers (1987) and Manley (1990) recognize that a lack of education and knowledge, together with inexperienced staff, causes a breakdown within the primary nursing system. 'The quality of nursing care can be no better than the competencies of the persons actively giving direct care to patients' (Felton, 1975). **Binnie (1989) states that education is a necessity not a luxury and as such should be built into the organizational management of the practice area.**

Table 27.1 Pre-conditions for the acceptance of accountability (Adapted from Bergman, 1981)

1. The necessary knowledge, skills and ability
2. The acceptance of responsibility being limited to the quality of care – an individual cannot be held responsible for the decisions of colleagues
3. Autonomy–independent decision-making
4. The acceptance of accountability is subject to being given the authority

---

Reflections of a primary nurse: Demonstrate confidence in decision-making

Long-term cachectic patient with multiple trauma and problems which resulted in repeated transfers to ICU. Hurriedly discharged from ICU at night to accommodate a ventilated patient. ICU had nursed the patient on a hired low-air-loss bed. ICU nurse very keen to impose her beliefs and ideas onto me and insisted I accept the patient on the hired bed (also because of lack of time to transfer patient to another bed due to incoming emergency). However, I had known patient for 3 months and had confidence in our ability to prevent damage to patient's skin integrity. Three months previously the patient had been transferred in from another hospital suffering from necrotic heels and a sacral sore. All pressure sores had healed while in our care. Patient arrived on hired bed from ICU. One sore had reappeared on a heel. I made the decision to transfer the patient to an Alpha X-Cell mattress, the patient's previous pressure-relieving surface. I was confident in the decision made.

Although this patient scored high on the pressure sore risk assessment scale, clinical judgement was used to inform choice of surface.

In time, the sore healed with regular nurse intervention and adequate nutrition.

Research into the effectiveness of primary nursing versus team nursing, patient allocation

or task allocation is, to date, rather subjective (Giovannetti, 1980; Ciske, 1981; Macguire and Botting, 1990; Johns, 1993) (Table 27.2).

Experience suggests that many of the negative aspects of primary nursing can be alleviated through support and discussion with colleagues. **A clearer understanding of the roles and contributions of others is essential for effective teamwork**. Multidisciplinary functioning depends on decisions being made by the whole team. A clearer understanding of roles can reduce power play and traditional rivalry, aiding collaborative practice (McMahon, 1989).

Reflections of a primary nurse: Effective teamwork and decision making

A trauma consultant had prescribed the application of oxygen therapy applied to a wound in a patient's groin in order for it to produce a scab quickly, prior to internal fixation of the patient's pelvic fractures.

Some nurses gave the care as prescribed by the consultant, aware that by the United Kingdom Central Council's Code of Conduct (UKCC, 1992) nurses must carry out the care prescribed. However, this must not be detrimental to the patient. The UKCC Code of Conduct (1992) states that nurses 'should work in a collaborative and co-operative manner with healthcare professionals and others involved in providing care and recognise and respect their particular contributions within the care team'. This was upheld by the nurses caring for this particular patient. However, the UKCC also states that 'no action or omission on your part, or within your sphere of responsibility, is detrimental to the interests, condition or safety of patients and clients'. By providing the care prescribed by the doctor, the nurses were perhaps delaying the patient's wound from healing.

The nurses had treated this wound for 3 months. It had progressed from a cavity 2 inches (50 mm) wide by 2 inches deep, to a superficial wound very nearly healed, but continuing to exude too much for a scab to form. Gould (1985) highlights that oxygen therapy is detrimental to the healing of wounds. Winter (1962) proved that the formation of a scab would remarkably hinder the healing of a wound.

Two days of oxygen therapy to the wound and no scab had formed, only a groin full of exudate. I approached the consultant in question on a ward round and explained my dilemma with rationale, including the infection risk his method posed. The consultant eventually accepted my rationale and expressed to the other doctors present that this should be a learning experience for them; also, that they should remember 'never to interfere with wounds and dressings, as the nurses' knowledge far exceeds that of the doctors!' He concluded by allowing the nurses to regain responsibility for wound management.

The therapeutic relationship has been highlighted as the key to understanding the needs of the individual and therefore the success of nursing assessment, intervention and outcome (Savage, 1995). Savage points out the link between the continuity of care (afforded through primary nursing) and the nature of the nurse–patient relationship – noting that knowing the patient fosters a closeness from which the therapeutic potential emerges. Manley (1990) suggests that this closeness may have negative effects, such as increasing stress and burn-out among nurses, and encouraging an over-dependence in patients.

Reflections of a primary nurse: Stress

Stress, as defined by the *Concise Oxford English Dictionary*, is a 'demand on physical or mental energy'. However, it is important to remember that the same event may have different effects on different individuals. Hans Selye (1956), a world authority on stress, defined it as 'any circumstance which causes a particular measurable physiological response'.

My personal feelings are that the older I get, the more aware I become of stress; what causes it, how it manifests itself and how to avoid it or treat it. From the stress of my O-level exams where my body's response was psoriasis, to coping with full-time nursing, in sometimes desperate conditions, and part-time studying – inducing more headaches, migraines and sleepless nights than I care to remember.

I do not recall having coping mechanisms when I was younger – perhaps smoking. My recent

Table 27.2 Outcomes considered to be associated with primary nursing as a system of care delivery

Positive	Negative
An enhancement of therapeutic nursing and the nurse–patient relationship (McMahon and Pearson, 1991)	Increased stress and burnout of staff (Holmes, 1987)
Increased continuity of care resulting in increased patient/family gratitude (Pearson, 1988)	Supernurse syndrome (Manley, 1990) – feeling the need to be all things to all patients
Increased quality of care delivery (McFarlane, 1976)	Over-dependence by patients (Manley, 1990)
The development of professional maturity (Binnie, 1989)	Reduced teamwork (McMahon, 1989)
Enabling environments and increased creativity (Sturt, 1989)	Some doctors may find primary nursing threatening as they are not *in charge* of nurses (Sparrow, 1986; Wright, 1987)
Improved patient satisfaction (Ciske, 1981) Reduced overall cost of nursing and reduced length of stay (Felton, 1975)	
Increased staff retention, especially those with more education (Binnie, 1989)	
Perceived to have increased knowledge, improved communication skills and gave greater consideration to discharge planning (Macguire and Botting, 1990) Increased staff support for each other (Ciske, 1981)	
A reduction in the stereotyping of patients as difficult or demanding (Pearson, 1988)	
The generation of interest and the uptake of ideas throughout associated hospitals and community	
Increased learning opportunities for staff (Binnie, 1989)	
Clear definition of role and contribution of nurses within the multidisciplinary team (Wright, 1987)	

ways of coping have been by giving up smoking and taking up dancing, Pilates and aromatherapy, along with getting more sleep and drinking less alcohol!

I try to enjoy the good things in life more these days, when I have the time, and I never let the sun go down on bad feelings.

Helping others to manage their stress can be more complicated – or easier – depending on the person. Perhaps the most important point is to remember that each person is an individual, with individual coping mechanisms. Sharing ideas, thoughts and feelings and trying to listen and understand are high on my list of priorities.

Benner (1984) analysed observational data of nurses in practice, identifying five levels of competency in clinical practice. These levels – novice, advanced beginner, competent, proficient, expert – allow performance characteristics at each level to be identified which in turn can help inform the identification of learning needs. Benner indicates that it is only at the competent stage, where nurses have experienced 2–3 years practising in the same or similar area, that nurses pass from a stimulus-response performance level to that of a holistic practitioner, demonstrating an ability to perceive the patient's needs in the light of long-term goals.

These findings hold significance for nurses working within the speciality of trauma where frequently the period of hospitalization is just the beginning of the long road of rehabilitation and reintegration into society.

Primary nursing and the organization

Primary nursing as a system for organizing the delivery of nursing care has been advocated by the Department of Health (1989) and the Audit Commission (1991, 1992).

In order to maintain primary nursing as the system of care delivery, the organizational philosophy needs to support innovative practice and value the contribution of nursing (Marran, 1974; Hegyvary, 1982). Wright (1989) reinforces this belief when stating that 'to ensure the success of any change in nursing practice, education or management, the nurse must negotiate with other healthcare groups and be able to convince others of the benefits of the change in attaining the goals set out in the

organisation's strategic plans'.

The recommendations of the British Orthopaedic Association (1989, 1992) regarding the management of skeletal trauma within the UK highlighted the need for specialist trauma centres (where senior medical staff are available 24 hours a day) to reduce the morbidity and mortality associated with major trauma. In response to these recommendations, consultant medical staff in the Oxford Trauma Service operate a 24-hour resident on-call system to ensure that patients receive expert medical care on arrival. During the planning stage of this reorganization it became clear that the development of a consultant-led, but nurse-managed service would aid interdisciplinary communication and maintain continuity. Thus, restructuring of the medical service complemented and further supported primary nursing as the system of organizing nursing work. Mutual support during the restructuring process has led to enhanced collaborative practice to the benefit of patients.

In Oxford, individuals are admitted to the trauma unit through a variety of routes and consequently have differing physical and psychological needs on arrival:

- directly from the accident and emergency (A&E) department
- from theatre recovery following initial surgical intervention
- from ICU
- increasingly from other orthopaedic/trauma units for specialist surgical intervention
- from trauma clinics for further operative management.

The primary nurse uses knowledge, skills and experience to assess and prioritize the immediate needs of the individual on arrival at the unit. Frequently during this initial assessment, physical needs will dominate.

Expertise and its application in primary nursing

Savage (1995) notes how experienced nurses employ a variety of strategies, e.g. touch, humour and body posture, to promote and manage closeness with patients. Experienced nurses are able to elicit relevant information without the use of rigid frameworks which can stifle the natural direction of the interaction (Pearson, 1988). Benner (1984) highlights that expert nurses develop trust from the outset. The identification of a primary nurse gives the individual a point of contact within the frightening, unfamiliar environment into which they have been thrust.

Maslow (1968) depicted human needs as falling into five categories – physiological, health and safety, belonging, self-esteem and self-actualization. When lower level needs are met, then the needs at a higher level become prominent and require attention. This is a useful framework for nurses to use when assessing and prioritizing the needs of their patients. The expert nurse incorporates prior experiences, so that assessment of physical and psychological needs becomes fluid and intuitive (Benner, 1984).

As interventions dealing with physiological needs such as pain relief, fluid replacement and maintenance of function are performed, psychosocial needs can be identified and the planning of longer term goals can commence.

Benner (1984) describes how expert nurses have difficulty articulating what they know because they operate from 'a deep understanding of the total situation'. Their practice is tacit in nature and therefore difficult to describe or research (Kitson, 1987).

Primary nursing affords expert nurses greater opportunity to use their experience to form therapeutic relationships simply through increased contact with their patients. The therapeutic relationship allows communication at a higher level through already knowing (Savage, 1995). Through 'knowing' the patient, the primary nurse is well placed to detect subtle changes in condition, often before vital signs or other indicators are affected (Benner, 1984), for example slight changes in pallor without changes in blood pressure and pulse heralding impending hypovolaemia.

More and more credence is being given to the importance of psychological factors in relation to physical recovery and well-being (McMahon and Pearson, 1991). Stress can have a profound effect on the body, and can lead to high blood pressure, breathlessness, nausea, sweating, muscle spasms, insomnia, tiredness, constipation, diarrhoea and poor appetite (Cooper *et al.,* 1988). Identifying stress reactions enables the nurse to diagnose accurately the underlying

problem and carry out appropriate therapeutic interventions. **Knowing the patient, clinical knowledge, experience and a holistic approach to care will enable the nurse to reframe the problem within the context of that individual's experience (Powell, 1991).**

The primary nurse is responsible for planning the individual's care from admission to discharge (Manthey, 1980). Central to this process is the identification of factors which could potentially hinder progress towards recovery. Within a nurse-managed system of care supported by primary nursing, it is the nurse who is well placed to access colleagues with specialist knowledge in order to aid holistic management of identified problems. Trauma as a speciality overlaps with neurosurgery, spinal surgery and plastic surgery, all of which can be viewed as discrete specialities. The recruitment of nurses with specialist interests in such areas of practice aids in the delivery of expert practice. Creating an environment where nurses feel comfortable asking for advice enables the dissemination of knowledge to occur to the benefit of the patients.

Reflections of a primary nurse: Clinical supervision

Impromptu teaching session to junior registered nurse. She expressed anxiety regarding the number of spinal patients on the ward with varying degrees of paralysis and potential problems regarding respiratory arrests.
Updated colleague on most recent changes to resuscitation guidelines. Discussed emergency procedures and what her role would be, including what to do if the senior nurse on duty was off the ward. Explained the potential risks and associated problems. Explained signs and symptoms, i.e. oxygen desaturation, increase or decrease in respiratory rate, difficulty in breathing, abdominal or diaphragmatic breathing and bradycardia or tachycardia.
Allayed fears and anxieties and reassured.
Reinforced availability for further impromptu sessions.

Sellick *et al.,* (1993) felt that the clearer lines of accountability evident within the primary nursing system of care delivery encouraged nurses to question and reflect on their practice, enabling

them to mature professionally and develop a greater knowledge base.

Reflections of a primary nurse: Personal critique

Twenty-five-year-old morbidly obese male, involved in RTA. Multiple injuries, mainly complex fractures of pelvis. Transferred from another hospital 4 weeks after injury for management of pelvic fractures. Bowels not opened for 4 weeks. At the time I, as primary nurse, was focusing on main problems of patient, i.e. loss of appetite, feeling unwell. The significant problem of constipation included how to manage the situation and what treatment options to consider.

All remedies had previously been tried by transferring hospital, but to no avail.

I felt the best solution would be to perform a manual evacuation in theatre while under a general anaesthetic. I discussed this with the consultant, who agreed.

However, at the time I failed to focus on the huge infection risks concerned with faecal matter being dealt with immediately prior to or following pelvic surgery. I was thinking of the main problem facing me and the patient, but not of the implications of my choice of solution. Instead, we decided that we should tackle the problem a few days after the pelvic surgery to ensure the wounds had reached the homeostatic phase. The process of eliminating 5–6 weeks' worth of faecal matter began, so a visit to theatre for this purpose alone was no longer necessary.

At the time of this incident there was not sufficient time for me to reflect in action. I was perhaps too focused on other problems, which clouded my ability to isolate specifics. Schon (1983) presents the notion of framing and reframing. He emphasizes that thinking and action are linked. Individuals change the way they perceive a problem by way of new understanding and interpretations gained through talking to and working on the problem with others.

The reasons why intervention was to be at a later date were pointed out to me by my mentor. I knew the reason why before I was told, but had kept it in my subconscious. This proves that, although I may learn new things, I may not necessarily use them at the appropriate time. This has taught me to force myself to think more on the go, of surrounding issues and implications and to discuss my feelings, ideas and findings with colleagues.

The impact of trauma and its wider implications

The impact of traumatic injury is felt not only by the victim, but also by the victim's family. A change in one individual has an impact on the dynamics of the whole family (Braulin *et al.*, 1982).

The initial focus of care following trauma will inevitably be towards the victim, but the family will also be experiencing feelings of fear, loss of control, helplessness, shock and disbelief (Gardener and Stewart, 1978). The primary nurse is well placed to assess not only the psychological effects of trauma on the individual, but also on the family. Psychosocial support for the families of trauma victims is crucial in order to maintain the family as a functional unit (Youngblood and Hines, 1992).

Epperson (1977) recognized that family members of accident victims passed through phases of anxiety, denial, anger, remorse, grief and reconciliation as they adjusted to the changes imposed on them following the traumatic incident. He highlighted that without appropriate help family members might become arrested in one or other of these stages. Families require support through the crisis so that they are able to support the patient emotionally; they have a vital role to play in outcome and long-term adjustment to disability (Youngblood and Hines, 1992).

Modern trauma care is characterizd by the increasingly aggressive management of skeletal and soft tissue injury, the result of which is earlier mobiliztion and a shorter length of stay in hospital. Victims of traumatic injury are discharged into the community where they are supported in essence by their families and community health workers. Follow-up is provided in outpatient clinics. The psychosocial implications of shorter length of stay is that primarily there is far less time to assess the victim and their family's reaction to the trauma. The full impact may not be realized until after discharge from hospital, where currently there is little professional support. It is therefore essential to begin supportive interventions early and to plan comprehensive discharge packages.

If the primary nurse is to instigate the process of discharge planning in order to 'reintegrate the individual into society' through assessment and planning, he or she must not view the individual outside the context of their family

and previously held societal roles. Early identification of potential problems can aid referral to
appropriate agencies to provide help and
support during the adaptation phase of recovery. The therapeutic relationship between the
primary nurse and the patient is the key to
understanding the individual's needs in both a
physical and psychosocial context (Savage, 1995). Trust and confidence in the ability
of the nurse is central to its development.
Research by Ersser (1991) demonstrated that
conflicting advice from health professionals
increases nervousness and anxiety.

The medical management plan may be complex and subject to alteration depending on the
outcome of initial surgical interventions. Emotional reactions following the traumatic incident may affect the individual's ability to
assimilate and retain information (Wilson-
Barnett, 1979). Benner (1984) notes that expert
nurses are not only able to recognize the
learning needs of the patient, but also the time
at which the patient is most ready to learn.
Information may need to be reiterated many
times before the patient and their family gain a
true understanding of the situation and its
implications for the future. Through knowing
the patient and the family, the nurse can act as
advocate, enabling treatment plans to be
tailored to individual needs in a way which is
acceptable to both parties.

---

*Reflections of a primary nurse: Identifying
barriers to learning*

Middle-aged man involved in serious road
traffic accident. Sustained multiple injuries
which resulted in restricted mobility for a
significant time and hospital admission of many
months. The patient also lost his sight as a result
of injuries sustained in the accident, was
suffering a degree of post-traumatic stress and
became colonized by methicillin-resistant *Staphylococcus aureus* (MRSA), requiring him to
be nursed in isolation.

The losses to this patient were unimaginable.
They included his job, income, status, independence, home, sight, recreational activities (such
as reading and walking), his sense of belonging
and his place in society.

The multidisciplinary team (MDT) needed to
have a holistic understanding of this patient. We
needed to understand his individual demands
and to anticipate his needs. Time was of the

---

essence, as capturing a patient's readiness to
learn is as important as it is difficult. Benner
(1984) stresses the importance of timing in this
situation. We needed to teach him how to:

- regain his independence in activities of daily
  living (ADL)
- function without sight
- maximize control over his life
- utilize social, emotional or spiritual help and
  support.

However, there were a number of problems in
trying to establish a supportive learning environment:

- reduced occupational therapy and physiotherapy input from prioritizing care delivery
  to more acute fellow patients
- constant interruptions
- lack of motivation and energy due to patient's
  depression
- patient's anxiety and embarrassment regarding inadequacies and insecure future
- staff shortages and the care needs of fellow
  patients
- patient sometimes only allowed certain people into his room, criticizing staff he perceived
  to be of a lower class, about their tone of
  voice, approach and standards of care, thereby causing an increase in stress levels for
  both him and the staff
- staff became defensive and found it difficult
  to accept his criticisms.

Being aware of problems that can affect a
learning environment is important. However, it
is of equal importance to be able to do something about it.

The learning environment needs to accommodate the needs of the staff as well as the
patients, as we are all learners in what can be
busy and threatening surroundings.

Teamwork and the balance of power

Advocacy has many definitions. Allen (1984)
defines an advocate as 'a person who pleads for
another'. Kohne (1982) describes advocacy as
the act of 'defending or pleading the case of
another', implying that the other cannot do this
for themselves. Kendrick (1994) asserts that if
power in healthcare was equally balanced
between patient, nurse and doctor, the need

for advocacy would be greatly diminished. He goes on to state that 'health care is so laden down with issues of power and politics that it raises doubts about whether nurses are actually in a position to act as the patient's advocate'; however, evidence presented in the following passage would seem to contradict this view.

Reflections of a primary nurse: Advocacy

A patient suffering from multiple injuries had been transferred from another hospital. He arrived at 1700 hours. At 0200 hours the following morning the on-call registrar was insisting on waking the patient to examine a wound.

The wound was a fasciotomy over the left tibia which had been slow to heal and was covered with an occlusive dressing. I felt that as this was not a critical injury the Registrar could wait 6 hours until the wound was seen on the ward round the following morning.

I acknowledged the importance of the Registrar's assessment, but felt that the timing was inappropriate for the patient.

Knowing that the patient needed his sleep, I acted as his advocate (UKCC, 1992).

Multidisciplinary team functioning depends on decisions being taken by the team as a whole, not exclusively by one or two powerful members. For primary nursing to function effectively, the contributions of nursing and medicine need to be perceived as being of equal importance and value, enabling holistic discussion involving the patient, in relation to the most appropriate treatment for that individual.

Murphy and Hunter (1984) state 'the professional, while obliged to act in the patient's best interest, is not permitted to define that interest in any way contrary to the patient's definition; it is not the professional but the patient who shall define what best interest shall mean'.

The giving of accurate, unbiased information enables the patient to make an informed choice about their healthcare needs. Allowing individuals to make decisions about their health increases their autonomy and fosters independence (Matson and Brooks, 1982). This, in turn, helps individuals maintain a more positive self-image (Robson, 1988), thus decreasing their vulnerability.

Rehabilitation and reintegration

Currently, rehabilitation facilities within the National Health Service following skeletal injury are run primarily on an outpatient basis. Davidson (1987) states that the worst-funded specialities are those furthest away from the curative process. Modern trauma care advocates aggressive medical management, resulting in a shorter length of stay in hospital. Research by Border *et al.* (1990) in Switzerland revealed that the cost of permanent impairment following injury was 44% of the total cost of trauma care and, as a result, recommended that further investment in effective rehabilitation was essential. In the last decade, trauma care in the USA and Germany has focused on the development of trauma and rehabilitation centres in an attempt to improve outcome following injury (Driscoll, 1992).

At present there remain no such facilities for the management of trauma within the UK. Audit has revealed that one-third of trauma deaths after arrival in hospital are preventable (Anderson *et al.*, 1988). Recommendations from the British Orthopaedic Association (1992) addressed problems encompassing pre-hospital care and the acute management phase of treatment. Interestingly, provision for rehabilitation scarcely warranted a mention. The relationship between rehabilitation and outcome has been poorly researched. It is estimated that, world-wide, across all ages, 15% of disability is caused through injury (World Health Organisation, 1982).

Management of severe injury and return to optimum functioning is a long process. Readmission to hospital for further surgical intervention is frequently necessary to achieve healing and acceptable outcomes. Psychological adjustment to trauma typically may not occur until long after the individual's physical scars have healed (Strohmyer *et al.*, 1993). Research by Rhodes *et al.*, (1988) reported that even 6 months post-injury was too soon to assess the full emotional consequences of trauma and its effect on the individual's lifestyle, roles and relationships.

Experience would suggest that patients find the transition from hospital to home stressful and frightening. Hospital is viewed as a safe environment where professionals assist them to make decisions about their health needs. Exploring the fears that individuals have during the transition from hospital to home will help the primary nurse to plan a comprehensive discharge package to alleviate or highlight areas where difficulties may arise.

A liaison service directed towards victims of traumatic injury where potential problems are identified by the primary nurse while in hospital might serve to ease the transition from hospital to home. It is suggested that such a service may lead to the early detection of both physical and psychological difficulties and could aid referral to appropriate agencies, resulting in positive outcomes.

The relationship developed between primary nurses and their patients enables a greater understanding of the effects of trauma on the individual. Through this knowledge practitioners are recognizing that a gap in the service exists. Steps need to be taken to redress the balance in order to ensure that individuals are adequately supported in the community.

Conclusion

Within a nurse-managed service where medical colleagues have, to some extent, relinquished control over both patients and nurses, collaborative practice is essential in order to achieve positive patient outcomes. For such a situation to be maintained, nurses require highly developed interpersonal skills and an ability to demonstrate their clinical credibility through expert practice. Interdisciplinary conflict is, to some extent, inevitable, but it need not be destructive. All parties can develop a deeper understanding of each other's roles for the benefit of patient care, through negotiation and discussion.

The therapeutic relationship between the nurse and patient is seen as the key to unlocking the significance of injury for the individual and those close to them helping them in the journey to recovery. Primary nursing, with its emphasis on the development of this relationship, is advocated as the most appropriate system for care delivery within the speciality of trauma.

References

Allen, R. E. (ed.) (1984) *The Pocket Oxford Dictionary.* Clarendon Press.

Anderson, I., Woodford, M. and de Dombar, F. (1988) Retrospective analysis of 1,000 deaths from injury in England and Wales. *British Medical Journal,* **296,** 1305.

Audit Commission (1991) *The Virtue of Patients: Making the Best Use of Ward Resources.* London: HMSO.

Audit Commission (1992) *Making Time for Patients – A Handbook for Sisters.* London: HMSO.

Baskett, P. (1990) Anaesthetists and trauma. *Anaesthesia,* **45,** 805–807.

Benner, P. (1984) *From Novice to Expert: Excellence and Power in Clinical Nursing Practice.* Addison-Wesley.

Bergman, R. (1981) Accountability – definition and dimensions. *International Nursing Review,* **28**(2), 53–59.

Binnie, A. (1989) Primary nursing – Where to start. *Nursing Times,* **85**(4), 43–44.

Border, J. R., Allgower, M., Hanson Jr, S.T. and Ruedi, T. P. (1990) *Blunt Multiple Trauma, Comprehensive Pathophysiology and Care.* Marcel Dekker.

Bowers, L. (1987) Who's in? *Nursing Times,* **83**(22), 36–38.

Braulin, J., Rook, J. and Sills, G. (1982) Families in crisis: the impact of trauma. *Critical Care Nursing Quarterly,* **5**(3), 38–46.

British Orthopaedic Association (1989) *The Management of Trauma in Great Britain.* BOA.

British Orthopaedic Association (1992) *The Management of Skeletal Trauma in the United Kingdom.* BOA.

Ciske, K. L. (1981) Primary nursing: an organisation that promotes professional practice. *Journal of Nursing Administration,* Jan./Feb., 28–31.

Cooper, C., Cooper, R. and Eaten, L. (1988) *Living with Stress.* Penguin.

Davidson, N. (1987) *A Question of Care: the Changing Face of the National Health Service.* Michael Joseph.

Department of Health (1989) *A Strategy for Nursing.* London: DOH.

Department of Health (1992) *The Health of the Nation.* London: HMSO.

Driscoll, P. A. (1992) Trauma: Today's problems, tomorrow's answers. *Injury,* **23**(3), 151–158.

Epperson, M. M. (1977) Families in sudden crisis. Process and intervention in a critical care centre. *Social Work,* **2,** 265–273.

Ersser, S. (1991). A search for the therapeutic dimensions of nurse–patient interaction. In *Nursing as Therapy* (M. McMahon and A. Pearson, eds), Chapman and Hall.

Ersser, S. and Tutton, E. (1991) *Primary Nursing in Perspective.* Scutari Press.

Felton, G. (1975) Increasing the quality of care by introducing the concept of primary nursing. *Nursing Research,* **24**(1), 27–32.

Ford, P. and Walsh, M. (1994) *New Rituals for Old.* Butterworth-Heinemann.

Frese, S. (1985) Coping with trauma. *Rehabilitation Nursing,* **4**(2), 58–60.

Gardener, D. and Stewart, N. (1978) Staff involvement with families of patients in critical care units, *Heart Lung,* **7**(1), 105–110.

Giovannetti, P. (1980) A comparison of team and primary

nursing care systems. *Nursing Dimensions*, Winter, 115–121.

Gould, D. (1985) Pressure for change. *Nursing Mirror*, **161**(9), 28–30.

Hegyvary, S. T. (1982) *The Change to Primary Nursing: A Cross Cultural View of Professional Nursing Practice*. Mosby.

Holmes, S. (1987) Managing the stress of primary nursing. *Nursing Management*, **18**(3), 62–66.

Johns, C. (1993) Professional supervision. *Journal of Nursing Management* **1**, 9–18.

Kendrick, K. (1994) An advocate for whom – doctor or patient? How far can a nurse be a patient's advocate? *Professional Nurse*, **9**(12), 826–829.

Kitson, A. (1987) Rising standards of clinical practice – the fundamental issue of effective nursing practice. *Journal of Advanced Nursing*, **12**, 321–329.

Kohne, M. F. (1982) Advocacy: What is it? *Nursing and Health Care*, **3**(6), 314–318.

Maas, M. L. (1973) Nurse autonomy and accountability in organised nursing services. *Nursing Forum*, **12**(2), 237–259.

Macdonald, A. M. (ed.) (1972) *Chambers Twentieth Century Dictionary*. W & R Chambers.

Macguire, J. and Botting, D. (1990) The use of the ethnograph programme to identify the perceptions of nursing staff following the introduction of primary nursing in an acute medical ward for elderly people. *Journal of Advanced Nursing*, **15**, 1120–1127.

Manley, K. (1990) Intensive caring. *Nursing Times*, **86**(19), 67–69.

Manthey, M. (1980) *The Practice of Primary Nursing*. Blackwell.

Marran, G. D. (1974) *Primary Nursing: a Model for Individualised Care*. Mosby.

Maslow, A. (1968) *Towards a Psychology of Being*. Van Nostrand.

Matson, R. R. and Brooks, N. A. (1982) Social-psychological adjustment to multiple sclerosis: a longitudinal study. *Social Science and Medicine*, **16**, 2129–2135.

McCaffery, M. and Beebe, A. (1997) Pain. In *Clinical Manual for Nursing Practice* (Latham, J., ed.), Mosby.

McFarlane, J. K. (1976) A charter for caring. *Journal of Advanced Nursing*, **1**(3), 187–196.

McMahon, B. (1989) Teamwork – a complete service with specialist skills. *The Professional Nurse*, June, 433–435.

McMahon, R. and Pearson, A. (1991) *Nursing as Therapy*. Chapman and Hall.

Morse, J. and O'Brien, B. (1995) Preserving self: from victim to patient, to disabled person. *Journal of Advanced Nursing*, **21**, 886–896.

Murphy, C. and Hunter, H. (1984) *Ethical Problems in the Nurse–Patient Relationship*. Alwin and Bacon.

Pearson, A. (1988) Primary nursing. In *Primary Nursing: Nursing in the Burford and Oxford Nursing Developments Units* (A. Pearson, ed.).

Powell, J. (1991) Reflection and the evaluation of experience: Prerequisites for therapeutic practice. In *Nursing as Therapy* (M. McMahon and A. Pearson, eds) Chapman and Hall.

Rhodes, M., Aronson, J., Moerkirk, G. and Petrash, E .(1988). Quality of life after the trauma centre. *The Journal of Trauma*, **28**(7), 931–935.

Rice, D. P. and Mackenzie, E. J. (1989) *Cost of Injury in the USA – A Report to Congress*. San Francisco.

Robson, P. J. (1988) Self-esteem – a psychiatric view. *British Journal of Psychiatry*, **153**, 6–15.

Savage, J. (1995) *Nursing Intimacy. An Ethnographic Approach to Nurse–Patient Interaction*. Scutari Press.

Schon, D. (1983). *The Reflective Practitioner: How Professionals Think in Action*. Basic Books.

Sellick, K. J., Russell, S. R. and Beckmann, J. L. (1993) Primary nursing: an evaluation of its effects on patient perception of care and staff satisfaction. *International Journal of Nursing Studies*, **20**(4), 265–273.

Selye, H. (1956) *The Stress of Life*. McGraw-Hill

Sparrow, S. (1986) Primary nursing. *Nursing Practice*, **1**(3), 142–148.

Strohmyer, L., Noroian, E., Patterson, L. and Carlin, B. (1993) Adaptation six months after multiple trauma: a pilot study. *Journal of Neuroscience Nursing*, **25**(1), 30–37.

Sturt, A. (1989) Myth and method. *Nursing Times*, **85**(85), 33–34.

UKCC (1992). *The Professional Code of Conduct*. UKCC.

Wilson-Barnett, J. (1979) *Stress in Hospitalisation: Patients' Psychological Reactions to Illness and Healthcare*. Churchill-Livingstone.

Winter, G. (1962) Formation of the scab and the rate of epithelialisation of superficial wounds and the skin of the young domestic pig. *Nature*, **200**, 377–379.

World Health Organisation (1982) *The Epidemiology of Accident Traumas and Resulting Disabilities*. Report on a WHO symposium, Strasbourg, 19–21 March 1981. Euro Reports and Studies 57. Copenhagen: WHO Regional Office for Europe, 1992:28.

Wright, S. (1987) Patient centred practice. *Nursing Times*, **83**(38), 24–27.

Wright, S. (1989) *Changing Nursing Practice*. Edward Arnold.

Youngblood, N. and Hines, J. (1992) The influence of the family's perception of disability on rehabilitation outcomes. *Rehabilitation Nursing*, **17**(6) 323–326.

28

Physiotherapy following injury

Liz Ellis and Sallie Lamb

Introduction

This chapter gives an overview of the role played by the physiotherapy team in the overall management of the trauma patient. The case study approach illustrates the following:

- Life sustaining interventions.
- Soft tissue management.
- The effects of disability.
- The process of physiotherapy for the hospitalized patient.
- Techniques and equipment.

The physiotherapist plays a pivotal role in the management of the trauma patient at all stages of care until the optimum level of function has been achieved. The three key situations in which physiotherapists are involved are:

1. Interventions to sustain life.
2. Interventions to manage soft tissue injuries not requiring surgery.
3. Interventions to prevent disability and facilitate rehabilitation.

Life-sustaining interventions

In the early stages of the management of patients who have sustained severe trauma, the most pressing concern is the preservation of life. Physiotherapists are often involved at this stage, not in the resuscitation process, but in providing respiratory therapies to ensure that

adequate ventilation can be maintained. This includes ventilated patients and those needing assistance with breathing.

Case study

A 45-year-old man sustained multiple right-sided rib fractures falling from a ladder. He smoked and normally had a productive cough. The main problems to consider were:

- high risk of developing lobar infection, as pain inhibits breathing and coughing
- secretion retention
- reduced lung expansion
- anxiety.

Aims of treatment:

- to assess
- to provide adequate analgesia
- to position the patient so as to facilitate maximal lung ventilation
- to teach breathing exercises and assisted coughing techniques to clear secretions
- to provide health education and advice
- to stand and mobilize the patient as soon as pain permitted to improve lung ventilation.

Management of soft tissue injuries

Certain minor injuries, strains and sprains, do not require admission to hospital. However, they can be debilitating to patients and are often treated by physiotherapists, either in the accident and emergency department or in the physiotherapy outpatient department. The mainstay of soft tissue injury management is RICE:

R Rest
I Ice
C Compression
E Elevation

together with early movement, which aims to control the inflammatory process and limit damage (Hunter, 1994).

Disability and rehabilitation

As medical technologies advance, the number of people surviving trauma is increasing (Pope and Tavlov, 1991). The efforts of the trauma team are focused not only on saving and sustaining life, but also on minimizing disability.

The environment in which we live and work is challenging. We take for granted that we can walk around, climb stairs, communicate with others, make and action thoughts. If these skills are removed, we become unable to cope in hitherto familiar environments. This is referred to as disability and is a mismatch between our ability to function and the difficulties posed by our environment (Pope and Tavlov, 1991). To minimize disability we can either improve our ability to function, change the characteristics of our environment, or aim to achieve a mixture of the two.

Many disciplines are involved in rehabilitation, a term used to describe the journey that patients undergo in order to minimize the disabling effects of trauma. Physiotherapy is a particularly important component of rehabilitation in the speciality of trauma as so many injuries have significant physical sequelae; for example, losing the ability to walk or the ability to move limbs independently. The physiotherapist uses a range of techniques to maximize the physical ability of the patient as part of this collaborative approach.

Case study

A 50-year-old woman attends the physiotherapy outpatient department for assessment within 2 weeks of being discharged from hospital following an ankle fracture.

Aims of treatment:

- to assess pain, swelling, ligamentous stability, range of movement, muscle power, gait and foot biomechanics
- to reduce swelling
- to restore optimum mobility of all foot joints using mobilization techniques
- to teach a home exercise and management programme
- to administer electrotherapy where appropriate
- to teach weight-bearing exercises and proprioceptive re-education in response to the rate of fracture healing
- to build up to end-stage strengthening and a return to normal activity as fracture union occurs.

The physiotherapy process

Physiotherapy starts within the first 24 hours of admission, during which the physical consequences of the injury or injuries are noted and specific pathological and functional deficits are identified. Deficits of muscle strength, range of movement, neurological functions such as sensation and reflexes, balance, mobility, dexterity, respiratory function and cardiovascular condition are documented. Comparisons are made with the patient's uninjured limbs, or to published reference values for normal physiological function (Jones and Barker, 1996). The emphasis of the assessment will depend on the type of injuries sustained. A detailed history of the injury, pre-injury abilities and the normal social and working environment of the patient is taken. From this point on it is possible to begin to form an opinion about an individual patient's prognosis and their potential for recovery, ideally with no residual disability. The amount and type of physiotherapy treatment needed to restore maximum function will be determined, together with the patient's requirement for aids, appliances or environmental modifications that can substitute for function (e.g. a wheelchair). The end-point of the assessment is a series of treatment goals which, whenever possible, is agreed with the patient and the rest of the team. The assessment is repeated regularly and progress is documented, the treatment goals being adjusted according to patient need and progress. A summary of physiotherapy treatment aims which are common to all injuries is provided in Table 28.1.

Table 28.1 Common aims in the physiotherapy management of any traumatic injury

To reassure the patient and increase confidence
To explain the nature of any injuries, anticipated recovery time and management plan
To assess for concurrent injuries
To assess and treat respiratory problems
To minimize the effects of soft tissue trauma
To maintain or increase range of joint movement
To maintain or increase muscle power and strength
To control pain
To reactivate balance
To restore normal function and movement as much as possible
To provide aids, or appliances in the case of fixed disability
To provide advice to the multidisciplinary team on specific aspects of management

The physiotherapy process is affected by a number of factors, most importantly the underlying pathology. The majority of fractures will heal naturally, although patients increasingly undergo some type of surgery to maximize the chance of healing, to ensure that the fracture segments are held in good alignment, and to speed up recovery by giving stability to fractures. This last point is particularly important as the longer a patient stays in bed, the more likely they are to develop secondary complications such as loss of muscle bulk, pressure sores and depression (Webber, 1998). All of these complications contribute to the likelihood of the patient developing permanent disability.

The physiotherapist has to give careful consideration to the type of fixation before mobilizing or instigating specific treatments, and this is done through close liaison with the surgical team. If there has been extensive brain damage or injury to the spinal cord, the input of specialist neurological rehabilitation services is advised. These physiotherapists have trained specifically in the assessment and management of complex problems arising from brain and spinal cord dysfunction, e.g. hypertonic muscles, abnormal movement patterns, balance problems and soft tissue adaptations. In these circumstances careful and specific handling techniques are required in order to treat the patient. Incorrect handling will be detrimental to recovery as it may accentuate problems, such as hypertonicity, pain, and loss of range of movement.

Some patients also have soft tissue injuries – damage to ligaments, tendons or muscles – and these are not treated surgically unless complicated by an open wound. The physiotherapist will assume responsibility for the treatment of soft tissue injuries using a variety of techniques to reduce swelling and pain and accelerate the healing process.

Patient motivation and compliance are important components affecting the success of physiotherapy interventions. It can take many months for a fracture to repair and remould to a level where normal function is safe. In the interim period, the patient has to bear the frustrations of limited activity. For example, patients who use elbow crutches often experience marked fatigue, as the physiological cost of crutch-walking is much greater than normal locomotion (Jones and Barker, 1996). Also, many of the treatments used in physiotherapy have a naturally slow and incremental effect. In a normal muscle it takes up to 3 months for the fibres to strengthen, and although this time course is probably quicker in damaged or weakened muscle, there is often a time delay before improvements are seen (Sale, 1991). It is important that exercise programmes are updated regularly. Patients should be counselled carefully about the natural time course of recovery and the efforts they will be required to make in order to improve physical function. A balance must be found between ensuring that the exercise programme is progressed sufficiently to ensure improvements, but is not so hard that it is uncomfortable or disheartening – a principle known as overload (Jones and Barker, 1996). In some cases injuries are such that full recovery is an unrealistic goal. This is a challenging situation in which the physiotherapist has to make every effort to ensure that the patient reaches their maximum potential while not giving false expectations.

Case study

A 25-year-old man sustained a fractured tibia in a motorcycle accident. Surgical fixation involved the use of an intramedullary tibial nail.

Aims of treatment:

- to maintain elevation of the limb until evidence of wound healing is apparent
- to assess for compartment syndrome
- to assess for knee and ankle ligament damage
- to assess leg length, alignment and rotation
- to control oedema and pain by the use of foot pumps, cryocuff and active exercises
- to teach an appropriate active exercise programme to restore knee and ankle mobility within 3–4 days
- to teach calf and hamstring stretches
- to ensure splinting of the ankle joint in a plantigrade position (90 degrees) until the patient is adequately weight-bearing and controlling ankle position with their own muscles
- to re-educate standing balance in accordance with required weight-bearing status (partial or full depending on fracture pattern and integrity of fixation)
- to re-educate gait, aiming for normal movement
- to educate about the fracture and its fixation, together with any activity restrictions such as driving, work or sport
- to increase weight-bearing as fracture healing occurs
- to re-educate proprioception (joint position, sense and balance mechanisms).

Following discharge from hospital the physiotherapy process usually continues in the outpatient department in combination with a home treatment programme.

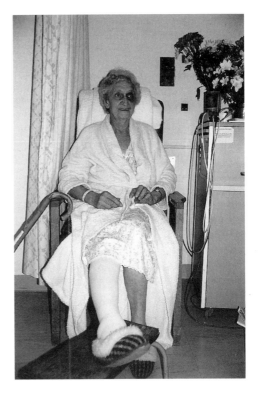

Figure 28.1 Patient with fractured neck of femur

spinal cord injuries, older adults with multiple pathologies, and chest trauma is also required. They need to develop a positive yet realistic approach, together with the ability to communicate with patients, their families and the multidisciplinary team. Physiotherapists are essential in the process of multidisciplinary goal-setting, advising on movement and mobility restriction in preparation for safe discharge to the community.

Skills needed in the physiotherapy team

Trauma is unpredictable and patients present with a wide range of injuries and problems. Many, but not all, will undergo surgical fixation of their fractures. Physiotherapists who work in the speciality of trauma require a broad range of skills and experience, including a sound knowledge of anatomy, mechanisms of injury, fracture healing and methods of surgical fixation. The ability to assess and treat head and

Case study

A 75-year-old woman fell sustaining a femoral neck fracture and as a result she required a hemiarthroplasty (Figure 28.1). Her post-operative management includes:

Main problems:

- fear of falling
- fear of pain
- lack of confidence
- multipathology
- disturbed balance mechanisms

Aims of rehabilitation:

- to assess for additional pathology, especially musculoskeletal, respiratory and neurological problems
- to assess social circumstances
- to maintain optimal respiratory function
- to teach early bed-to-chair transfers with nursing staff as part of a functional rehabilitation programme
- to restore ability to stand – re-educate static and dynamic standing balance
- to re-educate the ability to stand up from a chair – antigravity activity
- to restore confidence in walking with appropriate walking aids
- to assess for discrepancies in leg length and ensure provision of necessary orthotics
- to liaise with members of the team for effective discharge planning.

Overall objectives:

- to restore independent mobility via a functional approach to rehabilitation
- to restore independence in daily living activities.

Remember that the elderly patient responds well to the following:

- clear instruction, with one person at a time giving instructions
- encouragement and positive feedback
- reassurance and a calm approach

Advice on sitting to standing and walking with a Zimmer frame:

- ensure patient is wearing flat, non-slip footwear
- help them to the edge of the chair
- bend the knees as far as is comfortable, with the affected leg further forwards
- place hands on the chair arms – do not let the patient pull up on the frame, as this is poor technique
- lean well forwards so the head is over the feet or beyond
- push up to stand, emphasizing pushing up from the knees, looking ahead not down
- once in standing position, keep feet slightly apart and placed just behind the frame
- stand tall
- to commence walking place the frame forwards
- take two steps up to the frame
- before sitting, feel for the chair behind
- bend in the middle and slowly lower to the seat, sitting as far back as possible.

Techniques commonly used by physiotherapists in the treatment of trauma patients

Respiratory treatment (Webber, 1998)

Patients at risk from chest infection

- Those with pre-existing respiratory disease.
- Those who smoke.
- Those experiencing difficulty with breathing and coughing due to the pain of thoracic trauma, e.g. fractured ribs.
- Patients on bedrest.

Patients with respiratory problems:

- Positioning, e.g. upright sitting.
- Breathing exercises.
- Assisted coughing.
- Hands-on treatment.
- Mobilization and exercise.
- Positive pressure breathing apparatus, e.g. CPAP.

Strengthening exercises

Strong muscles are essential for normal movement. Muscles will only strengthen if they are exercised against resistance. Resistance may be applied using the weight of a limb, strap weights, elastic bands or springs. Strengthening exercises are often prescribed while the patient is bed-bound, in order to preserve as much strength as possible in the injured and uninjured parts of the body. When limb segments cannot be moved static exercises are prescribed, in which the patient holds the limb in an acceptable position and braces the muscles without moving any joints. Proprioceptive neuromuscular facilitation is a specialized method that utilizes reflex activity to stimulate muscles that are very weak (Jones and Barker, 1996).

Joint mobilisation

Sometimes joints become limited in their range of movement because the muscles around them are not strong enough to pull the joint through its entire range. At other times joint capsules or other soft tissues can become thickened and contracted, thus limiting range. In this situation joint mobilization techniques are used. These include passive stretching, in which the physiotherapist gently stretches the joint out, and serial plastering, in which joint range is gradually increased over a period of weeks by reapplication of plasters through an increasing joint range. Joints are complex structures, and to achieve normal movement they have to be able to move in many planes (often referred to as accessory movements). Manipulation or mobilization (a gentle form of manipulation) is often applied to increase accessory movement and thereby normal movement.

Mobility aids and gait re-education

Mobility is defined by the World Health Organisation (1980) as the ability to move from one posture to another; for example, standing up from a chair or walking around. Our ability to move around is determined by several factors which include volition, central and peripheral nervous system activation, joint range, muscle strength and a stable skeleton. The body also has to counteract the effects of gravity when moving and this involves a complex system of balance reflexes. Physiotherapists spend a great deal of time trying to restore mobility after trauma. After surgery or injury patients often have to learn to walk again. Frequently this involves the use of crutches, frames or sticks, and patients have to be taught how to use these safely and correctly. Sometimes they have to learn to walk with artificial limbs or permanent impairments of balance, sensory systems (hearing, sight, feeling), strength and range of movement, and walking aids are used to provide additional support. Other patients require walking aids as they are not allowed to take full weight through a limb until fracture repair is well under way. Gait re-education is the process of learning to walk again, and starts with learning to balance.

Walking aids in trauma are used to protect the affected limb from full loading until the fracture has healed sufficiently to allow full weight-bearing. The weight-bearing status is dependent on fracture pattern, fixation integrity and the strength of the limb. It will vary according to the individual. The aim of the physiotherapist is to achieve a gait pattern which is as near the patient's normal gait as possible, thereby preventing new problems from occurring (Jones and Barker, 1996).

Electrotherapy

The beneficial effects of ultrasound, heat and electrical currents have been established for some time (Wadsworth and Chanmugan, 1988). Transmissive ultrasound (1–3 MHz) is used widely by physiotherapists to reduce swelling and promote healing. Electrical currents, such as faradism (10 Hz, direct current) and interferential (0–150 Hz, variable alternating current) can be used to activate muscle contraction and reduce pain. Transcutaneous nerve stimulation (TENS) is used to reduce pain only.

Pain relief

If physiotherapy is painful it demotivates the patient. The ideal must be to have pain well controlled with regular analgesia. The value of effective postoperative pain management should not be underestimated. In some cases, for example where drug therapy is contraindicated or other methods have failed, the physiotherapist will try to reduce pain using ice, TENS or heat.

Splinting

Some physiotherapists are trained in the application and use of splints. Splints are used to correct or maintain the position of soft tissues and joints in order to maintain optimal joint position and/or prevent soft tissue contractures; for example, in the postoperative management of ankle fractures where the ankle is supported in a plantigrade backslab for several days until the patient is able to control the joint's position using active muscle contraction. If a splint were not applied, a position of equinus (the ankle being turned down and in) could result and this would severely limit the restoration of normal gait. Sometimes splints are used to counteract severe muscle weakness. For example, the quadriceps muscle is essential for holding the leg straight; if strength is lost, as is often the case in trauma, the knee gives way and standing and walking are difficult. In this case, the backslab serves to hold the knee straight. Splints are often used in patients who have sustained neurological damage after trauma, to prevent or eliminate hamstring or Achilles' tendon shortening caused by muscle spasticity.

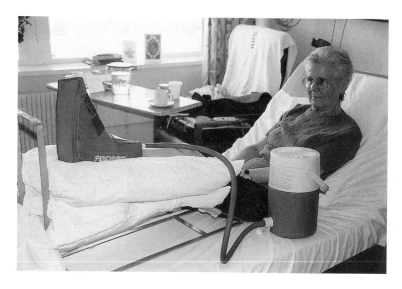

Figure 28.2 Cryocuff

Cryotherapy

The use of cryotherapy (cold therapy) is well documented in the management of soft tissue trauma. It is often used in conjunction with elevation and compression to reduce the amount of inflammatory exudate produced by localized soft tissue tearing. It can also be useful in the treatment of painful muscle spasm. Cryotherapy can be applied in a number of ways, including ice cube massage, ice packs and a cryocuff (Figure 28.2). The cuff is applied to limb segments and has the advantage of being easy to apply, contouring well to the affected area. With all such techniques care must be exercised to ensure patients do not receive ice or cold burns.

Continuous passive movement

Continuous passive movement (CPM) is applied using machines (Figure 28.3). It is useful in the treatment of various musculoskeletal conditions. The system is set up so that the limbs are elevated and the joints are moved repeatedly through a fixed range for up to 24 h. Effects of CPM include:

- reducing muscle spasm by mobilizing and stretching the soft tissues
- enhancing venous return and reducing oedema
- improving circulation and removing painful toxins
- enhancing the circulation of synovial fluid and aiding cartilage repair
- overcoming any natural reluctance to move the limb.

It is useful for intra-articular fixation, e.g. open reduction and internal fixation of tibial plateaux, acetabular fractures and intramuscular haematoma. The effectiveness of CPM is critically dependent on the correct positioning of the machine, slow movement and comfort. It is applied for long periods of time, often at night, and the involvement of nursing staff is integral to the success of the application (Coutts *et al.*, 1989).

Advice and education

The physiotherapist will educate the patient about their injuries and teach self-management programmes which should be maintained, where possible, in the absence of the physiotherapist.

Nursing staff may assist the rehabilitation process by ensuring the provision of regular effective analgesia, reinforcing treatment programmes and encouraging compliance with the following:

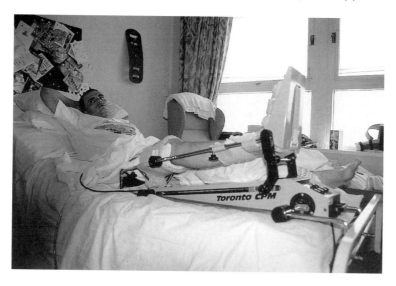

Figure 28.3 Continuous passive motion

- ongoing continuous passive motion and cryotherapy
- maintenance of exercise programmes prescribed by the physiotherapist
- maintenance of upper and lower limb elevation where indicated
- inclusion of mobility practice in daily routine.

Conclusion

The physiotherapist makes an important contribution to the multidisciplinary team by working closely with the trauma patient throughout his period of recovery. Emphasis should be placed on education, self-awareness and motivation with the aim that the injured person accepts ultimate responsibility for their own circumstances and recovery programme.

References

Coutts, F., Hewetson, D. and Matthews, J. (1989) Continuous passive motion of the knee joint. *Physiotherapy*, **75**(7), 427–430.

Hunter, G. (1994) Specific soft tissue mobilisation in the treatment of soft tissue lesions. *Physiotherapy*, January, **80**(1), 15–17.

Jones, K. and Barker, K. (1996) *Human Movement Explained*. Oxford: Butterworth-Heinemann.

Pope, A. M. and Tavlov, A. R. (1991) Disability in America: towards a national agenda for prevention. *Institute of Medicine*. National Academy Press.

Sale, D. G. (1991) Neural adaptation to strength training. In *Strength and Power in Sport* (P. V. Komi, ed.). Blackwell Scientific.

Wadsworth, H. and Chanmugan, A. P. P. (1988) *Electrotherapy Agents in Physiotherapy*. Science Press.

Webber, J. A. (1998) *Physiotherapy for Respiratory and Cardiac Problems* 2nd edn. Churchill Livingstone.

World Health Organisation (1980) *The International Classification of Impairments, Disabilities and Handicaps*. WHO.

29

The role of the occupational therapist in trauma care

Heather McDowell

Introduction

Occupational therapy is the art and science of helping people carry out the day-to-day activities that are important to them, despite impairment, disability or handicap. 'Occupation' in occupational therapy terms refers to 'all of the activities which occupy people's time and give meaning to their lives' (Neistadt and Crepeau, 1998).

The occupational therapist (OT) evaluates an individual's occupational performance and prescribes or adapts activities to improve the quality of that performance. Occupational performance is 'a meaningful sequence of actions in which the person enacts and completes a specified task that is relevant to his or her culture and daily life roles' (Fisher, 1997). Tasks fall into three areas (Reed and Sanderson, 1992):

1. Self-maintenance – maintaining one's own health and well-being.
2. Productivity – providing support to the self, family and society through the production of goods and services.
3. Leisure – for enjoyment, e.g. games, sports and hobbies.

Deficits may then be defined within each area under categories such as sensorimotor, cognitive and psychosocial.

Depending on the nature of the trauma sustained, and specific considerations relating to the individual affected, the OT will select different treatment approaches in isolation or in combination. One of three techniques may be used:

1. Remediation.
2. Compensation.
3. Education.

Any of these approaches may be used in order to enable the individual to achieve the desired task (Holm *et al.*, 1998). In order to be effective, occupational therapy intervention must address the needs of the individual, the nature of the injury, the phase of recovery and the context. The context of occupational therapy in trauma care may range from the intensive care unit (ICU) to an individual's home or even workplace. This eclecticism is a unique strength, but can also make occupational therapy an enigma to those outside the profession.

'Independence' is a key word often connected with occupational therapy. There can be a tendency by the health and social services systems to oversimplify independence, defining it merely in terms of 'needs/does not need assistance'. This definition only refers to the cost of caring for an individual and does not take into account the complexity and qualities of human behaviour which OTs can evaluate and enhance. The OT seeks to enhance effectiveness, efficiency and safety of task performance (Fisher, 1997).

This chapter aims to give an overview of the role of the OT, explaining how trauma patients can benefit from effective occupational therapy input. The use of specific examples is limited in order to illustrate the broad nature of the work.

The occupational therapy process

The four stages in the occupational therapy process are as follows:

1. Gather and analyse information.
2. Plan intervention.
3. Carry out intervention.
4. Evaluate outcomes.

The process is cyclical, and one or more cycles related to different problems may occur simultaneously (Hagedorn, 1995). The process is preceded by referral.

Referral

The nature of trauma is such that admission to hospital is unexpected. It is important therefore that referral to the OT is timely and appropriate. If not, effective intervention will be delayed, resulting in additional costs to the NHS (see also section 'Equipment Provision', below). Problems with referral systems should be investigated and addressed by the team. If appropriate, referral forms should be used in order to avoid omissions or confusion which can result from telephone and verbal referral systems.

Table 29.1   Examples of appropriate patient referrals

Older patients living alone, with decreased function due to fracture (with or without confusion)
Patients with postoperative precautions, e.g. non-weight-bearing
Patients who have sustained traumatic brain injuries
Patients with upper limb injuries requiring orthotics and/or rehabilitation
Patients who have sustained limb amputation or spinal cord injury – for full assessment of needs

---

Checklists and care pathways assist in the timing of referrals. If referrals seem inappropriate or the referral of some clients is overlooked, steps should be taken to raise the profile of the OT's role. This can be achieved by being proactive – participating in (not just attending) ward rounds and case conferences, and getting involved in regular informal discussions with the rest of the team regarding current cases. The team should be encouraged to seek advice about whether an individual would benefit from occupational therapy input. It can be helpful to draw up a list of indications for occupational therapy intervention as a guide, including any particular local variations (Table 29.1).

Accident and emergency department

Occupational therapy services are offered in some A&E departments to help reduce the number of patients admitted to acute wards who do not need inpatient surgical or medical intervention. If staff in A&E identify that an individual might not be able to carry out basic activities at home without some further input, a referral is made. The OT may be able to offer an alternative technique or a piece of adaptive equipment, as well as an opportunity to practice an activity in a supportive environment. They can also make a recommendation for Social Services input to enable the patient to achieve an activity safely, albeit not necessarily independently. It could be argued that this mode of intervention is inferior to an inpatient stay, and it is fair to say that the OT often faces the dilemma between a cost-driven system and the client-centred nature of the profession. However, if the patient is supported by flexible community services, including further occupational therapy input if indicated, hospital admission can be avoided in many instances (Sikorski *et al.*, 1985).

Gather and analyse information

On receipt of an appropriate referral the OT will gather relevant background information such as demographic and social details, past medical history and history of present admission.

Having been introduced, the OT will explain their role to the individual (and their carers if appropriate). An initial assessment will be conducted to establish an outline of the individual's pre-morbid and current life roles and level of occupational performance; also their expectations and aims (including those of their carers) regarding recovery. Questions such as 'What do you do normally?' 'What can you

Table 29.2 Examples of standardized tests

Standardized test	Description
Cognitive Assessment of Minnesota	Consisting of 17 sub-tests covering skills such as attention span, memory, orientation, mathematics, visual neglect, following directions, object identification, judgement, reasoning and safety (Golisz and Toglia, 1998). Assesses person doing task in a very controlled context.
Jebsen–Taylor Hand Function Test	Evaluates fine motor ability by timing the subject carrying out various sub-tests, including card turning, picking up specific objects, simulated feeding, stacking chequers (Kohlmeyer, 1998). Assesses person doing tasks in a controlled context.
Assessment of Motor and Process Skills – AMPS	Measures motor and process skills during specific tasks of daily living in terms of effectiveness, efficiency and safety. It uses an ordinal scale which mathematical analysis (via computer software) translates into an interval scale (Fisher, 1997; Wright and Linacre, cited in Rogers and Holm, 1998). Assesses person doing controlled tasks, but context can vary.

do now?' 'What do you want to do in the future?' are posed with regard to self-maintenance, productivity and leisure.

From the initial evaluation, and with the relevant model of practice in mind, the OT will select some more detailed assessments of the person, such as the tasks they wish to perform and the physical and social context. One of the core skills of an OT is to be able to assess all these elements in an integrated way in order to create individual solutions.

Assessments of task performance may be standardized or non-standardized. Standardized tests have been researched and reviewed to establish reliability and validity and may be norm-referenced or criterion-referenced (Table 29.2). They tend to be quantitative, using scoring systems which may be nominal, ordinal, interval or ratio.

Scores can be compared with normative data for a particular client group or between pre- and post-intervention assessments. Standardization on a large subject sample gives a test high in validity and reliability. In order to maintain the validity and reliability of a standardized assessment and interpret the results correctly, training is required. Therefore the OT carrying out the assessment needs to offer an interpretation of the results to the rest of the team, rather than raw scores.

Non-standardized assessments are widely used. Individual therapists and occupational therapy services develop their own tests to meet the needs of particular client groups or settings (Foster, 1996a). By observing an individual

carrying out a seemingly straightforward task such as washing and dressing or making a cup of tea (both common non-standardized assessments), the OT can identify (but not measure) sensorimotor, cognitive and psychosocial skills and deficits. These in turn are subdivided for the purpose of describing task performance. For example, sensorimotor skills include: touch, sight, hearing, pain response, spatial relations, reflex, range of motion, muscle tone, gross coordination, strength, endurance (AOTA, 1994 cited by Moyers, 1999). Each skill element can be described qualitatively for the task and context concerned, e.g. adequate or inadequate, safe or unsafe, thus enabling a global picture of performance to be obtained. This type of assessment is useful in informing plans for discharge from hospital, but does not offer valid and reliable data from which to evaluate a programme of intervention. Whether using standardized or non-standardized assessments, the OT uses core skills and experience to rate the individual's performance in other relevant areas.

'The environmental context is at least as powerful a determinant of the lives and functioning of persons with disabilities as their individual impairments' (Spencer, 1998). Following traumatic injury the initial context of occupational therapy assessment is likely to be the hospital setting. There will also be a target environment in which the individual will need to be able to perform certain tasks. This is often the home environment (existing or alternative), but may also include a place of work or study and the surrounding neighbourhood. Depending on the complexity of the case and the perceived quality of information available, environmental evaluation may be carried out through direct observation by the OT (with or without the patient) or by obtaining measurements and descriptions from the patient, carers and community professionals. Direct observation of the patient in their home environment is known as a 'home visit' or 'home assessment'. Home visits provide both a social and environmental context – who is available to help and what are their capabilities? A home visit utilizes a great deal of resource, therefore, as with any assessment or intervention procedure, the OT must use clinical reasoning to determine whether it is necessary. The OT should assimilate information offered by the team regarding the safety or medical stability of the patient, but it is ultimately the responsibility of the OT to decide whether a home visit is an effective and efficient medium.

Maslow's *Hierarchy of Needs* (1954, 1970, cited by Papalia and Olds, 1988) is a useful reference point when trying to establish priorities with a patient. In the hospital setting most people's 'physiological' needs are met and their 'safety' needs are at least partially met. Therefore most patients themselves are at the 'belongingness and love' stage of the hierarchy, and their main priority is to go home. This should be considered when trying to motivate patients, and while helping them prioritize their goals.

Plan intervention

The plan of intervention consists of an overall aim, and objectives designed to meet the aim. Goals must always be patient centred as this increases motivation. If the patient is unable to participate in the decision-making, it is even more important that conclusions are ethical and well reasoned (Hagedorn, 1995). Effective team decision-making should assist this process.

The OT requires the knowledge and ability to carry out, teach and adapt technical and creative activities of self-maintenance, work and leisure, in addition to having knowledge of adaptive equipment, environmental adaptations and the means to obtain them (Hagedorn, 1997a). 'Treatment involves participation by the patient which may be initiated or facilitated by the therapist' (Hagedorn, 1995). Other

actions, such as liaison, writing letters of referral, obtaining equipment, planning adaptations and conducting visits may also be essential in achieving the therapeutic goals. The term 'intervention' is used to encompass all actions aimed at eliciting a change in functional status (Hagedorn, 1995; Foster, 1996b).

Equipment provision

Equipment provision and environmental adaptations are a perpetual problem in many occupational therapy services. The assessment and recommendation for a piece of equipment may be straightforward, but the OT also needs to be aware of procedures and availability of equipment. An NHS-funded occupational therapy department may have its own short-term loan store from which it is usual to loan equipment free of charge on the basis that it will be returned. The range of equipment available for delivery and fitting is determined both by resources and the skill mix of staff in the occupational therapy department. If the patient lives locally, the logistics of delivering and fitting the equipment and collecting it again at the end of the loan period can probably be managed by the department. However, for patients whose injuries require treatment in regional referral centres the logistical problems of obtaining, fitting and collecting equipment promptly and safely out of area are significant. In many instances hospitals or community loan services do not loan equipment 'out of area'. An alternative source local to the patient must then be sought. As a result, the OT can spend more time chasing equipment than in face-to-face contact with the patient!

In some areas equipment may be funded by Health and/or Social Services, although there may be strict eligibility criteria for the issue of equipment funded by Social Services. Eligibility criteria are so strict for some areas that anyone who has sustained trauma is excluded, as it cannot be proved that they are 'substantially and permanently disabled' according to the words of the National Assistance Act 1948. In some areas, charities or private purchase are the only available options. This could be seen as a breach of the NHS Act 1977 (cited by Mandlestam, 1999) which states that NHS services 'shall be free of charge'. It may seem that a more consistent approach is needed to ensure adequate provision. Unfortunately, methods that work in one area may not necessarily translate to another, hence the continued variance.

Any source of equipment will require some period of notice in order that the patient receives the correct items. For example, following a femoral fracture a patient may be medically fit for discharge within a few days of surgery and progress rapidly from total bedrest to independence on crutches, but may still be unable to sit on a normal lavatory. If a prospective discharge date is set before the patient is fit to be fully assessed by the OT, the whole team must be consistent in ensuring that discharge is subject to satisfactory assessment and all necessary equipment being *in situ* at home.

Carry out intervention

The OT will have skills in some or all recognized treatment approaches. These fall into various frames of reference according to different texts (Hagedorn, 1997a), and may be categorized as shown in Table 29.3.

.

Table 29.3 Frames of reference applicable to occupational therapy in trauma care

Frame of reference	Application in trauma care
Biomechanical	Hand injuries, fractures, peripheral nerve lesions, amputations, burns
Neurodevelopmental	Traumatic brain injuries, spinal cord lesions
Cognitive-perceptual	Traumatic brain injuries

The treatment media in occupational therapy are meaningful activities (or elements of an activity) that are relevant to the individual receiving treatment. In order to use an activity therapeutically, the following process is used (after Hagedorn, 1997b):

- Select a task which offers potential to meet the therapeutic objective.
- Which elements have therapeutic value?
- What should the patient do/not do themselves?
- Is there a need for adaptation, materials and tools?

- Grade the task, e.g.
  - complexity/number of elements to the task
  - size of tools
  - position of materials
  - speed, duration, repetition
  - use specific movement patterns
  - strength required
  - instruction/prompts given
  - social context (support versus distraction)
  - perceptual and cognitive elements
  - environment – lighting, noise, temperature, furniture, visual cues, steps, rails.

Example: Cleaning windows

Easy task: e.g. part of a programme of short, meaningful activities to increase upper limb function (strength, coordination, etc.) or cognitive-perceptual function (scanning, attention, etc.).

- Well lit room without distractions.
- One small window at waist height to be cleaned with a light cloth.
- OT gives full instructions and may even facilitate the required movements by handing tools to the patient and applying window cleaner to the window for the patient.
- OT continues to give prompts as required.

Difficult task: e.g. work hardening for a patient whose job involves cleaning windows.

- Hot, noisy office with many windows and furniture, and people to work around.
- Work must be carried out in a defined time period.
- Many different tools to choose from (some heavy), use of ladder and crouching down.
- OT offers advice only.

Example: Personal care

Easy task: e.g. in the case of a patient requiring full care following traumatic brain injury.

- One element of personal care, such as brushing the hair, is chosen.
- Patient offered the brush.
- Patient given appropriate cues on how to use it and terminate the action appropriately.

> Difficult task: e.g. take a full bath or shower using appropriate adaptive equipment and techniques while adhering to orthopaedic restrictions.
>
> - Patient has to access the bathroom, set up the environment with any items they require, undress, run water, transfer safely into bath/shower, wash themselves to their satisfaction, transfer out, empty water, dry themselves to their satisfaction, complete any grooming and dress.
> - OT offers suggestions re technique or use of an aid.
> - OT monitors whether the restrictions are being maintained.
> - OT intervenes physically if safety is in question or the patient is unable to complete the task.

Application of frames of reference and treatment approaches

The following are examples of occupational therapy interventions for different categories of injury and context. They may overlap and are not designed to be exhaustive descriptions or treatment protocols.

A. Fractures and associated soft tissue injury

Depending on the fracture site, associated injuries and their pre-morbid level of function, the difficulties experienced by the client could be wide ranging as the following example illustrates.

It is identified that the client wishes to dress him/herself independently and that there is a deficit in a motor skill involved, such as bending to put on shoes and socks. The action of bending in this task is analysed in detail – whether seated or standing it involves flexion of the knees, hips, lumbar spine and glenohumeral joint, and protraction of the shoulder girdle, while stabilizing with one or both lower limbs. This level of detail enables the OT to identify the exact cause of the skill deficit.

Unless there are postoperative precautions to which the patient must adhere, the OT could choose a remedial approach. This would involve encouraging the individual to persevere with the challenging element of the task in order to achieve it. Through this activity the patient

will increase their range of movement, strength and activity tolerance, also increasing the overall confidence they have in their performance ability, thus ultimately achieving the goal of putting on shoes and socks.

Where the individual may be required to adhere to precautions, such as non-weight-bearing or a restriction on range of movement, the OT may educate the individual in a safe technique to adopt. Alternatively, introducing a piece of adaptive equipment to compensate for the constraint may allow the individual to complete the task effectively, efficiently and safely. The patient may of course not wish to work towards independence and choose to have assistance with the task until they wish to attempt it again. Depending on the expected recovery rate and the contribution of such activities to their progress, the patient may be encouraged more or less strongly to try the activity themselves.

> ### Case study
>
> A 22-year-old motorcycle courier involved in an RTA sustains a posterior fracture dislocation of the left hip. For 3 months following open reduction and internal fixation he is required to be non-weight-bearing on the affected leg and to restrict hip flexion in any activity to 60 degrees. He reports little pain and the team report that he is not fully adhering to restrictions. He lives with his mother in a two-storey house (bathroom and toilet upstairs, toilet downstairs) and has been with his girlfriend for two years. Hobbies include motorbikes, computers and socializing.
>
> *Model of practice.* Reed and Sanderson (1992) – adaptation through occupation.
>
> *Treatment approaches.* Cognitive behavioural and biomechanical, remediation, compensation and education (see Table 29.4).
>
> *Aim.* To facilitate safe discharge to the home environment, including resolution of the patient's priority problems, and ongoing recovery.

B. Traumatic brain injury

The brain-injured patient may be referred to the OT before being completely medically stable. Precautions to preserve basic body regulatory

Table 29.4 Case study (see text)

Objective	Problem areas	Treatment approach/intervention
• To be able to carry out all intimate care independently • To be able to carry out remainder of personal care tasks with minimal assistance • To be able to manage stairs with supervision	Self-maintenance: • Unable to sit on 17 inch high toilet due to restrictions • Unable to access bath or shower due to restrictions • Unable to reach below left knee for washing or dressing • Mobility limited to crutches on the level and stairs (unsafe)	• Assess for and arrange equipment, and practice technique to enable personal care tasks (biomechanical, compensation) • Practise activities which require mobility (biomechanical, remediation)
• To be able to get a drink and snack from the kitchen and take into living room • To be able to answer front door and telephone	Productivity: • Standing tolerance limited to 2 minutes, therefore domestic activities of daily living (ADL) restricted • Unable to carry items across room and around house	• Practice activities which require standing • Arrange perching stool (biomechanical, remediation) • Teach how to move items around house by rearranging environment (biomechanical, education)
• To return to a familiar, less restrictive environment and to be able to see friends and family at usual frequency • To be able to resume sexual activity at some level as soon as possible • To be more informed, hence less anxious about likely progress rate towards previous leisure pursuits	Leisure: • Anxiety re future functional ability, leisure and sexual activities 'Dying to go home' 'Hate hospital food' 'Can't smoke in here' 'Miles away from friends and family'	• Discuss how precautions affect leisure activity and allow patient to consider alternative pursuits for the next 3-6 months (biomechanical, education) • Advice about applying precautions to sexual activity • Patient to discuss with girlfriend and proceed carefully (biomechanical and psychological, education)

systems must be heeded by the therapist (Dow, 1989). Patients diagnosed as being in a vegetative state (VS) by a physician should be referred to occupational therapy for further assessment and intervention regarding sensory awareness (visual, tactile, auditory, olfactory and gustatory), level of wakefulness, and functional motor and communicative ability (Gill-Thwaites, 1997).

There are various definitions and assessment tools for VS, and the term itself continues to be debated. Evidence suggests that levels of arousal within VS can fluctuate, therefore the more opportunities there are to observe the patient's function, the more accurate the diagnosis (Gill-Thwaites, 1997).

The aim of occupational therapy intervention is to elicit increasingly localized, appropriate and consistent responses from the patient (Dow, 1989). In order to assess and treat levels of arousal the OT presents a sensory stimulus and observes the response. The patient's position may be altered to see if this alters the response, hence the use of supportive seating systems as an alternative to lying in bed.

Responses might include change in posture, facial movement, startle reaction, eye opening, or changes in heart rate, blood pressure or respiration. Electronic switches may also be used to magnify a response. Structured, graded stimulation enables the patient to interact with the environment and begin to become orientated in time and space. Emphasis is placed on forming a routine by the regular provision of stimuli through familiar activities (such as personal hygiene, grooming, listening to music or direct verbal stimuli).

In addition, the OT will address maintenance of joint range, skin integrity and control of oedema through retrograde massage, pressure garments, regular monitoring and adjustment of positioning and orthotics, ensuring collaboration with all relevant members of the multidisciplinary team.

As the patient's interaction with the environment becomes more consistent, occupational therapy intervention can turn towards more complex activities. A variety of approaches to traumatic brain injury may be used and eclecticism is favoured.

Rood, Brunstromm, Carr & Shepherd, Bobath and Peripheral Neuromuscular Facilitation are all examples of recognized treatment approaches for patients with motor control problems due to brain damage (Trombly, 1989a). Some of these complement one another well, others use opposing frames of reference. Team coordination is essential if the treatment programme is to be effective, as both the physiotherapist and the OT are likely to use principles from these approaches in their treatment sessions. Detailed discussion of these techniques is beyond the scope of this text – see references for further information (Trombly, 1989a, 1989b). In basic terms, all the approaches emphasize the importance of sensation to movement and the importance of repetition for learning. They differ on whether treatment should focus on the movement itself or the goal of the movement, whether spinal and brain stem reflexes should be used to elicit movement or inhibit it, and whether movement should be encouraged only in developmental order.

Following traumatic brain injury the individual may also have cognitive and perceptual deficits. Although the OT works with the psychologist and speech and language therapist to address these deficits, the unique role of occupational therapy is to assess and treat the *functional* cognitive and perceptual deficits which can sometimes outweigh their more visible motor problems when it comes to achieving everyday activities (Quintana, 1989). A functional problem may be due to one or more of a number of deficits, so detailed assessment is required. This is best done using standardized assessments to enable retesting and hence evaluation of treatment programmes.

Treatment may be remedial, compensatory or substitutive and involves the selective use of tactile, auditory and visual stimuli to retrain the patient in the required area through functional activities (Table 29.5). Almost any activity which requires the skill in question can be graded appropriately to become a treatment medium.

C. Traumatic amputation of a lower limb

Amputation following trauma, as opposed to amputation associated with chronic disease, often offers the patient a better functional prognosis – particularly the younger patient.

The absence of chronic disease and co-morbidity, e.g. peripheral vascular disease, diabetes, decreased cardiopulmonary function, cognitive or perceptual impairment leads to higher activity tolerance. The patient can therefore cope with more intensive rehabilitation, together with the additional energy demands of wearing a prosthesis. Although the psychological effects of a traumatic injury can be devastating, the amputee who has experienced chronic pain and disability or a concurrent loss, such as bereavement or unemployment, may be less able to overcome their problems (Raphael, 1984, cited by Colburn and Ibbotson, 1996).

The OT aims to assist the individual in coming to terms with the loss of the limb. Practical solutions to problems presented by everyday tasks are provided, with the individual being encouraged to create their own solutions. Equipment such as a wheelchair or grab rails may be used in order to overcome transfer and mobility problems. The individual is taught to use the equipment safely and efficiently on the ward in preparation for discharge to the home environment.

One of the most important applications of a pre-discharge home visit is to establish environmental access for a new wheelchair user. The OT assesses the individual performing a task, at the same time offering them coaching points or altering the environment in anticipation of a problem. In this way patients get a positive experience of carrying out the activity at the first attempt. The activity can subsequently be made more challenging as part of ongoing intervention if required. Collaboration with Social Services occupational therapy departments is essential to obtain necessary adaptations for the new wheelchair user to access their home. Occasionally rehousing will be required, although this is less likely for a traumatic amputee as they are more likely to wear a prosthesis.

During the rehabilitation phase the individual is given the opportunity to practise daily activities in a supported environment using the wheelchair and/or prosthesis and translate this to the home, work and leisure environments.

Desensitization of the remaining limb and management of phantom limb pain can be facilitated through graded stimulation, relaxation techniques and personal care activities. A grief process (Kubler-Ross, 1969, cited by Foster, 1996c) for the lost limb should be

Table 29.5 Examples of perceptual and cognitive deficits, together with some OT treatment options (Adapted from Quintana, 1989)

Deficit	Functional problem	Treatment example
Body scheme	• Lack of recognition of body parts or relationship between them • Difficulty dressing or transferring safely	• Tactile stimuli, accompanied by other cues depending on whether left or right brain injury
Unilateral neglect	• Shaves one side of face • Eats only one half of a plate of food • Bumps into objects on one side	• During tasks such as dressing, cooking and workbook tasks, offer visual prompts towards the affected side • When no further improvement, adapt environment • More easily treated for left than right brain injured patients
Figure ground	• Unable to find one object among others or against a similar background – more difficult if they are a similar shape, size or colour	• Grade tasks according to number of objects, similarity to each other or background • Carry out in a relevant context
Apraxia	Ideational • Does not know how to carry out a movement to achieve a goal or uses wrong tool for the job	• Generally seen in left brain damage, therefore may need visual clues rather than verbal to get appropriate response
	Ideomotor: • Cannot follow an instruction but can do the movement automatically	• Treatment sometimes not necessary • Options include guiding physically through the task, backwards chaining • Practise component parts of task then integrate into whole
Attention	• Easily distracted, therefore difficulties in learning and following instructions	• Environment with no distractions • Call attention specifically to the task • Use tasks which are interesting to patient
Memory	Decreased ability to learn/retain information	• Activities to 'improve memory' only effective if good attention span, therefore mainly compensatory strategies e.g. use of diaries, lists, labelling (use pictures as well as words for left brain injury)

expected and managed by OT, as well as issues regarding altered body image and the individual's preconceptions about using a wheelchair and/or prosthesis. In this type of intervention the 'therapeutic use of self' (Hagedorn, 1995) is most significant. In occupational therapy the therapeutic relationship is developed through meaningful activities – the way in which the activities are presented affects performance. Effective use of self can dramatically improve the patient's quality of life in the long term.

Traumatic amputation of the upper limb is normally treated within specialist units and is rare compared to lower limb amputation, therefore it is not included in this text. Following partial amputation of fingers, or transposition of fingers or toes onto the hand, the involvement of a hand therapist is recommended.

D. Upper limb injury

Following repair of damaged structures by the surgical team, the OT makes an assessment and goals of treatment are established, focusing around evidence-based treatment protocols as well as the patient's occupational aims. For example, following a tendon repair the OT forms a thermoplastic splint to prevent movements which could cause the surgical repair to rupture, while still allowing residual function to be maintained. The therapist instructs the patient in an exercise and scar management programme to carry out at home to prevent adhesions, maintain excursion of the tendons through the tendon sheaths, reduce oedema and maintain joint range.

If a nerve injury is reported by the surgeons, or altered sensation is experienced by the patient, sensation is assessed using a standardized test such as the Semmes–Weinstein Monofilament Test (Fess, 1993, cited by Kohlmeyer, 1998). If a deficit is identified, sensory re-education begins in order to protect insensate and altered areas from further damage, minimize hypersensitivity and achieve maximal function (Waylett-Rendall, 1998). A sensory re-education programme consists of graded stimulation of the affected area with different textured cloth, rice tubs, etc., and education of the individual to enable them accurately to locate and respond to stimulation of the affected area, thereby increasing their awareness of potential hazards. In a rehabilitation or community setting these activities can be translated into tasks of self-maintenance, productivity or leisure as appropriate to the individual.

The individual may have family or friends who are able to offer support while they are unable to use the affected hand. If support from Social Services is required and is acceptable to the individual, the OT should liaise with the appropriate service, monitoring the patient's progress and altering services accordingly.

E. Spinal cord injury

Whether the spinal cord injured patient is received into a regional specialist unit or a general hospital, the OT has the same aims of management – restoration of and compensation for lost function while addressing the psychological aspects of such a devastating injury (Trombly, 1989b). There are advantages and disadvantages to each setting. The regional unit might have advanced skills, experience and resources to deal with the injury and acute phase; however, it can be difficult for the OT at the regional centre to offer assessment of home and work environments, together with follow-up, because of the distances involved. Availability of resources is likely to define how much the team can achieve in either setting.

During the acute phase the patient may have restrictions imposed to protect the spinal cord from further damage, e.g. lying supine, log-rolling for pressure relief, restriction on shoulder and hip movement to prevent secondary movement of the spine. The OT seeks to enable the individual to participate in self-care activities to restore some independence within these restrictions.

The level of the lesion determines the techniques and equipment used in OT intervention. For a high-level lesion, e.g. C2, the aim will be to enable the patient to express their needs and preferences and have control over some of their environment, such as operating a book turner, feeding device and later a wheelchair, through switches and electronic devices.

For a mid-level lesion, e.g. C6, the aim will be to enable the individual to carry out basic personal hygiene and access activities within the ward setting, using orthotics and other specialist equipment. The OT may form splints to position the hands in order to develop a tenodesis grip. This position selectively shortens flexor and extensor tendons to enable a grip achieved by active wrist extension in the absence of innervation to the finger flexors, and release of the grip by active wrist flexion.

For a low-level or incomplete lesion, the OT will primarily be concerned with maintaining functional independence in the acute phase, ensuring at first that the patient can access their surroundings while lying flat in bed, progressing to efficient wheelchair or calliper mobility in various environments.

F. Burns

For a patient whose primary injury is a burn, the aims of occupational therapy intervention will be to

- prevent loss of joint mobility, e.g. with orthotics
- maintain and improve strength and endurance through patient-centred purposeful activity, e.g. for a burn covering the elbow joint and axilla the activity of cleaning a window would include all the necessary components and could be graded in various ways (see explanation of grading under section 'Carry Out Intervention', above)
- control oedema and scar development, e.g. through pressure garment provision and silicone gel
- promote self care skills
- assist patients in coming to terms with altered body image through therapeutic use of self
- ensure ongoing progress reviews until scar tissue has matured and optimum function

has been achieved in all three areas of daily life (Rivers and Jordan, 1998).

Evaluate outcomes

Many occupational therapy services use goal achievement as an outcome measure. It can work well where the multidisciplinary team sets goals together, but should be monitored for objectivity. It acknowledges the individuality of patients and can be especially useful in situations where standardized assessments are not yet available or are not flexible enough to be used and remain standard. In order to increase validity and reliability of goal-orientated outcome measures the goals should be specific, measurable, achievable, relevant and time limited. They need to be regularly reviewed and updated, and the treatment plan adjusted according to progress made. Accurate documentation is necessary in order to evaluate progress and enable audits of effectiveness to be conducted.

A standardized assessment of occupational performance, such as AMPS (Fisher, 1997) can highlight small differences in outcome, particularly in later stages of recovery when many outcome measures are not sufficiently sensitive to show small changes over time or between individuals. Some assessments simply do not consider the problems which the individual continues to face in sufficient detail, namely problems in achieving desired occupations which contribute to quality of life. AMPS is useful because is measures task performance as relevant to the patient. It can be used as an outcome measure pre- and post- intervention as there is no learning element. All tasks assessed are already familiar to the individual.

The occupational therapy profession, through clinical interest groups, is encouraging wider use of valid and reliable outcome measures in order to increase the efficacy and credibility of occupational therapy intervention. Through the use of integrated care pathways and treatment guidelines which are regularly audited, the evidence base for occupational therapy can be strengthened and clinical effectiveness can be increased.

Integrated care pathways for trauma are being developed and implemented following successes in reducing length of stay for elective surgery. For occupational therapy this success seems to stem from consistently early referral, a programme which allows time for more regular, quality patient–therapist contact and a well coordinated discharge. This is made possible through the closer teamwork which care pathways require. The patient is made aware of their potential recovery process early on and becomes an active participant in increasing their activity levels. Confidence in their ability to cope after discharge from hospital is increased through opportunities to practise daily living skills, and earlier discharge has been shown to benefit the patient's recovery (Ceder *et al.*, 1980; Jensen and Bagger, 1982, cited by Meeds and Pryor, 1990) and they are more likely to achieve their potential. Through evaluation of occupational performance the OT can provide feedback to the team regarding the overall progress of an individual towards their chosen lifestyle.

Conclusion

The aim of occupational therapy in trauma care is to enable the individual to regain satisfying life roles in order to maximize their quality of life.

Occupational therapy intervention will be as individual as the patient receiving it, will take into account the nature of the injury and the patient's cultural, social and environmental background. OTs use detailed understanding of task performance to make integrated assessments and form effective solutions through functional activities. Within models of practice, OTs use remediation of deficits, compensatory strategies and education to increase occupational performance. Indirect actions to secure equipment, social support and ongoing intervention can be just as important in the process. In order to realize its aims, OT intervention needs to be a continuum stretching from the hospital setting to the individual's target environment, the first step of which is referral.

Therefore, timely and appropriate referrals to occupational therapy are the key to an effective service. Occupational therapy offers unique skills to the multidisciplinary team, enabling the patient to step out of the injured role and resume their place in society.

For further information contact:

The College of Occupational Therapists
106–114 Borough High Street
London SE1 1LB.

Specialist sections and interest groups relevant to trauma care within the College are:

Occupational Therapy in Trauma and Orthopaedics (OTTO)

Clinical Interest Group in Orthotics, Prosthetics and Wheelchairs (CIGOPW)

National Association of Occupational Therapists in Neurology (NANOT)

Occupational Therapy for Elderly People (OCTEP)

References

Ceder, L., Thorngren, K. G. and Wallden, B. (1980) Prognostic indicators and early home rehabilitation in elderly patients with hip fractures. *Clinical Orthopaedics*, **152**, 173–184.

Colburn, J. and Ibbotson, V. (1996) Amputation. In *Occupational Therapy and Physical Dysfunction*, 4th edn. (A. Turner, M. Foster and S. E. Johnson, eds). Churchill Livingstone.

Dow, P. W. (1989) Traumatic brain injuries. In *Occupational Therapy for Physical Dysfunction*, 3rd edn. (C. A. Trombly, ed.) Williams & Wilkins.

Fisher, A. G. (1997) *Assessment of Motor and Process Skills.* Three Star Press.

Foster, M. (1996a) Assessment. In *Occupational Therapy and Physical Dysfunction*, 4th edn. (A. Turner, M. Foster and S. E. Johnson, eds). Churchill Livingstone.

Foster, M. (1996b) Process of practice. In *Occupational Therapy and Physical Dysfunction*, 4th edn. (A. Turner, M. Foster and S. E. Johnson, eds). Churchill Livingstone.

Foster, M. (1996c) Introduction to musculoskeletal and vascular problems. In *Occupational Therapy and Physical Dysfunction*, 4th edn. (A. Turner, M. Foster and S. E. Johnson, eds). Churchill Livingstone.

Gill-Thwaites, H. (1997) The sensory modality assessment rehabilitation technique. A tool for assessment and treatment of patients with severe brain injury in a vegetative state. *Brain Injury*, **11**(10), 723–734.

Golisz, K. M. and Toglia, J. P. (1998) Evaluation of perception and cognition. In *Willard & Spackman's Occupational Therapy* (M. E. Neistadt and E. B. Crepeau, eds). Lippincott-Raven.

Hagedorn, R. (1995) Case management. In *Occupational Therapy – Perspectives and Processes*. 157–174, Churchill Livingstone.

Hagedorn, R. (1997a) Applied frames of reference which focus on physical dysfunction. In *Foundations for Practice in Occupational Therapy*, 2nd edn. Churchill Livingstone.

Hagedorn, R. (1997b) Core skills and processes. In *Foundations for Practice in Occupational Therapy*, 2nd edn. Churchill Livingstone.

Holm, J. B., Rogers, J. C. and James, A. B. (1998) Treatment of occupational performance areas. In *Willard & Spackman's Occupational Therapy*, 9th edn. (M. E. Neistadt and E. B. Crepeau, eds). Lippincott-Raven.

Kohlmeyer, K. (1998) Evaluation of performance components. In *Willard & Spackman's Occupational Therapy*, 9th edn. (M. E. Neistadt and E. B. Crepeau, eds). Lippincott-Raven.

Mandlestam, M. (1999) Printed notes from training day for St George's Healthcare NHS Trust Occupational Therapy Department, 8 July (unpublished).

Meeds, B. and Pryor, G. A. (1990) Early home rehabilitation for the elderly patient with a hip fracture. The Peterborough hip fracture scheme. *Physiotherapy*, **76**, 75–77.

Moyers, P. A. (1999) The guide to occupational therapy practice. *American Journal of Occupational Therapy*, **53**(3), 247–322.

Neistadt, M. E. and Crepeau, E. B. (1998) Introduction to occupational therapy. In *Willard & Spackman's Occupational Therapy*, 9th edn. (M. E. Neistadt and E. B. Crepeau, eds). Lippincott-Raven.

Papalia, D. E. and Olds, S. W. (1988) Motivation and emotion. In *Psychology International Student Edition*, 2nd edn. McGraw-Hill.

Quintana, L. A. (1989) Cognitive and perceptual evaluation and treatment. In *Occupational Therapy for Physical Dysfunction*, 3rd edn. (C. A. Trombly, ed.). Williams & Wilkins.

Reed, K. L. and Sanderson, S. N. (1992) Glossary. In *Concepts of Occupational Therapy*, 3rd edn. Williams & Wilkins.

Rivers, E. A. and Jordan, C. L. (1998) Skin system dysfunction: burns. In *Willard & Spackman's Occupational Therapy*, 9th edn. (M. E. Neistadt and E. B. Crepeau, eds). Lippincott-Raven.

Rogers, J. C. and Holm, M. B. (1998) Evaluation of activities of daily living and home management. In *Willard & Spackman's Occupational Therapy*, 9th edn. (M. E. Neistadt and E. B. Crepeau, eds). Lippincott-Raven.

Sikorski, J., Davis, N. and Senior, J. (1985) The rapid transit system for patients with fractures of proximal femur. *British Medical Journal*, **290**, 439–443.

Spencer, J. C. (1998) Valuation of performance contexts. In *Willard & Spackman's Occupational Therapy*, 9th edn. (M. E. Neistadt and E. B. Crepeau, eds). Lippincott-Raven.

Trombly, C. A. (1989a) Neurophysiological and developmental treatment approaches. In *Concepts of Occupational Therapy*, 3rd edn. Williams & Wilkins.

Trombly, C. A. (1989b) Motor control therapy. In *Concepts of Occupational Therapy*, 3rd edn. Williams & Wilkins.

Waylett-Rendall, J. (1998) Sensory re-education. In *Willard & Spackman's Occupational Therapy*, 9th edn. (M. E. Neistadt and E. B. Crepeau, eds). Lippincott-Raven.

30

Collaborative practice

Jane Christie

Introduction

The aim of this chapter is to discuss the nature of collaborative practice in trauma care. Collaboration is defined as the ability 'to work jointly with others' (Swannell, 1992). Hamilton (1991) argues that using collaborative practice reduces hospital stay, despite higher patient acuity, lowers mortality rates, increases staff satisfaction and promotes cost containment (Kerfoot, 1989).

Healthcare professionals work together at each stage of the continuum of trauma care. At the site of an accident paramedics, doctors, nurses, firemen, police and recovery teams attend to the victims. On arrival in the emergency department nurses and doctors make assessments and carry out immediate care. Receptionists collect details for the purposes of documentation and identification, porters help to transport the injured person to x-ray, onto a ward or, in severe cases, to the intensive care unit. These are just a few of many roles. The injured person meets a variety of healthcare professionals during the course of their recovery, all of whom strive to adopt a collaborative approach in helping the patient to achieve their potential. But what does this collaborative approach involve?

Collaboration requires teamwork (Johnson, 1992). West and Field (1995) argue that care can be delivered more effectively where professionals work together in a coordinated, coherent way, but indicate that effective teamwork is very difficult to achieve. Barr (1993) identifies the characteristics of effective and ineffective teams (Table 30.1).

In trauma care, teams are not always as clearly defined as this. Following traumatic injury the situation is highly charged as members of the healthcare team work swiftly to save life or limb. As the injured person's condition stabilizes, the pace slows and a different style of teamwork ensues to aid support, rehabilitation and reintegration.

Examples
- The accident and emergency setting – the trauma team work together following agreed protocols with the aim of resuscitating the injured person.
- The acute ward environment – the team continue to stabilize the situation, enabling and supporting the injured person to make the transition from the impact of injury to the realization of the effect that it may have on their lifestyle. This team begin the rehabilitation process and provide a link to the next stage.
- The rehabilitation phase – the team membership is more fluid. The care required has to be flexible to meet the needs of the individual and those close to them – the outcome is not only survival, but quality of life in terms of role and relationships.

The following issues are considered to be important if teams are to work effectively (Barr, 1993) and will provide a framework for this

Table 30.1 Effective and ineffective teams (Adapted from Barr, 1993)

Effective teams	Ineffective teams
Team goals are clearly understood	The goals of the group are imposed on the members
Members coordinate the use of their knowledge and skills to achieve common tasks	Communication is usually one way, from member in high authority
Members contribute accurately, both content and feelings, by effective two-way communication	Delegated leadership is based upon authority and there is unequal participation by members
Knowledge of the whole task is shared and members have responsibilities for the whole as well as individual parts	Obedience to authority is the rule
Decisions are made according to the situation	Decisions are made by the highest authority
Conflicts are not ignored and are seen as positive and necessary for members' involvement	Conflict is ignored, avoided or suppressed
It is acceptable for team members to take calculated risks and there is support for team members who do	Conformity is the rule
Those who desire creativity and innovation	Those who desire order, stability and structure

chapter:

- identifying a shared purpose
- clarifying shared values and beliefs
- the role of the leader
- relationships within the team
- communication.

Identifying a shared purpose

To achieve multidisciplinary care, an organization needs to become people friendly and focused, service orientated, empowered, expert in systems thinking, involved and dedicated to goal achievement (Lenkman and Gribbins, 1994). However, Hilton (1995) argues that care is often compromised due to tunnel vision caused by a lack of knowledge of the roles of others, differing concepts and different goals. Since the introduction of Advanced Trauma Life Support, emergency teams are ready and prepared to manage the unexpected. This preparation is essential when the victim, initially shocked, vulnerable and helpless, is dependent on the team to manage their care while they cope both physically and emotionally with the impact of their injury. As the injured person recovers they become more knowing and potentially more powerful, demanding rights and participation in decision-making. Due to the disparate differences in the relationship and power base between that of the team and the injured person, it is not surprising that Meyer

(1993) finds there to be a lack of professional commitment to lay participation in care. Lay participation acknowledges a change in relationship between the professional and lay person, emphasizing partnership. The difficulties in the relationship between the professional and the lay person are highlighted in Table 30.2. Forming this partnership is an essential part of coming to terms with the injury and realizing the implications for their own lifestyle. The team of healthcare professionals needs to work closely together to support and guide the injured person back to recovery, extending the team into the domain of the victim and those close to them.

Table 30.2 Problems with lay participation in care (Adapted from Meyer, 1993)

Difficult to articulate and conceptualize

Patients may not wish to get involved

Healthcare professionals might abrogate their responsibilities

Not high-status work, therefore delegated to juniors who lack skills to deal with it competently

Limitations of interprofessional work to foster change in practice

Reluctance to change – dynamic conservatism

Inadequate information available to share with lay person

Transience, e.g. rotational posts lead to a lack of commitment and coping by being busy behind a screen of tasks

These problems can be overcome through the development of shared goals and expectations, so that team members know what it is they are working towards and can support each other in the process. Rowe (1996) argues that a team that works towards specific goals develops respect and understanding within the group. However, to achieve this shared aims need to be discussed, agreed and put into practice. Time and effort must be invested in ensuring that team members have time to achieve this away from the responsibilities of managing care.

West (1994) concludes that interprofessional care is about collaboration – the coming together of different health and welfare professionals as partners to develop a collective understanding. This implies a flattened hierarchy and shifting of leadership within a team (Thompson, 1983). The feelings of each team member are very important and can provide an outcome by which success can be measured:

- individuals should feel that they are important to the fate of the group
- individual tasks should be meaningful and intrinsically rewarding
- individual contributions should be identifiable and subject to evaluation and comparison
- teams should have intrinsically interesting tasks to perform
- there should be clear group goals with inbuilt performance feedback.

Temkin-Greener (1983) reported that characteristics associated with teamwork did not feature in practice. Teams failed to function as units with set goals and objectives, individuals were not designated as team members nor evaluated for their performance in a team, and conflict existed over decision-making. This disconnection was a result of the disparate and contradictory goals of the various professions, fuelled by an emphasis on professional loyalty. Those who work in trauma care, regardless of setting, will know of situations where this is commonplace. However, it is important when working in a highly charged and emotionally draining environment that leaders offer stability and support, negotiating and agreeing parameters and giving unconditional and non-judgemental feedback. Responsibilities of each team member need to be recognized and teams should feel able to

manage themselves knowing they have clear lines of accountability to a supportive leader.

Self-managed teams are very creative in generating complex and sophisticated solutions to problems, and can rise to any challenge that the future holds (Blancett, 1994). However, this is a risky business for those in positions of authority who like to maintain control, as it involves a whole new set of value systems.

Clarifying shared values and beliefs

Values are those beliefs and behaviours that are prized, freely chosen and acted upon (Simon *et al.*, 1978). Wilmot (1995) suggests that professional values present problems of definition and evidence. There are good arguments for accepting the differences between professional values as being unavoidable and perhaps desirable, and concentrating on optimizing the quality of interprofessional dialogue around these values rather than seeking to remove the differences. Blancett (1994) suggests that people need freedom, with the insight and understanding that values and principles order their behaviour.

Hilton (1995) investigated the attitudes, experiences and perceptions of experienced physiotherapists through interviews and small group discussion and brainstorming sessions. He subsequently generated data about the failure of teamwork. The following are examples of the attitudes and behaviours that were found:

- team process will fail if one professional adopts an authoritarian approach, as this is learned by juniors and perpetuated
- thinking that your word is law
- feeling insecure in your job
- believing that what you do is more important than someone else
- wanting to be the most important person rather than accepting that everyone has something to contribute
- resenting other professionals
- being a solitary individual who does their own thing regardless of what is going on around you
- unwillingness to communicate – too busy, too angry, too stressed
- doing separate things.

Any of us who work in a team will recognize that some of these attitudes exist within and between professions and lead to problems in collaboration.

Working in a team while recognizing and valuing one's own contribution and professional boundaries, is a skill that comes with knowledge and experience. It is the stressed and ill-informed who aggressively challenge the work of other disciplines, rather than accepting that their contribution may give a different perspective and therefore be of great benefit.

The role of the leader

Effective group leadership is the result of a number of features including flexibility of the leader, adaptability of the leadership style to various situations, the extent to which feedback is acknowledged and accepted and the use of disclosure between the group leader and group members (Yalom, 1985). This involves leadership qualities which inspire and facilitate empowerment and teamwork, such as the ability to coach, negotiate, communicate and network (Blancett, 1994). Effective leadership also involves taking risks (Gilmore, 1993) but at the same time (Table 30.3):

- treating others as you would wish to be treated
- communicating what and why in terms that people can understand
- helping motivate others by teaching them
- being an equal player in the organization and not letting personal initiative impede the growth of an organization or the success of peers
- maintaining a sense of humour to keep things in perspective.

Time needs to be invested in facilitating team development with the aim of helping members to gain an understanding and active commitment to the concept of collaboration. Without this, role boundaries will continue to be blurred, team members will conflict in their approach and the injured person will get unnecessarily involved in the mixed messages and political wrangling of poor working relationships.

Competitiveness within a team is very destructive. The danger of individuals trying to be the best or the most popular, rather than working towards shared goals, can increase conflict and stress in some individuals, leading to isolation and unhappiness. This can happen within a discipline or between professional

groups. A way of overcoming the problem of conflicting interests is outlined by Ovretveit (1994) who describes a framework that divides a patient's journey into eight phases. The aim is for the team to describe what happens in each phase, then to list the common problems from the patient, staff and management perspectives. This approach reduces the risk of personal criticism by keeping the focus on the patient. It facilitates team building, standard setting and helps other members of staff see their contribution to the process.

Table 30.3 Factors which facilitate the development of teams (Adapted from Barr, 1993)

Identify the need for a team

Mutual trust and respect for fellow team members

Understanding how the organization works as a whole

Understanding of the dynamics of teamwork

Appropriate support and autonomy from senior managers outside the team

Preparation and orientation of new team members to teamwork and the shared aims

Acceptance by team members of the grey areas which exist in professional roles

Active commitment to the concept of multiprofessional teamwork, accountability and interdependence

Operational policies for the team: reaching agreement on team values, philosophy, aims, objectives, priorities, roles, responsibility and working relationships

Resolution of conflict

To shift a unit from being competitive to collaborative, leaders must (Horder, 1992):

- openly address psychologically uncomfortable issues relating to organizational and personal values and beliefs
- evaluate and reward staff for being team players (furthering the organizational mission and contributing to the team's success in meeting its goals)
- identify and remove systems that encourage unproductive competition rather than collaboration and networking
- identify broad roles needed for a unit to function and allow team members to rotate through these roles as required
- let the team develop and monitor its own productivity and quality standards
- give the team access to and control over the resources it needs to do its work
- facilitate team development through

Table 30.4 Helping or hindering roles (Adapted from Hersey and Blanchard, 1988)

Readiness level	Helping roles	Hindering roles
1	Establishing: Help start the group along new paths. Propose tasks and goals. Define problems, help set rules and contribute ideas by: • getting started • clarifying purpose • defining goals • maintaining direction	Aggression: Assert personal dominance and attempt to get own way regardless of others by: • criticizing • attacking personality • dominating • name calling
2	Persuading: Request facts and relevant information on the problem. Seek out expressions of feelings and values by: • questioning • encouraging and guiding responses, advocating • developing alternatives	Manipulating: Respond to a problem rigidly and persist in using stereotypical responses by: • topic jumping • masking statements as questions • selective interpretation • gatekeeping
3	Committing: Help to ensure that all members are part of the decision-making process by: • facilitating involvement • synthesizing/summarizing • gaining commitment • problem-solving	Dependence: React to other people as authority figures, abdicate problem-solving to others, expect others to lead the solution by: • agreeing with everything • avoiding decisions or closure through sarcasm • seeking sympathy • expressing futility, resignation or helplessness
4	Attending: Demonstrate a willingness to become involved by: • listening • showing an interest • monitoring and observing • taking notes or recording • division of duties • regular attendance at meetings • free exchange of ideas and suggestions	Avoidance: An emotional retreat in thought, or physically by: • withdrawing psychologically • withdrawing physically • reflecting boredom • escaping the group

planned programmes, negotiation skills and an open mind towards the view of others.

Achievement of this change takes determination, consistency, the ability to facilitate team development and the confidence to take a measured risk.

Group decision-making can be seriously impeded if leadership style and group cohesion interact in such a way that dissent is suppressed. This is described as 'group think' (Janis, 1982). Undoing group think can be a difficult process, as powerful pressure exhibited by the group members prevents the situation changing. Challenging the group view through cooperative problem-solving is one of the most difficult but effective approaches to managing conflict (Morrison, 1993). Collaboration evolves from

an environment that promotes a sense of trust and commitment; it involves an open and honest discussion of facts and feelings. Trust and integrity are not established overnight; the process takes time and patience. Husted *et al.* (1990) suggest that to promote integrity and trust the leader should:

• always tell the truth
• keep their word
• encourage others
• practise excellence.

Teamwork implies cooperation rather than conflict, but conflict can act as a motivator and stimulator if appropriately channelled (Rowe, 1996). The readiness to develop a collaborative approach is recognized by the group's capacity to experience and manage competition, conflict, risk, stress and their willingness to communicate. Hersey and Blanchard (1988) describe the behaviour of individuals in terms of helping or hindering roles associated with four levels of readiness. For a team to be functioning effectively the players should be aware that their behaviour may affect others and the overall performance of the team. The aim should be to achieve the helping roles outlined in Table 30. 4. Moving from hindering to helping behaviours involves leadership that promotes self-awareness and a team that is ready to change and learn from others.

The Department of Health (1998) feels that there is a pressing need to work effectively together towards clinical governance, describing an environment that includes a flattened hierarchy with equal respect and mutual understanding for other members in the team (Kneale, 1994). Mutual cooperation allows the group to utilize the expertise within a service. However, it is recognized that these changes could be a threat to traditional authority where power may be used to protect established positions, creating barriers that limit the ability of healthcare professions to work together. It could be argued that collaboration is not only about working together, but the process that brings about collective understanding.

No one profession should be seen as the fount of all knowledge or having automatic right to leadership; the interprofessional approach should be power sharing (Thompson, 1983). 'Shared leadership' is misunderstood to mean that every member has equal input into every decision. Rather, it is having confidence in one's roles and responsibilities and the freedom to practise without fear of reprisal, thus encouraging patient centrality and good communication between team members.

Promoting collaboration involves a change in management style to facilitate and enable rather than direct and control (Jones, 1994). This does not mean organizational anarchy. Success is defined by the group and organizational position is no longer the reward for a job well done. Success as well as failure is shared. Implementation involves readiness on the part of the:

- Organization – to flatten bureaucratic pyramids and value staff as the experts, offering rewards for creativity
- Leaders – who must have a strong sense of self in order to know when to let go

- Practising clinicians – who must:
    - recognize and accept reality and respect staff as they are
    - share open relationships with others
    - be able to judge situations efficiently using innovative thinking
    - be creative and realize that there is no one right way to do things
    - be self-reliant decision-makers
    - be open-minded, especially to change, and willing to learn from anyone
    - give credit where credit is due, often conceding the spotlight to staff
    - coach without controlling the game plan
    - maintain and stimulate high levels of enthusiasm
    - communicate well, especially during times of controversy and stress
    - stimulate a sense of trust, and implement successful team-building strategies
    - demonstrate keen negotiation skills in problem-solving
    - be patient.

Brown and Chamberlain (1996) conclude that professional groups have a positive perception of quality and cost of care provided by teams, but little empirical study had been done on the organizational and behavioural issues that improve team functionality. Kneale (1994) suggests that an interprofessional approach to care is not simply health and welfare professionals working in teams, but a philosophy based on a collaborative partnership, thereby developing an explicit understanding of the roles of other professions.

Relationships within the team

Relationships within a team involve shared values, mutual respect and an understanding of each professional perspective (Rowe, 1996). Traditionally, group dynamics and interactions have been hampered by struggles for authority. Negative personality traits such as self-doubt, shyness, ego vulnerability, lack of assertiveness and lack of interpersonal skills training have resulted in the inability to work in a group (Beatty, 1987; Pihl and Spiers, 1977). It has become widely recognized that the collaborative relationships between members of the healthcare team may affect outcomes for the patients, staff and the organization (Jones, 1994).

Kneale (1994) describes interprofessional discrimination to be where one profession uses power, authority and position to limit the scope of other health and welfare professionals, creating barriers to change which are subtle, covert and difficult to detect. Several studies found a lack of mutual power control in the interactions of nurses and physicians (Fieger and Schmitt, 1979; Tellis-Nyack and Tellis-Nyack, 1984; Weiss, 1985; Katzman and Roberts, 1988).

Traditionally, the medical profession has authority over the other professions, including cultural authority whereby medical definitions and judgements are generally accepted as true and valid, right and proper (Gabe *et al.*, 1991). Katzman and Roberts (1988) confirm that nurses saw their professional judgement of patient care to be subservient to the decision-making power of the physician. This is explained by doctor dominance and nurse compliance enhanced by the gender issue that is so part of the education system and often seen in leadership positions (Alimo-Metcalfe, 1993). This medical dominance is perceived to inhibit multidisciplinary team collaboration. One reason for this might be that throughout their training, physicians are socialized towards independent thought and action. Historically they occupy the dominant position in the healthcare team, and due to this position they have not had the need to be been trained in the art of collaboration (Brown and Chamberlain, 1996). The more cynical amongst us know that there are still some who would not wish to relinquish this dominating approach. However, Jones (1994) argues that times are now changing and most nurses and physicians achieve equal levels of assertiveness and co-operation; the nurse is beginning to claim more practice and patient goal areas as sole responsibility and the physician is willing to delegate more shared areas to the nursing domain.

Power in a collaborative relationship remains fluid and is bestowed on those with an area of interest, shared equally with intention, and trusted not to be abused. It is linked to a dynamic decision-making process of communication and negotiation. Collaboration involves decision-making, accountability and problem-solving. There is a collective ownership for the achievement of goals and sharing

failures (Gomberg and Sinesi, 1994).

External factors that work against interpro-

Example

A particularly good example is afforded by a model of trauma care in which consultants lead a resident on-call service. This system ensures that there is a consultant trauma surgeon resident within the hospital 24 hours a day to assess and treat injured people, while providing support and training for the junior members of the surgical trauma team. Following this period the consultant has 24 hours off duty. The continuity and coordination of care is provided by a system of primary nursing with the support of physiotherapy 7 days per week and technicians 7 days per week, who carry out cannulation, phlebotomy and ECGs; together with surgical advice provided by the on-call trauma team.

This multi-professional approach to trauma care works because the trauma consultants are willing to delegate more areas of responsibility to other disciplines, but this not something that can be achieved over night. Lenkman and Gribbins (1994) identify that a collaborative approach requires a substantial commitment to education, empowerment and autonomy in decision-making at all levels throughout an organization. Changing roles and processes in this way aims to achieve clearer lines of responsibility, better communication and improved outcomes for the patient.

---

fessional collaboration are organizational structures (location or ideology), education and development (different orientation value systems) and perceived social standing (reluctance to communicate with those in a perceived lower social group or carers not bound by professional frameworks that guide practice).

Communication

Sharing information between professional groups is an essential feature of achieving collaborative working (Allison and Ewens, 1998). It involves communication and this is the key to optimizing outcomes (Roberts, 1987). It requires an exchange of knowledge and a challenge to traditional roles through professional interaction (Johnson, 1992). This professional interaction needs cooperation,

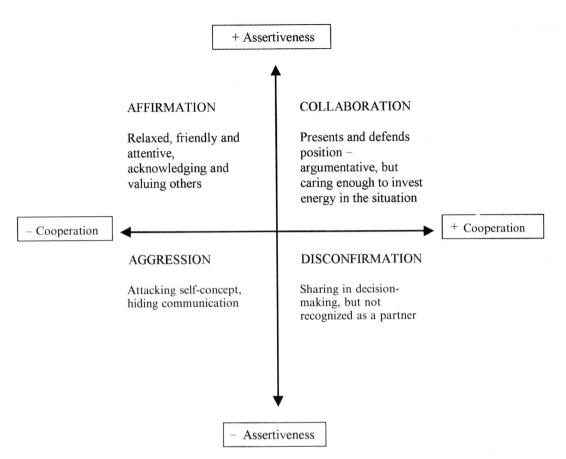

Figure 30.1 Message can carry four different behaviours (Adapted from Gordon and Infante, 1991; Johnson, 1992)

assertiveness and constructive problem-solving.

Coeling and Wilcox (1994) liken collaboration to ballroom dancing – hearing the same music and dancing the same step. Gomberg and Sinesi (1994) identify that communication becomes the mechanism to share perceptions with others. The ability to share perceptions and to perform different but chosen roles influences self-confidence. Behaviours and roles that are reinforced by successful interactions and feedback from professional colleagues are internalized. Also, behaviour choices can be altered, repeated or abandoned based on the outcome of the situation.

Figure 30.1 illustrates that messages can contain one of four behaviours. Varying degrees of assertive and/or cooperative behaviour lead to different outcomes. Openness is required to present and defend one's position and to appreciate the perspective and contribution of

other groups (Humphris and Littlejohn, 1995). Thus the issues of liability, loneliness of perceived responsibility and the time to practise as one would like to practise can be resolved (Coeling and Wilcox, 1994). Mutual trust can develop allowing relinquishment of control (Puta, 1989), leading to cooperation.

Good information is a fundamental requirement of good communication and care. The integration of information technology systems to manage patient care requirements can be achieved to utilize time more efficiently. One of the barriers to collaboration is that of each discipline possessing its own language and 'shorthand' (Patterson and Hayes, 1977; MacKinnon, 1984; Beatty, 1987). Swayne (1993) suggests that collaboration requires the use of a shared language with common terminology; for example, expressions like 'home visit' or 'wound care' mean different things to different disciplines. Each discipline needs to learn to be more specific, avoiding ambiguity, woolliness, inconsistency and jargon, and creating documentation that is acceptable, useful and effective (Swayne, 1993).

Traditionally, each discipline has written their own record of care. This is seen as a legal and professional requirement and, more recently, a tool to monitor and audit the quality of care. Through the need to improve clinical management, patient knowledge and the evaluation of care, the care pathway has developed. Critical pathways involve the identification and documentation of the sequence of standardized interdisciplinary processes or critical events that must occur for a particular case type. These critical events allow the patient to move along a continuum towards a desired outcome in a defined period of time (Newman, 1995). The development of pathways involves a collaborative effort, led by a credible expert experienced in coordinating care (Hewitson, 1992). The aim is to involve the team in the development of an action plan to act as a guide both for the injured and the team members involved in the care. An education programme is required for those giving the care, introducing the purpose and the benefits, the aim being that it becomes part of the culture. Progress is only documented if it varies from the agreed pathway. An analysis of this variance may be one way to examine practice and question interventions. The long-term aim is to generate action-based research to improve outcomes of care (Capuano, 1995). An example of a care pathway developed in an acute trauma service can be seen in Figure 30.2. Newman (1995) recognizes that pathways can foster collaboration and teamwork, as the responsibilities of each discipline are clearly defined.

The most valuable aspect of care pathway development is the opportunity for all the team members to contribute to a tool that aims to expedite the injured person's discharge from hospital. The individual and/or those close to them can become partners in care by knowing the overall care plan and by increasing their understanding of teamwork in the progress of planned treatment. It is an opportunity for each discipline to explain what it is that they do. The team can openly discuss overlaps, misunderstandings, responsibilities and priorities, streamlining rather than duplicating care in an effort to facilitate an effective service. Any

deviation from the pathway can be identified and costed, particular healthcare processes can be analysed and outcomes at different hospitals with similar cohorts of injured people can be compared. Pathways can improve accountability when specific professional idiosyncrasies in relation to particular events are exposed. Hours of care can be estimated and effective planning can aim to reduce variances in treatment.

Unfortunately, there are drawbacks. Pathways are time consuming to develop, and require commitment. This commitment must be from the whole team, as gaining cooperation from those who have not been part of the potentially powerful planning process is not easy. It is not something that the team can be told to do; facilitation and ownership has to cascade through the team, within disciplines and across professional boundaries. There is also a risk that a pathway can become a checklist, used routinely with little explanation, rather than a guide to inform practice.

Professionals are guided by the statutory and professional requirements of record-keeping, therefore guidance from the legal department is essential. This should be linked with an education programme that allows team members to explore the benefits and difficulties of this alternative approach. The documentation of variance becomes a shared experience, avoiding repetition and aiding communication between disciplines (Newman, 1995). Compiling separate professional records conflicts with the collaborative approach and the notion of continuity and efficiency. Effective collaboration requires a core identity and a language which can be provided by multiprofessional audit, but this must involve the team and the patient (Humphris and Littlejohn, 1995).

The care pathway is just one method of planning and recording collaborative practice. The power of the collaborative process involved in the development of a pathway cannot be underestimated, but poor implementation can lead to duplication and frustration. For successful implementation, all team members need to be involved from the beginning and have the opportunity to reflect upon the strengths and difficulties of adopting this process. The pathway becomes a guide for the healthcare team and those they are caring for, rather than another piece of paper to store in the healthcare records. The documentation of variance replaces the traditional record and a shared

CARE PATHWAY - Closed Ankle Fracture

	PRE-OP.	OP.	POST-OP.	DAY 1	DAY 2	DAY 3	DAY 4
AIMS	Accurate preoperative assessment of health and injury	Surgery is fully documented	Recover from anaesthesia and surgery	Management plan is understood	No oozing from wound	No oozing from wound following exercise	Leave hospital with discharge plan satisfied
	Skin is not taut around the injury site	Postoperative management plan is explicit	Recovery is fully documented	Splintage, rest and analgesia is understood	Mobility commences	Splintage is: effective, safe and comfortable with no pressure points, secured to prevent ankle movement	Community is informed
	Prepared for surgery		Informed about surgical event	Initial discharge plans are commenced	Patient takes responsibility for daily activities	Can mobilize independently with correct weight-bearing status	Ongoing care is arranged
	Initial discharge problems are anticipated				Discharge date is confirmed	Independent in daily activities	Knows who to contact if there are any difficulties
						Patient had the opportunity to talk about the accident and air fears	
						Can explain post-discharge plan and lifestyle changes	
ACTION							
Doctor	*Take history and examination including: x-ray, neurovascular status*	*Antibiotics given*	*Neurovascular obs.*	*Neurovascular obs.*		*Write up TTOs including DVT prophylaxis protocol*	
	Plan treatment	*Check x-ray*	*Explain the surgery and management plan*	*Reinforce explanation of: injury, result of surgery, possible complications, rehabilitation timetable*		*Complete audit sheet*	
	Discuss treatment plan	*Audit sheet*		*Order check Hb*			
	Complete audit sheet						
Physio.	*Make assessment including: present and past medical history, neurovascular status, respiratory function, pain and swelling*		*Ensure ankle is elevated and joint position is appropriate*	*Ensure ankle is elevated and joint position is appropriate*	*Provide exercise sheet and bandage*	*Check that definitive removable cast is fitted*	*Explain follow-up arrangements and assess understanding*
	Ensure ankle is elevated and joint position is appropriate		*Explain and assess understanding*	*Reassess splintage and adjust or change if indicated*	*Explain and assess understanding*	*Check patient understanding of: exercise plan, correct splintage and ankle position, balance between exercise and rest*	*Check able to do exercises, can remove and apply own cast, can explain the importance of good ankle position, knows where and when to remove the cast*
	Consider cryotherapy				*Provide walking aid and teach mobility*	*Assess safety at stairs/steps practice*	
	Explain and assess understanding				*Order appropriate cast*		

Figure 30.2 Care pathway

Nurse	Orientate to situation	Prepare for theatre (following protocol)	Record vital signs and neurovascular obs. 1/2 hourly > tds	Assist with transfer from bed to chair	Neurovascular obs. and TPR tds	Encourage to mobilize independently	Assess wound and apply appropriate dressing— follow protocol
	Give opportunity to talk about the accident	Escort to theatre	Advise to report changes in pain or sensation	Assist with hygiene needs	Assess wound, reapply dressing, repad backslab	Reinforce joint mobilization and gait re-education	Give and explain cast instructions and check understanding
	Encourage contact with family member or close friend	Collect from recovery	Elevate ankle above heart level	Encourage to dress in day clothes	Explain signs of infection and check understanding	Elevate ankle when at rest	Give and explain TTOs and check understanding
	Ask family/friend to bring in wash kit, towels and clothes		Observe dressing and redivac for excess oozing	Assess and record effects of injury on lifestyle and complete standard discharge screen	Encourage a balanced diet	Ensure bowels have worked - follow protocol	Reinforce advice re coping at home
	Elevate ankle above heart level at all times		Record and report any changes in condition	Refer to OT and SW if required	Assess pain and give analgesia if required. Record effect.	Give DVT prophylaxis	Explain follow-up arrangements and check understanding
	Record neurovascular assessment x3 daily		Record management plan and adapt care plan	Begin to discuss coping at home	Help to shower, keeping wound and cast dry	Assess pain— give analgesia	Give a record of follow-up arrangements
	Advise to report changes in pain and sensation		Follow anaesthetist's instructions	Remove redivac drain unless plan instructs otherwise	Encourage to dress in day clothes	Daily TPR and neurovascular assessment	Check that goals for discharge have been met
	Give analgesia if required and record effect		c/o IVI	Assess wound dressing, change if saturated and repad backslab	Encourage movement from bed to chair unaided	Observe wound dressing for oozing, change if necessary	
	Explain complications of bedrest and establish understanding		Record fluid intake and output for 24 hours	Liaise with physio. re plans for splintage	Explain the importance of a balance between exercise and rest	Report any wound oozing or pyrexia	
	Give DVT prophylaxis		Reinforce information about treatment and potential complications	Assess sleep pattern— give sedation if required	Help to walk, reinforcing agreed exercise plan	Ensure independent in washing and dressing	
	Record fluid balance if indicated		Liaise with family		Elevate ankle above heart level when at rest	Liaise with physio. and plaster room re cast fitting	
	Consider need for night sedation		Assess pain and give analgesia as required. Record effect.		Check wound for swelling or oozing following exercise	Confirm transport arrangements to get home	
	Ensure hygiene needs are met		Give DVT prophylaxis		Reinforce joint mobilization and gait re-education	Order medication to take home	
	Give advice re relieving pressure, exercise and fluid/dietary intake		Encourage pressure-relieving and limb exercises		Give DVT prophylaxis	Make outpatient appointment	
	Reinforce treatment plan and prepare for surgery		Offer an assisted wash		Assess bowel function -- give aperient if required	Ensure plans are discussed with family/friends	
			Assess nutritional score -- follow protocol		Discuss discharge plans	Make arrangements for suture removal at 14 days pos-op.	
			Assess new sleep pattern -- give sedation if required		Agree a discharge date	Write nursing letter	
			Identify, agree and record goals that need to be achieved by that date				

format promotes continuity, and aids audit and evaluation of the variance. Finally, the health-care team must have ownership of the audit process and be able to act upon the findings of their analyses. Without this the pathway becomes another bureaucratic tool that leads to conformity, order, and the suppression of open communication – death to collaborative practice.

Care pathways have the potential to generate action research and improve the outcomes of practice. They are one answer to planning and recording care and are a tool that can facilitate partnership and teamwork.

Conclusion

The aim of this chapter was to explore the nature of collaborative practice in the trauma setting. From the discussion it is evident that many have explored the nature of collaborative practice and have expressed similar views about successful teamwork. In summary, this involves shared goals values and beliefs, empowering leadership, relationships that are based on openness, trust and professional integrity and a method of written communication that allows for audit and evaluation of outcomes.

Many will argue that these ideas are not new, nor are they specific to trauma care. However, in a climate of clinical governance, developing roles, and increased consumer participation, collaboration can no longer be avoided. There is no question that the pressures of the work environment make it difficult to achieve. This may be due to the pressure of other priorities, lack of desire, or perceived lack of time. It is hoped that this chapter will provide inspiration for those who wish to reflect on their current practice in trauma care, question traditional systems and facilitate the development of collaborative practice through positive pro-blem-solving, openness and creativity.

References

Alimo-Metcalfe, B. (1993) A woman's ceiling: a man's floor. *Health Service Journal*, 14 October, 25–27.

Allison, A. and Ewens, A. (1998) Tensions in sharing client confidences while respecting autonomy: implications for interprofessional practice. *Nursing Ethics*, 5(5), 441–450.

Barr, O. (1993) Reap the benefits of a co-operative approach. Understanding interdisciplinary teamwork. *Professional Nurse*, April, 473–77.

Beatty, P. R. (1987) Attitudes and perceptions of nursing students towards preparation for interdisciplinary health-care teams. *Journal of Advanced Nursing*, **12**, 21–27.

Blancett, S. S. (1994) Self-managed teams: the reality and the promise. *The Health Care Supervisor*, 12(4), 48–55.

Brown, G. F. and Chamberlain, G. D. (1996) Attitudes toward quality, costs and physician centrality in health-care teams. *Journal of Interprofessional Care*, 10(1), 63–72.

Capuano, T. (1995) Clinical pathways. Practical ap-proaches, positive outcomes. *Nursing Management*, **26**(1), 34–37.

Coeling, H. V. and Wilcox, J. R. (1994) Steps to collaboration. *Nursing Administration Quarterly*, **18**(4), 44–55.

Department of Health (1998) *A First Class Service: Quality in the New NHS*. London: HMSO.

Fieger, R. M. and Schmitt, M. H. (1979) Collegiality in interdisciplinary healthcare teams: its measurement and its effect. *Social Science and Medicine*, **13A,** 217–219.

Gabe, J., Calnan, M. and Bury, M. (1991) *The Sociology of the Health Service*. Routledge.

Gilmore, V. L. (1993) Insight, initiative and imagination in nursing administration. *Holistic Nursing Practice*, 7(3), 15–20.

Gomberg, S. and Sinesi, L. (1994) A collaborative interac-tion model and implementation of shared governance. *Holistic Nursing Practice*, 8(3), 12–21.

Gordon, W. I. and Infante, D. A. (1991) *Test of a Communication Model of Organisational Commitment*.

Hamilton, S. (1991) Collaborative practice is necessary in ICU. *Nursing Management*, **22,** 96J–96L.

Hersey, P. and Blanchard, K. H. (1988) *Management of Organisational Behaviour*. Prentice Hall.

Hewitson, P. (1992) Collaborative care planning: a team approach to care. *International Journal of Health Care Quality Assurance*, 2(2), 12–16.

Hilton, R. W. (1995) Fragmentation within professional work. A result of isolationism in healthcare education programmes and the preparation of students to function only in the confines of their own disciplines. *Journal of Interprofessional Care*, 9(1), 33–40.

Horder, J. (1992) Interprofessional co-operation: the vision and the challenge. *Journal of Interprofessional Care*, **6,** 73–75.

Humphris, D. and Littlejohn, P. (1995) The development of multiprofessional audit and clinical guidelines: their contribution to quality assurance and effectiveness in the NHS. *Journal of Interprofessional Care*, 9(3), 207–225.

Husted, G., Miller, M. and Wilozynski, E. (1990) Five ways to build your self-esteem. *Nursing*, 20(3), 152.

Janis, I. (1982) *Victims of Group Think*. Houghton Mifflin.

Johnson, N. D. (1992) Collaboration – an environment for optimal outcome. *Critical Care Nursing*, **15**(3), 37–43.

Jones, R. A. P. (1994) Nurse–physician collaboration: a descriptive study. *Holistic Nursing Practice*, 8(3), 38–53.

Katzman, E. M. and Roberts, J. I. (1988) Nurse–physician

conflicts as barriers to enactment of nursing roles. *Western Journal of Nursing Research*, **10**(5), 576–590.

Kerfoot, K. (1989) Nurse–physician collaboration: a cost/quality issue for the nurse manager. *Nurse Economist*, **7**, 335–336.

Kneale, S. J. (1994) Discrimination – a hidden barrier to the development of interprofessional practice. *Journal of Interprofessional Care*, **8**(2), 151–155.

Lenkman, S. and Gribbins, R (1994) Multidisciplinary teams in the acute setting. *Holistic Nursing Practice*, **8**(3), 81–87.

MacKinnon, J. R. (1984) Health professionals' patterns of communication: cross purpose or problem-solving? *Journal of Allied Health*, Feb., 3–13.

Meyer, J. (1993) Lay participation in care: a challenge for multidisciplinary teamwork. *Journal of Interprofessional Care*, **7**(1), 57–66.

Morrison, M. (1993) *Professional Skills for Leadership. Foundations of a Successful Career*. Mosby.

Newman, B. (1995) Enhancing patient care: case management and critical pathways. *Australian Journal of Advanced Nursing*, **13**(1), 16–24.

Ovretveit, J. (1994) Pathways to quality: a framework for cost-effective team quality improvement and multiprofessional audit. *Journal of Interprofessional Care*, **8**(3), 329–333.

Patterson, H. and Hayes, S. (1977) Verbal communication between students in multidisciplinary health teams. *Medical Education*, **11**, 205–209.

Pihl, R. O. and Spiers, P. (1977) Some personality differences among the multiprofessional team. *Clinical Psychology*, **33**(1), 269–272.

Puta, D. F. (1989) Nurse–physician collaboration towards quality. *Journal of Nursing Quality Assurance*, **3**, 11–18.

Roberts, S. L. (1987) The role of collaborative nursing diagnosis in critical care. *Critical Care Nurse*, **7**, 81–86.

Rowe, H. (1996) Multidisciplinary teamwork – myth or reality. *Journal of Nursing Management*, **4**, 93–101.

Simon, S., Howe, I. and Kirschenbaum, H. (1978) *Values Clarification: A Handbook of Practical Strategies for Teachers and Students*. Dodd Mead.

Swannell, J. (1992) *The Oxford Modern English Dictionary*. Clarendon Press.

Swayne, J. (1993) A common language for care? *Journal of Interprofessional Care*, **7**(1), 29–35.

Tellis-Nyack, M. and Tellis-Nyack, V. (1984) Games that professionals play: the social psychology of the physician–nurse interaction. *Social Science and Medicine*, **18**(12), 1063–1069.

Temkin-Greener, H. (1983) Interprofessional perspective on teamwork in healthcare: a case study. *Millbank Memorial Fund Quarterly/Health and Society*, **61**(4), 641–658.

Thompson, D. (1983) Coalitions and conflicts in the National Health Service: some implications for general management. *Sociology of Health and Illness*, **9**, 127–153

Weiss, S. J. (1985) The influence of discourse on collaboration among physicians and consumers. *Research in Nursing and Health*, **8**, 49–59.

West, M. (1994) *Effective Teamwork*. BPS Books.

West, M. and Field, R. (1995) Teamwork in primary care. Perspectives from organisational psychology. *Journal of Interprofessional Care*, **9**(2), 117–122.

Wilmot, S. (1995) Professional values and interprofessional dialogue. *Journal of Interprofessional Care*, **9**(3), 257–266.

Yalom, I. D. (1985) *The Theory and Practice of Group Psychotherapy*. Basic Books.

31

Discharge planning

Claire Granville

Introduction

Jackson (1994) defines discharge planning as 'a process and service where patient needs are identified and evaluated and assistance is given in preparing the patient to move from one level of care to another, hospital to home, or hospital to another facility'.

Effective discharge planning following injury is an essential part of care.

There have been several papers published suggesting guidelines for discharge planning (Department of Health, 1989; HMSO, 1993; Scottish Office Home and Health Department, 1993).

Despite these guidelines being available, studies still show that discharge from hospital is often poorly planned (Bowling and Betts, 1984; Waters 1987; Worth *et al.*, 1994) and that room for improvement still exists.

Hospital stays have been reduced and rates of discharge have increased by 25% since the 1970s as the emphasis of care moves into the community (Social Trends, 1989; Government Statistical Service, 1986). It is imperative that discharge arrangements are organized in a timely fashion in order to prevent delays.

The aim of this chapter is to consider:

- Why planning should occur.
- The benefits of planning discharge.
- The people involved in the planning process.
- How effective planning can be achieved.
- The problems encountered during the planning process.

- How to overcome potential problems.
- The financial and emotional costs of delayed discharge.

Why plan discharge?

Those admitted to hospital following injury have a variety of individual needs and home circumstances; therefore planning is essential in order to ensure a smooth transition between hospital and the community (Ryan, 1994). The patient may be discharged to one of a number of places:

- home (with or without additional care)
- the home of a relative
- a community hospital
- a hospital in another area
- a speciality hospital/department
- a nursing/residential home.

The choice of placement is dependent on:

- the patient's condition
- the patient's prognosis
- the age of the patient
- the family network
- the availability of community services
- the financial circumstances (personal and government funding).

The majority of people admitted to hospital will need greater care on discharge than prior to admission (Victor and Vetter, 1988). Mistiaen *et al.* (1997) showed that 90% (of a sample size of

145 patients) had more than one physical complaint after discharge, such as 'easily tired' and 'unsteady', and that housekeeping tasks were found to be difficult. Following injury, individuals are often discharged with a walking aid, making everyday activities more difficult to cope with. The benefits of discharge planning are shown in Table 31.1

Table 31.1 Benefits of planning discharge following injury (Adapted from Nazarko, 1998)

Early agreement on placement clarifies the expectations of both patient and relatives, reducing confusion and anxiety

An agreed timeframe allows the patient's family and all relevant community staff time to prepare

If the planning process begins soon after admission, the costs associated with delayed discharge can be avoided

Efficient planning can reduce readmission rates due to poorly coordinated discharges

Early and regular communication with all involved helps to reduce the incidence of complaints

Clear documentation minimizes confusion and duplication between different members of the multidisciplinary team

People involved in the planning process

Discharge planning is a multidisciplinary process (Table 31.1) and includes:

- medical staff
- nursing staff – primarily the primary nurse
- physiotherapist
- occupational therapist
- social worker
- patient
- patient's next of kin and other significant family members or carers
- general practitioner
- community staff, including district nurse, practice nurse and other carers
- other specialist practitioners, such as speech therapist and dietician.

The medical team carry out surgical procedures and prescribe treatment; however, it is primarily the nursing and therapy staff who are in contact

with the patient and family. Medical criteria for discharge are set, and it is then the nursing and therapy staff who agree the discharge date, the planning process being coordinated by the primary nurse (Ryan, 1994). Occupational therapists and physiotherapists have a key role to play in the rehabilitation of trauma patients. Helping the patient to regain mobility, the provision of equipment and adaptations to the home are all within this remit. Coordinating the involvement of additional specialist services and facilitating the sharing of information is the role of the primary nurse. It is also vital to involve community staff early on in the planning process, as they may need to access specialist equipment or services, and adequate notice needs to be given.

Some patients will require input from social services and social workers in relation to funding or the provision of temporary sheltered placements in the community prior to returning home. In some parts of the country local initiatives have been developed to aid in this transition period. In the Oxfordshire area, in addition to community hospitals, other services are available to support people in their own homes, one example being the Oxford Intensive Care Support Team (OICISS). The scheme provides healthcare workers who assess patients in hospital in order to determine and organize support services prior to discharge, providing carers from services other than social services and community nursing. Although this is usually a short-term service, it facilitates early but appropriate discharge from hospital.

Another example is a scheme funded by the Health Authority, known locally as a 'progressive care' facility (PCF), based in Oxford Community Hospital. In general, only those patients whose general practitioners have admitting rights to specific community hospitals are eligible for admission. The PCF scheme affords patients who would otherwise not have access to a community hospital the opportunity to benefit from rehabilitation in an environment more suited to their needs. It also enables better use of beds in acute care wards. Patients suitable for the PCF scheme are referred by ward staff to a liaison nurse who confirms their suitability, explains the care provision arrangements and medical cover, together with projected length of stay – not usually in excess of 4 weeks. All patients who are referred must be capable of returning to their original place of residence within the agreed time period.

National schemes such as 'Hospital at Home' are familiar to many. Hospital at Home is a generic term referring to home-based nursing and rehabilitation services aiming to prevent admission or to facilitate early discharge from care in an acute hospital (Coast *et al.*, 1998). In many areas the Red Cross provide services where volunteers visit patients soon after discharge in order to assist with domestic tasks and offer companionship.

Traumatic injury can lead to complex discharge requirements. An injury may be of such severity that the patient may not be able to return home and will require care in a residential or nursing home environment; for example following serious head injury. In such circumstances a case conference, to which the patient, family and carers must be invited, is the preferred option for discussion of the salient points. A variety of other participants may also be involved in the decision-making process:

- patient
- next of kin
- social worker
- hospital doctor
- primary nurse
- residential home representative
- nursing home representative
- physiotherapist
- occupational therapist
- clinical psychologist
- general practitioner
- community nurse.

It has been suggested that involving the patient and carers more in decision-making would place control back with those who are affected by a change in health status and thereby increases their ability to cope (Wiffin, 1995).

How effective planning can be achieved

The discharge planning process involves assessment, planning and implementation. An assessment of the patient's abilities prior to injury is a prerequisite and should include activities of daily living, particularly mobility, and whether any support services are already in place. The assessment should start on, or shortly after, admission (Nixon *et al.*, 1998). This informa-

tion is vital in order to inform both treatment goals and discharge criteria. Unrealistic expectations in relation to a patient's functional abilities act not only as a demotivator, but may also delay the planning process.

Complex discharges frequently involve the requirement for an individual to be rehoused, or funding accessed in order to secure residential or nursing home placement. The following case studies illustrate such complex circumstances.

Case study

Mrs King, an 87-year-old lady, was admitted to hospital following a fall at home in which she sustained an open tibial fracture.

Medical history. Arthritis, hypertension and cardiac failure. She had made a good recovery from a CVA some years ago. Her recent falls were thought to be due to medication for hypertension.

Social history. She lived alone in a large semi-detached house, her husband having died some years previously.

Family. Daughter and son-in-law. Daughter severely disabled through multiple sclerosis; her husband was her main carer and had help from social services, respite care and day care. Son-in-law also looked after Mrs King.

Family stress. Son-in-law had suffered a nervous breakdown 18 months previously, largely due to the pressure of caring for his wife. He was becoming increasingly stressed due to the demands made on him by Mrs King who phoned him for help following a fall, or when she generally could not manage.

Problem. On admission Mrs King agreed with her family that she could no longer cope at home. Unbeknown to hospital staff, she agreed to her house being sold, assuming she would be able to move into warden-controlled accommodation. The house sold quickly and she was therefore left homeless.

Discharge planning. Problems due to homelessness:

- family unable to care for Mrs King
- finding an appropriate house – a big problem
- complex multidisciplinary liaison – hospital and community

- no access to community hospital bed as no discharge destination.

There were practical difficulties associated with taking Mrs King to view properties as occupational therapy assistance was needed for each visit. A telephone alarm system needed to be installed, appropriate care organized and arrangements made for furniture removal.

Emotional support. Mrs King had lost confidence, due to the loss of her home, independence and control. Support for the family was required and reintegration into a new environment had to be facilitated. Links were established with:

- local authority housing departments
- housing association
- physiotherapist
- occupational therapists
- community liaison nurse
- general practitioner
- home care team
- benefits agency and Department of Social Security.

A care manager was also arranged for Mrs King's daughter.

Outcome. Mrs King settled into a new home with a warden, and received home care each morning. The new home was near her family and was wheelchair-friendly, therefore her daughter could visit easily. The family's stress was relieved due to the availability of a warden and a security system, and Mrs King enjoyed the new social contacts she made.

Once Mrs King's house had been sold and she became homeless this immediately became her main problem – her injury becoming almost a secondary consideration. In this case an extremely large amount of time and effort was needed to achieve a satisfactory conclusion for all concerned. Effective communication between all parties was paramount, as there have been many studies to show that communication in discharge planning is poor (Worth *et al.*, 1994; Mistiaen *et al.*, 1997; Nixon *et al.*, 1998). In Mrs King's case the key coordinator regarding discharge was the hospital care manager, who continued to assume responsibility for her for 4 weeks post-discharge prior to handing over to community colleagues. Mrs King's hospital stay ended up being 10 weeks, although she was medically fit for discharge after only 2 weeks.

In contrast to housing being a problem, the next case study shows how the injury can be the root cause of the problem.

Case Study

Mr Brown, a 42-year-old gentleman, was admitted to hospital with a severe head injury, having been assaulted in a public house. Despite the severity of his injury, he eventually made a good physical recovery.

Family history. Mr Brown was one of four children; he and a sister were abused by their father as children. His mother died from cancer a few years previously and he is still unable to grieve for her death. His mother had also suffered violent attacks from her husband. He had sporadic contact with two of his sisters – usually for emotional support. Although divorced in his early twenties, he had some contact with his ex-wife, their daughter and grand-daughter, all of whom lived together. He had had many relationships since the divorce, all of which had proved unsustainable due to the emotional 'damage' caused by his father.

Accommodation. Bedsit with own kitchen and bathroom in a shabby multi-occupied house which was controlled by an aggressive landlord. He was on benefits, including housing benefit and had mounting debts.

Problems. As his condition started to improve he required more specialist neurological input. He developed severe anxiety post-head injury, low self-esteem and required intense emotional and psychological support. He had also been left with some memory problems. His landlord was demanding rent payment.

Liaison was required with:

- Care manager
- Occupational therapists and physiotherapists
- Housing department
- Family
- Landlord
- Friends and acquaintances
- Home care
- Neurological rehabilitation centre
- Victim support
- General practitioner
- Department of Psychological Medicine
- Criminal Compensation Board.

Discharge problems:

- high level of anxiety (due to head injury), compromising ability to cope with independent living
- previous accommodation unsuitable for discharge
- aggressive landlord – patient unable to cope psychologically with pressure
- finances – very difficult to control – care manager providing assistance
- no half-way house to help reintegration into community
- fearful of assailants and further assaults.

Outcome. Mr Brown was discharged into his previous housing, but with an application under way for rehousing. He received care 4 days a week in a neurological rehabilitation facility as an outpatient. Assessed as being 'highly anxious', weekly sessions were arranged with a psychologist to teach him coping strategies. A care manager provided continuous assessment and ongoing support with finances, running his home and coping in the community.

In Mr Brown's case, his head injury had a marked effect on his psychological and cognitive abilities, and exacerbated his anxiety and lack of self-confidence. As a result it was very difficult to discharge him safely into the community. He was an inpatient for 6 months, his care in the latter 3 months being almost exclusively concerned with discharge planning. Support in the community for this gentleman was required for many months.

Traumatic injury can have a great psychological effect on people, and they also have to contend with the prospect of their physical injuries. Although an individual may have been through much physical pain, knowing that one is going to be confined to a wheelchair for months or will have to rely on the use of crutches for a long period of time, may be a lot more disheartening and depressing. Imminent discharge home may heighten the awareness of this altered body image and in turn the patient may lose confidence and become frightened of going outside.

Following injury, the majority of people are only too keen to return home. However, the reality of moving from a safe hospital environment, where help is always at hand, to a home environment where independence has been replaced by total or semi-dependence can be daunting.

Verbal communication with all healthcare professionals involved in discharge planning should be backed up with written confirmation. This is particularly important where information regarding medication, wound care and restrictions on activity are involved. The patient and family should also be provided with written information regarding exercise programmes and arrangements for outpatient appointments. It is also helpful to provide a contact name or telephone number in the event of problems or queries arising post-discharge. Each part of the planning process should be clearly documented in the patient's records.

Problems encountered during the planning process

Despite the best efforts of all concerned, discharge planning may not always run smoothly. Table 31.2 summarizes several problems which may occur.

Table 31.2 Discharge planning problems

Failure to commence planning early, leading to patient/family feeling ill-informed and frustrated

Inaccurate assessment of discharge needs, leading to deficiencies in discharge arrangements

Delays in timely discharge, leading to poor resource utilization and increased costs per patient

Poor documentation, leading to confusion and duplication of effort

Lack of coordination exacerbating the already significant difficulties associated with complex discharges

How to overcome potential problems

In order to prevent some of the potential problems that discharge can create, planning should start on or shortly after admission (Nixon *et al.*, 1998), or when the decision to admit to hospital is made (Nazarko, 1998). This latter point is especially relevant now that the length of time patients spend in hospital is decreasing. Length of hospital stay following trauma varies widely: 'minor' injuries such as wrist and hand fractures can be treated quickly and patients are frequently discharged within 24–48 hours; an older person following fixation of a femoral neck fracture could be ready for transfer to a community hospital within 4 days. Early notice of discharge from hospital allows the community staff sufficient time to arrange necessary services and access equipment (Lim, 1998).

The financial and emotional costs of delayed discharge

Every admission to hospital has a cost. Coast *et al.* (1998) have investigated an interesting comparison between costs incurred at home as opposed to hospital, and suggested that home is the most cost-effective place to be. However, they also concede that these are not the results of other studies (O'Cathain, 1994; Hensher *et al.*, 1996). A patient who remains in an acute bed because a more suitable placement is unavailable represents an inappropriate use of NHS resource. The terms 'bed blockers' and 'delayed discharges' are commonly used as labels for such patients. Another term is 'inappropriately located patients' – where patients have been in hospital for 1 month or more and, in the opinion of medical and/or nursing staff, no longer require hospital specific services (Koffman *et al.*, 1996).

Reasons for delayed discharges have been cited as:

- lack of community or rehabilitation beds
- lack of specialist rehabilitation units, e.g. for head-injured patients
- lack of half-way houses for patients whose head injuries have resulted in varying degrees of cognitive impairment
- difficulties in transferring patients to rehabilitation facilities because of perceived problems in providing ongoing specialist care for injuries
- poorly coordinated discharges.

Nazarko (1998) highlights the emotional cost of delayed discharge, particularly in relation to the older person: 'emotional costs are borne by older people, their families and professionals struggling to provide a service in the absence of strategic planning.'

Conclusion

This chapter has given some insight into discharge planning and the complications that can arise when caring for an injured person. In many instances the process can be extremely complex, requiring effective and timely coordination of the efforts of a wide range of professionals. It is imperative that early assessment occurs and appropriate plans are made. 'The discharge of patients is an integral part of care that requires specific preparation to increase coping ability at home' (Wiffin, 1995). Communication between all interested parties helps to aid a smooth discharge, ensuring that no aspects have been overlooked. Discharge planning is a team effort, its success dependent on early assessment, collaboration, realistic goal-setting and accurate documentation.

References

Bowling, A. and Betts, G. (1984) From hospital to home: communication on discharge. *Nursing Times*, Pt 1, **80**(32), 31–33; Pt 2, **80**(33), 44–46.

Coast, J., Richards, S. H., Peters, T. J. *et al.* (1998). Hospital at home or acute hospital care? A cost minimisation analysis. *British Medical Journal*, **316**, 1802–1806.

Department of Health (1989) *Discharge of Patients from Hospital Health, Circular*, **89**(5). London: HMSO.

Government Statistical Service (1986) *Annual Abstract of Statistics*. London: HMSO.

HMSO (1993) *RCN Community Care UK*. London: HMSO.

Hensher, M., Fulop, N., Hood, S. and Ujan, S. (1996) Does hospital at home make economic sense? Early discharge versus standard care for orthopaedic patients. *Journal of Social Medicine*, **89**, 548–551.

Jackson, M. F. (1994) Discharge planning: issues and challenges for gerontological nursing. A critique of the literature. *Journal of Advanced Nursing*, **19**, 495–502.

Koffman, J., Fulop, N. and Hudson, M. (1996) Assessing the impact of delayed discharge on acute care. *Nursing Standard*, **10**(20), 41–43.

Lim, D. (1998) Joint effort. *Nursing Standard*, **12**(37), 20.

Mistiaen, P., Dunijnhower, E., Wijkel, D. *et al.* (1997). The problems of elderly people at home one week after discharge from an acute care setting. *Journal of Advanced Nursing*, **25**, 1233–1240.

Nazarko, L. (1998) Improving discharge: the role of the discharge co-ordinator. *Nursing Standard*, **12**(49), 35–37.

Nixon, A., Whitter, M. and Stitt, P. (1998) Audit in practice: planning for discharge from hospital. *Nursing Standard*, **12**(26), 35–38.

O'Cathain, A. (1994) Evaluation of a hospital at home scheme for the early discharge of patients with fractured neck of femur. *Journal of Public Health Medicine*, **16**,

205–210.

Ryan, A. (1994) Improving discharge planning. *Nursing Times*, **90**(20), 33–35.

Scottish Office Home and Health Department (1993) *Guide to Good Practice on Discharge from Hospital*. SOHHD.

Social Trends (1989) Number 19. Central Statistical Office, HMSO.

Victor, C. and Vetter, N. (1988) Preparing the elderly for discharge from hospital. *Age and Ageing*, **17**, 155–163.

Waters, K. R. (1987) Outcomes of discharge from hospital for elderly people. *Journal of Advanced Nursing*, **12**(3), 347–355.

Wiffin, A. (1995) An assessment of procedures. *Nursing Times*, **91**(28), 31–32.

Worth, A., Tierney, A. and Lockerbie, L. (1994) Community nurses and discharge planning. *Nursing Standard*, **8**(21), 25–30.

Part V

Political, environmental and organizational issues

32

Trauma Centres or Trauma Systems?

Keith Willett

The history of trauma services in the UK

'*In general, trauma care is fragmented, disorganised and has an unacceptably bad outcome. Pre hospital care of the accident victim is sub-optimal ... The patient is usually taken to the nearest hospital without regard to surgical ability*' Professor D. D. Trunkey, *British Journal of Surgery* Travelling Fellow (1987).

The magnitude of the cost of dealing with the injured in Britain should not be underestimated. There is a personal and tragic loss of 40 lives a day as a result of accidents, and over 100 each week in road traffic accidents alone. It has been shown that 20–25% of the population attend an accident and emergency department each year; 70% of these attendances are for injury and accidents. So, for a city such as Birmingham with a population of 3.1 million, its five accident and emergency departments will see an average of 68 000 patients each year. In socioeconomic terms the financial cost is often under-appreciated. It has been estimated that in 1995 the total cost of the results of accidents to Britain was £1.4 billion, of which £460 million was spent directly on the healthcare costs. When there is death or severe disablement there is also a greater unquantifiable personal cost as a result of the tragedy.

One of the major cost implications of trauma and its treatment is that it is a disease of the young. Under the age of 40 years it represents the most common reason for a male death or admission to hospital. There are more lost years of useful working life as a result of accidents than any other single disease. For the future, the only route to a major impact on the personal and financial costs of injury will come through accident prevention. Notwithstanding that, it is in contemporary practice, dealing with the care of the injured patient, where substantial benefit can be achieved. Sadly, the inadequacy of treatment, resulting in preventable death and disability in 25% of patients, demonstrated by Hoffman and Coll (1976), was shown not to have substantially improved by the time the Royal College of Surgeons of England reported on the management of patients with major injuries in 1988.

Although in recent decades the UK has lagged behind European and American countries in the organization of its trauma services, it was in the UK that much of the pioneering work was done. It was Robert Jones, the surgeon to the Manchester Ship Canal, who first developed a comprehensive accident service to support the canal's construction in 1888. He divided the 35-mile construction area into three zones, each served by a hospital supporting a chain of first aid stations and a transport system to evacuate the injured. Unfortunately, this organization was not mirrored in the massive expansion of hospital services that occurred in the mid-1930s, hospitals being sited more on the basis of wealthy benefactors' desires and, in particular with the accident and emergency services, attracting little attention in the layout of the hospitals. At the commencement of the

National Health Service in 1948 there was no discernible plan for emergency services.

Acceptable sites did exist; foremost was the Birmingham Accident Service directed and developed by Professor William Gissane. That pioneering centre was based on three principles:

- to separate the injured from the ill
- to provide continuity of care
- to do this under the close supervision of an experienced surgeon.

That unit set standards of treatment covering all grades of injury severity and all body systems. Teaching and research was central to the unit's philosophy, with particular experience in the fields of industrial injury, burns and road accidents. The Birmingham Accident Service, intended by Gissane to be a model for a national system of care of the injured, was not adopted and was abandoned after 50 years. Its uniqueness (particularly of its surgeons) and its failure to conform to the evolution of sub-specialization in surgery and the formation of the Accident and Emergency speciality were the professional reasons for its ultimate demise. Perhaps it was the medical political policy, opposed to specialist units not attached to larger general hospitals, that proved the model's greatest challenge.

The development of accident and emergency (A&E) departments was spawned of the Accident & Service Review Committee (ASRC) in 1961 chaired by Sir Henry Osmond-Clarke, and a Ministry of Health inquiry, chaired by Sir Henry Platt (Standing Medical Advisory Committee, 1962). They agreed on the development of A&E departments under the direction of orthopaedic surgeons. The government-initiated Platt Report was actually adopted, omitting the Regional Accident Units proposed by the ASRC. These were to have served a population of 1–2 million and deal with the most complex and demanding injuries. A later review (1971) of the implementation of A&E departments proposed the further development of a separate A&E medical speciality which was to become the norm. The limited number of consultants for these A&E departments fell woefully short of the 24-hour senior cover required.

The reception and emergency surgery of the seriously injured patient in Britain remains predominantly the charge of unsupervised junior medical staff.

Overseas models

North America

In the USA, similar concerns to those identified in the UK led to the development of the Emergency Medicine speciality. Pivotal research by Trunkey showed that the survival of patients with multiple injuries was markedly improved if they were taken to one central hospital rather than the nearest department offering an emergency service. The critical factor was the treatment of imminently remedial injuries by resuscitation and prompt surgery, such injuries being haemorrhage from organs, extradural haematoma and severe skeletal injuries.

In the USA, such centres are now designated 'Trauma Centres' by the American College of Surgeons to guidelines set in 1976. In the UK, in 1999, perhaps only a handful of units meet some of those service criteria. In the USA, full implementation has been patchy, with very few adopting the full recommendations of the American Committee of Trauma, but the three-level hospital structure is mostly implemented. Delivery of care in the Level 1 Trauma Centres is to a very high standard, senior staff presence being generated by the medico-legal requirements, billing system and education needs. Opposition to Trauma Centres has come predominantly from hospital administrators who have found that the high demand, unsociable hours and expensive service requirements result in adverse economic consequences – particularly as a significant proportion of the casualties are uninsured. The high volume of cases, particularly of penetrating injuries, has promoted the development of creditable rapid treatment systems. These have formed the basis of working protocols and promoted progress. These methods, such as Advanced Trauma Life Support (ATLS) have subsequently been adopted in many other developed countries, including the UK in 1988.

West Germany

In response to a high death toll from road traffic accidents in Germany in the 1960s, the ADAC aeromedical system was developed. This was part of the government welfare system, with an accident rescue service organized provincially around government-run hospitals, supported by ambulance and helicopter retrieval vehicles. These are manned by intensive care doctors. By the early 1980s the results of the ADAC system were impressive, with rapid accident scene attendance times, high on-scene treatment intervention rates and very low transfer mortalities. The geography of the country and fast road transport systems are advantageous to the system, but its limitation in daytime helicopter flights remains a problem. The Air Rescue Units, with a medical crew on each flight – a doctor and a paramedic – are usually located at hospitals. A Regional Control Centre, coordinating all emergency service calls, dispatches the rescue flights. Fifty aeromedical systems cover West Germany, each with a limited operation area of 70 km. In the 1970s the system averaged 1000 missions a year and initially retrieved predominantly accident victims (75%), but this has now fallen to 31%. The development of the pre-hospital rescue structure was naturally paralleled by the formation of regional hospital trauma centres capable of receiving such patients. The German medical system has dedicated trauma surgeons who deal exclusively with trauma, including all aspects of injured body systems. This is in contrast to the split loyalties in the UK, with elective speciality practice.

France

The Services de L'aide Medicale Urgente en France, known as SAMU, has been running since 1972 and is another example of pre-hospital care organization. Its development has paralleled that of the UK ambulance services, the major difference being a substantial medical contribution into the control and provision of the pre-hospital care. There is constant medical support in the control room triage and designation of response teams, including constantly available A&E doctors to attend the scene by rapid ambulance or helicopter.

The place of trauma centres in the UK

A number of studies have shown that up to 25% of deaths as a result of injury can be considered preventable when the severity of injury, appropriateness and quality of care is analysed. This alarming rate of preventable deaths has been shown to be greatly reduced by the institution of Trauma Care Systems. While similar studies do not currently exist for preventable disability, it can safely be assumed that the rate of disability and impact of Trauma Care Systems is similar in this regard. It would seem logical to conclude that the success of any trauma system capable of dealing with the continuing care needs from prevention through acute care to rehabilitation and a patient's return to society, would have equal place in British society. There is certainly substantial evidence to indicate the same rate of preventable deaths was present in Britain, as indicated by the retrospective study of 1000 deaths from injury (Anderson *et al.*, 1988). A further report by the British Orthopaedic Association in 1992 presented evidence that it was not just suboptimal care leading to death that was a national problem, but that the inadequate treatment of isolated limb injuries presented an even greater cost burden to society. Despite the perceived logic, the historical arrangement of British hospitals has fragmented pre-hospital care. The traditional working practices of consultants, established at the National Health Service's conception, have resulted in only moderate steps being taken in the improvement of trauma care. Arguably, the biggest impact on trauma care delivery in the UK in the last 10 years has not been a major reorganization of its services, but provision of a simple ABC system of educating junior doctors to respond, in the absence of senior support, to the presentation of a seriously injured patient. The ATLS course proved remarkably successful and popular and was rapidly followed by similar courses for nursing staff (ATNC) and pre-hospital paramedical staff (PHTLS). These systems at last gave a common language, and methods for assessment and resuscitation for the patient's triage, transfer and initial treatment.

The geography of Britain, with its high-density populations supported by district general hospitals every 10–30 miles, has not promoted development of the regional structure of trauma care. As a result in Britain, with few exceptions, the injured person is taken to the nearest A&E department, irrespective of its receiving capabilities. The British public is comparatively poorly educated in medical matters, and consider that as they pass through the doors of any hospital they are now 'safe'. The advanced and medically supported pre-hospital services, SAMU and ADAC in France and Germany respectively, are expensive but strongly supported by the people and, as such, are hallowed institutions.

In Britain, as indicated earlier, the Accident Service at Birmingham did possess many of the features of a successful service, but its unique personnel and structure did not match the plan for the development of acute speciality services and was therefore not copied.

British trauma experiments

In more recent years there have been professionally-led experiments, direct consequences of the recognized inadequacy of care, that will shape the development of trauma services in the UK. Examination of the current models in Britain and worldwide suggests that systems broadly fall into two types. The majority, based on the North American model, are considered *exclusive*, and involve the rapid transport of patients and the bypass of local hospitals which are not identified as Trauma Centres, despite the fact that they may be closer to the scene of the injury. Many urban practitioners of trauma medicine espouse this type of system. It may be applicable to populated areas, but even in this setting it has met with the problems of healthcare politics and evaluation, prestige and finance. Hence, for a number of reasons, there has been a shift to the concept of *inclusive* systems, recognizing the capabilities of all the care facilities; the role of every provider of healthcare is agreed, establishing lines of communication, transfer protocols and policies between the facilities offering different levels of care. The Trauma Centre, as exemplified by this model, is supporting, rather than dictating. However, the latter seems to be more applicable to the need in Britain.

Self-proclamation of Trauma Centre status, in the absence of a regionally agreed system, will not work.

Developing and sustaining the trauma system is a major challenge and will require redistribution of patients as well as medical and healthcare resources. Without the support and education of the public, and the necessary legislation, it is unlikely that any system will be successfully established. The Department of Health, as a result of the 1988 Royal College of Surgeons of England Report, established an experiment based at the North Staffordshire Royal Infirmary (NSRI) in Stoke-on-Trent. With three comparative sites, it sought to compare a North American style Trauma Centre with the then current District General Hospital practices. Two other experiments started in London and Oxford, the former prompted by the acquisition of an emergency aeromedical helicopter facility, the latter by a professionally-led manpower and training service restructuring.

Stoke-on-Trent experiment

An evaluation of this experiment was commissioned by the Department of Health with the principal aim of measuring the cost-effectiveness of a North American Trauma Centre system against the effectiveness of surrounding and comparative hospitals. Although prospective, it was not a randomized study; it examined the changes in cost, outcomes for trauma patients, and development of the system. Comparative units were used to control for secular trends, national changes in trauma care, and to enhance the scope for generalization of the results. The main developments of the trauma system in the North West Midlands were at the NSRI Trauma Centre. The medical staffing was increased to allow a resident consultant to be present to receive multiply-injured patients, and nursing staff were increased in A&E and the intensive care unit to deal with an increased number of patients who were being transferred directly to the Trauma Centre. Prior to the experiment, the reception and resuscitation procedures were considered to have been fully developed, with all the necessary specialities on site.

An independent review by the Medical Research Unit from Sheffield University at the end of the study period found that there was no evidence of reduction in avoidable death rate in either the Trauma System or the comparative regions. They also reported that there was no evidence of a difference in the changes in the Trauma Centre and changes in the comparative regions over the period studied (1990–93). The total operating costs and cost consequences of the Regional Trauma Centre were estimated to be greater by approximately £0.5 million per year. Overall, no reliable evidence of benefit was found for major trauma patients and the North West Midlands Trauma Centre experiment was not cost-effective in these terms. These findings were seen by many to be a product of the experiment design and measurement tools. The trauma system in the North West Midlands lacked two key features identified in American studies:

- there was no system in place for directly triaging appropriate patients to the Trauma Centre in Stoke
- the volume of major trauma treated in the Centre was less than 20% of the volume recommended for a Level 1 Centre in the USA.

It is also recognized that, in the development of a Trauma Service, senior specialist expertise in the supporting surgical specialities must be identified in the initial model design.

Royal London Hospital

The Helicopter and Emergency Medical Service (HEMS) was introduced in August 1990 and flew over 5000 missions, transporting more than 1000 patients in its first 5 years of operation. Run by the London Ambulance Service, it was initially mainly funded by commercial sponsorship, but with the medical, paramedic and nursing staff funded by the NHS. The HEMS system was designed to be a daytime rapid pre-hospital medical response unit and patient transfer system to the Royal London Hospital (RLH), with the appropriate facilities. It was set up in response to the transportation difficulties within the urban environment and the previous prevailing requirement for ambulance crews to take patients to the nearest receiving facility, irrespective of the patient's medical or surgical needs. Analysis of the outcome and costs of the HEMS system has been difficult because of its uniqueness. A comparison with the Stoke-on-Trent experiment showed that HEMS, in the same comparison period, between 1992 and 1996 received an average of 145 multiply-injured patients (ISS greater than 15) per year, compared with Stoke-on-Trent which averaged 180 patients per year. Of the Stoke patients, 35% were inter-hospital transfers, unlike the HEMS patients. The higher incidence of death in the HEMS patients may be explainable by the lack of pre-selection and the rapidity of the transfer. On balance, the patient outcomes were probably similar in the two units.

The cost–benefit analysis of such a system is very difficult. There are many ways of measuring 'value for money'; an economic evaluation must take into account the direct average costs as well as marginal costs, plus some measure of the health quality derived. A simple cost consequence analysis would be misleading. A public and high-profile review of the HEMS service, at the request of the purchasers for healthcare in London, concluded that HEMS was cost-effective at approximately £1.5 million a year, plus additional hospital costs. To date, the continuing funding of the HEMS system has been agreed, and it remains operationally unchanged from its inception. This is unlike the Stoke-on-Trent experiment, where there is no longer a resident consultant at the main receiving Trauma Centre.

The Oxford Trauma Service manpower experiment

This experiment, conceived in 1993, approached the issues around delivering trauma care and training from a different perspective. This experiment recognized the professional changes occurring in both medicine and nursing. It was built on two philosophies:

- A philosophy of care – that all trauma care should be delivered by, or under, the direct supervision of a fully trained surgeon.
- A philosophy of training – that every clinical experience should be a learning opportunity.

This was a direct response to the recognized poor quality of trauma care that was being delivered nationally, in that emergency medical services were dependent on predominantly inexperienced doctors in training. A worsening of that problem was anticipated, with the recent enforced reduction in junior doctors' working hours and the shortened surgical training to bring Britain in line with Europe.

The main elements of the Oxford experiment were to make dedicated consultants in orthopaedic trauma resident in the hospital to lead the service, providing 24-hour senior assessment and teaching on all trauma patients. This was only possible by a major change in the culture of nursing care on the Trauma Unit. The continuity of patient care and patient management became the responsibility of the primary nurse. The immediate results of this system were a reduction in the length of stay, fewer admissions (by better 'gatekeeping') and a higher proportion of those admitted undergoing surgery. The secondary elements of the system were the separation of medical specialist services for hand, spine, pelvic and acetabular trauma surgery. The presence of a 24-hour referral facility for these groups of patients, and those with complex or multiple injuries, was a facility taken up by the surrounding hospitals in the region.

In the first 5 years of the study there has been a year on year rise in complexity of the case mix received by the Oxford system. The service changes, as indicated by average costs, were cost neutral. Marginal costs have risen with the case mix change. The study is prospective and includes staff activity analysis, supervision rates for surgery, occupational psychology assessments for the staff, patient satisfaction surveys and patient outcome assessments. An interim report at 2 years indicated supervision rates for surgery changing from 15% to 70% and lengths of stay falling from 8 to 5 days. The objectives of reducing junior doctors' hours and improving quality of care had been met. The 5-year study is due to report following completion in 1998. The model continues to run in its original form. It is an example of an *inclusive* trauma system. It is in many ways similar to the Birmingham Accident Hospital design, but recognizes the multidisciplinary nature of surgery and nursing in its structure and is based on a large teaching hospital site. Its weakness remains for national rollout in the recruitment of orthopaedic surgeons with a primary interest in trauma. Recent polls of consultants and orthopaedic trainees indicate that only 15% would consider this long-term career option.

The future of trauma care in Britain

Pressures on current trauma practice in Britain come from increasing patient expectation, the medico-legal consequences of sub-optimal care, professional recognition of advances in the speciality and the increasing demand placed on seniors by the inexperience of their junior staff; these will effect change. Much time has

been spent debating the appropriate management of the multiply-injured patient in Britain. The argument for a one-site regional multi-speciality trauma centre is strong, but it is unclear in the wider perspective of emergency care whether the advantage to the few justifies designing the whole system around their needs. The same expertise, technology and senior input that advantages the polytrauma patients is equally recognized to benefit a greater number of patients with the more severe, often isolated injuries. The transfer of such complicated cases, however, remains very variable and unusual in Britain. This failure of centralization has resulted in the training of very few trauma specialists and a failure to develop the trauma expertise and reconstruction techniques that have occurred in the USA and other parts of Europe. This has occurred, despite contemporary wisdom, and has already identified several areas in orthopaedic trauma where specialist care is recommended for patient outcome and effective resource use. In some regions of the UK this process has begun to evolve, creating regional units staffed to receive complex injuries, such as open fractures, spinal injuries, pelvic and acetabular fractures, replantations and complex hand surgery, and limb injuries with associated vascular damage. This practice has developed around individual expertise rather than by an agreed regional system.

However, many hospitals remain isolated. The political consequences of imposing a regional structure with the possibility of bypass of hospitals or closure of A&E departments has fuelled the debate and stalled progress. Pride, prestige and lack of public education remain the hurdles to be negotiated.

More recently, a working party of the British Orthopaedic Association and British Association of Plastic Surgeons developed guidelines for the management of the severe open tibial fracture. It was easier to achieve a professional consensus on the optimal care of one such severe injury than to address the complexities associated with regional restructuring.

It seems most likely that progress will be made with trauma care in general by first agreeing professionally defined standards of care for those injuries where there is good published evidence for improved outcomes by referral to specialists or a specialist unit. A precedent has already been set in the UK by the Calman Hine Report, in providing a national structure for cancer services. It is now timely and appropriate to apply this methodology to trauma care. It will be the responsibility of the receiving consultant, working in conjunction with the Regional Specialist Units, to effect the agreed standard of care within their geographical region. The ability to deliver that standard should determine the capability of the hospital to receive such a patient, to deliver the definitive care, or institute bypass transfer policies. The selection of the appropriate policy should be individualized to the local unit based on personnel availability, skills, resources, transfer options and regional geography. The hospital size, catchment population or new attendance numbers should not be seen as the key markers of the standard of care; rather it should be the ability of the consultant sited in the hospital, working within a regional system, to return the right quality.

It is far more likely that we will achieve professional agreement and consensus for the appropriate structure and system of trauma care by focusing on the patient. This statement is not made without recognizing the limited financial resources available to the NHS and the cost-effectiveness of any one receiving hospital. The creation of a Regional Audit System, to which receiving primary and secondary units contribute, would be the indicator of performance and provide the route to remedy substandard practice. The creation of

Trauma Systems based on standards of care would be professionally acceptable and less threatening. Whether or not a unit is commissioned to receive patients would be less dependent on its size and more dependent on its performance.

Trauma care will change, but for those working at the leading edge, the rate of change has been frustratingly slow.

References

Anderson, I. D., Woodford, M., de Dombal T. and Irving M. A. (1988) Retrospective study of 1000 deaths from injury in England and Wales. *British Medical Journal*, **296**, 1305–1308.

Hoffman, E. and Coll, A. R. (1976) Mortality and morbidity following road traffic accidents. *Annals of the Royal College of Surgeons*, **58**, 233–240.

Standing Medical Advisory Committee (1962) *Accident and Emergency Services*. London: HMSO.

Supplementary Reading

Accident Services Review Committee of Great Britain and Ireland (1965) *Accident Services of Great Britain and Ireland Second Report*. London: British Medical Association.

West, J., Trunkey, D. D. and Lim, R. C. (1979) Systems of trauma care. *Archives of Surgery*, **114**, 455–460.

33

Leadership in the context of acute care

Deborah Langstaff

Introduction

The concept of leadership is multifaceted and prevailing environmental influences will, in part, determine leadership style. The *Collins English Dictionary* defines leadership as 'the position or function of a leader'. This seemingly simplistic interpretation belies the complexities that contribute to the successful enactment of the role.

The role of a leader is becoming increasingly convoluted. The variations which may be encountered in both the public and private sector continue to grow. The external and internal influences to which all organizations are subject in an increasingly global economy often demand a chameleon-like response from those in positions of leadership. Indeed, in the face of such challenge one of the defining characteristics of a successful leader might be the continued ability to achieve, despite an atmosphere of uncertainty and change – constant features within the National Health Service (NHS).

Many complex organizations (in particular those in which professionals make up a large proportion of the workforce) promote structures which support teamwork and collaboration. In such an environment of equals, the qualities required for successful leadership will invariably include the ability to empower, facilitate and communicate (Morgan 1988). Stewart (1996) offers the concept of shared leadership – a collegiate model. In support of this ideal and in contrast to the somewhat dated

view that a ship cannot have two captains, such a model has proved to be very effective in the author's place of work (Figure 33.1).

Adair (1983) suggests that successfully managing the tension between group needs, task needs and individual needs is a key leadership function, as there will seldom, if ever, be a perfect match. How true this is. The management of such conflicts, real or potential, can consume a significant amount of the 'leadership resource'.

McCoy (1983) discusses the individual versus the group ethic in his 'Parable of the Sadhu'. He described a dilemma of some complexity where, in the absence of preconditions and guidance, the group involved reacted instinctively as individuals, resulting in an outcome which was both unsatisfactory and contentious. In this particular example it was debatable whether leadership or facilitation would have been preferable. However, the fact that lack of direction was a contributory factor was incontrovertible.

Despite the many, and sometimes seemingly overwhelming, obstacles that every leader encounters, the rewards can be great. The opportunity to create a vision and energize others in the pursuit of collective achievement should be prized. It is as a result of such endeavours that we learn to value what is good and strive to emulate those leaders for whom we have respect and in whom we place our trust.

'Where there is no vision, the people perish'
(Proverbs 29, v.18).

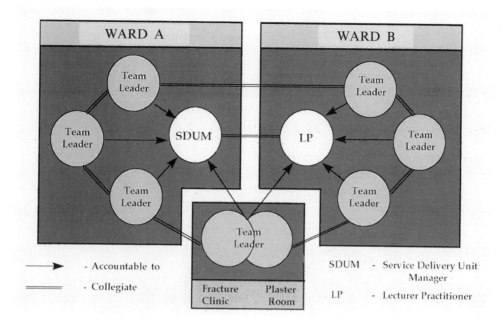

Figure 33.1   Trauma service delivery unit – nursing structure

The characteristics of leadership

Leadership qualities

The characteristics of a good leader are legion. However, success in any one particular work situation may well be determined by the leader focusing on those qualities which complement the environment in which he or she operates (Figure 33.2). Those who hold positions of leadership in acute care settings for example might consider flexibility, stamina and responsiveness to be key qualities.

Neubauer (1995a) states that the major role of leaders is to be passionate about the product (= nursing, physiotherapy, medicine) and the customer (= patients). Such passion may well exert a positive influence on the workforce, but conversely its effect may well be detrimental to those who perceive themselves to be less able than their peers. Those infused with a passion akin to missionary zeal may prove too demanding for the aforementioned group. Living under an umbrella of constant expectation can lead to a withdrawal from the cause.

Linked with 'a passion for excellence' is the value system which the leader displays. Simon *et al.* (1978) suggest that values are those beliefs and behaviours that are prized, freely chosen

and acted upon. There must therefore be a degree of mutual acceptance between the leader and his or her subordinates in relation to the values that the group as a whole have chosen to cherish. It is important that these values are made explicit, in order that new members may be clear in their expectations and that the potential for any future conflict is minimized. Mission statements and philosophies of care provide examples of group values being made explicit – provided that they are kept up to date.

Moss-Kanter (1988) emphasizes the importance of personal and interpersonal skills. She identifies three stages associated with the role of change-master/leader:

1. Formulate and sell the vision.
2. Find the power to advance the idea.
3. Maintain the momentum.

Another characteristic which Moss-Kanter states is an integral part of this leadership style is a trait she describes as 'kaleidoscope thinking' (experience not associated with one's own field or department). This style of leadership involves communication and conviction, and is energized by commitment. Following this principle, vision must be articulated and communicated

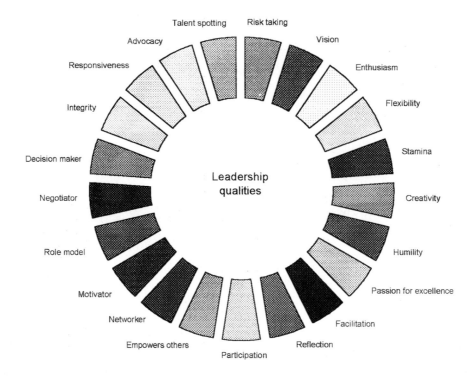

Figure 33.2 The qualities of leadership

repeatedly in order for new staff to understand and share the philosophy which underpins the service.

How do leaders acquire their own set of values? We all hold a set of moral views, often gained from personal experience, events, familial/peer influences and religious persuasion. In an American study, Dunham-Taylor (1993) suggests that being acknowledged and valued by influential persons affected the values that some leaders subsequently prized. Mentorship plays a significant part in the development of a leader's portfolio of qualities.

Mentorship: Reflections of a senior nurse

Lessem (1987) and Lievegoed (1979) concur, in so far as they each describe intrapreneurial (development of oneself) development in terms of phases and transitions. The realization of one's full creative potential is influenced by our passage through these phases, enabled and facilitated by personal vision, effective mentorship and the development of competency within one's own professional niche. I was lucky

---

enough to have an influential mentor who recognized my potential early in my career, but I believe that my creative abilities have been maximized as a direct result of my MBA studies. As Kolb *et al.* (1984) state: 'The establishment of alliances between business (= hospitals) and higher education promises to increase the effectiveness of both.'

The climate in which groups of staff are expected to perform is in dynamic equilibrium with the quality and outcome of care/treatment – the leader acting as a catalyst (Figure 33.3). Neubauer (1995b) argues that in the world of the twenty-first century, creating a climate with the proper balance between support and challenge is crucial. Freedom without structure is anarchy, yet structure without freedom is imprisonment. The difficulty in maintaining a balance between these two extremes in order to facilitate professional and organizational growth is perhaps influenced by the emotional climate which surrounds the

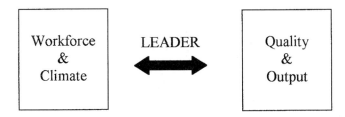

Figure 33.3 Dynamic equilibrium

working group. Ekvall (1991) makes explicit the distinction between climate, which he describes largely in behavioural terms as attitudes and feelings which are relatively easily observed, and culture, comprising deep-rooted assumptions, values and beliefs, which frequently exist on a pre-conscious level. Leaders cannot create optimal environments for others unless they are part of one themselves. Gilmore (1990) suggests that, in nursing, an effective leader creates a climate: 'You can walk into an effective unit and feel its tone and esprit. Conversely, chaos and disorder are equally palpable.'

Mentorship is commonly linked to the clinical supervision by senior staff of their junior colleagues. The needs of the clinical leader/manager in relation to this kind of support seem to attract less attention. Being a leader can be lonely, but the individual need not become isolated. One advantage of the collegiate model described earlier is that it allows for mutual mentorship; when one party is struggling, the other is at hand to provide the necessary support and help, thereby restoring the balance. Another advantage is the provision of a critical but friendly ear; someone with different yet complementary skills who shares the same values and, importantly, whose judgement one can respect.

The ability to act as a role model is often cited as an important leadership quality. Whether a leader can be deemed to have been successful in this area can only be determined by the behaviour and actions of those who choose to follow their example.

Leadership: The role model

An experienced team leader was recounting to her manager (also a practising nurse) details of

a particularly complex clinical dilemma. She described how she had discussed the issue with colleagues on duty at the time. The consensus was summarized thus: 'What would Sally (the aforementioned manager) do in this situation? She would probably. ... That's what I'll do then.' It is via routes such as these that the influence of an effective role model affects the practice of others. The outcome was successful!

As Manthey (1990) confirms, leaders are people who influence others by how they act and what they say.

Decision-making features prominently on the agenda of any leader. A humorous, but perceptive view of good decision-making is quoted by Agor (1986) and although originating from a senior executive in private industry, it has universal relevance: 'I believe that good, intuitive decisions are directly proportional to one's years of challenging experience, plus the number of related and worthwhile years of training and education, all divided by lack of confidence or the fear of being replaced.'

Neubauer (1993) links decision-making with trust. She argues that the goal should not necessarily be to be liked, nor indeed disliked. Leaders inevitably have to make difficult decisions – the test is whether staff can trust that you will be consistent, fair and that your values will be visible in your decisions. How many of us would pass such a test?

The impact of the organization

Within the NHS there are a variety of institutional models responsible for the provision of inpatient care. In the acute sector, most familiar will be organizations such as the Teaching

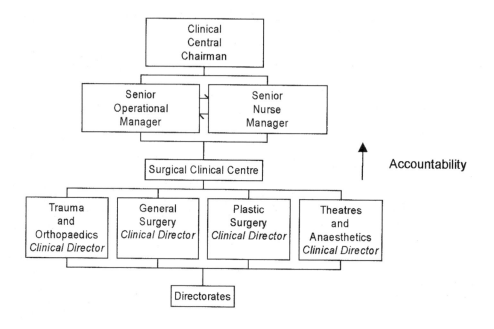

Figure 33.4 The directorate structure

Hospital, the District General Hospital and the Community Hospital – all now functioning as independent Trusts. Mintzberg (1989) describes the structure of complex organizations, such as hospitals, as professional bureaucracies. He explains that, due to the nature of the operating tasks (i.e. patient care and treatment), the organization surrenders much of its power, not only to the professionals themselves, but also to the associations and institutions that select and train them. Such organizational complexity requires a degree of decentralization to these highly trained individuals. However, the resulting autonomy can lead to conflict. The objectives and value systems of professionals may well be at odds with those of their colleagues in general management positions. In many instances the debate is focused around the thorny issue of resourcing. The organizational challenge must lie in the creation of a management structure for multidisciplinary teams which allows an appropriate degree of autonomy for practitioners from different professions and with different levels of seniority (Ovretveit, 1996).

Rather than attempt to control professionals *per se*, Harrison and Pollitt (1994) refer to the government and management tactic of 'incor-poration', whereby professionals are encouraged to become active participants in management processes and, as a result, exert some degree of control over their professional colleagues. In NHS Trusts the most commonly encountered organizational model is that of the Directorate. Services of a similar or complementary orientation are grouped together and operate as discrete functional units under the overall umbrella of what may conveniently be called a 'Clinical Centre'. In many such directorates, especially those whose primary function is clinical care rather than support or facilities, the Director will usually be a member of the consultant medical staff. A Clinical Centre Chairman will also be appointed to represent the interests of the different directorates at Board level. A Senior Operational Manager and a Senior Nurse Manager complete the triumvirate (Figure 33.4).

What impact does this type of structure have on leadership and its effectiveness, where does the power lie and whose values will predominate? Despite the best efforts of both government and Trust executives, it is unlikely that those holding clinical directorships will develop an overwhelming managerial bias, putting clinical prerogatives in jeopardy. If this holds true for medicine, can the same be said for other disciplines, nursing for example? Possibly not, and if not, why not? The answer may well be inextricably linked to clinical practice. Consultant medical staff, irrespective of seniority, continue to practise medicine despite the acquisition of management responsibilities. The practising clinician maintains credibility amongst peers and colleagues and is responsive to service/patient needs in a way that only those who actively participate can. Hewlett (1987), one of the founders of Hewlett Packard (a company familiar to the majority of clinicians), stressed the value to be gained from leaders/managers who are situated close to the problem, i.e. the workplace, thereby retaining credibility and first-hand knowledge.

The vast majority of nurses who hold operational management positions no longer have clinical practice as an integral part of their role, with the exception of Ward Sisters and Charge Nurses. These staff, despite their extensive clinical experience, are still relatively junior in organizational terms. They provide leadership within the context of their own domain, the ward, yet where is their inspiration, where are their role models? As a profession, should nursing not strive to afford equal value to the commitment to practise at senior level as that which is demonstrated by fellow disciplines? Despite its inadequacies, one of the objectives of the clinical grading system introduced in 1989 and currently under review, was to address this very issue – the need to retain the experienced nurse in clinical practice beyond the level of Ward Sister/Charge Nurse, i.e. the emergence of the H and I grade nurse. Regrettably, many organizations considered this option to be a luxury they could ill afford. Senior nurses were therefore obliged to take up management positions when in search of promotion and, as a result, many were able to avoid the dichotomy of management versus practice. Progressive establishments which place a high value on clinical nursing and the intellectual capital invested in those leaders contributing to and participating in service development, will reap the rewards for both staff and patients alike. 'Managers have tended – and still tend – to underrate the contribution of the nursing viewpoint to decision making' (Stewart, 1996).

Nurses must ensure that this sentiment becomes a thing of the past.

The effect of leadership style on service delivery and practice

The historical perspective on leadership supports the view that a leader should lead from the front; in military terms this style is undoubtedly one of the most effective – not so in the organizational jungle of today's healthcare systems. McGregor (1960) first presented his now familiar Theory X and Theory Y, in which these terms were used to describe two different views about what makes people work well. Theory X suggests a carrot and stick approach, i.e. incentives are required in order for individuals to perform well. Theory Y suggests that, essentially, most individuals want to perform well, but need a favourable environment in which to do so. Leaders who favour an enabling and empowering approach (Theory Y) rather than that of control (Theory X) are undeniably more in tune with the environmental requirements of most professionals. More recently, devolvement of responsibility, trust and support are key features of a management approach described by Walker (1991) as 'creative empowerment', the purpose and outcome of which is to draw out the hidden talents and skills of the workforce.

Harwood (1997) suggests that leaders need to become advocates for their professional services, and in many respects this view is to be supported, but is it consistent with the current focus on collaborative practice? Ten years ago Reich (1987) argued that we needed to honour our teams more, our aggressive leaders and maverick geniuses less. He supported the notion of the 'team as hero' and described the commitment and achievements of such teams as collective entrepreneurship. The core task of the leader in this type of environment is to manage uncertainty and create conditions of 'safety' in which the team can continue to work effectively (Gilmore, 1990). Henry (1991) suggests that the leadership style most conducive to fostering creative endeavours is participative leadership, in which the leader becomes more of a facilitator and mentor.

A leadership style which recognizes and values what Jelinek and Schoonhoven (1990) describe as 'local knowledge' (the specialist expertise exhibited by a discrete team or group of staff) will ensure that the advantages and quality associated with that expertise will be passed on to the recipient of the service; in the case of healthcare – the patient. The York study findings regarding skill mix and the effectiveness of nursing care relate cost and quality to good managers (Carr-Hill *et al.*, 1992), and by virtue of being a manager, Manthey (1990) argues that one must also be a leader. Conway (1995) posits that quality is linked to the reflective ability of the practitioner, which is in turn linked to their 'world view' (cumulative, educational and experiential inputs). Nursing Development Unit criteria (King's Fund, 1995), cite reflective ability as a key attribute. Reflective practice is an integral part of educational programmes for professional registration for nurses. It has yet to gain formal recognition within the medical profession and professions allied to medicine, as a skill which contributes positively to collaborative practice and teamwork.

The psychological profile of a leader will inevitably influence the way in which leadership skills are manifest, and indeed experienced by others. There are a number of tools available which can provide such profiles. One of the more familiar typologies is that developed by Myers-Briggs (1987), the Myers-Briggs Type Indicator (MBTI). This tool is primarily concerned with the valuable differences in people that result from where they like to focus their attention, the way they like to take in information, the way they like to decide, and the kind of lifestyle they adopt. People with preferences opposite to yours tend to be opposite to you in many ways. They are likely to be weak where you are strong, and strong where you are weak, each type has its own set of inherent strengths. Haley and Stumpf (1989) present the hypothesis that different personality types use certain cognitive trails and fall prey to predetermined biases inherent within these trails. This would suggest that following the determination of a leader's personality type predictions could be made in relation to the decision-making behaviours and performance of particular individuals.

'Critical thinking leaders are creative' (Gilmore, 1990). Therefore those whose style encompasses the development of a vision which can be communicated to others may well achieve greater success than those who cannot. Vision comes alive only when it is shared (Moss-Kanter, 1988; Westley and Mintzberg, 1989). Leaders of innovation persist in an idea; they keep at it. To some extent everything can look like a failure in the middle, but without persistence, important changes never take place.

Conclusion

'Leadership has to be earned and won' (Calman, 1994). The qualities which allow individuals to achieve positions of leadership are many and varied. Bespoke leadership styles need to be developed in order to complement the environmental diversity within the health service today and in the future. Multidisciplinary collaboration, teamwork and the ability to empower others are all recognizable features in the delivery of healthcare and the pursuit of excellence. In the words of Martin Luther King, recognized as one of the world's great leaders:

'I have a dream'

. . . so should we all.

References

Adair, J. (1983) *Effective Leadership*. Gower.

Agor, W. (1986) The logic of intuition: how top executives make important decisions. *Organisation Dynamics*, **14**, 5–18.

Calman, K. (1994) Working together, teamwork. *Journal of Interprofessional Care*, **18**(1), 95–99.

Carr-Hill, R. *et al.* (1992). *Skill Mix and the Effectiveness of Nursing Care*. Centre for Health Economics, University of York.

Conway, J. E. (1995) *Expert Nursing Knowledge on an Evolutionary Process*. PhD thesis, Warwick University (unpublished).

Dunham-Taylor, J. (1993) Experiences, events, people – do they influence the leadership style of nurse executives? *Journal of Nursing Administration*, **23**(7/8), 30–34.

Ekvall, G. (1991) The organisational culture of idea management: a creative climate for the management of ideas. In *Managing Innovation* (J. Henry and D. Walker, eds). Sage Publications.

Gilmore, T. (1990) Effective leadership during organisational transitions. *Nursing Economics*, May–June, **8**(3), 135–141.

Gilmore, V. (1993) Insight, initiative and imagination in nursing administration. *Holistic Nurse Practice*, **7**(3), 15–20.

Haley, U. and Stumpf, S. (1989) Cognitive traits in strategic decision making: linking personalities and cognitions. *Journal of Management Studies*, **26**(5), 477–497.

Harrison, S. and Pollitt, C. (1994) *Controlling Health Professionals*. Open University Press.

Harwood, A. (1997) What kind of leader are you? *Nursing Times*, **93**(12), 66–69.

Henry, J. (1991) Making sense of creativity. In *Creative Management*. Sage Publications.

Hewlett, W. (1987) The human side of management. In *Managing Design* (D. Walker and R. Roy, eds.). Open University Press.

Jelinek, M. and Schoonhoven, C. (1990) Strong culture and its consequences. In *The Innovation Marathon*. Blackwell.

Kings Fund (1995) *Nursing Development Unit Leadership Criteria*, Kings Fund Centre, London.

Kolb, D., Lubin, S., Spoth, J. and Baker, R. (1984) Strategic management development: experiential learning and managerial competencies. *Journal of Management Development*, **3**(5), 13–24.

Lessem, R. (1987) Developing in phases. *Intrapreneurship*, Gower.

Lievegoed, B. (1979) *Phases*. Rudolf Steiner Press.

Manthey, M. (1990) The nurse manager as leader. *Nursing Management*, **21**(6), 18–19.

McCoy, B. (1983) The Parable of the Sadhu. *Harvard Business Review*, Sept./Oct., 103–108.

McGregor, D. (1960) *The Human Side of Enterprise*. McGraw-Hill.

Mintzberg, H. (1989) The structuring of organizations; cited in Asch, D. and Bowman, C. (eds) (1991) *Readings in Strategic Management*. Macmillan.

Morgan, G. (1988) Emerging waves and challenges: the need for new competencies and mindsets. In *Creative Management* (J. Henry, ed.). Sage Publications.

Moss-Kanter, R. (1988) Change-master skills: what it takes to be creative. In *Managing Innovation* (J. Henry and D. Walker, eds). Sage Publications.

Myers-Briggs (1987) *Myers-Briggs Type Indicator*. Consulting Psychologists Press.

Neubauer, J. (1993) Redesign: managing role changes and building new teams. *Seminars for Nurse Managers*, **1**(1), 26–32.

Neubauer, J. (1995a) The value of nursing. *Journal of Nursing Management*, **3**, 301–305.

Neubauer, J. (1995b) Thriving in chaos: personal and career development. *Nursing Administration Quarterly*, **19**(4), 71–82.

Ovretveit, J. (1996) Five ways to describe a multidisciplinary team. *Journal of Interprofessional Care*, **10**(2), 163–171.

Reich, R. (1987) Entrepreneurship reconsidered: the team as hero. *Harvard Business Review*, May/June, 77–83.

Simon, S., Howe, L. and Kirschenbaum, H. (1978) Values clarification: a handbook of practical strategies for teachers and students; cited in Wilmot, S. (1995) Professional values and interprofessional dialogue. *Journal of Interprofessional Care*, **9**(3), 257–266.

Stewart, R. (1996) *Leading in the NHS, A Practical Guide*. Macmillan Press.

Walker, D. (1991) Creative empowerment at Rover. In *Managing Innovation* (J. Henry and D. Walker, eds). Sage Pulications.

Westley, F. and Mintzberg, H. (1989) Visionary leadership and strategic management. In *Managing Innovation* (J. Henry and D. Walker, eds). Sage Publications.

34

Strategic and operational issues in service delivery

Deborah Langstaff

Introduction

This chapter aims to give an overview of the issues which affect service delivery, both from a strategic and an operational perspective. It is important for clinicians at all levels to develop an understanding of the political and socio-economic imperatives affecting the provision of healthcare today. At the inception of the National Health Service in 1948 its objective was simple – the provision of healthcare for all, free at the point of delivery. Naive assumptions were made in the early days; the notion that as the health of the population improved largely due to improved access, the requirement for healthcare might well diminish. The picture today is very different. While the early recipients of NHS care were no doubt grateful for what they considered to be state benevolence, the expectations of today's consumer display little of this early passivity. Advances in technology, media hype, patients' rights and rationing all feature prominently in the healthcare debate.

For those clinicians and managers who bear responsibility for service delivery and development within a climate of increasing economic constraint, the task becomes ever more challenging. Efficiency and effectiveness are the universal criteria with which service providers must wrestle, while attempting to maintain quality of care. The issues which impact on service delivery are multifactorial and will be explored during the course of the chapter. Consideration must be given to the organizational environ-

ment itself, together with the internal and external influences affecting healthcare provision. Stakeholder issues, the impact of change and technology and the dilemma of defining need in the face of limited resources will also be discussed. Finally, the experience of the workforce in the acute care setting will identify some of the key issues and pressures which affect the functional ability of clinical teams. Although many of the topics under discussion will have generic applications, trauma specific examples will be given where relevant.

The organizational environment

It is pertinent to begin this section by giving a brief outline of key organizational developments in the NHS over the past 20 years. After the election of the Conservative government in 1979 there was a growing Treasury preoccupation with the funding of the health service. In 1980 almost 90% of the national health bill was met by the Treasury (Office of Health Economics, 1982). Initial attempts to encourage the development of a 'private sector' concluded that it was unlikely to offer financial support of any significance. The notion was then put forward that productivity could be increased and savings made by virtue of better management. The Griffiths Report (1983) proposed a fundamental restructuring of the NHS organization, duties, responsibilities, accountability and control. The era of general management had arrived. Despite these new arrangements, resource allocation

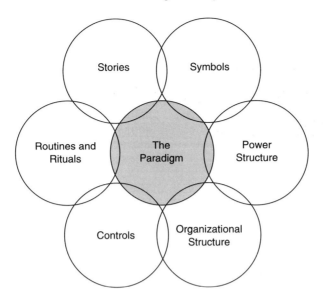

Figure 34.1 The cultural web of an organization (Adapted from Johnson and Scholes, 1993)

was still a significant issue. Throughout the 1980s the Resource Allocation Working Party (RAWP) formula was applied which allocated funds to regions, ostensibly taking account of need rather than as a result of some historical accident in the location of hospitals (RAWP Report, 1976). In broad terms, the formula was based on the size and composition of the local population.

Eventually, in 1989, further radical reform of the healthcare system was proposed. The White Paper *Working for Patients* (Department of Health Report, 1989), (together with the NHS and Community Care Act) promoted the establishment of internal markets – hospital services being a specific target. The advent of the purchaser-provider split coincided with the formation of NHS Trusts in 1991–93. The potential shift in the balance of influence from consultants towards purchasing authority managers and fund-holding general practitioners was felt in part to be the key to increased control. Finally, the most recent reforms have centred around the creation of so-called 'primary care groups' (PCGs).

Wrigley and McKevitt (1994) argue that it is the responsibility of professionals and managers to understand, and respond to, the character of the core public service; to attend to its purpose rather than to tinker with its structures and organizations.

It is against such a turbulent background and accelerating pace of change that professionals and managers strive to deliver a service. The potential for conflict between a chief executive's objective – to meet the legal and financial obligations of the Trust – and the clinicians' objective – provision of quality healthcare – is ever present. However, Rowe (1996) argues that conflict appropriately channelled can act as a motivator-stimulator for ideas and proposals within a team. The expectations of an increasingly aware and informed public, together with the pressure to meet government imposed targets, require increasingly sophisticated skills and attributes from the workforce.

Audit, risk management and, latterly, clinical governance are all tools with which to improve quality of care and reduce the financial impact of litigation. The Clinical Negligence Scheme for Trusts (CNST) was introduced in 1995 to provide a framework for risk management. The programme comprises three levels of attainment, with a time frame for achievement. A discount in insurance premiums for Trusts is the reward for those who meet the stated criteria.

This then is the 'global' environment within which NHS Trusts must function. What are the environmental characteristics of individual organizations? The cultural web described by Johnson and Scholes (1993) is a useful conceptual tool for understanding the way in which beliefs and assumptions, linked to the political symbolic and structural aspects of an organization, guide and constrain the development of strategy. The organizational paradigm central to this model is subject to influences located within the six satellite functions and as such can become a variable dynamic (Figure 34.1 and Table 34.1).

Table 34.1 The cultural web of the trauma service (Adapted from Johnson and Scholes, 1993)

Stories	• Macho personalities
	• Conflict between organization and professional objectives
	• Shroud waving
Symbols	• Technical jargon
	• Association with university of world reknown
Power structure	• Traditional power of medical profession
	• New power of nursing and management
Organizational structure	• Decentralized
	• Non-hierarchical
	• Central 'support' function (indirectly exerting power and influence)
	• Professional versus organizational accountability
	• Communication
Controls	• Targets and budgets
	• Monitoring at clinical centre level
	• Quarterly reviews of SDU against business plan by CEO
Routines and rituals	• Long working hours
	• Project groups
	• Endless 'meetings'

CEO, Chief Executive Officer; SDU, Service Delivery Unit

Ekvall (1991) makes a distinction between climate and culture. He regards organizational climate as an intervening variable which affects the results of the operations of the organization, most notably through influencing processes such as communication, problem-solving, decision-making and the psychological process of learning and motivation.

How then do individuals respond within the context of their own organizational mêlée? Flynn (1993) suggests that rigid control makes service delivery units (SDUs) insensitive to the needs and wishes of their users. He argues that the organizational structure should be designed to ensure that the SDU has sufficient support to be able to do its job. Rowe (1996) concurs, stating that those managers who err towards

control rather than flexibility stifle the ability of teams in their response to changing patient needs. Cavanagh (1996) holds the view that in order to create an environment which fosters a new psychological contract between employee and employer leading to trust, commitment and mutual benefit, there must be opportunities for employees to become more self-managing as opposed to being subject to direct central control.

Beer *et al.* (1990) offer a somewhat contradictory perspective. They suggest that in order for individuals to become more responsible they must be put into a new organizational context, resulting in the imposition of new roles, responsibilities and relationships, arguing that individual behaviour is powerfully shaped by the organizational roles people play. Although a seemingly brutal tactic, the author has experience of a change process achieved via this somewhat direct approach.

Case study

Environmental change had led to the need for reorganization of the trauma service at local level. Changes in clinical practice, the introduction of a resident consultant-based service, an increase in the number of surgical procedures, and reduced length of stay had all contributed to the need for a review. These factors had resulted in an under-utilization of bed capacity. At the time, the service consisted of three 20-bedded wards and an outpatient department. The plan was to downsize, maintain current capacity with inbuilt scope for expansion, and offer financial savings. The wards were reconfigured into two 24-bedded areas and the traditional role of the ward sister was abolished and replaced by three team leaders per ward. Senior nurse input was provided via the collegiate relationship of the lecturer practitioner and the service manager, one based on each ward (see Figure 33.1).

Although the new service model was presented as a *fait accompli* and was non-negotiable, the facilitation of the change process, reconfiguration of teams, the identification of those who would assume new roles and responsibilities and the clarification of lines of accountability were all managed using a participative process. The time-scale was short. Implementation (which included a rebuild), from inception to the unit becoming fully operational, took 7 months. Bringing together different people with different styles and backgrounds has

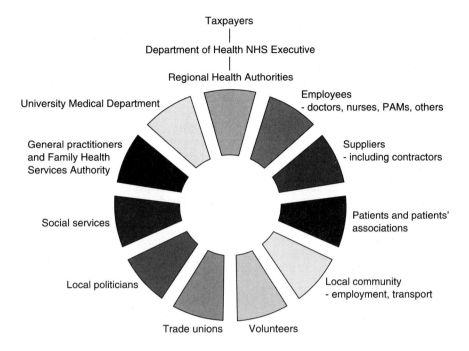

Figure 34.2 Stakeholder groups for the Chief Executive of a teaching hospital (Adapted from Stewart, 1994)

culminated in our departmental philosophy of collaboration, commitment and trust. The non-hierarchical management style, nurses managing care, and a high priority afforded to education, all contribute to the intellectual capital invested in the staff – the return being manifest in quality of care and auditable outcomes. The service has functioned in this way for 5 years, and its structure and operational strategy is unique. The environment continues to change and as a learning organization we are still attempting to find perspectives and practices which can cope with such turbulence (Moss-Jones, 1995).

As Mintzberg (1976) states, 'organisational effectiveness does not lie in that narrow-minded concept called "rationality"; it lies in a blend of clear-headed logic and powerful intuition'.

Internal and external influences in service provision

Stakeholders

All stakeholder groups are potentially in conflict with management, because managers may interpret the organization's or their own interests differently from those of particular stakeholders (Stewart, 1994). The complexity of the stakeholder issue as applied to the health service is highlighted in Figure 34.2.

The perspectives of the various stakeholders are many and varied. It could be argued that there is a degree of inevitability in the fact that individual groups will focus on those issues with which they most readily identify. If this is taken as a given, then interested parties may never display a truly altruistic outlook. Skelton (1994) believes that existing powerful groups, consultants for example, are not going to hand over resources, information or decision-making responsibilities to the less powerful unless they can see a tactical advantage in so doing. Winship (1995) suggests that empowerment is arguably the central therapeutic task of a system of healthcare and that empowerment of the most vulnerable members of society is a yardstick of the commitment to equality and democracy. How is this perceived by patients? Is the degree of reciprocity acceptable and how valuable an indicator of consumer perspective are tools such as patient satisfaction surveys? Loughlin (1993) argues that as patients consult to gain access to medical knowledge they do not

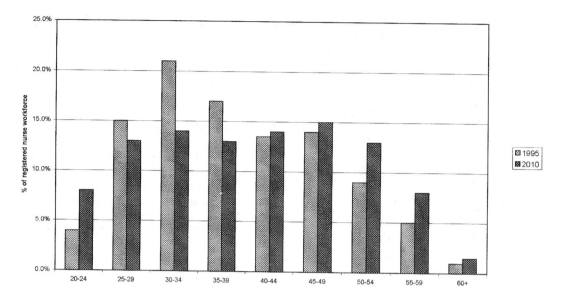

Figure 34.3   Registered nurses – actual (1995) and forecast (2010) age distributions (GB) (From Buchan *et al.*, 1998)

have, should not clinicians and managers consult about experiences they do not have in order to find out how their service is perceived? Wrigley and McKevitt (1994) use the term 'differential information' to describe the information deficit that exists between health professionals and their patients. When buying bananas, for example, we can make personal judgements as to whether the fruit is ripe, attractive and affordable, based on our intrinsic knowledge of the product. Not so in healthcare. How can patients be sure that the treatment or advice they are being offered is the most appropriate for them – and indeed are other options available which have not been presented?

Gaster (1995) explores the issue of power in relation to knowledge and collectivity. Collective power applied to public services and consumer groups has been gaining momentum over the last 30 years. She argues that this is an important development as it can help to combat the fragilities of some stakeholder groups who inherently have less power than others.

Demographic change – some key issues

When Dr Jonathan Miller was asked 'What is the greatest leap in medical science in the twentieth century?', he replied 'Nursing' – not great technology as was expected. This may be considered by some to be a controversial statement. Why should nursing be afforded this special recognition? Many have a very simplistic view of a nurse's role and consider it to be merely meeting the physical care needs of patients. Gilmore (1993) states that the health needs of today's patients are often associated with an increase in complexity, severity and co-morbidity, resulting in heavier utilization of human and material resources within acute care. While other disciplines, such as medicine or physiotherapy, have intermittent contact with patients, nurses are the one group whose presence is constant. They provide the cohesion which binds a service together. Miller's statement reflects the metamorphosis that nursing has undergone in order to meet the challenges of healthcare provision today.

However, despite advances in practice and an increased recognition by some of the role, impending demographic change will further test the resilience and responsiveness of the nursing profession. In the wake of falling recruitment, Freeman (1996) reported the difficulties associated with gaining a national overview of nursing requirements, particularly since the inception of NHS Trusts – no central remit being in existence. The prediction was that ultimately the NHS would fall apart in nursing terms. A survey carried out by Smith and Seccombe (1998) for the Institute of Employment Studies on behalf of the RCN highlights the problem of an ageing workforce. Projections demonstrate that by the millennium almost half the nursing workforce will be over 40 years, and by 2010 one-fifth of all nurses will be over 50 (see Figure 34.3). In order to maintain the registered nurse workforce at its current size, intakes to pre-registration education would roughly have to double. A sobering thought for the future.

On the demand side, one of the most significant features of demographic change relates to an increase in the numbers of older people within the UK population, both in absolute terms and as a percentage of the total. The proportion of the population aged 75 years and over will have almost doubled from 4.2% in 1961 to 7.4% in 2001, where it will plateau, although the 85 years and over age group will continue to increase (Office of Population and Census Surveys, 1992). The significance of this in government terms is the increase in expenditure associated with the escalating healthcare needs of this group. For the speciality of trauma, the significance lies in the provision of increased resources to care for patients who have sustained femoral neck fractures in addition to other fractures commonly associated with falls. The challenge for the future will be to ensure how an increase in demand can be met by a diminishing workforce.

Rationing, need and the implications of technological advances

In the public domain many services are rationed, the NHS being a case in point. Wherever limited services meet unmet demand, rationing takes place, consciously or unconsciously, by political will or by bureaucratic inertia, by budgetary choice or under work pressure, by frustration or idealism (Stewart and Ranson, 1988). Although rationing *per se* does not affect emergency services in the way that long waiting lists and purchasing authority decisions affect those patients requiring elective procedures, a type of rationing does exist.

With the advances in technology and surgical techniques, the management of patients with complex fractures and multiple injuries is now highly sophisticated. For those patients who

have sustained complex pelvic fractures or unstable spinal injuries, for example, surgical management is most appropriately carried out in so-called 'tertiary referral centres'. Here, the multidisciplinary team have developed specialist expertise as a direct result of their continued exposure to such case mix complexity. Their role, in addition to providing a service to the local population, is to offer advice and a service to district general hospitals (DGHs) within the region, when patients' treatment requirements exceed the capabilities of staff in the referring hospital. The dilemma for the clinician arises when, due to local pressures on bed capacity, management intervention denies the acceptance of such patients in favour of those already 'within' the system, whose injuries may in comparison be relatively minor. As a result, some multiply-injured patients cannot access the treatment they require, and when timescales for definitive surgical intervention could be crucial, this may lead to sub-optimal outcomes for these individuals. This then is a form of rationing. In the author's experience, managing the admissions of a number of such patients can almost be considered analogous to the role of an air traffic controller – several patients in a holding pattern in peripheral DGHs, bringing them in to land according to whose fuel will run out first! The consequence of greater expectation (both from patients and medical colleagues) has resulted in an increased demand for this type of specialist service, a fact recognized and described by Flynn (1993). He suggests that in this type of scenario, unless there is an open-ended budget, rationing is inevitable. The argument here in terms of access to services must surely hinge on the definition of the 'local' population.

How then are choices made? The distinction between priority needs (what people must or ought to have) and wants (what people might like) according to Rose (1989) is a matter of political debate. The Oregon Experiment in the USA has received much publicity, and indeed censure, for the introduction of healthcare rationing. The rationing process was developed according to a 'formula' which takes account of public perceptions of the relative importance of treatments, clinical judgements, 'quality of life' and the money available to the state for spending on medical services. Seedhouse (1994) would argue though that unless a person has knowledge or experience of a thing or process, they cannot possibly judge whether it is a thing or process of quality. A scheme suggested by Callaghan (1987), also in the USA was to set an age limit on eligibility for Medicare (the federally supported insurance plan for those over 65 years old). His argument was that beyond a certain chronological period no treatment should be offered to those who could not pay for it. Although reluctant to say what the age should be, he maintained that such a proposal was not as harsh as it sounded, arguing that many older people may not necessarily want to go on living, and that some treatments do not produce more fulfilling life – just more of it. Despite the fact that these two proposals originated in the USA (where health-care must be paid for) the problems of resourcing and choice apply equally in this country. There are no easy answers.

> *Example*
>
> Consultant surgeon sets the medical criteria for the discharge of a patient who has sustained an open tibial fracture, reduced and stabilized with an intramedullary nail. These criteria having been met, the patient enquires of the doctor: 'When may I go home?' The response is: 'That's not up to me now. When your nurse, physiotherapist and occupational therapist are happy with your progress and feel that you will be able to cope, then you may go home. The decision lies with them.'

Management style and the workforce

Creativity and expertise

Creativity comes from people. Machines and computers cannot be creative in themselves, because creativity requires something more than the processing of existing information – it requires human thought, spontaneous intuition and a lot of courage (Morita, 1986). Drawing on the talent and creativity of staff is the key to developing services in response to environmental need. Ovretveit (1995) suggests that the real benefit of a team approach comes not just from coordinating the activities of separate professions, but from moulding them in new and creative ways, thereby producing a sum which is greater than the parts. The view held by Nolan (1995) is that the diversity and complexity of the healthcare environment reinforces the fact that no profession has hegemony across all contexts. Castledine (1995) suggests that nursing and medicine are part of a continuum in which cure and care have a reciprocal relationship, with the relative emphasis shifting depending on context. Such a view requires the recognition of intellectual equality in relation to decision-making within clinical teams.

Simon (1988) contends that expertness is the prerequisite to creativity, but not every expert can use that knowledge creatively. The challenge then is how to manage our creative teams in order to support their endeavours. The determinants of success are multifactorial. Certain elements are worth emphasizing: the value of experience and its contribution to the creative process, the need to encourage lifelong learning and an awareness of self within the context of the groups to which we belong.

Teamwork

'To be effective, a team needs to have a number of qualities. These include shared aims, a recognition of the distinctive roles of individual members, leadership, measure of performance and team structure' (Calman, 1994). We all belong to a variety of teams – the domestic team, the work team, a team of volunteers, a sporting team. Do we exhibit similar behaviours and attitudes within the context of each individual group setting? Unlikely. While Smith-Blancett (1994) suggests that the ideal team member should be creative, flexible, inquisitive, energetic and capable, Belbin (1981) offers an alternative perspective on such universality. He proffers that individuals have a dominant preference for one of the eight different roles he identifies as existing within the context of a team. Successful teams are those where diversity of membership and skill result in an increased creative and functional potential. This is not to say that with such a complementary membership the risk of conflict is eliminated. Neubauer (1993) believes that mutual respect within teams does not require agreement on every issue; however, it does require a willingness to trust the skills and expertise of others. In the opinion of Rowe (1996), conflict – appropriately channelled – can act as a motivator and stimulator for ideals and proposals within the team. The risk associated with too 'democratic' a team, however, is that with an operational tactic such as informal consensus, instead of allowing greater commitment it may allow people quietly to ignore decisions, thereby undermining teamwork (Ovretveit, 1995). In the words of a former Israeli Foreign Minister: 'Consensus is something agreed in public and ignored in private.' This need not always be the case.

Example

In the author's workplace, consultant trauma surgeons provide a 24-hour resident on-call service – this system is not operational elsewhere in the UK. The significance of this method of practice lies in the fact that, irrespective of the time that a patient presents to A&E, there will always be an on-site consultant available to make decisions about treatment. Under the direction of the admitting consultant, a management/treatment plan will be made following discussion with the patient, and a time will be scheduled for surgery. If surgery has to be postponed or delayed for any reason, that management plan will be followed by the medical team on call at the time. Although the surgeon actually carrying out the operation might have favoured a different method of management, despite considering both options to be equally acceptable, the original plan will be adhered to, the only exception being a deterioration or change in the condition of the patient. This consensus approach to the management of trauma patients is a necessary corollary to the institution of the residency programme. The constant presence of the 'team' leads to an element of discontinuity for the individual consultant; however, the benefits of such senior on-site personnel are undoubtedly advantageous to the patient.

Performance

There are two elements to consider here: the performance of the individual/workforce; and performance in relation to activity and quality.

What affects the quality of a service? Maxwell (1984) proposed six dimensions of quality for health services which have subsequently been reviewed (Maxwell, 1992):

- effectiveness
- acceptability
- efficiency
- access
- equity
- relevance.

The application of one or more of these components to elements of service provision can be problematic and the evaluation of outcomes via audit is often a time-consuming task. Brown and Chamberlin (1996) state that the quality of the service rendered depends a great deal upon the level of interprofessional collaboration occurring within teams. A key factor in the pursuit of quality according to Coote (1993) is the motivation of the workforce. Government initiatives, such as league tables and charters, though envisioned as mechanisms by which to improve quality, may well act as disincentives for staff when like is not compared with like.

Example

One centrally determined indicator was the 30-minute wait to consultation with a doctor in the outpatient clinic. In the speciality of trauma, for example, seeing the doctor first and without the benefit of x-rays and/or removal of plaster prior to examination and assessment would only serve to lengthen the wait, inconvenience the patient and frustrate the staff. This particular anomaly has now been addressed, having been replaced by the 30-minute wait to consultation with *any* health professional.

Flynn (1993) warns against the moral pressure which league tables rely on. There is strong evidence in support of the view that health status varies considerably with social class (DHSS, 1980; Whitehead Report, 1987). This means that measurements of performance must be corrected for the differences in expected outcomes due to social class. The reliability and validity of many performance indicators in the

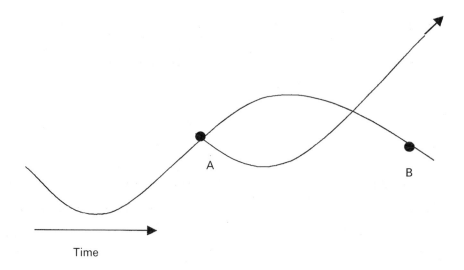

Figure 34.4 The sigmoid curve

health service must therefore be open to question.

Skill mix and its effect on quality of care has long been debated. Carr-Hill *et al.* (1992), who examined the relationship between skill mix and quality of care – currently the definitive study – found that higher nursing grades gave better quality care. This finding must surely be pertinent to other disciplines. Keen (1995) argues that one would not choose to have one's car repaired by an unqualified mechanic, so why then do some experts feel that it is acceptable to care for patients with less qualified staff? Aitken (1998) believes that there is no managerial substitute for an expert nurse clinician's judgement. Kramer and Schmalenberg (1988) studied major hospitals in the USA and identified those that were good places to work (so-called 'Magnet' hospitals). They had a variable skill mix, 67–94%, and demonstrated low turnover. Findings included values such as quality of care, nurse autonomy, innovation, education and non-rigid communication. These are all process measures, but these hospitals also had lower mortality rates – an example of processes contributing to outcomes. Similar work to the US Magnet studies is set to take place in Europe and the UK (Aitken, 1998). Although the utilization of high skill mix is associated with higher fixed costs, the increase in productivity contributes significantly to lower unit costs, as has been the experience of the author.

What then is the cost of increased performance expectations in human resource terms? Managers must guard against the effects of emotional overload and burn-out among staff. The personal and contextual resources that an individual draws from will have a significant effect on their experience of care-giving. Across the disciplines, continued exposure to the 'crises' encountered by staff caring for trauma patients can create a cumulative burden. Leppanen-Montgomery (1997) suggests that caring is not a heroic, independent act; instead it arises from within the context of a community or a team. Greiner (1972) describes the continued exposure to such crises as a state of 'psychological saturation'. He also clearly argues for the notion of a sabbatical as temporary respite from the unremitting demands of stress in the workplace. The chance to reduce clinical commitment and the opportunity to reflect, research and evaluate in 'work time' rather than 'borrowed time' would appeal to many.

Handy (1993) offers us the concept of the sigmoid curve (Figure 34.4) which he suggests is applicable to almost every aspect of life. The accelerating pace of change shrinks every sigmoid curve and the way to ensure constant growth/regeneration is to begin another curve 'A' while there is still enough energy, resource and time to ensure success. To wait until point 'B', with disaster looming, is frequently too late.

The management task must be to ensure the development and the implementation of strategies which promote the wellbeing and longevity of staff in the workplace. As the proportion of economically active young people in the population is diminishing, such a precious resource is also deserving of care.

Conclusion

This chapter can address only briefly the complexity of service provision in the acute sector of the NHS. The objectives of clinicians who hold management positions are frequently at odds with those who hold executive positions. Political and financial imperatives abound, risk management and the penalties for negligent or sub-optimal performance are an ever-present threat. Increased expectation and the dilemmas associated with rationing services create pressures for all those responsible for healthcare provision, most notably clinicians. The value of strong leadership and effective teamwork cannot be underestimated. It is the development of such strategies which will give not only the individual a chance to survive in the turmoil of today's working environment, but also offers a lifebelt to colleagues and teams who are less well equipped to ride the storm. Must the philosophy of *Animal Farm* still burden us in the twenty-first century?

'All animals are equal, but some are more equal than others' (Orwell, 1945).

References

Aitken, L. (1998) Powerful nurses protecting patients. *Nursing Standard*, **13**(7), 30–31.

Beer, M. Eisenstat, A. and Spector, B. (1990) Why change programs don't produce change. *Harvard Business Review*, Nov./Dec., 158–166.

Belbin, M. (1981) *Management Teams – Why They Succeed or Fail*. Oxford: Butterworth-Heinemann.

Brown, G. and Chamberlin, G. (1996) Attitudes towards quality, costs and physician centrality in healthcare teams. *Journal of Interprofessional Care*, **10**(1), 63–72.

Buchan, J., Seccombe, I. and Smith, G. (1998) In Smith, G. and Seccombe, I. (eds) *Changing Times: a survey of registered nurses in 1998*. Institute of Employment Studies.

Callaghan, D. (1987) *Setting Limits: Medical Goals in an Ageing Society*. Touchstone.

Calman, K. (1994) Working together, teamwork. *Journal of Interprofessional Care*, **8**(1), 95–99.

Carr-Hill, R., Dixon, P. and Griffiths, M. (1992). *Skill Mix and the Effectiveness of Nursing Care*. Centre for Health Economics. University of York.

Castledine, G. (1995) Defining specialist nursing. *British Journal of Specialist Nursing*, **1**, 264–265.

Cavanagh, S. (1996) A 'new' psychological contract for nurses: some management implications. *Journal of Nursing Management*, **4**, 79–83.

Coote, A. (1993) Understanding quality. *Journal of Interprofessional Care*, **7**(2), 141–150.

Department of Health Report (1989) *Working for Patients*. London: HMSO.

DHSS (1980) Inequalities in health. *The Black Report*. London: HMSO.

Ekvall, G. (1991) The organizational culture of idea management: a creative climate for the management of ideas; cited in Henry, J. and Walker, D. (eds) (1994) *Managing Innovation*. Sage.

Flynn, N. (1993) *Public Sector Management*. Harvester Wheatsheaf.

Freeman, H. (1996) Trusts offer 'golden hellos' for angels. *British Journal of Health Care Management*, **2**(2), 95–96.

Gaster, L. (1995) *Quality in Public Services*. Open University Press.

Gilmore, V. (1993) Insight, initiative and imagination in nursing administration. *Holistic Nurse Practice*, **7**(3), 15–20.

Greiner, L. E. (1972) Evolution and revolution as organisations grow. In Asch, D. and Bowman, C. (eds) *Readings in Strategic Management* (1989), pp. 373–387. Macmillan.

Griffiths Report (1983) *NHS Management Inquiry Report*. London: DHSS.

Handy, C. (1993) *The Empty Raincoat*. Random House.

Johnson, G. and Scholes, K. (1993) *Exploring Corporate Strategy*. Prentice-Hall.

Keen, A. (1995) Political influences in nursing. In *Nursing, Beyond Tradition and Conflict* (M. Jolley and G. Brykczynska, eds). St Louis, MO: Mosby.

Kramer, M. and Schmalenberg, C. (1988) Magnet Hospitals: Part I and II: Institutions of excellence. *Journal of Nursing Administration*, **18**, 11–19, 13–24.

Leppanen-Montgomery, C. (1997) Coping with the emotional demands of caring. *Advanced Practice Nursing Quarterly*, **3**(1), 76–84.

Loughlin, L. (1993) Involving patients in the planning and delivery of care: working towards a common goal. *Journal of Interprofessional Care*, **17**(2), 161–166.

Maxwell, R. J. (1984) Quality assessment in health, *British Medical Journal*, **228**, 1471–1472.

Maxwell, R. J. (1992) Dimensions of quality revisited: from thought to action. *Quality in Healthcare*, **1**, 171–177.

Mintzberg, H. (1976) Planning on the left side and managing on the right. In *Creative Management* (J. Henry, ed.). Sage.

Morita, A. (1986) Selling to the world: the Sony Walkman story; cited in Henry, J. and Walker, D. (eds) (1994) *Managing Innovation*. Sage.

Moss-Jones, J. (1995) Learning organizations: an emerging paradigm? In *Creative Management*, Readings 1. Open University Business School.

Neubauer, J. (1993) Redesign: managing role changes and building new teams. *Seminars for Nursing Managers*, **1**(1), 26–32.

Nolan, M. (1995) Has nursing lost its way? *British Medical Journal*, **311**, 304–307.

Office of Health Economics (1982) *Compendium of Health Statistics*. Office of Health Economics.

Office of Population and Census Surveys (1992) *Population Trends*, **67**, 41.

Orwell, G. (1945) *Animal Farm*. Secker and Warburg.

Ovretveit, J. (1995) Team decision making. *Journal of Interprofessional Care*, **9**(1), 41–51.

RAWP Report (1976) *Sharing Resources for Health in England*. Resource Allocation Working Party Report. London: HMSO.

Rose, R. (1989) Charges as contested signals. *Journal of Public Policy*, **9**(3), 261–286.

Rowe, H. (1996) Multidisciplinary teamwork – myth or reality? *Journal of Nursing Management*, **4**, 93–101.

Seedhouse, D. (1994) *Fortress NHS*. Wiley.

Simon, H. (1988) Understanding creativity and creative management. In *Handbook for Creative and Innovative Managers* (R. L. Kuhn, ed.). McGraw-Hill.

Skelton, R. (1994) Nursing and empowerment: concepts and strategies. *Journal of Advanced Nursing*, **19**, 415–423.

Smith-Blancett, S. (1994) Self-managed teams: the reality and the promise. *The Health Care Supervisor*, **12**(4), 48–55.

Smith, G. and Seccombe, I. (1998) *Changing Times: A Survey of Registered Nurses*. Institute of Employment Studies.

Stewart, J. and Ranson, S. (1988) Management in the public domain. In *Public Sector Management* (D. McKevitt and A. Lawton, eds). Sage.

Stewart, R. (1994) *Managing Today and Tomorrow*. Macmillan Press.

Whitehead Report (1987) *The Health Divide: Inequalities in Health in the 1980s*. Health Education Council.

Winship, G. (1995) Patient empowerment – individualism versus collectivism. *Therapeutic Communities*, **16**(2), 113–116.

Wrigley, L. and McKevitt, D. (1994) Professional ethics, Government agenda and differential information. In *Public Sector Management* (D. McKevitt and A. Lawton, eds). Sage.

35

Creating the optimum learning environment

Jane Christie

Introduction

This chapter aims to explore the issues which help to promote a positive learning environment when caring for the injured person. Following injury, the victim and those close to them are vulnerable and anxious. Caring for these people is often a painful business, and the pain experienced by those doing the caring often goes unacknowledged, and at great personal cost (Butterworth *et al.*, 1998). Additional stress is created in the pursuit of collaborative teamwork, and in striving to value the contribution of each discipline, while meeting the needs of the injured.

Promoting a positive learning environment, in both the physical and the psychological sense, is one way to develop self-awareness in staff and those for whom they care. It allows for the exploration of internal feelings and anxieties created by caring for the vulnerable and injured. It allows healthcare professionals the space to explore their feelings and relationships, and this can inform practice.

Butterworth *et al.* (1998) identify the following prerequisites which might need to be met before self-awareness can be fully developed:

- organizational culture
- a structured way of thinking about relationships and interaction
- constant and consistent supervision.

These prerequisites provide the framework for this chapter.

Organizational culture

It is not possible to develop self-awareness in a culture that is not receptive. A successful learning organization is one that is continually expanding its capacity to create the future. Learning is a way of life and taps into people's natural curiosity and motivation to learn. Senge (1990) identifies that an organization requires core competencies for thinking and interacting based on five disciplines:

1. Shared vision – where projects are linked to this vision.
2. Team learning – mastering the practice of discussion and team learning, suspending assumption, entering genuine thinking and discoverinh new views.
3. Personal mastery – focusing energies, developing patience and seeing reality.
4. Mental models – explore thinking, and make thinking open to the influence of others.
5. Systems thinking – fusing other disciplines by creating networks used to identify problems, move solutions and improve solutions.

The dominant culture in healthcare that still exists is that emotion and feelings should not be expressed. This is no longer acceptable practice when the amount of work and the intensity and severity of injury is ever increasing. Change is the responsibility of everyone, and empowerment is the aim, achieved through the valuing of personal feelings, experiences and emotions. In the right learning environment healthcare professionals are able to reflect on their experiences, to build on their repertoire of skills and to understand the meaning of practice (Saylor, 1990; Temple, 1991). Those who are self-directed acquire sensitivity and competence in social interaction, and have the skills and competencies to master productive tasks involved with controlling and manipulating the environment (Mezirow, 1981).

Developing a research agenda that supports the generation of new knowledge from practice can contribute to this change process. Glennie and Cosier (1994) discuss a method used to facilitate interdisciplinary learning and professional development. Collaborative inquiry is a method of cooperative research which challenges the assumption that it is necessary to separate the subject and the researcher in order to establish objectivity and therefore 'truth'. These often mutually exclusive roles give way to relationships based on bilateral initiative and control, so that all of those involved work together as co-researchers and co-subjects. The method was first developed by Heron (1971) and has been promoted and extended by others, notably Reason and Rowan (1981) and Reason (1991). The model of work echoes Schon (1987) and is based on the concept of experiential learning (Kolb, 1979). Collaborative inquiry sets experiential learning in a group context. This process needs a facilitator with vision, who has the ability to motivate others and can teach and guide the process.

Collaborative inquiry empowers those experts, giving them a voice in forums where the nature, pace and direction of change is being debated. It can be testing and time consuming, but outcomes are rich and multifaceted (Glennie and Cosier, 1994). Multiprofessional learning is effective and valued when it is the product of an iterative process which moves, over time, between action and reflection. Ownership of the research agenda, process and outcomes, and its correlate empowerment, is a highly effective catalyst for professional development and collective change across agency boundaries. The generation of emergent data, preoccupying here and now issues which practitioners face daily, is critical to the process of improvement in cooperative practice. The facilitator needs to:

- examine their relationship with power and control, to know it and to manage it

- genuinely believe in practice expertise, to encourage its expression and honour its validity.

Trauma care is a relatively new speciality and could benefit from the generation of collaborative inquiry which would promote sharing of ideas and the testing of new theories (Table 35.1).

Table 35.1 The process of collaborative inquiry (Adapted from Glennie and Cosier, 1994)

Step 1	Definition	Agree ground rules, context and methodologies
Step 2	Conscious observation	Of themselves and others
Step 3	Intuitive observation	The need to be absorbed and in touch with deep knowing (tacit knowledge)
Step 4	Reflection, analysis and planning	Reconvene, gather data and develop generalizations. Plans need to be made to test theories or avoid unsuccessful strategies or unrewarding behaviours

A structured way of thinking about relationships and interaction

Those working with injured people encounter many situations of suffering, uncertainty and conflict, and these require appropriate responses. In the move away from manipulation and control to more humanistic practices, healthcare professionals need a process that allows interpretation of the clinical situation and the resolution of complex phenomena (Johns, 1997).

Reflection has emerged as a significant learning process (Johns, 1997). It is not a new concept, Aristotle mentions its use in his work on practical judgement and moral action (Coutts-Jarman, 1993). More recently Schon (1987) writes extensively on the reflective practitioner. He argues for a curriculum that educates professionals to move away from the positivist philosophy to the artistry of reflection-in-action. This would allow for confusing problems that defy technical rationality to be solved in practice (Schon, 1987).

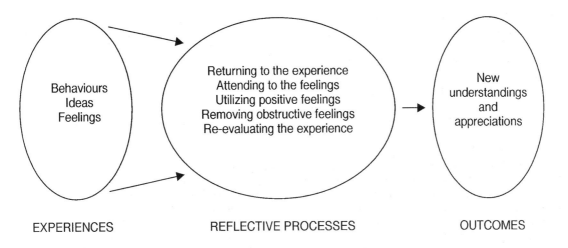

Figure 35.1   The reflective cycle (Adapted from Boud *et al.*, 1985)

Reflection as a psychological process involves thinking quietly, mulling over events in our mind and making sense of experiences (Boud *et al.*, 1985). It is not a flawless process as it depends on accurate recollection of an event or experience (Newell, 1992). It involves reconsideration; an idea rising in the mind (Swannell, 1992); stopping to think (Flaherty, 1983); stillness (Keegan, 1988); and thinking on your feet (Schon, 1991). Knights (1985) argues that reflection cannot occur without the aware attention of oneself or others; it requires a listener as a reflector. Reflection can also be a spiritual process that is achieved through meditation and prayer (Boud *et al.*, 1985).

Reflection involves the consideration of an unexpected event and the knowing-in-action that led up to it – our thoughts turn back on the surprising phenomenon and at the same time back on ourselves (Schon, 1987). It involves learning through conflict which, with guidance, leads to empowerment.

Professionals reflect in the midst of action and without interruption, their thinking shaping what they are doing while they are doing it; the key to success is to bring past experience to bear on present activity (Cervero, 1988). During action there is a conscious awareness of performance (Giddens, 1979; Jarvis, 1992) and review of one's repertoire of clinical experiences (Saylor, 1990). Reflection provides data for self-evaluation (Saylor, 1990) and for the understanding of one's own value system (Phaneuf, 1976; Barnett and Wainwright, 1987).

Reflection can be a social and philosophical method of analysis that investigates the collective experience of a group of people in a social system (Ziechner, 1981; Kendall and Roddy, 1991). It involves the integration of attitudes and skills in methods of inquiry (Ziechner, 1981). It acknowledges feelings, values and beliefs (Boud *et al.*, 1985). It is a method of problem-solving through the recognition of patterns, making sense of complexity and resolving the difficulty (Flaherty, 1983; Goodman, 1984; Schon, 1987; Saylor, 1990; Schon, 1991; Jarvis, 1992).

Reflection involves exploring, analysing, reviewing and questioning what is known, and the subjective feelings and actions of individuals and others (Dewey, 1933; Barnett and Wainwright, 1987; Schon, 1987; McDaniel, 1990; Gandy and Jenson, 1992; Newell, 1992). This enquiry often leads to very unexpected outcomes (Boud *et al.*, 1985) (Figure 35.1).

Reflection can also be deliberate (Munby and Russell, 1989). It is a cognitive process that depends on the retrospective review of past events (Schutz, 1970; Phaneuf, 1976; Flaherty, 1983; Shulman, 1987; Saylor, 1990). It can also involve looking back to see if goals have been achieved in order to decide a plan for the future (Flaherty, 1983; Hall, 1983; Boud *et al.*, 1985; Leipo-Kilpi, 1990; Parse, 1990). It can also lead to the development of new knowledge and skills to increase richness and value in life (Ziechner, 1981; Keegan, 1988; Jarvis, 1992). It is a learning tool where learning results from experience (Dewey, 1933; Ausabel, 1968; Kolb, 1984; Boud *et al.*, 1985; Munby and Russell, 1989).

Reflection increases awareness of why we attach the meanings we do to reality (Mezirow, 1981) and it enables one to view an issue from a different perspective (Kendall and Roddy, 1991). It clarifies the meaning of experience in terms of self (Boyd and Fales, 1983), thus helping to explain our actions (Clarke, 1986) and providing the opportunity to correct what is wrong (Flaherty, 1983) and identify what has been achieved (Boud *et al.*, 1985).

Despite its high profile, there is little critical examination of either the theoretical or practical problems of reflection in trauma practice. Schon (1991) argues that the practice of reflection involves preparation for performance in a range of professional situations. Practice is a repertoire of expectation, images and techniques which might be taught if they were constant, but instead it is characterized by unique events that are always changing (Schon, 1991). These situations are the triggers for reflection (Boud *et al.*, 1985).

Trauma care is full of complexities, uncertainty and conflicting value judgements. The work is characterized by unique events that are always changing. Often the team caring for injured people in any setting rarely have time to carry out their work, let alone the time or energy to reflect on what they have done. Informally, groups of healthcare professionals may meet socially and discuss the events of the day, but this is often an emotional discussion of the stresses and frustrations, and tends not to lead to positive problem solving or increased self-awareness. Reflection helps to alleviate anxieties and share problems with one's peers by finding positive solutions to situations (Green, 1997).

Lack of reflection is an adaptive response and a natural consequence of the fast-paced and unpredictable nature of trauma care. Schon (1991) argues that, in professional practice, reflection remains private and inaccessible, preventing others learning from the experts.

Experts view their situations holistically, and much of their knowledge is embedded in practice (Polyani, 1967). This is known as tacit knowledge, which Meerabeau (1992) argues is a positive asset and the hallmark of a profession. However, there is a mismatch between forms of professional knowledge and the changing characteristics of practice settings (Schon, 1991). Healthcare professionals find it difficult to learn from experience because it is rarely valued by their peers, management or the organization; it is the technical, rational type of knowledge that is of greatest importance (Powell, 1989) and is rewarded as such. This is strongly influenced by the increasing technology and power of the medical model. If experienced healthcare professionals do not learn from practice or learn negative aspects then this may make their practice static and unperceptive (Powell, 1989). As practice becomes more routine they fail to think about their work and fall into rigid repetition (Powell, 1989). It then becomes much safer and more secure not to reflect, because they do not have to change what they do not see as being wrong (Saylor, 1990). This ultimately results in an increased gap between theory and practice.

In response to this rigidity and ritualistic practice, and in an attempt to narrow the theory/practice gap, nursing education has begun to focus on reflection as a method of improving personal and professional awareness. This is no bad thing, as reflection can be intentionally taught (Boyd and Fales, 1983) and could be developed during shared education (French and Cross, 1992). However, in their usual haste to change practice, educationalists have jumped on the bandwagon and implemented reflection in the easiest way. In the safe haven of the educational establishment, journals and critical incidents are discussed and analysed. Writing can help to develop critical thinking (Hahnemann, 1986) as writing skills and thinking skills are a mutually interactive process (Allen *et al.*, 1989). Therefore a clinical log or diary offers the opportunity for reflection (Sedlack, 1992). Journals, fieldwork, seminars, small group work and games are all strategies for experiential learning and may address provocative issues and provide insights into alternative methods of solving clinical problems (Gandy and Jenson, 1992; Newell, 1992). However, the skill of experiential learning in which people are most deficient is still reflecting in practice (Boud *et al.*, 1985). There is no question that these are some of the successful ways to promote reflection, but it can also be argued that professionals can only be taught through experience and close association with expert practitioners (Meerabeau, 1992).

The other issue is that although reflection has

been advocated as the way that the healthcare practitioner enhances the application of research-based practice (Lamb and Huttlinger, 1989), there is no guarantee that knowledge learned in the classroom will be transferred to practice or that it will improve the quality of care (Dewing, 1990).

As time spent on courses is very short in relation to an entire career, it would be of great benefit if reflection was used in practice deliberately to promote learning from experience (Powell, 1989). Although experience is vital for learning, just having experience is not enough – it needs to be observed and reflected upon (Schon, 1991).

Management of practice is a highly skilled occupation, as an environment suitable for reflection must be created (Jarvis, 1992). This involves helping adults construe experience in such a way that they more clearly understand the reasons for their problems and understand the options open to them in order that they may assume responsibility for decision-making (Mezirow, 1981). Good managers need to recognize when performance is in danger of becoming presumptive or ritualistic, and must create a situation where reflection can occur (Jarvis, 1992). Friere (1972) argues that an ethos of support, encouragement, non-judgemental acceptance, mutual help and individual responsibility can be created.

Alternative perspectives are presented with different value systems and ways of seeing, a premium being placed on personalizing what is learned by applying insight to one's own life and works as opposed to mere intellectualization (Mezirow, 1981). Professional expertise increases through the act of reflection and the ensuing increased self-confidence, rather than through the factual content of the reflections (Newell, 1992).

Managers need to seek and be responsive to feedback and advice. They must be able to recognize mistakes, make change, and accept that cycles of learning and action should be permanent features of their job (Campbell, 1991).

Social skills can be taught by action and then reflection (Clarke, 1986), and time for thinking and group discussion needs to be created (Schon, 1987; Saylor, 1990). The task is to help the team enhance their understanding of, and sensitivity to, the way others perceive, think and feel while involved in common endeavours (Mezirow, 1981).

The fact that, for some, reflection may be the cause of intense stress cannot be ignored (Campbell, 1991). If, through reflection, an individual identifies that change in personal thoughts, feelings or behaviour is needed, then a great deal of inner conflict may be created (Boyd and Fales, 1983). This can result in a sense of failure, unnecessary criticism and development of new problems (Schon, 1991) which may sometimes be as destructive as ignoring the issue in the first place. Inner conflict cannot always be avoided as it is an experience characteristic of change (Boyd and Fales, 1983). However, support networks, discussion groups and supervision can help reduce negative results of reflection, increase self-esteem and identify learning from experience (Boyd and Fales, 1983). Those who are unfamiliar with reflection would benefit from pairing up with at least one other whom they trust, and together they could utilize reflection in their own practice (Dewing, 1990). They must be helped to identify real problems involving reified power, relationships rooted in institutionalized ideologies which one has internalized in one's psychological history (Mezirow, 1981).

To achieve a change in perspective they must consequently be led to understand the reasons embedded in the cultures, myths and concomitant feelings which account for their needs and wants, as well as the way they see themselves in their relationships (Mezirow, 1981). Access must then be given to alternative perspectives (Schon, 1991).

In the present culture of the health service this requires an enormous shift in attitude towards the management and practice of care. Friere (1972) demonstrated how this is possible by placing emphasis on equality and reciprocity in building a support group through which learners can share experiences with a common problem and come to share a new perspective. Responsibility needs to be devolved downwards so that individuals have to explain their own practice (Darbyshire, 1991) and develop creativity, insight and empathy (Goodman, 1984).

Corporate commitment will help provide support for the manager, but also create the right atmosphere for reflection (Schon, 1991). Managers must be prepared to share their knowledge and experience, to demonstrate the characteristics of open-mindedness, wholeheart-

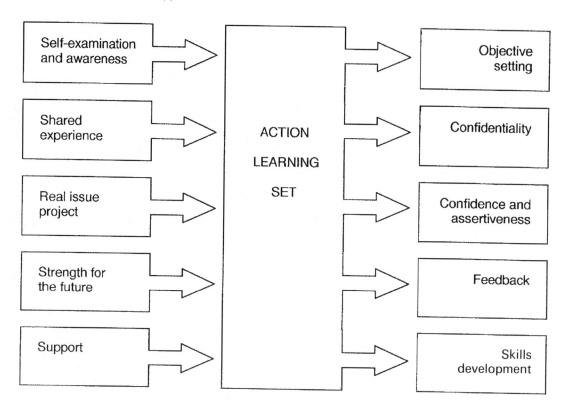

Figure 35.2   The processes involved in action learning

edness and responsibility in order to promote those features in others within the team.

Structured reflection through action learning sets encourages understanding, allowing reflection and time to find an effective solution (Figure 35.2). The approach allows for different learning styles and ensures that the participants complete the learning cycle time after time as they act on, reflect on, reframe and test their subsequent actions to enhance the potential of their day-to-day work. This process has demonstrated its value in improving collaboration and interprofessional working by reducing competitiveness and generating knowledge from practice (Curtis Jenkins and White, 1994).

Constant and consistent supervision

Clinical supervision is the process whereby a healthcare practitioner reviews with another person their ongoing clinical work, as well as aspects of or reactions to that work (Sever-

insson, 1996). This may involve sharing responsibility and assessing the level of anxiety by sharing personal feelings, thoughts, concerns vulnerabilities and actions (Farkas-Cameron, 1996). Supervision is believed to emphasize practical knowledge, making results visible and reflected upon (Hallberg and Norberg, 1993). Hawkins and Shohet (1992) suggests there are three elements to consider in the context of clinical supervision: normative, restorative and formative:

- Normative addresses those issues in practice which relate to quality control and the demands of the organization. Evidence to further inform this process may come from staff satisfaction scales, sickness and absence rates, and numbers of patient complaints.
- Restorative relates to supportive help that must be available for professionals working constantly with stress and distress. Clinical supervision is seen by some as a proactive, protective device to assist cop-

ing, and has more value than waiting for reactive solutions, measured through coping, stress and burn-out questionnaires.

- The formative component of clinical supervision relates to the educative process of developing life-long learning through the opportunity to observe and reflect upon their practice. Evaluation may be carried out by assessing the progress of those being supervised.

Callion and Baxter (1995) argues that this supervision should be an exchange between professionals to enable professional development, but then describes the process as a list of managerial tasks related to improving performance, suggesting rigidity and control. Arguably its success is dependent on the development of an environment where reflection, challenge and support are part of the culture. The question is not how expensive is this process, but what is the cost of not offering this opportunity as part of the working ethic? The principles of supervision can be explored in theory, but the practice of supervision can only be taught by example.

Hughes and Pengelly (1997) fear that the misuse of supervision through mechanistic checklists can focus anxiety and stifle learning. Managers who fail to value creative questioning fail to appreciate that rapid change may lead to deskilling and regression, failure to allow uncertainty, and failure to acknowledge mistakes with openness and in the confidence that they can be learned from, and will be unlikely to sustain the practice of supervision, let alone a happy, innovative developing team.

Butterworth *et al.* (1998) carried out evaluation research demonstrating that true clinical supervision has a beneficial impact on staff. When done well by those who are adequately trained and have adequate support themselves, it provides a forum for the preservation or restoration of integrity (de Raeve, 1998). Strong leadership, clear lines of accountability and adequate resources all play an important part, but the ability to guide reflection and promote initiative, imagination and creativity are a vital contribution to good supervision.

In an environment where there is considerable pressure on staff, it could be argued that any opportunity for 'time out' would be greatly received. However, staff don't always see clinical supervision as 'time out'. When carried out effectively, supervision can involve discomfort and anger when issues are raised for exploration and interpretation. The realization of another perspective is not always easy to understand. When sensitively managed, the outcome is evidence of learning and achievement. Investing this time, effort and support in team members can only help increase self-esteem and in turn improve team work.

Conclusion

This chapter has briefly explored the main contributory factors in promoting a positive learning environment. In trauma care, at any stage of the continuum, individuals, their loved ones and those caring for them are dealing with intensely emotional situations and complicated transitions. Dealing with this using a positive problem-solving approach involves the development of self-awareness. With a supportive, receptive culture as a backdrop, the following key actions are essential for shared learning, personal development and the generation of new knowledge:

- mastering collaborative discussion and utilizing critical thinking to explore complex issues
- generating collaborative research
- promoting reflection in practice
- maintaining leaders in practice to role model expert supervision
- investing time and effort in staff to reward and retain expertise and develop practice.

References

Allen, D. G., Bowers, B. and Diekelmann, N. (1989) Writing to learn: a reconceptualisation of thinking and writing in the nursing curriculum. *Journal of Nursing Education*, **28**(1), 6–11.

Ausabel, D. P. (1968) *Educational Psychology: a Cognitive View*. Holt, Rinehart and Winston.

Barnett, D. and Wainwright, P. (1987) The right reflection. *Senior Nurse*, **6**(5), 33–34.

Boud, D., Keogh, R. and Walker, D. (1985) *Reflection: Turning Experience into Learning*. Kogan Page.

Boyd, E. M. and Fales, A. W. (1983) Reflective learning: the key to learning from experience. *Journal of Humanistic Psychology*, **23**(2), 99–117.

Butterworth, T., Faugier, J. and Burnard, P. (1998) *Clinical Supervision and Mentorship in Nursing*. Stanley Thornes.

Callion, H. and Baxter, T. (1995) Clinical Supervision. *Nursing Management*, **1**(9), 20–21.

Campbell, I. (1991) The reflective practitioner. *Nursing Standard*, **5**(19), 34–35.

Cervero, R. (1988) *Effective Continuing Education for Professionals*. Jossey Bass.

Clarke, M. (1986) Action and reflection: practice and theory in nursing. *Journal of Advanced Nursing*, **11**, 3–11.

Coutts-Jarman, J. (1993) Using reflection and experience in education. *British Journal of Nursing*, **2**(1), 77–80.

Curtis Jenkins, G. and White, J. (1994) Action learning, a tool to improve collaboration and promote change: counsellors, general practitioners and primary care team. *Journal of Interprofessional Care*, **8**(3), 265–273.

Darbyshire, P. (1991) Nursing reflections. *Nursing Times*, **87**(36), 27–28.

De Raeve, L. (1998) Maintaining integrity through clinical supervision. *Nursing Ethics*, **5**(6), 486–496.

Dewey, J. (1933) *How We Think*. DC Health.

Dewing, J. (1990). Reflective practice. *Senior Nurse*, **10**(10), 26–28.

Farkas-Cameron. M. (1996) Clinical supervision in psychiatric nursing. *Journal of Psychosocial Nursing*, **33**, 31–37.

Flaherty, M. J. (1983) A time for reflection and redirection. *Nursing Management*, **14**(3), 45–46.

French, P. and Cross, D. (1992) Interpersonal and epistemological curriculum model for nurse education. *Journal of Advanced Nursing*, **17**, 83–89.

Friere, P. (1972) *Pedagogy of the Oppressed*. Harmondsworth: Penguin.

Gandy, J. and Jenson, G. (1992) Group work and reflective practicums in physical therapy education: models for professional education behaviour development. *Journal of Physical Therapy Education*, **6**(1), 6–10.

Giddens, A. (1979) *Central Problems in Social Theory*. Macmillan.

Glennie, S. and Cosier, J. (1994) Collaborative inquiry: developing multidisciplinary learning and action. *Journal of Interprofessional Care*, **8**(3), 255–263.

Goodman J. (1984) Reflection and teacher education: a case study and theoretical analysis. *Interchange*, **15**(3), 9–25.

Green, S. (1997) Reflection of an experience. *British Journal of Theatre Nursing*, **6**(12), 27–29.

Hahnemann, B. K. (1986) Journal writing: a key to promoting critical thinking in nursing students. *Journal of Nursing Education*, **25**(5), 213–215.

Hall, C. (1983) A time for reflection. *Journal of Advanced Nursing*, **8**(6), 457–466.

Hallberg, I. R. and Norberg, A. (1993) Strain among nurses and their emotional reactions during one year of systematic clinical supervision combined with the implementation of individualised care in dementia nursing. *Journal of Advanced Nursing*, **18**, 1860–1875.

Hawkins, H. and Shohet, R. (1992) *Supervision in Helping Professions* (H. Hawkins and R. Shohet, eds). Open University Press.

Heron, J. (1971). *Experience and Method: An Inquiry into the Concept of Experiential Research*. Guildford: University of Surrey Human Potential Research Project.

Hughes L. and Pengelly, P (1997). *Staff Supervision in a Turbulent Environment*. Jessica Kingsley.

Jarvis, P. (1992) Reflective Practice and Nursing. *Nurse Education Today*, **12**, 174–181.

Johns, C. (1997) Reflective practice and clinical supervision. Part 1: The reflective turn. *European Nurse*, **2**(2), 87–97.

Keegan, L. (1988) Self-care. *Official Journal of the Association of Operating Room Nurses*, **4793**, 715, 717, 719.

Kendall, J. and Roddy, A. (1991) Radical reflection as a theoretical framework in nursing using acquired immunodeficiency syndrome as an example. *Journal of Professional Nursing*, **7**(5), 283–292.

Knights, S. (1985) Reflection and learning: the importance of a listener. In *Reflection: Turning Experience into Learning* (D. Boud, R. Keogh and D. Walker, eds). Kogan Page.

Kolb, D. A. (1984) *Experiential Learning*. Prentice-Hall.

Kolb, D. (1979). *Organizational Psychology: an Experiential Approach*. Prentice-Hall.

Lamb, G. S. and Huttlinger, K. (1989) Reflexivity in nursing research. *Western Journal of Nursing Research*, **11**(6), 765–772.

Leipo-Kilpi, H. (1990) Self-reflection in nursing teacher education. *Journal of Advanced Nursing*, **15**, 192–195.

McDaniel, C. (1990) Nursing administration research as a paradigm reflection. *Nursing and Health Care*, **11**(4), 191–193.

Meerabeau, L. (1992) Tacit knowledge: an untapped resource or a methodological headache. *Journal of Advanced Nursing*, **17**, 108–112.

Mezirow, J. (1981) A critical theory of adult learning and education. *Adult Education*, **32**(1), 3–24.

Munby, H. and Russell, T (1989) Educating the reflective teacher: an essay review of the two books by Donald Schon. *Curriculum Studies*, **21**(1) 71–80.

Newell, R. (1992) Anxiety, accuracy and reflection: the limits of professional development. *Journal of Advanced Nursing*, **17**, 1326–1333.

Parse, R. R. (1990) A time for reflection and projection. *Nursing Science Quarterly*, **3**(4), 143.

Phaneuf, M. C. (1976) *The Nursing Audit: Self Regulation in Practice*. Appleton-Century-Crofts.

Polyani, M. (1967) *The Tacit Dimension*. Routledge and Kegan Paul.

Powell, J. H. (1989) The reflective practitioner. *Journal of Advanced Nursing*, **14**, 824–832.

Reason, P. (1991) Power and conflict in multidisciplinary collaboration. *Complementary Medical Research*, **5**, 485.

Reason, P. and Rowan, J. (1981) *Human Inquiry: A Sourcebook of New Paradigm Research*. Wiley.

Saylor, C. R. (1990) Reflection and professional education: art, science and competency. *Nurse Educator*, **15**(2), 8–11.

Schon, D. (1987) *Educating the Reflective Practitioner*. Jossey Bass.

Schon, D. A. (1991) *The Reflective Practitioner: How Professionals Think in Action*. Avebury.

Schutz, A. (1970) *On Phenomenology and Social Relations*. University of Chicago Press.

Sedlack, C. A. (1992) Use of clinical logs by nursing students and faculty to identify learning needs. *Journal of Nursing Education*, **31**(1), 24–28.

Senge, P. (1990) Building learning organisations. *Journal of Quality Participation*, **15**(2), 30–38.

Severinsson, E. I. (1996) Nurse supervisors' views of their supervisory styles in clinical supervision: a hermeneutical approach. *Journal of Nursing Management*, **4**, 191–199.

Shulman, L. S. (1987) Knowledge and teaching: foundations of the new reform. *Harvard Educational Review*, **57**, 1–22.

Swannell, J. (1992) *The Oxford Modern English Dictionary*. Clarendon Press.

Temple, A. (1991) Reflection and the charge nurse. *Nursing Standard*, **5**(26), 32–34.

Ziechner, K. M. (1981) Reflective Teaching and Field-Based Experience in Teacher Education. *Interchange*, **12**(4), 1–22.

36

Risk management

Mary Burrows

Introduction

Risk management is a process of identifying, assessing and controlling risks which lead to improving the quality of care for patients and staff. The spectrum of risk management covers three areas: the organization, the environment and the individual. Understanding individual and collective responsibilities in the risk management process and learning to work as a team are important in order to ensure the delivery of effective healthcare. Objectives for this chapter are to:

- establish an understanding of risk management
- define the scope of risk management
- establish a framework for putting risk management into practice.

Understanding risk management

Risk management uses a number of approaches in managing activities within an organization. Carter and Crockford (1994) defined risk management as a process of bringing together many functions such as finance and insurance, traditionally dealt with separately, into one management function. This allows an organization to develop a comprehensive approach to managing risk. At its simplest, risk management is the application of good management principles.

The main types of risk are business risk and pure risk. Business risk, classified as manage-

ment science, has four components:

1. Technical – new technologies, impact on organizations, competencies.
2. Social – changes in expectations.
3. Economic – inflation, budgetary constraints.
4. Political – government ideologies, philosophies, policies.

These components are applicable in the healthcare setting and impact on the development and direction of not only a hospital in its entirety, but locally in clinical areas such as wards. The Patient's Charter, which has increased the expectations of patients and the perceived ability of hospitals to meet demands, is a good example of social influences on business risk.

The second type of risk, pure risk, also has four components:

1. Physical effects of nature – weather, floods, fire.
2. Social deviations from expected standards of conduct – theft, violence, negligence.
3. Technical issues – breakdown of equipment.
4. Personal issues – sickness and injury.

In understanding and putting risk management into practice, recognition of the interrelationship between pure and business risk is important. They do not exist in isolation – sickness on a ward (pure risk) will have an impact on delivery of care affecting service delivery (business risk) (Figure 36.1).

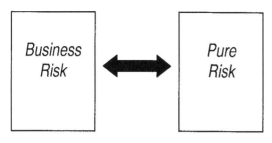

Figure 36.1   The interrelationship between the two types of risk

Defining risk and risk management

Risk has many definitions, the earliest provided by Willet (1901) as 'the objectified uncertainty regarding the occurrence of an undesirable event'. The classic definition of risk was provided by Knight (1921) who considered risk as:

- a knowledge of the problem (e.g. identified hazard)
- an understanding of the range of possible outcomes

- the ability to objectively assess the likelihood of each outcome occurring.

Defining hazard as the ability to cause harm (e.g. needles) and risk as the probability or likelihood that harm will occur (e.g. needlestick injury) is the simplest way of defining components of risk management. Table 36.1 lists some of the hazards that healthcare professionals face in the clinical setting.

Table 36.1   Hazards in the workplace

Equipment
Environmental (e.g. temperature)
Needles/sharps
Slips, trips and falls
Clinical waste
Substances/chemicals/drugs
Manual handling
Aggression and violence
Exposure to radiation
Exposure to microorganisms

Risk management has many definitions which differ based on the context of risk; for example

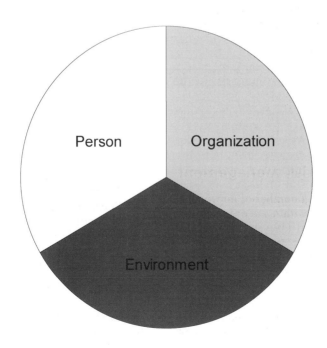

Figure 36.2   Elements of risk management

financial risk definitions are mainly concerned with assets of an organization, not about injuries to staff. Raz (1982) defined risk management in healthcare as 'a function of planning, organising and directing a programme of activities to identify, evaluate and take corrective action against risks that may lead to patient injury, employee injury and property loss or damage with resulting financial loss'. This definition encompasses elements of risk management – the organization, the environment and the individual (person) (figure 36.2). The five key elements of risk management are shown in Table 36.2.

Table 36.2   Key elements of risk management

1. Defining activities	Clinical activities, scope of service provided
2. Identifying hazards and risks	Organizational, environmental, those affecting people
3. Risk assessment	What is the level of risk based on frequency, outcome and probability
4. Reduction or minimization actions	Steps to control, reduce, minimize risks
5. Risk finance	Financial management, resourcing

There are many models for establishing risks, most related to finance and industrial health and safety. Health and safety risk analysis models have been used successfully to reduce staff injuries and damage to equipment. For healthcare, application of complicated models like those used in industry are useful, but often limited and narrowly focused. A process described by Bowden (1994) in Figure 36.3 is a workable model for risk management.

Healthcare staff must recognize that it may not be possible to avoid risks when delivering care and, in many cases, reducing or preventing risk is the most practicable option. Risk prevention is effected through the development and implementation of protocols and standards for patient care, together with systems for maintaining equipment and facilities. Risk funding is in two forms – assume the funding within budgets or, alternatively, via transference, usually associated with others carrying the risk. Examples of risk transference are con-

tracting out services and private finance initiatives.

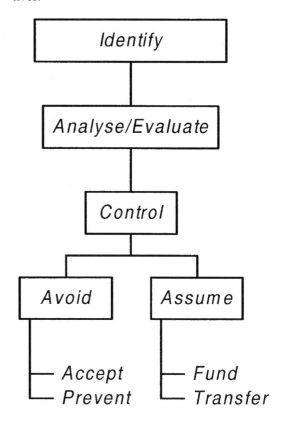

Figure 36.3   A model for risk management (Adapted from Bowden, 1994)

Identifying responsibilities and process

Risk management is everyone's responsibility. However, as with any organization the extent of how responsibility is delineated may vary. A chief executive will carry the largest responsibility in an organization, being ultimately responsible for the activities it undertakes. Many risks identified relate to identifying the person or persons responsible; therefore clarity of responsibility may help to minimize risks.

Corporate responsibility

Responsibilities are outlined in health and safety legislation, particularly the Health and Safety at Work Act 1974 (HASAWA) and the Management of Health and Safety at Work

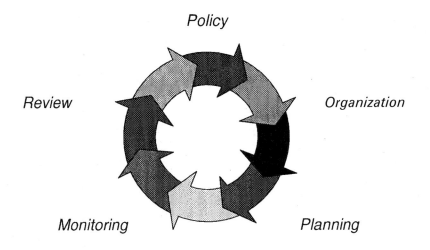

Figure 36.4 The five-step loop for health and safety management

Regulations, 1992. Other pieces of legislation, including the NHS Community Care and Reform Act 1990, also outline management responsibilities. In summary, the main responsibility in HASAWA lies with the employer to take all steps as are reasonably practicable to ensure the health, safety and welfare of staff and others (this would encompass patients and visitors). In hospitals, the chief executive and executive board carry this corporate responsibility. This is delegated and translated into operational duties for managers.

Managers

Managers discharge this operational responsibility by developing policies and procedures, being good communicators of information through instruction, supervision and training, ensuring that the workplace is suitable and that sufficient and appropriate equipment is provided. Spinks (1994) wrote about the responsibilities of nurses and problems that arise from not controlling risks in the clinical setting. She discussed how nurses and nurse managers must be made aware of their responsibilities and how they must apply effective risk management control methods to reduce risks to patients. This means being accountable for actions within the clinical setting, overseeing systems and people and ensuring that risks are identified and dealt with either through local management or by others such as directors. This accountability

applies to all clinical staff and is not unique to nurses.

Employees

Employees have a responsibility within HASAWA to work with employers on health and safety and to take due regard for their own safety. They also have a professional duty of care. Responsibility is individual, but also collective in organizational terms – the sum of all individuals. Greetham (1994) considered doctors and nurses and their responsibilities in the clinical arena. They can put patients at risk, but can prevent risks. Greetham focused on the culture of the NHS and the potential for having a culture that admits to nothing, even when fault is glaringly obvious. He put much faith in the development and use of effective communication systems in the hospital and with other hospitals, general practitioners and the community. Proper management systems are required to reduce risks and controlling them lies with management, but individuals must participate in this process by identifying risks. There are difficulties with accepting responsibility for managing risks irrespective of whether the individual is a doctor, nurse, physiotherapist or manager. Risk management requires a change in culture and that requires commitment, good communication and time. The implementation of clinical governance will help to address many of the issues discussed.

Process

The Management of Health and Safety at Work Regulations is legislation developed through the requirements of the European Union and directives on health and safety. It substantiates a framework piece of legislation, the Health and Safety at Work Act 1974, and focuses on management of risk as its primary aim. The five-step loop for health and safety management as defined by the Health and Safety Executive's publication entitled *Successful Health and Safety Management*, formalizes the management approach, as shown in Figure 36.4.

The establishment of a policy supported by organizational arrangements such as who is responsible for activities (i.e. manager, senior nurse, clinical director) is the first step. The plan should identify, reduce and control risks. Performance measurement is through monitoring and evaluation, reviewing findings and determining if policy needs revision to reflect outcomes.

Example: Infection control in clinical practice

Control of infection in a ward is a practical example which can be used to follow the process. By following the five-step loop, a policy on the control of infection would be developed. This is normally developed as a corporate policy with supporting procedures. Next, organizational arrangements are established for policy implementation (role of management, staff and/or infection control link nurses, medical, clinical and ancillary staff). The third and most crucial stage is to plan implementation to include training, staffing requirements, equipment and/or supplies needed. This stage can be quite complex and participation of clinical teams is quite important to ensure that implementation is successful. Stage four is defined as 'closing the loop'. Plans are monitored for outcomes and the review/ evaluation process is applied to test out the effectiveness of the infection control policy. Often this part of the loop is missed and the consequences of changing practices are not fully evaluated. This in itself can lead to other risks. Placing clinical waste bins in a ward corridor to ensure separation of clinical and domestic waste can impede evacuation of beds in a fire; the risk of this could be greater than the risks associated with clinical waste storage.

Example: Manual handling – improvements in clinical areas

Manual handling injuries account for the majority of sickness/absence in the nursing profession today, as identified in the publication by the Royal College of Nursing (1996). It must not be forgotten that other healthcare professionals – physiotherapists, healthcare assistants, ancillary support workers (i.e. porters, domestics and engineers) and medical staff – are all at risk of back injuries, although extensive research into the extent and frequency of injuries for these groups has yet to been done. The Manual Handling Operations Regulations 1992 encapsulated in law the requirement to apply risk management principles to protect the health, safety and welfare of individuals, in this case those involved in the manual handling activities within a hospital setting. The results have been dramatic in many hospitals where there has been considerable investment in hoists, slides and other aids to reduce manual handling operations. Investment in the training and development of staff in safe methods of handling, and developing patient care plans that identify risks to staff and detail preventative measures, together with a general increase in awareness, have all been factors contributing to improved conditions for staff.

Example: Use of risk profiling for patients who may exhibit threatening behaviour in a trauma setting

The following risk profile method illustrates how the process outlined earlier in the chapter for determining and controlling risk can be applied.

Risk identification
Potential for unpredictable aggressive behaviour from patients who are brain injured. Outcomes include physical and/or verbal assault on staff members, relatives or other patients.

Risk assessment
Ascertaining the frequency of occurrence, severity and probability that aggressive behaviour will occur. This can be done by looking at previous information, such as incident reports, and behaviour of patients related to their medical condition:

- frequency – how often episodes of aggressive behaviour occur
- severity – what is the potential outcome, e.g. no injuries, minor injuries, lost time, long-term sickness, severe injuries
- probability – the chance that it will occur, e.g. daily, weekly, infrequently.

These are usually expressed in terms of low, medium or high for each category. The combination of all three will give you a judgement on risk which can be used for the next step.

Risk control (reduction/minimization)
Based on the risk assessment level of low, medium or high, a plan to minimize risks can then be established. Examples of this may be: improving the history-taking of a patient on admission; isolating the patient so as not to harm themselves and others; providing an extra member of staff with special skills to deal with threatening behaviour; providing training for multidisciplinary staff to recognize the signs of aggression or challenging behaviour.

Risk funding
This may entail additional funding for staff, isolation areas for safety (change of the built environment) and training initiatives.

Clinical risk management

The implementation of legislation which focuses on the identification, assessment and control of risk as a result of new legislation, coupled with the removal of Crown Immunity, has made a significant impact on improving the management of health and safety in the health service today. We will now reclassify health and safety management as non-clinical risk management and include it as part of the clinical governance framework.

Clinical risk management refers to the application of the risk management process to activities of direct patient care. It was first discussed in the Department of Health's guidance document entitled *Risk Management in the NHS*, originally published in 1992. Ascertaining risks to patients receiving medical care follows the same process outlined throughout this chapter – identification, assessment, control and funding. The illustration of risk profiling discussed earlier can be applied to activities associated with patient care in exactly the same manner.

Determining what risks patients face is quite broad and encompasses a range of indicators such as the following:

- return to A&E within 24 hours
- missed fractures
- inappropriate treatment
- medication errors
- return to surgery
- delay in treatment.

The difficulty with identifying risks related to direct patient care is getting healthcare professionals to recognize that clinical risks do exist and that, by the use of preventative techniques, they can influence the outcome for patients. The sensitivities surrounding clinical risk management may be presentational. The emphasis in this country began as a means of reducing potential legal claims, a defensive medicine approach, rather than by using risk management as a means of improving quality of healthcare. While effective risk management is useful in defending legal actions, it is not the reason for risk management. The emphasis must be on clinical teams working together to seek ways of improving procedures for diagnosis, treatment and care and recognizing risks throughout the process.

We discussed earlier the three elements of risk: organization, environment and individual (Figure 36.2). Clinicians must recognize that when harm occurs, all three elements are in play. This will move the NHS away from a blame culture and towards one of looking at the factors surrounding an incident and learning from an analysis of process and outcome.

There are a number of approaches used for identifying risk in clinical practice – models such as discussed earlier – but the use of indicators such as incident reporting, complaints and claims are good markers for risk identification.

Incident reporting

Incidents are defined as untoward events that have a detrimental short- or long-term effect on a patient, member of staff or member of the public. Clinical treatment and outcomes, patient care, working practices, health, safety, fire, security (including data protection) and incidents involving property are all examples.

There are legal requirements for reporting certain incidents which are outlined in the Reporting of Injuries, Diseases and Dangerous Occurrences Regulations, 1995. An employee off work for more than 3 days as a result of an incident at work (this includes violence) or a fracture sustained by a patient after falling, are two types of incident that fall within the reporting requirements of this regulation. Hospitals will have their own internal system for reporting incidents with a nominated person to notify certain incidents to the Health and Safety Executive, the government enforcement body.

Incident reporting is one of the most beneficial tools for risk management. At its simplest, it provides a record of events for a given point in time. This is useful for understanding incidents, how they occurred and the interaction of organization, environment and individuals. Incident reports also provide documentation for staff and patients if a complaint or claim is subsequently made. The challenge facing healthcare workers is changing behaviour to use the forms to identify untoward events which traditionally they have never reported or felt comfortable to report. In particular, medical staff are notorious for not using incident forms, even if they have sustained an injury to themselves, let alone an event which has occurred to a patient. Individuals need to see the benefit of highlighting issues, for they are often not unique. By reporting, changes can be made which may be beneficial to many as a result of improving systems, buildings or equipment. This is demonstrated in the following examples.

Example: Insertion of chest drain

In this particular example, the insertion of a chest drain into the wrong patient as a result of X-ray labels being mixed up illustrates how incident reporting can lead to changes in practice. Subsequent to the incident, an investigation took place and a number of changes were implemented:

- new checking procedures for identification and labelling of X-ray films as part of a quality assurance programme
- medical examination of X-ray results and clinical condition/findings to help confirm results

---

- better consultation with medical staff and their consultants where concerns of this nature are raised.

Example: Communication regarding surgical procedures

Valid consent given by a patient is extremely important before any investigative procedure or treatment can proceed. In this case a surgical procedure was discussed with the patient and consent was obtained. The patient did not communicate concerns about which doctor would carry out the surgery; however, post-operatively the patient was distressed to learn that it was not a consultant who carried out the surgery, but a registrar under clinical supervision. This was reported as an incident, but it could be classified as a patient complaint. As a consequence of the incident, the consent process now includes discussions with patients on who may perform the procedure and under what circumstances, so that any concerns can be raised prior to procedures being undertaken.

The major problem with effective incident reporting is engaging staff in the process and making sure that they feel safe using it. In other words, it cannot be used to blame individuals. Incident reporting can also produce rather high expectations by staff hoping to see improvements overnight, which in many cases does not occur. This can lead to apathy and people refusing to use a system as they see no benefit in doing so. If these issues are confronted and discussed openly with staff, incident reporting can indeed be effective.

Standards of clinical documentation and record-keeping

Adequate documentation in medical notes is the best indicator of events, but it tends to be poorly written, illegible and incomplete. Many in the legal community believe that if events are not written down, they did not happen. When clinicians discuss the risks and benefits of a procedure, patients may claim later that they were unaware of certain consequences of treatment and thus, if better informed, would not have opted for it. Medical staff will find it difficult to substantiate if no record exists of their discussions in patient records. A consent form in itself does not provide the necessary evidence that risks and benefits were explained.

It is also important that events are recorded, whether for a single patient episode or indeed for any clinical activity. Documentation, be it patient records, incident reports, audit reports, risk assessments, standards, complaints, claims or business plans, provides a wealth of information which helps teams to identify risks to staff and patients. It is by using available data and turning it into valuable and useful information that the foundation for an effective risk management programme can be established.

The main disadvantage seen by clinicians is the time required to write events down and, more importantly, to what extent information should be documented. There are no easy answers to this and it is best for clinical teams and individual practitioners to determine how information should be recorded, provided that it is clear and concise. Some clinicians use letters to patients after outpatient visits as a way of communicating precisely what was discussed, with a copy kept in the medical records for review at their next visit. This is a good example of using communication effectively while ensuring that discussions are recorded.

Complaints and claims

Information gathered from complaints and claims is another useful tool for identifying risks to patients, staff and the organization. The difference between complaints and claims is that the latter come into play a substantial period after the incident and thus it is more difficult for clinical staff to remember what took place. Complaints are recent, reflecting events as seen through the eyes of the patient, and can make an impact on improving care if listened to and dealt with appropriately by clinical staff.

It is important that legal claims are not seen as indicators of bad practice, but rather as opportunities for improvement, if needed. It must be remembered that claims regarding clinical practice are not synonymous with negligence and, in most cases, patients pursuing claims are looking for explanations as to the outcome of their treatment. Much of this could be prevented by improving communication between patients and clinicians and using incident reporting and complaints procedures to identify clinical practice and patient outcomes.

Conclusion

The main responsibility for risk management lies with the employer and starts with the executive directors thence through the management chain. Employees have a responsibility for themselves and how this affects their performance within an organization. Mayatt (1996) stated that there still remains a weakness within the NHS to emulate the effective management of risk as demonstrated by commercial organizations. This is the legacy of Crown Immunity, which previously protected healthcare providers from prosecution under health and safety legislation, but is now much wider and incorporates the issue of openness and honesty within the NHS sector, particularly regarding clinical practice.

Since the removal of Crown Immunity under the reforms of the NHS and the introduction of risk management as part of the clinical governance framework, a steep learning curve has been travelled with some success. However, many healthcare providers have a long way to go to achieve successful risk management in their organizations. Mayatt believes that a lack of accountability of individuals still exists in the healthcare sector today. This is based on the cultural attitude that still prevails, in that it is acceptable to subordinate one's own risk management in the interests of patient care and healthcare delivery. This reflects the views of Greetham, stated earlier, but attitudes are changing. Healthcare professionals are taking more account of their own welfare and that of their patients in the course of their duties. The two can exist together and clinical teams working together can make a difference.

References

Bowden, D. (ed.) (1994) *Managing Risk; Merret Health Risk Management.*

Carter, R. L. and Crockford, G. N. (1994) *Handbook of Risk Management.* Kluwer.

Greetham, J. F. (1994) Prevention and control of clinical negligence. In *Managing Risk: Merret Health Risk*

Management. (D. Bowden, ed.).

Knight, F. H. (1921) *Risk, Uncertainty and Profit.* Houghton Mifflin.

Mayatt, V. (1996) The management of occupational safety and health. *Health Care Risk Report,* **2**(20), 20–25.

Raz, D. (1982) Risk management in US hospitals. *Hospital and Health Services Administration.* Canada.

Royal College of Nursing (1996) *Hazards of Nursing – Personal Injuries at Work.* RCN.

Spinks, M. (1994) Risky business. *Nursing Standard,* **8**(40), 22–23.

Willet, A. H. (1901) *The Economic Theory of Risk and Insurance.* Irwin.

37

Legal issues

Mary Duncan

Introduction

A surprisingly small percentage of accidents lead to claims; it is not clear to what extent this is due to ignorance of a possible remedy or concerns about the cost of making a claim.

This chapter outlines the basic rules applicable to personal injury claims to help the practitioner to understand the patient or family's likely concerns about making and pursuing a claim. Details of referral agencies and sources of further help are suggested, with addresses, telephone numbers and websites at the end of the chapter.

Who can claim?

Liability

Civil claims

It is surprisingly common for potential claimants to look blank when asked to comment on who was to blame for their injury. It often seems to be felt that 'someone' will pay if a claimant has been injured. A self-employed tree surgeon who somehow managed to saw through the line which was securing him to a tree still thought he might have a claim, as did the farmer who was trampled by his own ram.

For a claim to succeed it must be proved that someone else was negligent (or in breach of statutory duty) and that that negligence caused the injuries and other losses. Negligence, in a legal sense, is careless conduct causing damage to others. The claimant must show that the defendant owed a duty of care to the claimant, i.e. to take reasonable care to avoid acts and omissions which would be likely to injure the claimant, that the defendant has not taken that care, and that the claimant has suffered damage as a result.

A duty is owed where the defendant could reasonably foresee that an act or omission would harm his 'neighbour'. A duty is broken when the defendant either does something that a reasonable person in that position would not do or omits to do something that a reasonable person in that position would do.

In a clinical negligence claim, the 'Bolam' test will normally be applied; that is, the claimant will need to show that the defendant followed a course of action that is not supported by any responsible body of medical opinion.

Insurance

Claimants may have their own insurance, whether motor insurance or a personal accident policy. If a claim is to be made under an insurance policy it is important that the insurer be notified as soon as possible, since delay may entitle the insurer to avoid liability under the policy. This chapter is primarily concerned with civil claims for damages rather than claims against any policy the claimant may hold.

Claimants

Generally

Someone who has suffered a physical injury

may have a claim. More technical rules govern claims for post-traumatic stress disorder (PTSD) and fatal claims.

Post-traumatic stress disorder

The courts have been concerned to avoid 'opening the floodgates' of PTSD claims, and strict rules have accordingly been developed which limit, sometimes rather artificially, who may bring a claim for damages for PTSD in cases where there has been no physical injury to the claimant and the claimant was not actually in the area of danger or did not reasonably think that he was. First the claimant must be suffering from PTSD as defined in the *Diagnostic and Statistical Manual of Mental Disorders* (American Psychiatric Association, 1994). Secondly, the claimant must be sufficiently 'proximate' in time and space to the accident and there must be a close relationship of love and affection between the claimant and the victim of the accident. For example, parents who see their child being injured in an accident can normally claim, whereas a brother might not be able to; the court would consider the closeness of the ties between the siblings. If parents are simply informed about an accident to their child, and they do not see the immediate aftermath, they cannot normally claim.

Fatal claims

The deceased's claim for damages for personal injuries and other losses may be pursued through his estate. Any dependants may have a claim for loss of support (dependancy) under the Fatal Accidents Act 1976. A 'bereavement award' of £7500 may also be claimed by the deceased's spouse, the parents of an unmarried legitimate minor or the mother of an unmarried illegitimate minor. The amount of the bereavement award does often cause offence and distress to claimants as it is perceived as wholly inadequate.

What can be claimed?

Generally
Quantum, or the amount a claim is worth, is generally separated into general damages, special damages and future loss. Interest may also be payable.

General damages

These cover items which cannot be quantified precisely. In most personal injury claims the main item of general damages is damages for pain and suffering, that is, compensation for the physical or mental injury itself. Claimants who have seen reports of million pound claims are often indignant at the relatively small amounts of money paid for the pain and suffering element. It helps to explain that the maximum award for pain and suffering for a quadriplegic is around £150 000 and the remainder of the large damages awards is mostly made up of loss of earnings and cost of care.

It is helpful if a claimant keeps a diary of problems encountered following an accident, as this will ensure that the details are not forgotten when it is time to prepare a statement. The defendant is thus made aware of the full extent of the claimant's problems.

Special damages

These are items of loss which can be calculated reasonably accurately. Examples are loss of earnings, travelling expenses for medical treatment, cost of medical treatment and medicines, personal effects damaged in the accident and excess on an insurance policy. It is helpful if a list is kept of all losses incurred, together with receipts and other documentary evidence where possible.

Future loss

The calculation of this is quite complex. Essentially, if there are losses that are likely to continue for the foreseeable future, the claimant will not simply recover the annual loss multiplied by the number of years for which the loss is likely to last. The court will apply a multiplier, that is, a discount to allow for the fact that the claimant will be receiving the money all at once rather than over a period of years and can therefore invest it and obtain interest on it.

Interest

The claimant may be entitled to interest on some of the damages. The rate payable and the period for which it is payable varies, depending on the type of damages. Interest on special damages runs from the date of the accident, generally speaking, whereas interest on general damages runs only from the date of service of proceedings.

Benefits

If the claimant receives state benefits as a result of the accident, these may be deducted from the damages at the end of the case. The Compensation Recovery Unit (CRU) calculates the benefits received and supplies a certificate to the defendant who has to pay the CRU the sum demanded when the case is settled. The calculation of exactly which benefits are deductible from the damages is quite complicated, but a claimant should be aware that a deduction is likely.

Provisional damages

Generally, once a claim is settled a claimant cannot bring a further claim if there is an unexpected deterioration in the injuries. A provisional damages award may be made if there is, at the time of settlement, a chance that at some definite or indefinite time in the future the claimant will develop some serious disease or suffer some serious deterioration in his physical or mental condition. The claimant will be given the opportunity to make a further claim within a specified period should the disease or deterioration occur. A classic example of a case suitable for a provisional damages award is where there is a small risk that a claimant will develop epilepsy following a head injury. Conversely, a risk of developing arthritis in the future will not normally be the subject of a provisional damages award.

How to go about a claim

Whom to consult

A solicitor should be consulted as soon as possible. Most specialist solicitors will give a free initial interview. A claimant should check whether the firm has solicitors who are members of the Law Society Personal Injury Panel, that is, true personal injury specialists. Only members of the Personal Injury Panel can offer conditional fee insurance through Accident Line Protect which is generally more attractive and cheaper than other schemes.

While legal aid remains available, the claimant should also check whether the firm holds a legal aid franchise for personal injury or clinical negligence work. This is an indication that certain quality procedures are in place as well as being essential from 31 July 1999 for new clinical negligence legally aided work.

Citizens Advice Bureaux may also help a claimant who is apprehensive about seeing a solicitor but, for all but the smallest claims, a solicitor will need to be seen sooner or later. Claimants should be wary of claims agencies who may take a significant 'cut' of the damages and may work out more expensive than a solicitor in the long run.

How to find a solicitor

The following sources of information will assist:

Accident Line

This is a referral scheme run by the Law Society which refers claimants to a local firm of solicitors which has at least one member of the Law Society's Personal Injury Panel and which has agreed to give a free initial interview. This should not be confused with other similar sounding agencies which do not necessarily give the same guarantees.

The Law Society

The Law Society will give details of all local solicitors and can say which are personal injury panel members and which are clinical negligence panel members.

Citizens Advice Bureaux

These are a good source of general advice on many issues arising from accident claims, including benefits and financial problems. They will also know local firms of solicitors and can recommend a selection to claimants.

Who may be sued

Generally, the person who was negligent or their employers will be sued. Effectively, the defence of most personal injury claims is dealt with by the defendant's insurers and solicitors, often with little or no involvement of the actual defendant. This can be helpful, particularly in tragic cases where a claimant does not wish personally further to upset the defendant, but needs to recover damages.

In road traffic cases, if a defendant is uninsured or untraced the Motor Insurers Bureau (MIB) will usually deal with and pay a claim. Detailed rules govern these claims and further information can be obtained from the MIB.

If injuries result from a criminal act, a claim may be lodged with the Criminal Injuries Compensation Authority. The address is given at the end of this chapter.

Process and time frame

Generally

The majority of personal injury claims (probably 95%) settle without the need for a trial. The advent of the Civil Procedure Rules on 26 April 1999, following the Woolf Report, should mean that claims progress faster once proceedings have been started.

There are, however, built in unavoidable delays in any personal injury claim. At least one medical report has to be obtained to prove the injuries. It is not sensible to obtain a report too soon, as an accurate prognosis will not be possible. It may be necessary to wait some years for the claimant to recover, or at least for a reasonably certain prognosis to be available. Children's claims, especially those involving damage to intellectual ability, may have to wait many years before the full effect of the injuries on the child's future prospects is clear.

Stages of a claim

A typical case will pass through the following stages:

Pre-action protocol

A period of exchange of information between claimant and defendant before proceedings are started. This will usually involve the claimant sending full details of the claim to the defendant. The defendant must acknowledge the letter within 21 days and the defendant then has 3 months in which to investigate the claim and decide whether or not to admit liability. If liability is denied, documents must be ex-

changed and the claimant may issue proceedings. If liability is admitted, the claimant must supply details of quantum and the defendant then has 21 days in which to make an offer. For details of the personal injury protocol see the Lord Chancellor's Department website.

Starting proceedings

A claimant's statement of case will be served, sometimes drafted by a barrister. This must be verified by a statement of truth, usually signed by the claimant. An untrue statement of truth will render a claimant liable to punishment for contempt of court.

Defence

This must usually be served within 28 days at the latest from the service of the proceedings, although extensions of time may be granted.

Allocation

The court will decide to which track the case should be allocated. Generally, personal injury claims where damages for pain and suffering are likely to be less than £1000 will be allocated to the small claims track and will be dealt with more informally by way of arbitration. Claims worth over £1000 up to £15 000 will be allocated to the fast track, and claims over that amount, to the multi-track. Procedures in the fast track are more streamlined than in the multi-track. The principle of proportionality (that costs should be proportionate to the amount in issue) is now considered very important by the court.

Disclosure

This is the exchange of lists of documents relevant to the case by the parties. Again the lists have to be verified by a statement of truth and it is important that a claimant understands the duty to tell his solicitor about all documents that may be relevant to a case, even if harmful to the claimant's own case.

Exchange of witness statements and reports

Any witness statements and expert reports on which the parties intend to rely must be exchanged at a time set by the court. In fast track cases there may well only be one agreed medical expert and the written report only will usually be put in as evidence; the expert will not be called to give evidence in person.

Case management conference

In multi-track cases there is likely to be at least one case management conference at which the claimant should be present. The object is for the judge and the parties to review the case, see whether the areas of dispute can be reduced, and whether there is any scope for disposing of the case without a full trial. Mediation will be considered.

Trial

Under the Civil Procedure Rules a trial is meant to be very much a last resort, and the parties will have been encouraged to settle throughout the case. In fast track cases, a trial 'window' will have been allocated near the beginning of the case so that a claimant will know in what month the case is likely to be heard should it go to trial. The aim is to hear all fast track cases within 30 weeks of directions being given. Arrangements for listing multi-track cases may be more variable, depending, for example, on when a prognosis is likely to be available.

Payment of damages and costs

This is not usually a problem with an insured defendant. In legally aided cases there may be delays with release of at least some of the damages pending assessment of the claimant's legal costs by the court. This is because if there is a shortfall on costs recovered from the defendant, this shortfall may have to come out of the claimant's damages. This is called the operation of the statutory charge and should have been explained to the claimant by the claimant's solicitor at the beginning of the case.

Interim payments

In long-running claims, interim payments (now known as 'Part 25 payments') may be obtained, provided that the court is satisfied that if the claim went to trial the claimant would obtain damages for a substantial amount of money against the defendant, and the defendant's liability will be met by an insurer, or the defendant is a public body.

Payments into court

These are now known as 'Part 36 payments'. A similar 'Part 36 offer' may be made before proceedings are started. These are important as, if a claimant fails eventually to beat a Part 36 payment or offer made by the defendant, the claimant may be penalized in costs. A claimant in those circumstances would normally be ordered to pay the defendant's costs from the date of the Part 36 payment or offer. Particularly in small claims, where the costs at risk may well exceed the value of the claim, Part 36 payments must be taken very seriously. Claimants may make Part 36 offers themselves, stating the amount they would be prepared to accept in settlement of their claim and a defendant who fails to beat such an offer will also usually be penalized in costs and have to pay a penalty rate of interest as well.

Limitation

Court proceedings must generally be started within 3 years of the date of the accident. Minors and people under a mental disability generally have longer. Shorter periods apply to some claims, longer periods to others, hence the need to consult a solicitor as soon as possible.

Inquests

The purpose of an inquest is not to establish or apportion blame, but to establish the cause of death. Strict civil rules of evidence do not generally apply, but Coroners will generally limit questions to witnesses that appear to be directed only to establishing fault. Evidence is given on oath.

The Coroner's jurisdiction is derived from the Coroner's Act 1988. When a Coroner is informed that a body is lying within his district and he has reasonable cause to suspect that the deceased died an unnatural or violent death, or the deceased has died a sudden death the cause of which is unknown, or has died in prison, the Coroner shall as soon as practicable hold an inquest. There will not, however, be an inquest where serious criminal proceedings result from the death, for example a charge of causing death by dangerous driving.

Sometimes a jury will be present, for example

if the death occurred in prison or in police custody, the death was caused by an accident, disease or poisoning, notice of which is required to be given under any Act to a government department or inspector, or if the death occurred in circumstances the continuance or possible recurrence of which is prejudicial to the health or safety of the public (Section 8 Coroners Act 1988).

Relatives of a deceased may be represented by a solicitor or barrister at an inquest. The Coroner should be told that this is desired early on. Interested parties have the right to question witnesses at the inquest either in person or through their legal representative. Relatives also have the power to request their own post mortem.

Possible verdicts at an inquest include unlawful killing, natural causes, industrial disease, lack of care, suicide, accidental death/misadventure, open. The most common verdict in road traffic accident cases is accidental death, which still leaves open the possibility of a civil claim. A verdict of lack of care may be relevant in a clinical negligence case.

Inquests can be helpful to the bereaved as a 'milestone' which they feel better for passing. Without forewarning, they can also be extremely traumatic, as some Coroners ask the pathologist to go through the whole post mortem report in considerable detail. Most Coroners' officers will now warn relatives in advance so that they have an opportunity to leave the court when this evidence is being given, but this does not always happen.

Legal costs

Generally

Many claimants are concerned about the risk of incurring substantial legal costs. Costs should always be discussed at the initial (usually free) interview and written details of a solicitor's terms of business should be provided to a claimant. If a claimant has a good personal injury claim, costs should not be a real problem; it may be different if a claim is not clear cut.

Legal aid

This is likely shortly to be unavailable for most personal injury claims, but remains for the present for medical negligence claims. If available, it is likely to be the best source of funding, subject to the question of whether any contribution is payable by the claimant. Applications for legal aid are subject to a merits and means test. Minors generally qualify in their own right financially for legal aid. Strict financial limits apply. Legal aid for personal injury claims is not generally available if an applicant's capital (excluding a dwelling house with equity of up to £100 000) exceeds £8560 and/or if disposable income (after deductions for housing costs, etc.) exceeds £8751 per year. (Figures given as at April 1999.)

Legal expenses insurance

Many people are not aware that they have legal expenses insurance. It is commonly added on to household and motor policies and such policies should always be checked promptly if a claimant may have a claim. There are often strict time limits within which a claim for cover must be made under the policy. Cover under a policy may be quite limited and the small print must always be checked.

Trade unions

Advice on and funding for a claim for damages for personal injuries may well be available from a claimant's trade union. Some unions also run schemes for members families as well.

Conditional fee agreements

This is an arrangement whereby a solicitor agrees not to claim any profit costs from the claimant unless the claim is won. Disbursements (e.g. cost of medical reports) may still be payable and the claimant will normally also have to pay for an insurance policy to cover the risk of being ordered to pay the other side's costs. In a claim covered by the Accident Line scheme, such insurance is likely to cost less than £165 as at March 1999. Clinical negligence claims are not covered by Accident Line and insurance policies for these claims generally cost some thousands of pounds.

Under a conditional fee agreement a solicitor, if successful in the claim, will take a success fee based on an agreed percentage of his basic costs. A claimant should always ensure that the conditional fee agreement is in the Law

Society's approved form. This should include an agreement by the solicitor to limit the total of the success fee, whatever the percentage of basic costs agreed, to a maximum of 25% of the damages recovered.

Conditional fees are complex. When considering a conditional fee agreement, a claimant should be given explanatory leaflets called 'Conditional Fees Explained' and 'Accident Line Protect' by the solicitor, and a detailed explanation. The attraction is that a conditional fee agreement removes the need to fund an action as it goes along (save possibly for disbursements) and the risk of paying the other side's costs may be removed by the appropriate insurance.

Private funding

If the claimant is reasonably well off and has a good personal injury claim which is very likely to succeed, privately funding a claim may be a better option than entering into a conditional fee agreement (depending on the solicitor's private charging rate and the extent to which the costs are likely to exceed costs allowable by the court against the defendant). The claimant has to fund the action as it proceeds, but should recover the bulk of the costs from the other side at the end of the case and will not suffer any deduction from the damages in respect of a success fee.

Small claims

These present particular problems, as where general damages for personal injury are likely to be less than £1000 a claim will be referred to the small claims court. Only limited costs will be recoverable and it is not likely to be worth while to instruct a solicitor accordingly. Staff at the local county court will help with formulating a claim and various explanatory booklets are available at court and on the court services website.

Practical help

Rehab UK is a registered charity. Its principal aim is to enable people with disabilities to become socially and economically independent in the community. There is a range of training and employment programmes for people dis-advantaged in the labour market, some particularly tailored for people with traumatic brain injuries. There is also a disability assessment unit to help in the rehabilitation and restoration of function of those who have become disabled.

NOTE: This chapter states the law as at 26 April 1999. It can only give a basic outline of the relevant principles and is no substitute for detailed legal advice.

Reference

American Psychiatric Association (1994) *Diagnostic and Statistical Manual of Mental Disorders*, DSM-1V.

Sources of further information

Accident Line

PO Box 61
London NW1 7QS
Tel: 0500 192939.

Citizens Advice Bureau Headquarters and Administrative Office

Myddleton House
115–123 Pentonville Road
London N1 9LZ
Tel: 0171 833 2181
Fax: 0171 833 4371
Website: www.nacab.org.uk

Court Services Department (Headquarters)

Southside
105 Victoria Street
London SW1E 6QT
Tel: 0171 210 2065
Website: www.courtservice.gov.uk

Criminal Injuries Compensation Authority (Head Office)

Tay House
300 Bath Street
Glasgow G2 4JR
Tel: 0141 331 2726

Law Society (personal injury and clinical negligence panels)

Law Society
Ipsley Court

Berrington Close
Redditch B98 OTD
Tel: 01527 517141
Website: www.lawsociety.org.uk

Lord Chancellor's Department

Selborne House
54-60 Victoria Street
London SW1E 6QW.
Tel: 0171 210 8500
Website: www.open.gov.uk/lcd

Motor Insurers Bureau

152 Silbury Boulevard
Milton Keynes MK9 1NB
Tel: 01908 240000

Rehab UK – Disability Assessment Unit

Windermere House
Kendal Avenue
London W3 OXA
Tel: 0181 896 2333
Website: www.rehabuk.org

The Hospital Series (Poems from the John Radcliffe Hospital, Oxford)

Peter Austin

One journey (6 April 1998)

i

Listless
Restless
Disturbed by the currents of the sea
I rise and fall at the mercy of the bed Pegasus
I am at its bidding
Confined to the journeys on which it will take me
A captain with no command
The swell takes me from front to back to side
A ceaseless ride to eternity

ii

With no warning
The bows begin to dip
Sliding deeper into the abyss below
And as it slid further
I sank with it
We sank together
Our voyages intrinsically entwined
Destiny awaits us on the ocean floor
I never arrive

iii

I am on a child's swing
High above the ground
Below me deeper still
The heady heights of a garden
Cold trees in ice light
Sweat running shadows
A frozen pond reflects the night darkly
I start to fall
Ground rushing up to eat me

iv

I am sitting in a time travel car
The first in a worms wax museum
Courtesy of hospital bed
I twist this way and that
Swing first left then right
Watch helplessly
A silver procession of lorries
Tanks
Static military displays pass by my eyes

v

Squashed until three inches wide
No pain
I study every bolt and rivet
Each engine wheel in microscopic detail
Rust covered base of filing cabinet
Standing on cracked lifted damp linoleum
Putrefied spider hangs weightless
Ignored by the black beetle
Crawling slowly to an unknown end

vi

I reach another brick wall
And dissolve through it
Rising swiftly on a reverse helter skelter
A swirling upwards ride
Fleeting images too fast to discern
In this giddy spiral

vii

I hear voices
The first since my journey started
Voices of reality
Tugging me back to my day wake hours

A view from a hill (13 April 1998)

Eating the day
Grey hills nourishing themselves
Gorging on welcome light
To return in road swathes of brown/green

Spring trees tickled the sharp air
As the laughter of hedgerows
Echoed reflections of silver streams

Glinting metal cages
Glide in silent distance
Morning journeys
Started from the spread of rooftops
I see below me
All overseen now by a white/blue sky

Confinement (16 April 1998)

The race is passing me by
As I remain inside
Time spans other dimensions
My own access is denied
To the speed and the hustle
Of everyday bustle

The routines have all been changed
Of which I have become part
I arrived unintended
(Help was by Descartes)
Now my contribution
Just lies in institution

The pace has just been dropped
An hour stretches for three
Inability to move
Reduces all I can see
Left to contemplate how I feel
As I await my next meal

The race is going ahead
Faster for some – I'm the cause
Increasing demands are now made
On time's more palpable laws
Constraints and restrictions
This life of contradictions

The phlebotomist (9 May 1998)

Man will conquer all
Then when all else fails
He will fall upon his fellow kin
A hammer killing nails

Beneath the forest of my skin
The wild veins have been raped
Pillaged by the point and phial
Neither arm escaped
   He retreats – I think I'm safe
   The battle surely over
   But he returns – I find it is
   Not safe in sanctuary cover
With no feelings of regret
Compassion or remorse
The sabre wielding Cossack comes
With butterfly not horse
He lifts the lethal weapon
Plunges it to land
Satiating his lust for blood
From my exposed upturned hand

The physios (14 May 1998)

All was quiet
All was still
Resting peacefully
As you will
Then in they come
Army of two
Leaves you wondering
What they'll do
'Lift that leg'
'Bend that knee'
'Off you go'
'One – two – three'
'Pump that weight'
'Up and down'
Stop too soon
See them frown
'Time to sit'
'Time to stand'
'We are here
To lend a hand'
'Take one step'
'Lean on that crutch'
Strange how soon
You lose the touch
Tiring walk
Shattered return
Getting there
You have to learn
Better each day
Now I've obeyed
Thanks to the physios
I've got it made

Commuter watching 19 May 1998

I am in the position now
To watch – not participate
Commuters queue across the bridge
Their cars almost stagnate
Glints of sun on bodywork
Betray a forward move
Inch by inch they shuffle on
Motion theory try to prove
Beneath the bridge another line
More vehicles standing still
Drivers left to contemplate
Views against their will
Sudden surge four car lengths long
Then quickly apply the brake
Collective through from all involved
'Get a move on for heaven's sake'
Magic trick or miracle
The queue's no longer there
Traffic has dispersed like breath
Just its fumes hang in the air.

Two sided conversation 22 June 1998

'Bear on me' my left side said
While my right side cried 'No weight!'
'Step right up' my left side said
'No time to hesitate'
  'Follow me' my left side said
  As my right side lagged behind
  'Wait for me' my right side said
  But the left side paid no mind
'I'm sorry' is what my left side said
'But my injury has now healed'
'That's not fair' my right side said
His resentment not concealed
  'Don't pick on me' my left side said
  'It's not my fault I'm fixed'
  'But you didn't have' my right side said
  'Plates, screws and bones all mixed'
'Is that so' my left side said
'I must therefore apologise'
'I'll help you then' my left side said
'Together we'll harmonise'

Index